362.1
GAR

Betrayal
of T

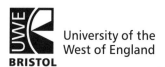

D0453332

Betrayal of Trust

The collapse of global public health

LAURIE GARRETT

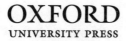
OXFORD
UNIVERSITY PRESS

OXFORD
UNIVERSITY PRESS

Great Clarendon Street, Oxford OX2 6DP

Oxford University Press is a department of the University of Oxford.
It furthers the University's objective of excellence in research, scholarship,
and education by publishing worldwide in

Oxford New York

Auckland Bangkok Buenos Aires Cape Town Chennai
Dar es Salaam Delhi Hong Kong Istanbul Karachi Kolkata
Kuala Lumpur Madrid Melbourne Mexico City Mumbai Nairobi
São Paulo Shanghai Taipei Tokyo Toronto

Oxford is a registered trade mark of Oxford University Press
in the UK and in certain other countries

Published in the United States
by Oxford University Press Inc., New York

A catalogue record for this title is available from the British Library

Library of Congress Cataloging in Publication Data
Garrett, Laurie.
Betrayal of trust: the collapse of global health/Laurie Garrett.
Includes bibliographical references and index.
1. World health.   2. Public health—Cross-cultural studies.   3. Epidemiology.   I. Title.
RA441.G37 2001   362.1—dc21   2001033910
ISBN 0 19 850995 2 (Hbk)
ISBN 0 19 852683 0 (Pbk)

10 9 8 7 6 5 4 3 2 1

Typeset by Integra Software Services Pvt. Ltd., Pondicherry, India
www.integra_india.com
Printed in Great Britain on acid-free paper by
T.J. International Ltd., Padstow, Cornwall

To Dr Jonathan Mann,
who dared to think boldly of a new public health
in which humanity held a place above technology

Contents

Acknowledgements

A book of this magnitude obviously owes a lot of debts. So many people have generously offered their ideas, assistance, and support over the five years of research and preparation of *Betrayal of Trust* that I scarcely know where to begin. I am overflowing with gratitude.

There are two groups of people without whose support this book would never have existed and so it is to them that I must express my most ardent thanks. I have had the pleasure of working for *Newsday* since 1988 where I have flourished under the editorial leadership of editor-in-chief Tony Marro and his management team of Charlotte Hall and Howard Schneider. I have been particularly fortunate in having uniquely supportive immediate editors and colleagues: Les Payne, Reg Gale, Marcy Kemen, Dele Olojede, Tim Phelps, Robert Cooke, Ridgley Ochs, Viorel Florescu, Delthia Ricks, Joe Dolman, and the staff of 2 Park Avenue, the Washington Bureau, and the *Newsday* library. And while I'm on the subject of *Newsday*, thanks, Ray, for standing up to L.A.

I have a unique situation at *Newsday*, affording me—and my readers—opportunity to see firsthand plagues in India and Central Africa, declining life expectancies in Siberia, policy debates in Washington and Geneva, and dying tuberculosis patients on the wards of Bellevue. I know of no other news organization in the English-speaking world that sends reporters on as many far-flung journeys in pursuit of public health news. And I am grateful to the readers of *Newsday* who have over the years praised and circulated stories that described suffering not in their suburban communities, but in far-off countries where people struggled every day to survive. Many news organizations today mistakenly believe that Americans aren't interested in, and don't care about, the day-to-day struggles of Chinese farmers, Ugandan AIDS workers, Ukrainian prostitutes, or Indian truck drivers. Thank you, *Newsday* and our readers, for proving them wrong.

The other group I must thank in ardent terms is a trio of brilliant, hard-working women who formed the invisible team behind *Betrayal of Trust*: Amy Benjamin, Jill Hannum, and Adi Gevins. Because I continue after ten years to suffer from repetitive strain injury, acquired through use of a lousy computer system, I cannot type. Hannum and Benjamin have been my fingers. But it would grossly understate their roles to label them transcribers, as both women have proved insightful, tireless editors whose feedback was invaluable every step of the way. Both faced tough personal challenges over the course of production of *Betrayal of Trust* and I thank them for their continued commitment to this project despite those diversions. In the final throes of production, Kathy Diamond lent her hands to the typing tasks, as well. Thanks, Kathy.

Gevins and I worked together as radio documentary producers (in former lives), and she has gone on to obtain a degree in library science and become one of the country's top researcher/archivists. I was, indeed, fortunate that her busy schedule allowed time for some digging for this book. Without her tireless tramping through obscure archives, most of the data that appears in Chapter 4 would never have been unearthed. Sad to say, public health archives in the United States are in shabby disarray. Gevins wishes to thank all of the librarians and staff that assisted her, particularly: Buddy Ferguson of the Minnesota Department of Health; the Reference staff of the School of Public Health at UC Berkeley; the Reference staff of the Bioscience and Natural Resources Library at UC Berkeley; The Urban Institute; Sandy Smith at the Centers for Disease Control.

I thank the families and significant others of Hannum, Benjamin, and Gevins for not squawking about how much of their time I was capitalizing. (And I thank FedEx for getting *nearly* all of our packages back and forth on time between New York, Oakland, Mendocino, Seattle, and Boulder.)

I gained additional research assistance from the staffs of the New York Academies of Science and Medicine, the New York City and State Departments of Health, the World Health Organization, the CDC, the NIH Office of AIDS Research, and the United Nations AIDS Programme. Particular thanks are owed to Peter Piot, David Heymann, Wendy Wertheimer, Malgorzata Grzemska, Anthony Fauci, Bill Paul, Jim LeDuc, Jim Hughes, and Bob Howard.

Chapters 3 and 5 and my work in the CIS and NIS owe tremendous debts of gratitude to a host of people, some of whom, for their own protection, I dare not name. Here in the United States I am grateful to Murray Feshbach; Jim Smith and his staff at the American International Health Alliance; Richard Stone at *Science*; Robert Steinglass of BASICS; Regina Napolitano and Howard Cohen of Coney Island Hospital; Ed O'Rourke of Children's Hospital in Boston; Lyle Conrad; and Alexis Shelokov. Overseas, I thank my marvellous translators: Irakli Gogorishvili in Tbilisi; Karin Keerdoo in Tallinn; Elena Frolova in St Petersburg; Vadim Belogolovin in Kiev; Petra Francova in Prague; and many others. And among professionals in the region I am particularly grateful to Brigg Reilly (MSF); Yuri Boshchenko (Odessa Plague Station); Archil Kobaladze (Atlanta-Tbilisi Health Partnership); Victor Aphanasiev (MOH, St Petersburg); Grigory Latyshev (MdM); Alla Soloviova (UNICEF); Edward Korenberg (Ivanov Institute); Boris Revich (Centre of Demography and Human Ecology); Sona Strbanova (AIHA); Elena Gurvich (USAID-Moscow); Yuri Komarov (MEDSOCECONOMINFORM); and the staffs of AIHA Moscow and Kiev.

In Bombay, a special thanks to Subash Hira.

In the Democratic Republic of Congo, I am deeply indebted to several scientists, doctors, and translators, particularly Dr Tamfum Muyembe. But because of the current civil war and repression in that country I fear that a kind word from me might do more harm than good for the rest of them. *Bonne chance, mes amis. Vous avez beaucoup de courage et j'espère qu'à l'avenir, la paix la justice règneront dans tout le Zaire.*

Thanks, of course, to Leigh Haber for her hard editing work on *Betrayal of Trust* at Hyperion.

And for ideas and encouragement, thanks to my family, close friends, and Joshua Lederberg, Peggy Hamburg, Steve Wolinsky, Phil Lee, Michael Osterholm, Mary Wilson, Doug Foster, D. A. Henderson, Jon Cohen, attorney Ed Burke, former student intern Robert Struckman, John Moore, and others who have generously shared their ideas and feedback.

Finally, there would be no book in your hands were it not for the tireless and energetic support of my good friend and agent, Charlotte Sheedy. Thanks for all of those soothing calls, Charlotte, that got me through the final phases of this mammoth project.

Introduction

Act, before disease becomes
persistent through long delays.
—Ovid, 43 B.C. to A.D. 17

When I am not travelling on some distant continent, I walk across the Brooklyn Bridge at least once a day. Usually I'm in a hurry, racing to my office or an appointment, and the trek is executed at a dash, slowed only by the throngs of gawking tourists. There are days, however, when I am so overcome by the beauty of my adopted hometown, by its breathtaking skyscape and historic harbour that, like the tourists I sometimes disparage, I am compelled to stop cold in my tracks and stare. And in those moments, as I gaze over Wall Street, the ferry building, Ellis Island, and the Statue of Liberty, my imagination invariably rolls backwards in time, to the mid-nineteenth-century days before the bridge anchorage upon which I stand was erected. In my mind's eye the harbour is packed, deck to deck with clippers and other sailing ships bearing cargo from all over the world. I can hear the shouting of stevedores and skippers. And I can see the great Brooklyn journalist Walt Whitman leaping from ship to ship as he crosses the East River from his *Brooklyn Eagle* offices, located just a few blocks from my home, to the bustling South Street Seaport of Manhattan. Nearly all of New York City was concentrated on that tiny tip of Manhattan Island, bordered by the harbour, the Hudson River, and the misnamed East River—actually no river at all, but a tidal basin.

There are few places on earth where the populace races forward in time at a pace as furious as that pursued by New Yorkers. There's no time to look. Progress: it's a Manhattan mantra each new generation of immigrants has chanted. Not all progress was achieved in a deliberate, sagacious manner. Indeed, much simply sprang from catastrophe, as disasters gave birth to long-neglected or serendipitous change. Such certainly was the case for the health of New Yorkers. And, in many instances, for their general lifestyle. No matter how sorry their own lot, the immigrants dreamed that the fortunes of their children and grandchildren would be better. Progress.

I can almost see them when I pause on my bridge perch long enough to allow my imagination to slow. From that vantage point I can take in all that once was New York City back in the days when fewer than half of its children lived to blow out the candles on their eighteenth birthday cakes. I see Governors Island in front of me and visualize clipper ships held there in quarantine during hot, sticky summer weeks while the populace of Manhattan cowered in fear of yet another devastating epidemic of cholera,

1

smallpox, or yellow fever. In dingy offices near City Hall scientists dutifully logged in the death tolls, using the latest statistical techniques to determine how many fewer, or more, New Yorkers succumbed in this year's plague, compared to the last. Progress then edged its way around the world at the pace of the winds in sails or of horses drawing wagons. Even so, its inexorable forward movement allowed the spread of microbes to new continents with such devastating results as the obliteration of Native Americans and the introduction of smallpox to every human niche of the planet.

In this city of immigrants, natives, and escaped slaves modern public health was invented. Certainly, elements of the science and policies that form the core of public health also arose in London, Paris, Berlin, and Boston, but it was in Gotham at the dawn of the twentieth century that bands of sanitarians, germ theory zealots, and progressive political leaders created the world's first public health infrastructure. From its inception New Amsterdam, and later New York City, was a global trading post, its very survival dependent upon its multilingual, diverse population. While other colonial outposts also shipped goods, New York surpassed colonial competition by opening its harbour to ships and immigrants from all over the world. And in so doing, New York also opened itself up to the world's diseases. The city, from its earliest seventeenth-century days, had only two options: close itself off and suffer economically, or open its arms to the world while creating systems within the city to control disease. For two hundred years New Yorkers fought off epidemics and pestilence, learning by erring how to create an enormous metropolis that was, from at least a disease perspective, safe. Vital statistics, clean water, pasteurized milk, mass vaccination, less hazardous workplaces, public sewers—these were the hallmarks, achieved one agonizing step after another, of Gotham's public health system.

In the mid-1990s I wrote *The Coming Plague: Newly Emerging Diseases in a World Out of Balance*, which looked at the reemergence of infectious diseases. It was clear to me then that the only dam that could effectively hold back the river of microbes and threatening pathogens was that very public health infrastructure.

To be effective, of course, a twenty-first-century infrastructure could no longer be confined to Gotham, or Los Angeles, or the United States of America: it had to be global in scale. The very measures that ensured longer lives for New Yorkers at the dawn of the twentieth century would have to be implemented planetwide a century later if disease in one earthly ecosphere could be held at bay, away from the other towns, cities, and suburbs of the planet. Such a global public health infrastructure would have to embrace not just the essential elements of disease prevention and surveillance that were present in wealthy pockets of the planet during the twentieth century, but also new strategies and tactics capable of addressing global challenges.

To prevent the sorts of pandemics predicted by scientists in *The Coming Plague* pharmaceutical, laboratory, government, and health forces worldwide would have to be marshalled as never before. The goal could not be a technological quick fix. Rather, society needed to take aim at a far more complex—and elusive—target, comprised not just of the fruits of scientific labour but also of politics, sociology, economics, and even elements of religion, philosophy, and psychology.

When *The Coming Plague* was published I was inundated with demands for solutions. As a journalist I felt uncomfortable: it wasn't my role to solve society's dilemmas, only to describe them. But as a global citizen I despaired. I could, indeed, see solutions, but they didn't fit into tidy sound bites—or bytes. And some of the answers appeared so complex that I felt inadequate to the task of elucidation.

I needed to know more.

To begin with, I had to understand what, exactly, was a public health infrastructure. I needed to see public health in action. I needed to comprehend fully how such an infrastructure worked—or, all too often—failed.

But how strong does such an infrastructure have to be? How much taxpayer money or international aid is needed to stave off disease? How vulnerable is the safety net that protects the health of New York City or any other society by providing for its most vulnerable and impoverished members?

To answer those questions, I went to the former Soviet Union in 1997, travelling across twelve time zones—from Western Europe to Eastern Siberia—for four months. I witnessed numerous epidemics, falling life expectancies, hospitals bereft of even the most fundamental supplies, physicians earning their livings as taxi drivers, and surging new health crises. It was abundantly clear that public health infrastructures were not terribly resilient; in the face of societal stress and economic difficulty they quickly collapsed. And the impact on human health was immediately observable.

It was also apparent that the Communist leaders of the Soviet Union had some bizarre notions of public health, based on ideologically inspired misinterpretations of biology. They rejected all notions of biological determinism, packing off to gulags and firing squads those geneticists who sought to prove that evolution was real, and that life began with the genetic molecules DNA and RNA. The staunch opposition to evolutionary theory of Joseph Stalin's reign left Soviet scientists and physicians intellectually crippled—a disability that still afflicted public health in that region of the world ten years after the collapse of communism.

In search of public health answers I also travelled extensively in sub-Saharan Africa and India, where public health crises abounded. Africa's struggle to catch up economically with the rest of the world was showing success in several countries, and public health improvements often—but not always—followed. But as the Ebola epidemic in Zaire illustrated, an unstable, corrupt society is inevitably a public health catastrophe. Many of the former Soviet nations shared with Zaire and other African nations deep-seated corruption that drained the life blood from their social sectors just as parasites suck the essence of life from the guts of infected children. The pandemics of drug-resistant tuberculosis and HIV further drained Africa's fragile economies, reversing their courses of progress and development, and commanding all of their public health resources. Every filled graveyard in Africa's plagued cities signalled another loss to the workforce and another step backward.

Progress: such an elusive pursuit.

In India's case economic progress brought worsening public health. The federal government, eager to spend its growing wealth on nuclear weapons and military efforts, relinquished all responsibility for the health of its one billion citizens. It turned public health over to the states, most of which lacked the resources and political will to do much more than create bloated, corrupt, inefficient bureaucracies. India had no real national public health infrastructure at the end of the twentieth century: no surveillance system, no reporting mechanism, barely a vital statistics registry.

But surely public health in the United States had witnessed bold progress during the twentieth century: as I stand on my beloved Brooklyn Bridge every day am I not gazing at a populace that is profoundly healthier than its great-grandparents?

To understand why America's public health leaders felt worried, cynical, and even besieged in the 1990s I focused on the history of the health of the peoples of New York City, the County of Los Angeles, and the State of Minnesota. The choice of New York City was an obvious one, as it had been the birth place of modern public health.

Los Angeles County is where I and four generations of my ancestors grew up. When my grandmother, Evelyn MacKenzie Garrett, worked in the early twentieth century as a public health nurse in the Clara Barton Hospital in Los Angeles, the region had 875 000 residents, and the needs of those individuals—Californians and Mexicans, alike—were, on the whole, met. Occasional epidemics of scarlet fever, measles, and other infectious diseases claimed hundreds of lives. But Los Angeles County's sparsely populated expanse, temperate climate, and high employment rate guaranteed comparatively long lives for its citizens.

By the time I finished college and graduate school, however, Los Angeles County boasted a 1980 population of 7.5 million people, and sharp political, cultural, and economic divides splintered the populace. A steady flow of Spanish-speaking immigrants from nations to its south ensured California a large, cheap labour force. But for Los Angeles County, which was responsible for the region's vast public health needs, the new Hispanic population only aggravated racial and economic tensions that already were high vis-à-vis the African-American population. During the aerospace industry boom of the early 1980s money flowed faster than Los Angeles water, for those fortunate enough to work in the proper economic sectors. And for the first time, amid wild property speculation, access to affordable housing reached crisis proportions. The public revolted, freezing property taxes.

And in the 1990s, with the county's population topping ten million and racial and class tensions genuinely explosive, the county struggled to pay public health bills with ever-decreasing property tax revenues. By 2001 Los Angeles County had eleven million residents, half of whom spoke Spanish in their homes, and the area's public health needs increasingly reflected those of the regions where the new immigrants come from: Mexico, Central America, Indochina.

Under its constitution California placed responsibility for public health at the county level, and gargantuan Los Angeles County struggled to meet its mandate. In the 1990s it nearly went bankrupt doing so, and as the twenty-first century dawned the county's ability to pay its health bills was tenuous.

The prairie state of Minnesota approached the millennium wealthy, healthy, and sassy. After World War II it built the strongest public health infrastructure in the nation. In 1997 Minnesotans were among the ten longest-living populations in the world, and their public health system was internationally admired. But political winds shifted at the close of the 1990s, and Minnesota set to dismantling its social systems.

A sound public health system, it seems, is vital to societal stability and, conversely, may topple in the face of political or social instability or whim. Each affects the other: widespread political disorder or antigovernmentalism may weaken a public health system, and a crisis in the health of the citizens can bring down a government.

The year 2000 found health in the old Superpowers endangered. And in the world's poor nations, where most of the planet's population resided, every improvement in health seemed to be smashed on the shores of underdevelopment. In 1996 Canadian scientist Joseph Decosas decried underdevelopment at a gathering of AIDS researchers in Vancouver. Holding an imaginary glass of water in the air Decosas grimly said that 'if the solution for AIDS would be to bring a glass of clean water to everybody in the world, we would *not* be able to bring that. We have not been able to stop children from dying from simple diarrhoea by providing clean drinking water.'

We have not, at the millennium, been able to bring clean water, food, or life's succour to the world's poor.

Every night in 1997 more than 200 million Indians went to bed hungry, officially malnourished—including half of the country's children. In China a smaller percentage of the nation's children—one out of every five—was malnourished, but 164 million Chinese went to sleep with hunger gnawing at their stomachs. As did some 25 million Pakistanis, 15 million Brazilians, and more than a third of all Africans. In the Democratic Republic of the Congo (formerly Zaire) and central Africa half the population was malnourished, and globally in the1990s nearly 800 million people on any given day were starving, or a population roughly two and a half times the size of that of the United States of America.

No wonder that AIDS researchers moaned about the seemingly impossible requirements for a viable HIV vaccine: 100 per cent efficacy, 100 per cent safety, stability in tropical heat, and a price of less than one dollar a dose. Even at that price such a vaccine might be as elusive for the world's poor as Decosas's clean glass of water. While science searched for technological solutions, what really stymied most of the world was frighteningly basic.

In Eastern Europe the 1990s saw a rocky road to economic recovery, but progress did, indeed, emerge in such countries as Poland, the old East Germany, and the Czech Republic, with average per capita incomes nearly doubling during the decade. Not so farther east in the Slavic, Baltic, and Central Asian nations of the former Soviet Union. There wealth concentrated in the hands of former Communist bosses, criminals, and bankers, leaving the populaces in despair. In 2000 Russia ranked as the number one riskiest economy for foreign investment.[1]

Progress for public health at the millennium seemed chained to economics. Nations could not advance so long as their populaces were debilitated by illness. And they lacked the financial abilities to build health infrastructures. Still, optimists drew satisfaction from the World Bank's strong commitment to public health and its increasing global recognition that healthy nations developed more rapidly than those impeded by an ailing populace. That message was the World Health Organization Director-General Gro Harlem Brundtland's battle cry in 1999.

But the new century finds experts at odds over the mission of public health. No two deans of the West's major schools of public health agree on a definition of its goals and missions. While one school—the University of California, Berkeley—selected a biotechnology executive in 1998 as its dean, another—Harvard—opted that year for a leader whose battle was against the most ancient—even traditional—scourge, tuberculosis. A schism appeared and widened in academia, pitting technologists and health managers against the more traditional advocates of disease prevention and epidemiology.

Regardless of the mission statements of academic centres, it was clear by the 1990s that public health, as a discipline, was changing radically. Whether its practitioners were running family planning clinics in Cairo, antibiotic import and distribution for Sri Lanka, drinking water surveillance in Moscow, or multibillion-dollar Medicaid programmes for the United States, their political clout was diminishing and cost-effectiveness was the watchword of the day. It was no longer sufficient to prove that a given intervention prevented disease and saved lives: now it had to do so *affordably.*

If an arsonist torches an office building the roles of the fire department and police are obvious. When they do their jobs—stop the fire and apprehend the arsonist—the community recognizes their achievements and applauds their actions. Because of this it is politically difficult-to-impossible to slash a police or fire department budget except in times of municipal bankruptcy.

If, in contrast, the workers in that office building are strong, healthy, and long-lived, it is next to impossible to prove that the efforts of local public health officials are responsible.

Public health is a negative. When it is at its best, nothing happens: there are no epidemics, food and water are safe to consume, the citizens are well-informed regarding personal habits that affect their health, children are immunized, the air is breathable, factories obey worker safety standards, there is little class-based disparity in disease or life expectancy, and few citizens go untreated when they develop addictions to alcoholic or narcotic substances. In the absence of failures in these areas, politicians faced with budgetary crises, or dictators eager to expand their local and regional power, may feel justified in hacking away at government health budgets. Even if epidemics emerge, such as those of HIV, Ebola, pneumonic plague, or drug-resistant tuberculosis, national leadership is often insulated from the danger, as they typically are far more wealthy than the imperilled citizens and have access to elite health coverage.

And public health advocates, fearing for their jobs or programmes, may be tempted to bend to political whims of the day, veering away from the voice of Science to back ideological or religious trends. Such was the case in the Soviet Union, where rational genetics and the medical social practices flowing from Darwinian evolutionary understandings were abandoned in favour of the absurd anti-genetics belief system of Lysenkoism. Only those Soviet scientists bent on perverting public health's mission, concocting ghastly biological weapons of mass destruction, were spared the shackles of Lysenkoism in favour of genocidal weapons based on the central dogma of DNA.

The scope of activities that fell under the rubric of public health by the end of the twentieth century was quite broad. In 1988 the US Institute of Medicine (IOM) struggled for a definition of public health,[2] arriving at the following: 'The committee defines the mission of public health as fulfilling society's interest in assuring conditions in which people can be healthy.'

Elsewhere in their report, the Institute of Medicine committee tried to justify their overbroad definition:

> Knowledge and values today remain decisive elements in the shaping of public health practice. But they blend less harmoniously than they once-did. On the surface there appears to be widespread agreement on the overall mission of public health, as reflected in such comments to the committee as 'public health does things that benefit everybody,' or 'public health prevents illness and educates the population.' But when it comes to translating broad statements into effective action, little consensus can be found. Neither among the providers nor the beneficiaries of public health programs is there a shared sense of what the citizenry should expect in the way of services, and both the mix and the intensity of services vary widely from place to place.[2]

In other words, there was no agreement about what constituted 'public health' other than assuring that people were healthy. In the absence of a coherent definition of the discipline it was no wonder its advocates were struggling to defend their budgets and policies. During the 1980s, the IOM found that every state lost funding and personnel in all areas except provision of clinical health care. Such vital services as drinking water and food quality control, environmental and occupational health, laboratories and disease control all lost money and personnel.

Even the prestigious Institute of Medicine found it difficult to distinguish medicine from public health. Though the two pursuits classically shared few interests and often were in direct conflict, political pressures over the course of the last half of the twentieth century had blurred the borders between the two. In the United States 'public health' had become—incorrectly—synonymous with medicine for poor people. Few

Americans at the millennium thought of 'public health' as a system that functioned in their interests. Rather, it was viewed as a government handout for impoverished people.

When Congress and the White House set out in 1990 to reduce the national debt public health suffered and the loss of federal funds was felt all the way down to the level of neighbourhood clinics. In its first term the Clinton administration tried to map out a new national health-care system, tightly linked with public health and able to absorb the then thirty-seven million uninsured Americans. Unable to find common ground with the Congress and the health insurance industry, the White House was soundly defeated.

By the end of the decade, more than forty-four million Americans were uninsured, the nation had no coherent health-care system, and the numbers of uninsured was swelling by 100 000 people each month.

In lieu of a national medical infrastructure, public health and curative medicine were provided by a hotchpotch of for-profit insurers, physician organizations (PPOs), county, state, and federal insurers, health maintenance organizations (HMOs), and managed care companies. With every passing day it became more difficult to decipher who, if anyone, was protecting the public's health. And government public health budgets continued to plummet, dropping 25 per cent between 1981 and 1993.[3] While the federal and some overall state health budgets increased between 1994 and 1998, the bulk of those funds were directed to provision of medical care. Most key public health programmes took substantial hits.[4]

By 1998 the states with the most people enrolled in HMOs and managed care plans had the weakest safety nets. In California, for example, which led the nation in HMO enrollment, one out of every four citizens was uninsured and the state's largest county health system repeatedly faced bankruptcy.

The health management perspective also found adherents in Europe, Latin America, and the developing world. Managed care advocates marched across Russia, the Baltics, Eastern Europe, and the Caucasus preaching the gospel of cost controls and team care. Western European governments, long the prime health providers in their societies, hung on to the managed care miracle in hopes of slimming down their budgets, a key component at play in the new global capitalism.

And the World Health Organization, once the conscience of global health, lost its way in the 1990s. Demoralized, rife with rumours of corruption, and lacking in leadership, WHO floundered. Other international agencies—notably the World Bank and UNICEF—stepped in to the breech. By 1997 the World Bank was the biggest public health funder in the world, bankrolling $13.5 billion worth of projects, primarily in developing countries.[5]

'The health of the world stands at a crossroads,' wrote an august group of international health leaders.[6] 'For half a century, most countries have achieved impressive progress in their health conditions. Yet the causes of ill-health do not stand still—humanity's very progress changes them. The past decade has witnessed a profound transformation in the challenges to global health; persistent problems have been joined by new scourges in a world that is ever more complex and interdependent. The idea that the health of every nation depends on the health of all others is not an empty piety but an epidemiological fact.'

It was time to face reality: as the vital statistics of the human race appeared to be improving, the threat, even materialization, of reversal was ever present.

It begs the question: what is public health?

It is not curative medicine. CT scans, open heart surgery, hormone treatments, fibre optic images—these are all great boons for medicine, but they are not public health. And, perhaps surprisingly, they have not been responsible for the vast improvements in the public's health. Even vaccines and antibiotics—both of them vital tools of the modern public health arsenal—have contributed comparatively little to population-based improvements in such key indicators of public health as life expectancy, infant mortality, and infectious disease deaths.

Vital statistics data from England, Wales, and Sweden show that in 1700 the average male in those countries lived just twenty-seven to thirty years. By 1971 male life expectancy reached seventy-five years. More than half that improvement occurred before 1900; even the bulk of the twentieth-century increases in life expectancy were due to conditions that existed prior to 1936. In all, 86 per cent of the increased life expectancy was due to decreases in infectious diseases.[7] And the bulk of the decline in infectious disease deaths occurred *prior* to the age of antibiotics. In the United Kingdom, for example, tuberculosis deaths dropped from nearly 4000 per million people to 500 per million between 1838 and 1949, when antibiotic treatment was introduced, an 87 per cent decline. Between 1949 and 1969 the TB death rate fell by only another forty million cases to 460 cases per million, or 9 per cent.

The same can be said for the United States, where less than 4 per cent of the total improvement in life expectancy since the 1700s can be credited to twentieth-century advances in medical care.[8]

It is a matter of considerable academic debate which factors were most responsible for the spectacular improvements seen in life expectancy and infant mortality in the United States and Western Europe between 1700 and 1900. Some of the following were key: nutrition, housing, urban sewage and water systems, government epidemic control measures, swamp drainage and river control engineering, road construction and paving, public education and literacy, access to prenatal and maternity care, smaller families, and overall improvements in society's standards of living and working. In the early twentieth century elimination of urban, overcrowded slums that lacked plumbing and toilet facilities clearly improved the health of tens of thousands of Americans and Europeans.

The critical dilemma for the twenty-first century was embedded in the disparity between the rich and poor, both within and among nations. In the wealthy world the twenty-first century was greeted by stock markets ebullient about biotechnology and protein-based public health—the alleged pharmacopoeia of future disease prevention. But in much of the world the core advances in public health pioneered between 1890 and 1920 in New York City had, even a century later, to take hold. Drinking water remained contaminated; human waste was dumped untreated; children went unvaccinated and malnourished; hygiene was ignored in hospitals and precious antibiotics were dispensed like sweets in black markets worldwide.

What New York public health pioneer Hermann Biggs and his colleagues demonstrated before World War I in Gotham was that public health not only had little to do with organized medicine, but that it might often be antagonistic to physicians. It would oppose schemes that placed individual health in primacy over the good of the public, as a whole. Biggs battled with doctors over the naming of tuberculosis patients, for example: doctors wanted discretion for wealthy clients while Biggs demanded safety for all New Yorkers. Public health fought on behalf of the community, placing special attention on the poorest, least advantaged elements of that community, for it was amid conditions of poverty that disease usually arose.

Public health is not an ideology, religion, or political perspective—indeed, history demonstrates that whenever such forces interfere with or influence public health activities a general worsening of the populace's well-being usually followed. As visualized by its American pioneers public health was a practical system, or infrastructure, rooted in two fundamental scientific tenets: the germ theory of disease and the understanding that preventing disease in the weakest elements of society ensured protection for the strongest (and richest) in the larger community.

As infectious diseases became less of a concern in the wealthy world, in the mid-twentieth century public health leaders struggled to apply those basic tenets, and the infrastructure upon which they were based, to non-microbial collective health issues, such as cancer and heart disease. The translation was not easy, and in some arenas it clearly failed. It proceeded most coherently where the cause of disease—the culprit—had an outside, threatening nature similar to the fear invoked by mysterious microbes. In the world of fin de siècle New York City in the1890s members of all social classes and ethnic groups were sufficiently fearful of germs to strive for communitywide solutions and support public health. Similarly, in the second half of the twentieth century public health benefited by characterizing the tobacco industry and polluters as sources of cancer threat to the community, fast-food distributors as heart disease promoters, and radiation emitters as creators of deformed babies. But the links were never as strong, either scientifically or politically, as those Biggs, France's Louis Pasteur, and their contemporaries made between germs and infectious diseases.

Public health in the wealthy world, therefore, struggled to maintain respect, funding, and self-definition in the late twentieth century.

It was no coincidence that one hundred years previously the precious concept of public health arose in New York City, as it was the world's centre of nineteenth- and twentieth-century globalization. The public health leaders of Biggs's day weren't uniformly progressive individuals—indeed, many were complete bigots. But they were a practical lot. They understood that the economy of Gotham thrived on globalism, and that such a vast economic reach necessarily held risks. Chief among those risks were the microbial hitchhikers carried inside the immigrants, travellers, and cargo from all over the world. When the immigrants settled into horrible, crowded tenements lacking toilets and running water, the risk to the community was compounded, as even rare and latent diseases could be amplified in such surroundings into terrible epidemics. Thus, they reasoned, it was in the interests of the community as a whole to address the health needs of those tenement dwellers, providing milk to the children, disease surveillance and epidemic control for all, food inspections, pure water, clean streets, shorter and safer work hours, and improved housing.

In the newly globalized economy of the twenty-first century no part of the planet is too remote, too exotic, or too forbidding for travellers or business development. The whole world is becoming New York City—a polyglot of multiple language-babbling traders, artists, social classes, religions, and tensions.

Even hatreds and community conflicts have globalized. A group of alienated individuals might fight its battles on home turf or, quite frequently, choose symbolic sites thousands of miles away to target with weapons of terrorism. A confrontation in Asia might play out in a series of bombings in Paris, Berlin, and Chicago. By the 1990s the US government was fixated on terrorism, recognizing not only foreign but also domestic forces capable and willing to resort to the use of deadly force against innocent civilians. Deadliest of all options—frightening beyond words—was the spectre of deliberate release of supergerms that would sweep around the world claiming tens of thousands of lives in man-made epidemics.

The US government once again turned to technology for answers, hoping some device could be invented that would sense such weapons of bioterrorism before their release. Once again public health—the *only* viable protection against epidemics, whether natural or man-made—was given short shrift.

If anthrax were released in Grand Central Station one morning, who would be the first in New York City to realize such a dastardly act had been committed? Surely it would not be some mythical sensory device, nor the law enforcement officials wielding the contraption. It would be members of the public health infrastructure, alerted by hospital reports of unusual illnesses cropping up from Brooklyn to the Bronx.

In the absence of such an infrastructure, Gotham would be doomed to an anthrax epidemic that could not be staunched by millions of dollars of high-tech military and FBI interventions. The saviours of the city could only be her public health warriors.

From my perch on the Brooklyn Bridge, I can see jet after jet circle out of John F. Kennedy International Airport: the ships are gone, and the new globalism is airborne. Time has collapsed, bringing risks and opportunities to every community within days. Tomorrow it will be hours. Perhaps by 2050 it will be minutes. Progress.

The challenges of public health have never been greater, either in counties like Los Angeles, prosperous states such as Minnesota, or former super powers like the Russian Federation. Each is now linked to the other. The community has expanded. Its membership is six billion human beings, more than five billion of whom live in the global equivalent of New York City's 1890s tenements.

For most of the world's population in 2000, the public health essentials mapped out in New York before World War I have never existed: progress, in the form of safe water, food, housing, sewage, and hospitals, has never come. An essential trust, between government and its people, in pursuit of health for all has never been established. In other parts of the world—notably the former Soviet Union—the trust was betrayed long ago.

Yes, scientific and medical tools invented in the twentieth century will form a vital basis to global public health efforts in the twenty-first century, as will bold innovations based on altering human and microbial genetics. But the basic factors essential to a population's health are ancient and non-technological: clean water; plentiful, nutritious, uncontaminated food; decent housing; appropriate water and waste disposal; correct social and medical control of epidemics; widespread—or universal—access to maternal and child health-care; clean air; knowledge of personal health needs administered to a population sufficiently educated to be able to comprehend and use the information in their daily lives; and, finally, a health-care system that follows the primary maxim of medicine—*do no harm*.

In the days of Biggs and Pasteur public health was local, manageable enough if backed with sufficient political support. Its infrastructure provided, first and foremost, communitywide prophylaxis against disease.

Now the community is an entire world. It watches, and squirms, as plague strikes Surat, Ebola hits Kikwit, tuberculosis overwhelms Siberian prisons, and HIV vanquishes a generation of Africans. The community grows anxious. Though it empathizes, it fears that what is 'over there' could come 'here.' Worse, as it bites into bananas grown 'over there,' the community collectively worries: what microbes or pesticides am I consuming?

Public health needs to be—must be—global prevention.

Now that would be genuine progress.

CHAPTER 1

Filth and decay

**Pneumonic plague hits India
and the world ill responds.**

*This town is coming like
    a ghost town
No job to be found
    in this country.
Can't go on no more,
    people getting angry.
This town is coming like
    a ghost town.
This town is coming like
    a ghost town.
This town is coming like
    a ghost town.
This town is coming like
    a ghost town.
This town is coming like
    a ghost town.*
From 'Ghost Town'
—The Specials, 1981

No one else got off the train. Thousands got on.

Even before the ageing Indian locomotive lumbered its way into Surat passengers began scouring their sacks and suitcases in search of rags or scarves to wrap around their faces. Protesting children wailed, but mothers, speaking Hindi, Tamil, Punjabi, Bengali, or English, sharply insisted.

'You must wear this, child. It will protect you,' they said. And as the train approached the city the children's dark eyes widened above their impromptu masks and the rocking passengers grew silent.

The only Westerner aboard gathered her bags and, to the obvious astonishment of fellow passengers, got off the train, stepping into the torrid September heat of Surat. Throngs of masked Suratis, encumbered with bags and infants, elbowed their ways onto the train, shouting and jostling for seats. Though they had tickets, most would gladly stand for hours if need be, relieved to get far away from the monsoon-soaked city.

Far away from the plague.

In less than a week 500 000 residents of Surat had fled, forming a diaspora of Suratis that, thanks to India's vast train system, now stretched from the Himalayas to Sri Lanka. An estimated 600 000 day workers and business travellers who normally visited the gem and fabric districts of Surat stayed away. Thus, less than half of Surat's typical daily census of 2.2 million remained. They were the poorest of the Gujarat State's poor: lower caste citizens who could no more conjure the seventy rupees (or $2.50) for a lower class train ticket than $500 for a seat on a jet.

As the chugging sound of the departing train dissipated, a near silence, punctuated by occasional motorbike rickshaws, reigned. Four train carriages remained, painted with large red crosses and signs saying ACCIDENT MEDICAL RELIEF. The ground around the carriages was chalk white with thick layers of DDT pesticide powder.

Rubbish blew about the streets, inspected by foraging cows sacred to the largely Hindu population. Roads that usually resonated with the high frequencies of diamond polishing devices and 300 000 power textile looms were silent. Boards, loosely hammered in place, sealed shut the pharmacies, private medical clinics, and nongovernmental hospitals. Those citizens who remained moved quickly, rags or masks wrapped about their noses and mouths.

Only the prostitutes near Ved Road flaunted their faces (as well as their figures), calling out from brothel balconies to would-be customers. And, perhaps surprisingly, there were customers, despite the plague.

'This came as a sudden grip, a blow from the sky,' declared Gujarat's Minister for Health Subash Shelad. 'I wish there weren't so much panic.'

But panic had, indeed, taken hold, and Surat was a ghost town. At the sprawling new Holiday Inn a visitor could have any room she pleased, as all of the rest were empty. Meals were a bit limited, as farmers were afraid to bring their goods into the plague-ridden city. And it took some time for the turbaned Sikh doorman to find a rickshaw taxi willing, even for the equivalent of a normal month's wages, to take a visitor about town.

Amid the squalor of open sewers, ramshackle crowded houses, and roaming livestock emerged a cluster of poor Surati men shouting, 'Plague! Plague! Plague!' The terrified men raced about madly, waving wooden clubs and shouting for all the world to hear. Kicking up a cloud of dust they settled into a tight circle, staring at the ground. And cowering in terror, trapped between human feet, was a brown rat, its beady eyes blinking in the bright sunlight.

'Plague,' a man reiterated, waving his club menacingly at the rat. Yet so great was the collective fear that the men of Ved Road dared not hit the sorry rat lest it might give its assailant a retaliatory bite. After a moment the rodent made its escape, scurrying down a refuse-strewn hillside and disappearing into a DDT-coated hole.

The men looked sheepish. When told that the fleas that may carry *Yersinia pestis* plague-causing bacteria usually inhabit *Ratus ratus*—black rats—the cluster feels its manhood restored, each man puffing up his chest and sternly vowing to kill the first ebony-coloured rat he sees.[1]

In September 1994 all of India resonated with plague panic, coupled with a near universal condemnation of a filthy Surat.

'Surat is perhaps the most decrepit, unlivable, and unmanageable Indian city of its size,' wrote the *Telegraph*.[2] The Calcutta newspaper was typical of India's major media as it decried the Surati 'bankruptcy of administration, the decadence of society and the collapse of basic civic amenities.'

Nothing shamed the nation's commentators and intellectuals as deeply as world attention to India's rats, and the urban filth in which they thrived. While politicians wagged their fingers scoldingly at Surat's local government, the nation's intellectual elite found in the symbolic rat reason to denounce the most fundamental aspects of Indian economics and politics. Typical of the perspective were the views expressed by Nikhil Chakravartty, who noted that the vast Indian nation was ruled by a strong federal hand during the decades of colonialism.[3] But since independence, Chakravartty continued, the centralized federal government had weakened and local administrations had taken over rule of every aspect of Indian life, with disastrous results.

'In short, a fearsome underworld has surfaced in all the metropolitan centres and larger municipalities. The plague menace, we are warned now, spreads through garbage piling up on which rats thrive,' Chakravartty wrote. 'Come to the best of our urban centres and you will see garbage-piling has become a common feature. In Calcutta, garbage reaches mountainous proportions before it is touched by municipal authorities. Bombay may be better off in the posh super-rich pockets, but things are no better in the densely populated areas.'

'It is fashionable nowadays to talk of globalization, of getting into the world currents. But if our municipalities and district boards are in a state of disuse and become the inevitable breeding ground of epidemics, what sort of economic miracle are we going to bring about?'

Like their American and European counterparts in the late nineteenth century, India's intellectuals in 1994 cried out for sanitation and hygiene, the absence of which they blamed not only for the plague, but also for every imaginable failure in their society.

On such a note of hand-wringing, J. N. Dixit wrote that 'this crisis should impel us to ruminate on the economic and social implications of such an epidemic. Speaking of crises, at times, one is pushed to superstitious apprehension, even para-psychological paranoia about India's fate!'[4]

But the focus of plague paranoia was nothing as surreal as parapsychology but rather the mundane, eyesore-inflicting, nose-offending filth that filled the streets and alleys of India, having long since become the single most familiar and reliable feature of her urban landscapes.

'It's as if a medieval curse is upon us. But the hex is self-inflicted. We are our own worst murderers. Because we are the practitioners of filth. The emperors of garbage,' read one editorial in *India Today*.[5] 'As in all societies that have made progress, a ground-swell of public opinion against dirt and disease has been the backbone of fundamental reform because it is a simultaneous upheaval against endemic corruption and fatalism. Ultimately, the health of a nation is also its wealth. There are dramatic movements in this country in the fields of entrepreneurship, economic modernization, science and technology. But unless this collective lurch toward progress is accompanied by a vision of a cleaner and more hygienic life, India will never quite qualify in the eyes of the international community as a modernising nation. Nobody wants to invest in the dark ages.'

And so by the fourth week of the epidemic, fires burned in every city in the nation, filling the air with the putrid smell of flaming refuse. Herds of day workers built mountains of incredible height made entirely of filth, doused them in petrol, and with these pyres hoped to set India on a course from Plague to Progress. In perhaps the most vivid symbolism of the day, city administrators in Bombay hired Irula tribes-men from the southernmost state of Tamil Nadu to hunt rats in the city of some fourteen million humans crammed so densely that an average of 130 000 souls lived in each square mile. Famed for their rodent-catching skills, the Irula tribesmen had for centuries eaten rats, which comprised their main daily source of protein. Bombay told the Irula they could eat all they wanted, and actually get paid for their feasting.

But, despicable as Surat's verminous filth was, the stench, waste, and rodents of the city played little, if any, role in the start or spread of the nation's plague epidemic. While it may have sparked a long overdue urban beautification campaign, the plague in Surat had much more to do with horrid housing, human panic, and bereft health care than *Ratus ratus*.

It didn't even start in Surat. And flea-ridden rats in the Gujarati city weren't responsible for its spread.

The epidemic began hundreds of miles to the south-east in a rural part of Maha-rashtra State, the capital of which is Bombay.

The earthquake hit while villagers slept, striking with a Richter force of 6.4: not enough to topple well-constructed motorway overpasses in Los Angeles, but quite suf-ficient power to level the mud and brick homes of the Beed and Osmanabad Districts. The September 30, 1993, earthquake's epicentre was the eastern Maharashtra city of Latur, in which tens of thousands of homes were levelled. Surrounding Latur some ten thousand villages were obliterated, one million homes destroyed, and more than ten thousand people killed.

For days afterward aftershocks of up to Richter scale 5.0 rocked the Osmanabad and Beed Districts, prompting a human exodus of survivors who fled the earth's rage. The peasants of Beed, being practical sorts, hastily harvested their crops and locked the food inside whatever structures had outlasted the earthquake before decamping the region.

The Indian government, with about $30 million in financial aid from the World Bank, erected prefabricated houses, sprinkling the structures where Latur's villages once had stood. And the residents trickled back into the region during the summer of 1994.[6]

No one in India had seen a case of plague in more than thirty years. During the 1980s, convinced that *Yersinia pestis* bacteria had disappeared from India, state governments one by one shut down their plague stations, stopped looking for cases, and eventually even ceased random rat and flea checks.

On August 26, 1994, Yashitha Langhe, a man from the village of Mamala, located near Beed, returned to his earthquake-ruined home. He opened doors sealed for months behind which he had hastily stored harvested grains before fleeing the tremors eleven months previously. And he was overwhelmed by a cloud of black fleas that seemed to leap from the decrepit storeroom, biting at every millimetre of his body. When he looked down it seemed that the very ground on which he stood was moving.

At his feet, and all about the Mamala man, were black rats, grown fat and populous, thriving on the stored grain bounty. The Mamala man's experience was repeated that week in village after village, in Beed, outside Latur, as earthquake refugees returned to their hamlets to lay claim to new government-built houses and retrieve their caches of grain.

Yersinia pestis is a bacterium that can survive for extended periods of time in an apparently dormant state in soil. This capacity was overlooked when Indian officials decided to abandon all plague surveillance programmes. In Maharashtra State, plague public health programmes were eliminated in 1987; the last officially certified human case appeared in nearby Karnataka State in 1966.

The bacteria can also hide in the guts of fleas, causing no harm to the insects, quietly reproducing and passing their offspring off to subsequent generations of fleas.

But when conditions change—in ways no-one clearly understood even by the end of the twentieth century—a genetic signal is triggered in the bacteria's DNA. A gene called *hms* (for hemin storage) switches on, causing the secretion of proteins that essentially shift the *Yersinia pestis* population from acting as a benign commensal thriving in the gut of a flea into a super dangerous bacterial collective that invades the insect's foregut. There, the microbes block the movement of food, and the flea begins to starve.[7]

The starving flea shifts its diet and, frantic, becomes far more aggressive. It will then in a frenzy assertively attack any warm-blooded creature, living off the blood that it extracts from the animal's body. Rats, particularly those of the black *Ratus ratus* species, are primary targets. And aboard the rats the fleas are protected by the rodent's fur and are highly mobile, carried energy-free by the scurrying creatures.

When humans come in proximity of the rats the plague-carrying fleas are capable of leaping distances that are orders of magnitude greater than their own size, landing on *Homo sapiens* skin to feast on 37°C blood.[8]

Yersinia pestis then has other tricks in its genetic bag. The bacteria have several special genes—at least twenty of them—that give the organism unique powers over the cells of humans and other animals. The instant *Yersinia* come in contact with human cells these genes switch on, causing production of a lethal cascade of chemicals.

The first set of chemicals drill a microscopic hole in the protective membrane of the human cell.[9] Then another set of genetically coded proteins becomes a transport tube carrying chemicals from *Yersinia* into the victimized cell. These chemicals swiftly incapacitate the targeted cell.

Meanwhile, *Yersinia* also secretes a set of proteins into its immediate environment that blocks defensive efforts of the human's immune system. Mighty macrophages—large immune system cells that usually gobble up invading microbes—are rendered impotent by the *Yersinia* chemicals. The effectiveness of this stunning and complex system of attack lies in the fact that these genes, and the proteins they encode, are not originally of bacterial origin. They are animal genes, stolen millennia ago through unknown means and put to deadly, effective purpose by the bacteria. Thus, a protein system originally intended to serve an entirely different purpose—a benign role—in animal cells has evolved into one of the most complicated and efficient offensive weapons apparatuses in the microbial world.

If *Yersinia* takes hold in cells of the skin and lymphatic system a disease called bubonic plague results. As colonies of *Yersinia* grow, the human's lymph nodes swell, often to enormous sizes, and ugly pustules form on the skin, oozing yellow, viscous liquid.

In the villages around Beed people began by late August to develop precisely these symptoms. And on September 14, 1994, Indian Union Health Secretary M. S. Dayal confirmed that there were four cases of bubonic plague in Mamala, Beed District, Maharashtra State.

Two days later the Maharashtra State authorities announced that 10 per cent of the village population of Mamala were suffering bubonic plague, and India's National Institute of Communicable Diseases issued laboratory confirmation that the ailments of the Beed District were caused by *Yersinia pestis*.

Although even a handful of cases of bubonic plague would have been justified cause for mass panic in India or anywhere else in the world six decades earlier, there shouldn't have been serious alarm in 1994. After all, *Yersinia* could be defeated with the cheapest and simplest of antibiotics: tetracycline and doxycycline. If administered in the first stages of illness, or simply after suspected exposure to infected fleas, these drugs were usually 100 per cent curative.

Once illness was established, however, treatment became more difficult. *Yersinia* could move into the red bloodstream, causing septicaemia and ravaging the heart and liver. Or it could colonize the lungs, producing pneumonic plague. That was the most contagious and dangerous form of the disease, for once *Yersinia* inhabited the convulsed, coughing lungs of a human being it no longer required rodents or fleas to spread, creating contagion. A microscopic mist of exhaled droplets was sufficient to pass the bacteria from one person to the next.

Untreated, or improperly treated, *Yersinia* easily claimed 50 per cent of all infected human beings. But it was inconceivable that any nation in the world at the end of the twentieth century would fail to stop a bubonic plague outbreak, preventing the less easily controlled pneumonic form from emerging.

So on September 16, the Beed District's Health Secretary R. Tiwari told local reporters that 'there is no need to panic'. Help, he insisted, was on its way. Maharashtra State Health Minister Subash Salunke further insisted that all Beed District plague reports were 'wildly exaggerated'. But he admitted that *Yersinia* might have surfaced after its long hiatus, because the bacilli, he said, 'could live in the soil for ten to fifteen years'.

In Bombay, Dr V. L. Yemul of the Haffkine Institute expressed the opinion that the region's earthquake had disrupted the ecological niches of long-hidden *Yersinia* colonies, opening up previously hidden soils. Further, he said, in the aftermath of the quake populations of rival rat species grew and fought over the stores of grain left by frightened villagers. Their blood fights attracted fleas, allowing for a surge in that insect population. Thus, he argued, what was seen in the tiny village of Mamala, population 375, was likely to also be occurring in earthquake-ravaged villages throughout the region.

The earthquake had disrupted the health-care infrastructure of the region, levelling clinics and driving physicians and nurses from their homes. So local authorities were hard-pressed to identify and treat all the bubonic plague cases. And further exacerbating the problem was the monsoon, which in 1994 was the most powerful one anyone could recall. Roads were washed out, turning even a short distance into a severe, lengthy journey. A reporter who attempted to travel the roughly 400 kilometres (or 240 miles) of roads from Bombay to Latur had to give up after fourteen gruelling hours of dodging elephants, diesel trucks, sacred cows, and other vehicles on a road frequently narrowed to less than a truck's width of passable road.

But in truth, India would have had difficulties no matter where *Yersinia* had surfaced, for the country's public health infrastructure was stretched beyond limits. At a time of record-breaking economic growth, India was slashing its public health expenditures, shifting responsibilities from the federal to state levels, and seemingly washing its hands of all responsibility for the people's health. By 1991 to 1992, federal public health spending, which included hospital services, was a mere 0.04 per cent of the national budget, or more than tenfold less than was spent in the previous decade.

Bad as that might have been, the 1992 to 1993 federal budget saw a 20 per cent further reduction in public spending. And few states compensated by increasing their local public health expenditures. None increased spending by more than 5 per cent.

In 1992 only three nations—Brazil, Mexico, and the Russian Federation—were carrying more than India's astounding external debt of $77 billion. Foreign investors had steadily increased their confidence in India, but even with annual growth during the 1990s, private foreign investment in the country was less than $1.5 billion in 1994.

The Indian economy grew steadily in the early 1990s by a rate of 4 per cent a year—a genuine speed demon pace for India, but a crawl by regional standards. Pakistan in contrast grew by 9 per cent annually, South Korea by 10 per cent.[10]

Despite its massive external debt and comparatively slow economic growth, India was considered a promising financial state, heading toward a free market and rapidly eliminating former laws that rigidly controlled its industries and limited outside investment. With an estimated 1994 population of 900 to 950 million people and a gross national product (GNP) per capita of $310 per year, every sector of the Indian economy was growing in the early 1990s at rates well above those seen in most of Africa, Eastern Europe, or the Americas. Value-added manufacturing in 1991 was an impressive $40 billion—one of the largest seen in the third world. So the country was easily able to service its national debt and still meet its annual expenditure needs.

The boom was felt especially strongly in India's southern and western states, where trade deregulation prompted entrepreneurial zeal. In Bangalore, for example, industrious Karnatakans created a vast computer software manufacturing empire. Bombay swiftly became the core of capitalistic enthusiasm in India. And to its north Surat almost overnight was transformed.

Between 1971 to 1991, the population of Surat grew by an astounding 151.61 per cent, with most of that increase representing impoverished migrant workers who toiled in the $600 million textile or $1 billion diamond industries. As the population grew, so did the number of horrendous slums—up from ninety in the 1960s to three hundred by 1994, inhabited by some 450 000 people. There were no formal sewage or water systems in these slums; housing was slapdash lean-tos, even tents; malaria and hepatitis were epidemic; and no one apparently enforced even India's weak labour and safety regulations in the businesses along Ved Road.

What drew industry to Surat was precisely the weakness of its government, lack of health and pollution enforcement, eager, unskilled labour force, and a virtual tax-free environment. By 1994, one out of every three diamonds mined in the world were polished in Surat.[11]

'Perhaps the greatest irony,' wrote the conservative *Business Standard* of Bombay, 'is that the epidemic has hit one of the economically most active areas of the country in a state which is considered to be the most business friendly. . . . What is more, the Gujarat government has gone out of its way to be more accommodating to business than most and has in turn been able to reap the benefits of a rapid industrialization which is not the case with the rest of the country. But somehow down the line, the need for good municipal services was forgotten. Businessmen who were busy making money cared little about minimum civic services or the basic quality of life that says no filth, mosquitoes, flies, fleas, and rats. And when the epidemic hit, they were the first to pack their Maruti 1000s and run. India today has clearly got its priorities wrong.'[12]

The problem, indeed, was priorities. In 1992 India spent twenty times more on its army than on health. And for a decade, India secretly toiled on a massive, hugely expensive effort to create nuclear weapons. The public health sector was at its lowest rank of any major spending category. Just ahead of it was education, which was so poor in India that only 50 per cent of adult men and less than a third of women were able to read, placing India below not just the global literacy average, but subaverage for the poorest nations on earth.

In 1994 nearly a quarter of all Indian children hadn't received their full battery of UNICEF-recommended vaccinations, infant mortality rates were more than ten times those seen in Europe and North America, life expectancy was about fifty-nine years, and more than three humans were born annually for every one that died, guaranteeing that the nation's population explosion would persist well into the twenty-first century.[13]

Meanwhile, India was eager to move swiftly towards a free market and away from its formerly state-regulated socialist economy. It was privatizing many sectors, including health. More than 75 per cent of all care was, by the mid-1990s, provided by private physicians, and the essential public health infrastructure was rapidly disappearing.

'Instead of moving forward to meet the newer health challenges, the situation is sliding backwards,' Dr Alok Mukhopadhyay, chair of the Independent Medical Commission on Health in India, said, noting that public health in his country was in a state of 'gradual but sure decay.'[14]

Against that backdrop, compounded by earthquake and monsoon, Maharashtra's key official, Salunke, and local Beed and Latur health officials struggled in mid-September to keep the bubonic plague epidemic under control. Quick surveys revealed a twentyfold increase in the Latur rat population, with similar rodent explosions counted in Osmanabad. A scouring of local records found that the first complaint of flea infestation was filed, but unheeded, on August 5, and the first human plague case occurred on August 26. Even more disturbing were national plague data released to the media: though India saw no human plague cases from 1966 to 1988, *Yersinia* did, despite prior claims to the contrary, make its comeback in 1989 with three human cases. And in 1991 with fifty. And in 1992 with 135 plague cases nationwide.

Given India's history with plague it seemed a substantial oversight to have dismissed this upward trend in cases. Plague broke out in Calcutta in 1895 and raged across India until 1918, killing more than ten million people. After that *Yersinia* was endemic in India for five decades, claiming more than two and a half million additional lives between 1919 and 1968.

Yet the state governments had all ignored plague surveillance for years. And amidst the outbreak in Maharashtra State, officials continued to downplay the situation, telling inquiring journalists that everything was under control.

A key exception was Dr Syamal Biswas of the Plague Surveillance Unit in distant Bangalore. After investigating the situation around the Beed District of Maharashtra, he pronounced conditions 'extremely favourable' for a pneumonic plague epidemic. His warning was ignored.

By that time 317 human bubonic plague cases had been identified in six districts of Maharashtra State. Though officials, including India's Minister of Health G. Shankaranard, continued to insist that there was 'no cause for concern', newspapers in Bombay began attacking Maharashtra Governor Sharad Pawar and his government, accusing them of neglect.

'But now that it has happened I say don't worry,' Maharashtra's Salunke insisted. 'We have beautiful antibiotics. This is not the Middle Ages. We have pesticides. We have surveillance. I promise you, there will not be one death in Maharashtra. Not one.'

But plague had already spread and was quietly erupting with lethal impact some six hundred kilometres to the north-west in Surat.

Filthy, ramshackle Surat reeled from the monsoon of 1994. For eighty-seven days rain poured on the city, dropping a record eighty-one inches. The Tapti River swelled and overflowed its banks, flooding the ghettos and slums of the city. Along the notorious Ved Road, considered Surat's most abominable slum, Tapti floodwaters rose perilously, reaching rooftops by the end of August. Tens of thousands of Suratis fled during early August, seeking housing in dry parts of the city. It was not uncommon during August to find a dozen people crammed into a shack that normally housed four, or to espy migrant workers sleeping on the floors between the textile looms or diamond polishing machines on which they worked during the days.

Even during the dry season Ved Road was a horror. Most of its residents were migrant workers, 10 to 20 per cent of them were usually from the Beed and Latur districts of Maharashtra. They crowded into houses and shared a handful of toilet facilities. There were 150 people per toilet, open sewers, and a constant stench.

Thanks to the August monsoon the Tapti waters didn't recede from Ved Road until the second week in September. As if to validate the miracle of Ganesh Chaturthi, the rains stopped on September 10, the Tapti receded below its banks, and the mud of Surat began to dry by September 15. It was cause for genuine joy and celebration, as befits the Festival of Ganesh.

Ganesh, the elephant-headed Hindu god, was a favourite of the poor and disadvantaged, for he had heroically overcome tragedy. Reunited after years of forced separation Ganesh greeted his mother, showering her with hugs and kisses. Upon seeing and mistaking the intent of their warm embraces, the mother's new husband flew into a rage, grabbed his sword, and sliced off Ganesh's head.

'What have you done,' cried the mother. 'You have killed my son!'

Shamed, the slayer searched frantically for a way to bring Ganesh back to life. Spotting a passing elephant, he chopped off the animal's head and placed it upon Ganesh's neck. And Ganesh became one of the greatest of gods, fun-loving, filled with great fortune, concerned about the poor.

Traditionally Ganesh's saga is celebrated on September 18 with jubilant festivals. Neighbourhoods and households compete, each trying to outdo the other with their elephant statues of Ganesh. Amid dancing, singing, and drinking, the statues are paraded about for hours, eventually dumped into a body of water. In Surat, the Ganesh statuary found itself in the Tapti River.

Weeks of monsoon had left much of the Tapti's banks unstable, so the usually spread-out celebrations were concentrated, the crowds of festive poor jam-packed into small spaces. They carried their elephant god high, his four arms and trunk waving to the masses.

Somewhere in those crowds was at least one person from Maharashtra. A plague carrier whose infection had gone untreated and moved into his lungs. He coughed as he celebrated.

And three days later, seven feverish, pneumonic celebrants sought help from Dr Pradeep Gupta and his staff in the emergency room of Surat Civil Hospital.

'By twelve-thirty we found that seven had been admitted,' an exhausted Gupta recalled three days later. 'Two had died. They all had bilateral pneumonia and blood in their sputum. And their history of illness was short—certainly less than four days. Then there were other admissions and by Thursday [September 22] by 11:00 a.m. we had thirteen. And seven of the first thirteen were dead.'

The first wave of patients all came from the slums of Ved Road.

By then, six weeks after Yashitha Langhe had come down with bubonic plague in far-off Mamala village in Maharashtra, the federal government was insisting that less than seventy people in India had plague, all of them suffering the easily treated bubonic form.

Gupta, a young, energetic civil service physician, suspected instantly that his dead and dying patients were victims of pneumonic plague, a disease he knew only from textbooks. He took his suspicions to Dr B. D. Parmar, who examined sputum samples from the dead under a microscope. A professor of medicine at the Medical College of Surat, Parmar was typically consulted when Civil Hospital physicians found puzzling infectious disease cases.

'I diagnosed the first case here on September 20,' Parmar recalled. 'The patient was admitted for malaria that developed suddenly. I ordered an X-ray which showed bilateral pneumonia. We treated that case as pneumonic plague, since there are some cases reported from Beed District of bubonic plague. We suspected pneumonic plague since the symptoms were fast-developing over a period of six hours. And the patients developed blood in the sputum and respiratory failure within no time, with bilateral pneumonia.'

Parmar's first case was a thirty-five-year-old migrant worker from Maharashtra.

'He had an X-ray done at a private hospital,' Gupta said of that first patient. 'That was at 8 p.m. It looked completely normal. Then he developed a high fever at midnight. On taking his X-ray here an hour later, we saw violent signs of pneumonic plague. Violent. He died that night. That indicates the virulence of the organism.'

'Was that frightening to you?' a visitor asked.

'Definitely!' Gupta exclaimed, his voice muffled by the three respiratory masks he wore, one of which was designed to protect workmen from chemicals.

'Definitely,' he repeated, shuddering.

On September 20, Parmar and Gupta cornered their new boss, the recently appointed medical supervisor of Civil Hospital, Dr Dinesh Shah. A middle-aged man accustomed to the reins of authority, Shah wanted to see the laboratory work himself. After examining under the microscope smear samples from the patients, he said, 'Yes, looks like pneumonic plague.'

Shah ordered smears sent to the National Centre for Infectious Diseases in New Delhi and contacted local authorities. But privately he was troubled by seemingly odd aspects of Surat's outbreak. There were no plague-dead rats in the city; all of the first cases were adult men, which seemed strange; there were no initial paediatric cases, which violated patterns seen historically.

'It's very surprising,' Shah told his staff. 'No ratfall. This just came in straight to the city in pneumonic form. Did someone from Beed come here? Maybe.'

'Or maybe,' he continued with a chill, '*Yersinia* has mutated.'

Professor Parmar was also concerned about the apparent oddities in Surat's epidemic. And he told Shah that without help from the city's 137 private physicians, 'This will spread like wildfire. It's a Black Death.'

The civil doctors, fully supported by the Gujarat State Minister of Health Subash Shelad, did their level best to spread word of the apparent plague outbreak calmly, hoping to solicit assistance from the city's private physicians.

They were totally unprepared for what followed.

The private doctors panicked. Eighty per cent of them fled the city, closing their clinics and hospitals and abandoning their patients. The fear in those physicians' eyes did not go unnoticed by the populace, and rumours of a great impending disaster spread swiftly among the largely illiterate masses. Surat's middle class discreetly packed their bags and slipped out of town.

Then, on September 22, Surati and Bombay newspapers carried banner headlines declaring, 'Surat Fever!'

'Over eighty people are feared to have died following the outbreak of a mysterious fever here last night,' read the lead of a typical Bombay newspaper article that morning.[15] 'Dr Mahendra Gandhi, a private practitioner in the city, has confirmed forty-five deaths and said the toll is likely to cross eighty'.

It was only the opening salvo of a barrage of wildly exaggerated reports that would hit the world's media, most of them relying on panicked private physicians for their information. The BBC, which is hugely popular in India, echoed these reports, saying on September 22 that a mysterious deadly fever had broken out in Surat.

The exodus began.

Within twelve hours of the BBC broadcast an estimated 100 000 Suratis boarded trains headed in every imaginable direction across the Indian subcontinent. Because Surat had no unemployment it had attracted workers from as far away as Bangladesh, Tamil Nadu, Delhi, Uttar Pradesh, Punjab, even Nepal. Now they fled homeward, potentially taking with them infectious microbes.

Friday, September 23, found an estimated 300 000 more Suratis, handkerchiefs wrapped about their faces, queued up for trains. By then the Civil Hospital had seen thirty-one pneumonic plague deaths and its wards were packed with plague and with the worried well. Officials declared Surat a 'ghost town,' and five states, including Gujarat and Maharashtra, went on emergency health alert status.

News reports across India ran the gamut from the *Times of India*'s calming headline that day ('Disease is infectious, but curable') to the *Daily*'s claim that more than 250 Suratis were dead, and 10 000 had the plague. One report had it that half the population of tiny Kattar village in rural Gujarat were dead, all plague victims. Still another account had it that *all* of Surat was 'disease affected'.

Bombay was in a frenzy. Most of the Surati exodus came south to India's huge Arabic Sea metropolis, and local radio, television, and newspapers buzzed with rumours of dead rats and people within the city limits. It was said that eight people had died of plague the previous night in the Bombay suburbs of Borivili and Dadar.

So far the only clear casualty of the epidemic was truth. So expansive was the misinformation, government prevarication, and media frenzy that Indians from the Himalayas to the islands of Goa were almost to a person convinced the plague was among them. The reality would later seem disappointingly mundane as most of the ailing were, at least at first, lying in Surat's Civil Hospital.

But the federal government took no action, made no effort to slow the Surati exodus, and did not offer any concrete assistance to the beleaguered medical staff of Civil Hospital. At the Bombay end the Maharashtra State government similarly lacked a clear strategy. It seemed helpless to stem the monumental flow of Suratis who poured out of Bombay's several train stations in enormous human herds, quickly disappearing into the suburban and slum crowds of the densely-packed metropolis.

Hysteria was further fuelled by India's unique perspective on medicine. Few societies on earth in the late twentieth century were as culturally complex as India. Outsiders often noted that India was like an onion: one peeled layer after layer, often finding cause to weep in the process, but upon reaching the core discovered another onion inside. Each of India's many religions demanded all-encompassing devotion from its followers, affecting every aspect of their lives. And India's experiments with democracy had to avoid granting dominance to any particular religious view. Failure to walk that delicate balancing act usually resulted in mass outpourings of violence.

Medicine and health are, in Western tradition, based primarily in a scientific tradition that requires proof not only of logical theorem but also of practice. The body is a physical set of bones, flesh and organs. Illness is reversed through a host of interventions which seek to repair failing systems or obliterate invading microorganisms.

Western medical discipline was widely practiced throughout India, and the Indian Medical Association adhered to scientific traditions that roughly mirrored those professional standards in place in England.

But on official, equal footing under Indian law were ayurvedism, homoeopathy, yoga, Tibetan treatments, and a host of other health-care traditions that viewed the human body and its illnesses in fundamentally different, usually spiritual, ways. Although plague might in 1994 be easily treated with tetracycline under Western allopathic care, antibiotics played little or no role in ayurvedic or other ancient Indian practices.

The result was that nearly anyone could hang up a shingle, declaring himself a physician, and the nation's medical providers represented a mind-boggling blend of genuine healers, crackpots, and exploitative charlatans. More than 75 per cent of all health care in India was delivered by 'private' physicians, most of whom lacked serious training in either allopathic or other healing traditions and were likely to offer treatments that would certainly be illegal in nations that practiced Western medicine. The new free market atmosphere that reigned over health care in 1994 only exacerbated the problem, pitting charlatans with no medical training in any tradition against legitimate physicians who had devoted more than a decade of their lives to the vigorous study of either allopathic or traditional medicine.

The competition was fierce, and the hardest-fought battles took place in India's largest cities, where physicians practicing all traditions of health care went after the hearts, minds, and rupees of the growing middle class. By 1994 it was glamorous to be an antigovernment physician who decried the stupidities and corruption of state and federal authorities. It was fashionable to declare as lies most government public health declarations. And intra-physician competition often echoed this antiestablishment theme, making the most outrageous of 'physicians' chic among the middle and upper castes.

Indeed, India's Minister of Health B. Shankaranand was not a physician, but a businessman who faced indictments on mishandling of public funds during his previous service as petroleum minister. Shankaranand and his predecessor in the Ministry of Health supported an unusual medical paradigm: daily consumption of one's own urine as treatment for cancer or AIDS.

So from the first moments of Surat's epidemic the Indian public was deluged with at least as much misinformation as actual facts. And while it was tempting to blame the media for its lack of accuracy and for yellow journalism, India's health-care establishment had to share credit. The information schism—between truth and fantasy, accuracy and exaggeration—would prove disastrous for India in coming days.

But in Surat itself there were few citizens left who could be misinformed, and nearly the entire medical profession, save the dedicated nurses and physicians of Civil Hospital, had flown the coop.

One exception was Dr Lalgibai Patel, who on the morning of Thursday, September 22, anxiously paced the halls of Civil Hospital, distraught. His wife, Durga Watideri, had come down during the night with a nasal drip. That seemed pretty minor, Patel said, but rapidly worse symptoms appeared as the night wore on. Her throat began to burn so badly she couldn't swallow.

'And then I discovered she had a serious problem,' Patel, who was at his wits' end, recalled. 'She had chest pain, vomiting. I took her to a hospital for treatment, a private hospital. But the hospital was closed. By then she was vomiting blood. So then I brought her here.' No sooner had twenty-eight-year-old Watideri taken to bed on the Civil Hospital plague ward than Patel's seven-year-old son and twenty-two-year-old brother also came down with the disease.

'Being a man of medicine I was confident of recovery,' Patel said. 'But then when I saw the horror of it I was terrified.'

It would be weeks before Patel's family would recover, though all would, thankfully, live to tell tales of the Plague of '94.

Throughout the hospital nervous families related similar stories, describing sudden illness marked by vomited blood, loss of breath, chest pains, stomach pains, and high fevers. They spoke from behind masks, careful to stay out of the way of exhausted medical personnel. Occasionally tempers flared among the small remaining staff of sleep-deprived doctors and nurses: loud shouts of disagreement rang out in sporadic, brief bursts of rage.

Along the hallway leading to the plague ward masked lower-caste women, dressed in colourful saris, swept the floor and scrubbed the walls as if such cleanliness would prevent spread of *Yersinia* inside the hospital. The ward, separated in half by a long curtain, contained about eighty steel beds, white paint peeling off their rusty frames. Female patients were on the left side of the curtain, males on the right. With all the beds full, additional patients lay upon trolleys. Despite the crowd, there was little sound, as most of the patients were too sick to talk or even moan.

Behind thick isolation doors in two sealed chambers were the most dangerous patients—those who were actively coughing up *Yersinia*-contaminated blood and sputum. The nervous Dr Gupta, still wearing three masks at a time, moved among the patients, checking their antibiotics, fevers, and pains. His manner betrayed three sleepless days as he stumbled and slogged his way from bed to bed.

The following Friday India began to pay what would eventually be an enormous price for its epidemic. The United Nations Security Council demanded a full accounting of India's plague control efforts amid quiet threats of boycotts of Indian goods. That put the plague on Prime Minister Narasimha Rao's agenda. He dispatched Health Secretary M. S. Dayal to Surat. Dayal, a greying, bespectacled civil servant, was the top bureaucrat in the Ministry of Health. He flew into Surat on Friday morning, returning that afternoon to Delhi, and telling journalists and Prime Minister Rao that 44 Suratis had died of pneumonic plague and another 174 cases were being treated.

'The situation in the affected area is well under control,' Dayal claimed, adding that Surat health officials were commencing door-to-door surveys throughout the city, searching for additional cases.[16]

But Dayal's pronouncement did little to vanquish public—and world—fear. All over India sales of tetracycline soared and pharmaceutical supplies were swiftly depleted by a public convinced that the danger was great in every corner of the nation. To assure adequate doses for genuine treatment use, India's Food and Drug Administration was compelled to warehouse caches of tetracycline.

On Saturday morning accurate newspaper headlines told the Indian people that Rao's government had officially declared Surat 'plague-hit' and dispatched the army's Rapid Action Force to the city in order to maintain quarantines and stop the exodus of potential *Yersinia* carriers to other parts of the nation.

By the time the bereted Rapid Action Force, clad in blue camouflage combat gear, arrived Saturday afternoon, Surat had already lost three-quarters of its population, or an estimated 450 000 to 600 000 people. Critics attacked the federal government for failing to act sooner. Railroad authorities, also drawing in a torrent of criticism, began to seal shut all trains as they passed through Surat, declining to stop in the city except to off-load medical supplies.

International concern rose. The World Health Organization called India's outbreak 'the most serious' seen anywhere in decades. Authorities all over the world called out for plague expertise and advice.

They were greeted by an embarrassed silence. India wasn't the only nation that had shut down its plague programmes, confident that *Yersinia* no longer posed a threat. The once vast plague infrastructure of the former Soviet Union was, three years after the collapse of the USSR, in complete disarray. Few European scientists studied *Yersinia* anymore. And representatives of the US Centers for Disease Control and Prevention nearly choked with embarrassment as they conceded that only one employee—a half-time scientist based in Fort Collins, Colorado—had expertise in plague. No one had sizable stockpiles of plague vaccine, nor could any be manufactured on a time-scale of less than six months.

World Health Organization Director-General Dr Hiroshi Nakajima was silent. The world, left on its own to decide how to react to India's calamity, joined in the panic. Airports began to screen incoming Indian jets, and talk of more restrictive policies was in the air. In Delhi officials thought such drastic international reaction could be forestalled so long as plague remained confined to remote Beed and the city of Surat.

But no such luck.

Over the weekend alleged plague cases surfaced in Delhi and Baroda. A patient who appeared to suffer from plague fled hospital captivity, prompting a hysterical search of the ancient slums of the capital. He would never be found.

As international pressure mounted, Minister of Health Shankaranand himself journeyed to Surat on Saturday. With an entourage of Delhi officials, Shankaranand toured Civil Hospital only to be mobbed outside the facility by an angry group of Suratis and journalists demanding to know what the federal government was going to do to save the city. Belligerent, Shankaranand shouted angrily at the mob, ordered protection from army troops, and fled the city.

Meanwhile, abandoned Surat reeled under the stench of uncollected refuse, unfed, dying animals, and rotting shipments of food. There were too few workers remaining in Surat to take care of business. With an estimated forty-five thousand diamond polishing units idle, in the city notorious for profit priorities, it was little wonder that basic civil needs went unmet.

Monday morning found the situation out of control. Nationwide use of tetracycline was so widespread that the World Health Organization issued warnings that India might breed tetracycline-resistant microbes, of all sorts. More than ten million doses of the drug were distributed in Gujarat State alone.[17]

'We are trying,' complained Gujarat State Minister of Health Subash Shelad. 'We are telling people that only those should take tetracycline who come into contact with a known plague case. Only if there are symptoms. That is the continuous statement of the government. We are very clear about that.'

Shelad, who had set up a command post inside Surat's Civil Hospital and worked round-the-clock coordinating the emergency plague response, patted the pocket of his tunic. 'I've got mine in my pocket. I've not taken it.'

But the public would continue to ignore such protestations from the government. Within a week Surat's much-depleted population consumed fifteen million doses of tetracycline. And drug companies, including American and European manufacturers, filled pages of newspapers advertising not just tetracycline, but also a long list of anti-biotics, cleansers, pesticides, and rat poisons that people living in Indian towns hundreds of miles from Surat would clamour to purchase.[18]

India marked Tuesday's World Tourism Day with the most drastic decline in tourist visits seen in more than a decade. Twenty per cent of all tour packages to India sched-uled for October were cancelled. Tourists already in country cut short their trips and fled. Such usually crowded landmarks as the Taj Mahal, Goa's beaches, Jaipur's 'pink city', and the mountain Buddha of Bodhgaya were deserted. Hardest hit were resorts and hotels that catered to high-end tourists and business travellers: luxury hotels were suddenly emptied.

As economic ministers sweated over how best to compensate for these losses, ten states, spread over a vast distance, declared that they had all identified suspected plague cases.

And that brought dire calamity: complete economic collapse. On Wednesday, September 28, the Gulf State Nations (Kuwait, Saudi Arabia, Qatar, Oman, and the UAE) banned all flights, goods, and citizens from India. Pakistan and Sri Lanka—both eager for long-standing political reasons to cripple India—immediately followed suit.

The Bombay stock market crashed, experiencing its worst one-day decline since the 1989 assassination of Rajiv Gandhi. Annually trade between the Gulf States and India usually amounted to $3 billion. Further, some 400 000 Indians worked in the Gulf, sending home hard currency remittances to support their families. This cash flow ceased abruptly because the Gulf States banned all postal communications to and from India—a move that certainly could not have any biological credibility for plague control but did succeed in striking another critical Moslem blow against the Hindu-dominated Indian economy. Air flights between the Gulf and India, usually carrying twelve thousand passengers a day, were cancelled. All Indian-produced goods and electronic goods were banned in the boycotting Islamic countries.

Within forty-eight hours other critical trading partners and sources of valuable tourism dollars would close all connections to India: the Russian Federation, China, Egypt, Malaysia, and Bangladesh. And most nations that did not go so far as to completely ban Indian personnel, flights, and goods, did insist upon inspection of Indian travellers.

On September 29 Nobel Laureate Mother Teresa was compelled to submit to a medical check-up at Rome's Leonardo da Vinci Airport. Before departing the aircraft *en route* to her meeting with Pope John Paul II the hunchbacked, tiny nun smiled at her fellow passengers and told them that they had nothing to fear from the plague.

WHO did little to stop this international stigmatization of India, save issuing press releases: 'There is no need for fear nor panic.... This is a treatable disease and the measures taken in India are considered to be wholly adequate.' All reasonable boundaries between sound public health and globalized panic had been crossed. WHO did little to slow the stampede toward hysteria or stifle the opportunistic shouts of boycott calls from India's ancient nemesis, the Islamic states. The worldwide community reeled under the weight of fear that dated to the fourteenth century, and few authoritative voices sought to remind the terrified humanity that science had long since conquered *Yersinia pestis*.

The Indian cabinet met hastily on September 29, including the country's United Nations delegate. By then there were 1463 suspected plague cases in the country and forty-seven deaths—all in Surat. Surat's Civil Hospital alone held 659 suspected plague cases. States reporting unconfirmed additional cases included Delhi, West Bengal, Rajasthan, Maharashtra, Gujarat—areas that spanned virtually the length and breadth of the nation. In Delhi, where suspected plague cases filled the beds of the All India Institute of Medical Sciences, panic drove closure of all public schools. Local authorities said that two people had died of plague in Delhi, one in Bombay.

The Ministers issued an assurance to the nation: 'India will be free of plague epidemic in three weeks.'

The Bombay stock market responded by dropping another 77.3 points in a single day's trading. States with no reported plague cases were, nevertheless, facing ruin. The southern state of Kerala, for example, witnessed cancellation of virtually every October tourist group.

In Europe and North America trade and travel with India remained open, though passengers were asked to submit to medical inspections. On October 1 an Indian traveller aboard Air India flight 101 was detained at London's Heathrow airport on suspicion of having plague.[19] The man was locked for hours in a windowless room at the airport while authorities scrambled to find appropriate quarantine facilities. But England no longer had quarantine rooms at its airports, having long since abandoned such procedures. The man's isolation sparked political outcry both in New Delhi and in England's House of Commons. After five hours the man—who did not, after all, have plague—was transported from Heathrow in a special airtight infectious diseases ambulance and placed in isolation at Northwick Park Hospital pending laboratory analysis of his blood and sputum.[20] Members of the Indian expatriate community in London decried the British action as racist. Whether racism, indeed, motivated the response, it remains impossible to justify such extreme measures on the basis of biology. Even if the unfortunate traveller had been infected with the bacteria, dispensing antibiotics to his fellow passengers would have been appropriate public health policy—*not* incarceration.

In Washington the plague drew considerable interest and concern. Though the US State Department issued repeated pleas for calm, there was quiet concern that a plague carrier might disappear into an urban centre, go untreated, and spark an American outbreak of the usually curable disease. Plague could easily be treated with antibiotics, but officials had little confidence that typical American emergency room physicians could properly diagnose the pneumonic disease, prescribing appropriate curative and preventive measures. A quick survey revealed that more than 90 per cent of all flights from India, arriving either directly or via a European city, landed at John F. Kennedy International Airport in New York City. Every day some 2000 to 3000 passengers from India arrived at the airport, many of them relatives of the estimated 100 000 Indian immigrants living in New York.

On September 27, the US Centers for Disease Control and Prevention and the New York City Department of Health devised a strategy aimed at spotting plague cases swiftly and preventing spread within New York. The plan hatched in New York and Atlanta was also implemented in six other American cities that served as lower volume ports of call for travellers from the Indian subcontinent.

The CDC set up a plague hot line which, between September 27 and October 31 received 2692 calls from concerned, sometimes hysterical, citizens.

In New York responsibility fell to the city's new chief of infectious diseases, Dr Marcelle Layton. The young, curly-haired Layton was a cool-headed individual widely respected by colleagues nationwide.

A month earlier (August 27, 1994) Layton had received a communication from the CDC concerning the outbreak of bubonic plague in the Beed District of Maharashtra State in India. As director of the New York City Department of Health's Bureau of Communicable Disease, Layton routinely received such notifications of unusual outbreaks. And most overseas reports prompted only minor interest, posing no real threat to New York.

But by September, as word spread of the pneumonic cases of the disease in Surat, American concern heightened. Of particular interest to Layton was word from the CDC that 'screening is not occurring of [airline] passengers in India'. That meant it would be up to authorities at passengers' destinations to identify possible plague carriers.

As Layton's staff prepared an ambitious surveillance effort to monitor all thirty-one flights from India daily at JFK Airport, and alert the metropolis's medical personnel, Health Commissioner Dr Margaret Hamburg met with Mayor Rudolph Giuliani. Hamburg convinced New York's mayor that, distant as India was, New York City health safety was at issue because JFK was America's main port of entry for visitors, tourists, and immigrants from the Indian subcontinent. Giuliani asked why planes from India couldn't simply be stopped—barred entirely from entry. And Hamburg laid out the biological and logistic reasons why such a politically sensitive measure would provide only false security: an estimated half million residents of the plagued city of Surat had already fled their city, reaching destinations all over the subcontinent—not just India; most passengers from India actually changed planes in Frankfurt, Amsterdam, Paris, and London and would still get into the United States one way or the other. Moreover, plague was completely curable with modern antibiotics, Hamburg reminded the mayor. Giuliani lent Hamburg's health department his support.

On September 27 Layton's plan of action went into effect. Working closely with scientists at the CDCs plague laboratory in Fort Collins, Colorado, she mapped out a three-pronged strategy. First, her staff set out to alert the health providers of greater New York City. A special fact sheet, detailing the signs and symptoms of plague, was faxed to the emergency rooms and infection control offices of 102 hospitals in the city and dozens of facilities in neighbouring Westchester, Suffolk, and Nassau counties. In addition, bulletins were sent to twenty thousand doctors practicing in New York City, and a Hindi-language flyer was distributed at an October 8 Indian festival in the borough of Queens.

Key to the city's efforts were activities at JFK Airport. The CDC gave all of the airlines pamphlets concerning plague, and airline personnel were expected to recognize symptoms of the disease. The CDC similarly informed representatives of the Immigration and Naturalization Service and US Customs, as it was employees of those agencies—not health officials—who routinely saw all international passengers. Thus, responsibility for spotting possible plague cases fell to employees of private airlines, the INS, and US Customs: none of them medically trained.

'If there were a suspect case, a New York City medical officer would go to the runway,' Layton later explained, 'and remove the suspect. All the other passengers would remain on the plane until diagnosis was confirmed.'

Under US law, if a plague case were confirmed aboard such a flight, all passengers would then be required to submit to an examination, provide officials with details regarding their future destinations, and make themselves available for a full week's follow-up medical surveillance.

'If plague cases weren't spotted until the passengers had disembarked, finding those people would be very problematic,' Layton said.

One suspected plague case was, indeed, identified aboard a flight from India, and Layton's plan was put into action. But all the remaining nine suspect cases were spotted after the passengers had disembarked; two were noted by observant US Customs officials; one by a JFK ticketing agent, and the remainder by emergency room physicians in the New York City area.

One customs agent looked up from an Indian passenger's bags to see red fluid dripping from the individual's mouth. Alarmed, and convinced the Indian was bleeding, the Customs agent triggered the plague alert to health officials at the airport. It turned out that the Indian was simply chewing betel nuts, which exude a bright red juice and stain the consumer's mouth and teeth with a fiery crimson colour.

But the other suspect plague victims were not so fortunate—all were suffering from serious illnesses; one died of malaria. Two others had malaria, four were ailing due to viral infections, one had chronic liver disease, and the last had typhoid fever.

It was fortunate, Hamburg said, that none of the cases were plague, as the exercise pointed up a number of deficiencies in America's disease safety net, some of which would be difficult, if not impossible, to correct.

Foremost, said Nobel Laureate Joshua Lederberg of Rockefeller University, was the vague and often contradictory nature of information from overseas. Typically, outbreaks that occurred in poor countries were inadequately characterized, even misdiagnosed. In the case of India's plague, valid laboratory confirmation that *Yersinia pestis* was the cause of the epidemic did not materialize until February, nearly six months *after* the outbreak. Diagnostic uncertainty overseas made Layton and her associates nervous. What if their entire alert system was directed toward the wrong microbial scourge, she asked, and some other disease managed to slip unnoticed into JFK? What if India was wrong, *Yersinia* wasn't the problem, and while all of Layton's resources were diverted some dangerous virus slipped into New York?

Although it was easy to point up failures in a poor country, Drs Ruth Berkelman, Jim Hughes, and Grant Campbell of the CDC retrospectively acknowledged severe shortfalls on the US side. Physicians in the United States were largely unable to differentiate between plague and other ailments. Most American medical schools had long since abandoned public health and infectious diseases training, confining such subjects to elective courses or advanced classes for would-be specialists. The links between medicine and public health in America were, at best, weak. And there were large lags between the times of recognition of those possible New York City cases and the isolation of pneumonically diseased individuals, thus potentially allowing large numbers of people to be exposed.

Containing exposure and tracking down secondary cases—particularly disembarked fellow passengers—proved daunting for New York City.

'The bottom line is we had a gigantic protocol based on recognizing people on board planes,' Layton said. 'But most potential cases weren't recognized until they were already in the community.' Even a single bona fide case of plague, spotted after the passenger desembarked, would have severely taxed the city's health resources and forced Hamburg to divert personnel from most other programmes. Had there been multiple cases, or if the ailment had been viral (and therefore untreatable) the situation would have quickly overwhelmed the health department's resources. Such had not always been the case in Gotham: in the early twentieth century plague control had been routine, and successful.

Nationwide, the US public health safety net caught thirteen potential plague cases related to the India outbreak: ten in New York City; one in Albany, New York; and two elsewhere in the country. Overwhelmed as the New York City Department of Health might have been, it did prove the most vigilant and efficient local agency in the country, CDC officials insisted.

'The recent plague experience in India provides a clear example of the high price of ignoring global microbial threats,' Hughes and Campbell concluded, noting that the US public health system had long since lost any sense of vigilance over outbreaks occurring overseas.[21]

But those conclusions would be reached in hindsight. During the first week of October 1994 every nation in the world was on some form of plague alert and India was a pariah.

In October all of India was suddenly overcome with a fit of mass hygiene hysteria. Rats were caught; streets were scrubbed; rubbish was piled high and set afire, thereby exuding eye-tearing stenches and a putrid smoke. Surat, alone, would burn up three thousand tons of waste during the next weeks, and spread hundreds of pounds of probably unneeded DDT. (As there was no ratfall or flea-carried bacteria in Surat there could be no logical need for the pesticide.) Someone put a huge surgical mask over the mouth of Mahatma Gandhi's colossal statue in New Delhi. In the town of Thane in Maharashtra State a terrified man denounced visitors from Gujarat who came to his village as plague carriers: on the night of October 2 he murdered all three of them, the youngest being a seven-year-old girl.

The Bombay stock market continued to plummet, falling a total of 213 points, or 5 per cent of its total value, since plague had struck Surat a month earlier. Stock market jitters reflected growing anxiety in circles of commerce about the government's ability to—frankly—*govern* in a crisis.

'Too many people in India, and abroad, are in near-panic,' complained the *Times of India*. 'Too few of our national and state leaders appear to be sufficiently agitated. It should be the other way around. To put it starkly: India's future is at stake.'

On October 2 New Delhi federal officials released startling new plague numbers: nationwide, they said, there were 4059 cases, 1297 in Gujarat State and 2105 in Maharashtra. With the release of those numbers came yet another plea for international calm.

But Oman responded by conducting an emergency airlift of all its citizens then in Bombay. By Tuesday October 4 there were, officially, 4780 suspect plague cases and forty-eight deaths. A five-year-old child in Old Delhi died: plague was blamed.

And then a sort of intellectual warfare broke out, pitting some of India's leading biologists and physicians against one another and fuelling ancient suspicions and hatreds.

First, India's National Institute of Communicable Diseases—the nation's large federal research centre in New Delhi—had possession of alleged plague samples from the nation's suspected patients. But the All India Institute of Medical Sciences also had samples. And the institutes locked horns in a seemingly bizarre turf battle. The AIIMS, which was handling all the suspected cases identified in Delhi, refused to release its blood and sputum samples to NICD on the grounds that the materials should remain within AIIMS labs and NICD microbiologists ought to come to AIIMS, rather than the samples leaving the hospital's grounds.

NICD, for its part, insisted it should act as the clearing house for all *Yersinia* samples. And in a case of possibly misplaced pride it declined laboratory assistance offered by the US Centers for Disease Control and Prevention, London School of Hygiene and Tropical Medicine, and Plague Laboratory in Odessa, Ukraine.[22]

At the NICD an *ad hoc* plague laboratory was erected on the top floor of an old cinder block building. Amid the blistering October heat of New Delhi laboratory workers from the Zoonosis Division toiled round-the-clock under humbling conditions. Well-trained microbiologists, some of whom had studied in the best universities in the West, worked with equipment that might be found in an American high school teaching laboratory. No air-conditioning relieved their discomfort as they sweated beneath protective plastic gear, gloves, and goggles. Samples of sputum and blood cooked on laboratory benches in the tropical heat.

At the plague control room Dr D. C. Jain and a team of epidemiologists struggled to keep track of the plague reports that were then pouring in from every corner of the country. Clearly sleep deprived, Jain nervously responded to a steady stream of phone calls, staff queries, and official interruptions. The exhausted epidemiologist could barely complete a sentence before another question was fired his way. To each he seemed to respond physically, recoiling, squinting, and tensing from head to toe. The key question levelled at Jain hourly by Ministry of Health officials was, 'Is this an epidemic of *Yersinia pestis*, and are all these illnesses nationwide due to plague?'

'The molecular epidemiology has not been done,' Jain sputtered, acknowledging that the sort of detective work that is essential in an epidemic hadn't been initiated in the Surat outbreak. 'We still do not say it is plague because our laboratory is finding the bacteria has morphology similar to plague bacilli. They do not say it *is* plague, they say it's *similar*. The basic thing is whether it's plague or not: it's not possible at this juncture for me to say. It is yet to be confirmed.'

But at New Delhi's Infectious Disease Hospital Dr K. N. Tewari was swamped with supposed plague cases. Most of the 749 people he tested were simply the worried well or individuals suffering from other, milder infectious diseases. Tewari placed those cases in general wards of the hospital.

But there were a few cases Tewari was convinced were genuinely caused by *Yersinia pestis*. His laboratory confirmed them.

'We have got definitely three cases without any history of going out of Delhi for that [plague] period,' Tewari insisted. 'All are from the slums of Delhi. And they have no history of contact with a person with plague. It *is* pneumonic plague. And we have thirteen more that need to be investigated.'

One of Tewari's confirmed cases was four-year-old Vijay Kumar, who for four days had been suffering from a high fever, respiratory difficulties, and a sharp pain in his neck. Skinny Kumar stared with wild, terror-struck eyes over the edge of his mask.

Near Kumar on the plague isolation ward lay twenty-two-year-old Harish. For five days he had been suffering fever and uncontrollable coughing. From behind his mask, worn to protect a visitor to the plague ward, Harish spoke between fits of coughing.

'I had a sudden onset of fever,' he related in Hindi. 'And I have no recall of being around anybody who was sick.'

Across the hall from the nearly empty plague ward was the crowded ward Tewari called 'the plague phobia room,' full of patients whom the doctor felt were fine. But the patients refused to leave, convinced that they had the dreaded disease.

Tewari was joined by a cluster of young colleagues who insisted that fear of plague was 'silly', and horribly exaggerated.

'There must be a uniform global policy on these plagues,' Dr Dinesh Gupta insisted loudly, out-shouting the rest of the physician cluster. 'No bans! No closed borders!'

While Delhi's Infectious Disease Hospital and the staff of Surat's Civil Hospital were absolutely convinced that they had laboratory-confirmed *Yersinia* cases on their hands, NICD officially vacillated, unable to produce definitive epidemiological or laboratory proof. Over at AIIMS doctors continued to hold on to samples. But they were in no position to settle the controversy. They were preoccupied with their own mysterious outbreak of hepatitis E, which was spreading through the facility, so far claiming sixty employees.

In Surat a group of four private physicians announced on October 1 that they had proof there was no *Yersinia* in the city. The epidemic, they said, was due to 'hantana virus', a mis-statement of a class of rodent-borne microbes called hantaviruses. Their claim drew rage from the hard-working physicians of Civil Hospital who on October 3 offered a substantial reward to anyone who could prove that their *Yersinia* diagnosis was invalid.

The critical quartet (Drs Bipin Desai, Sudhir Marfatia, Nainesh Parikh, and Balwant Mistry) had to back off from their 'hantana virus' claim in the face of overwhelming evidence that the ailing patients recovered when treated with antibiotics, which are only effective against bacteria. So on October 6 the group offered a new hypothesis: there was no plague; there was melioidosis. Admitting that 'we do not have any patient or his sputum' from which to draw samples in evidence, the quartet said, 'we request the doctors concerned to look into this theory and give the right solution of this disease to Surat, Gujarat, and the country'.

Another group of physicians from B. J. Medical College in Pune, Maharashtra, said their alleged bubonic plague cases actually suffered from *Burkholderia pseudomallei*, a bacterium that rarely causes illnesses in otherwise healthy individuals.[23]

Scientists from AIIMS eventually weighed in, further roiling the waters. They announced in late October that their 'attempts to culture *Yersinia pestis* from patients have failed so far, although it is not a difficult organism to grow.'

They went on to suggest that the hantaviruses, melioidosis or another bacteria—leptospirosis—might be causes of the epidemic. However, they failed to note a critical detail: they hadn't isolated any of these organisms from their samples.

Digging further into the obscure possibilities the same group of Pune physicians that originally proposed *Burkholderia* was the problem switched their bets, backing the species *Pseudomonas pseudomallei* as the epidemic's agent. The group claimed to have cultured the melioidosis-causing bacteria from lymph nodes drawn from 30 per cent of the patients diagnosed with bubonic plague.

The stakes in this fight, both medical and political, were high. If the critics were correct, physicians in Surat—*government employees*—had erred shamefully, bringing disgrace and economic ruin to the nation. If the critics were incorrect, the federal government could claim credit for alerting the world to the epidemic, and get off the hook for its public health failures in response to the outbreak. Either way the Civil Hospital physicians were too busy battling their epidemic, and too powerless—far too lowly in the government hierarchy—to effectively leap into the fray. And scientists in Delhi seemed unable to conjure convincing data rapidly enough to nip the debate in the bud.

Melioidosis is a disease rarely seen on the Indian subcontinent; it is more typically found in South-east Asia. The bacteria are usually transmitted through skin wounds via exposure to contaminated water. There were no known epidemics of melioidosis ever reported, even in South-east Asia. The microbe was never known to be passed from person to person. And most carriers of *Pseudomonas pseudomallei* were never taken ill, but became lifelong carriers of the generally harmless bacteria. It might not, therefore, seem surprising that 30 per cent of the residents of an earthquake-torn rural area had the microbes in their lymph nodes. It would, based on known history of human melioidosis cases, be nothing short of medically astounding if upwards of 10 per cent of a village population developed acute symptoms analogous to bubonic plague as a result of exposure to the agent.

Tularaemia—another suggested explanation for the epidemic—was a more severe bacterial disease whose symptoms more closely resembled those of pneumonic plague, including fevers and enlarged lymph nodes. But most tularaemic patients also developed terrible skin ulcers, which were not seen on the Beed or Surat patients. Further, the bacteria were not endemic to the Indian subcontinent and were usually carried by species of ticks found only in much colder climates such as the North American plains and the Russian Steppes.

'I wish these so-called Senior Scientists had taken the time to talk to the laboratory at NICD,' an exasperated Health Secretary Dayal exclaimed. 'In Beed there is *no doubt* it's plague. We saw antibodies in serology. There was no doubt it was bubonic—the symptoms were clear and distinct. We have cultured samples from the blood! We have isolated the bacteria! True, the molecular epidemiology has not yet been done. But combined with all this evidence—sputum, PHA, high titres, antibody responses—we do *strongly* suggest it's *Yersinia pestis*.'

But the common people of India were all too willing to believe virtually anything except the government's position. In Bombay they spoke on street corners of a Pakistani conspiracy.

'Look who was first to call for a boycott of India,' they would knowingly tell a visitor. 'Pakistan! There is no plague. It's all a big lie Pakistan used to bring down our economy.'

Conversely, in Calcutta they spoke of a government cover-up: 'Thousands are dying of plague every day, but they are hiding it! And now they say it's something else. It's a lie.'

With each day the distrust grew, NICD's credibility fell, and more nations carried out punitive actions against India. The Dutch airline KLM sprayed pesticides throughout its plane cabins as they disembarked from India. North Korea denied docking privileges to all ships, of any nationality, that had previously been in Indian waters. Sudan placed all travellers from India in jailed quarantine for six days. China barred all Indians. Hong Kong informed all Indians that they would face two days mandatory quarantine or immediate deportation. The Ukraine placed one hundred passengers from India under armed guard, refusing to allow them to disembark from their aircraft.

The world was behaving in an utterly irrational manner over an entirely preventable and curable bacterial disease whose greatest threat was from the historic collective memory of the human species. India's domestic responses were obviously confused, contradictory, and inadequate. Yet the World Health Organization took no strong action on India's behalf until October 7, nearly two months after the Beed outbreak began. That morning, WHO Director-General Hiroshi Nakajima flew with an Indian government entourage to Surat, examined cases at Civil Hospital, and then returned to New Delhi to face the Indian media. Citing article 11, paragraph 3 of the International Health Regulations, Nakajima said he had come at the request of the Gulf State Nations to assess India's epidemic.

Speaking with a thick Japanese accent that Indian journalists were at pains to decipher, Nakajima criticized the 'very large gap between so-called suspect cases and confirmed cases' in Surat, but said that there were, indeed, 'a large number of pneumonic plague cases'.

And then he added a puzzling statement: 'Concerning Surat I would say today there is a plague in Surat. But if you compare the number of confirmed cases—192—in a city of I think 1.8 million population we cannot say there is an epidemic. I prefer to say there is a plague in Surat. But I'm not prepared to say there is an epidemic in Surat.'

As Nakajima spoke tension and whispers spread among the journalists. Not knowing the cause of the Indian media's agitation Nakajima nervously continued, his accent thickening and the press corps' inability to comprehend growing worse.

'As for laboratory work,' Nakajima began, obviously flustered, 'NICD technology is good. But working conditions are so bad that I recommended to the minister of health to provide better working conditions. The laboratory is oversaturated. I'm a little afraid the NICD laboratory isn't able to perform in such a way.'

The WHO director-general severely condemned the quality of laboratory facilities in Surat, recommended large-scale epidemiology and rat surveillance, and called upon the Indian government to conduct serious scientific studies.

As for international boycotts, Nakajima was evasive. Official WHO policy called for no such action, he said, but article 7 of the International Health Regulations stipulated that an epidemic couldn't be declared over until twice the organism's average incubation time, or twelve days in the case of plague. Therefore, India's epidemic—an 'epidemic' he'd already refused to grant even existed—would officially persist until November.

The room erupted.

'You are coming here like Caesar to judge!' shouted one reporter.

'You are reaching hasty conclusions!' another cried.

'What will you tell the Gulf States about this boycott?' asked another.

'There is no plague in India! You are a liar,' shouted a chorus of reporters. Chaos replaced order and the distressed WHO entourage left in haste.

It was another two weeks before India's international woes ceased. By then the outbreak would have proven disastrously expensive. Dr Ann Marie Kimball of the University of Washington in Seattle estimates tourism and trade losses, alone, amounted to $1.3 billion.[24] That is close to other published estimates for tourism and trade losses.[25] None of the published estimates of the cost of India's plague included the nearly two-week-long cessation of textile and diamond industrial activity in Surat, loss of agricultural production in Maharashtra, panic purchasing of antibiotics, or direct medical costs.

Certainly when these issues are considered a toll approaching $2 billion seems reasonable: an extraordinary price to pay for what eventually was a total of fifty-six deaths and fewer than 6500 cases of an antibiotic-susceptible infection.[26]

India continued to pay a political price for its epidemic long after all the plague wards were closed and the last *Yersinia*-carrying rat was exterminated. It was the cost of inadequate government attention to public health.

The lack of rapid, definitive evidence of *Yersinia pestis* infection in the sick and dying patients and a clear epidemiological explanation for the two separate outbreaks of bubonic and pneumonic diseases left wide open a door for the entry of fanaticism, conspiracy theories, crackpot ideas, and general antigovernment sentiments. Though the US Centers for Disease Control and Prevention was eventually invited to examine available Surat samples and confirmed the presence of *Yersinia*, most of the sputum and blood extracted from the initial flurry of cases in September was destroyed through lack of proper handling and refrigeration in either Surat or Delhi. Thus, it wasn't possible to match case by case the presence of symptoms with laboratory evidence of *Yersinia* infection. That left plenty of room for other, often conspiratorial, interpretations.

The CDC did a full genetic analysis of the Surat strain, concluding it was a *Yersinia* strain not previously seen. Similar conclusions were reached by scientists at the Pasteur Institute in Paris and the Plague Laboratory in Stavropol, Russia. Though the agency meant simply that it didn't match any strains in their archives, the finding fuelled a large number of conspiracy theories. In particular, the *Hindustan Times* claimed that the strain was manufactured in a biological warfare laboratory in Kazakhstan and sold to a Kashmir rebel group called the Ultras.[27] That was enough to prompt the Ministry of Defence to lay claim to all remaining *Yersinia* samples, thus removing them forever from public health analysis.

Before the Ultra theory hit newsstands in mid-1995, WHO and the Indian government had requested epidemiology assistance from the US Centers for Disease Control and Prevention. Dr David Dennis, the only plague expert on the US payroll, led a small team of investigators that examined cases in Surat, Delhi, and the Beed District during the last two weeks of November 1994. They concluded that the epidemic was genuine, but were unable to isolate *Yersinia* from most samples, partly because mass use of antibiotics was widespread and may have eliminated some evidence of the bacteria. Nevertheless, in March of 1995, with assistance from the CDC, the NICD published definitive evidence of *Yersinia pestis* in samples from both Beed and Surat. A few months later researchers from the Central Public Health Laboratory in London published evidence that the microbe responsible for melioidosis absolutely was *not* present in disease victims, utterly refuting claims made in October 1994 by the doctors in Pune.

But just as it seemed controversy over *Yersinia*'s culpability in the outbreak was settled and the book might be closed on India's epidemic, PCR (polymerase chain reaction) genetic sequencing reports released by the United States, France, and Russia fuelled an entirely new set of accusations aimed directly at the United States. PCR sequencing revealed that the Surat *Yersinia* strain was of comparatively low virulence and contained a unique set of genes not seen previously with plague. The role of these genes was unclear, but not thought to be worrisome, as Russian tests showed the strain to be highly susceptible to a broad range of readily available antibiotics. Within days of the release of these reports the US embassy in New Delhi found itself under siege, as local scientists and reporters claimed that the mysterious extra gene segment in the Surat *Yersinia* could only have been man-made. It was, they said, a product of genetic engineering. And the engineers were either Americans, or, in an alternative theory, Kazakh scientists working at the behest of the US government. US Ambassador Frank Wisner came under personal attack, accused of crafting the entire scheme.

The logic was deeply conspiratorial and ultimately US-paranoid.[28]

That the logic defied basic tenets of microbial evolution and was patently incorrect made no difference. And conspiracy theorists insisted that only the US government possessed adequate technology to create such superbugs. Some Indian news publications during the summer of 1995 claimed that the United States had a massive biowarfare programme under way. To back up their allegations they pointed to $300 million allocated by Congress that year for production of defensive bioweapons measures such as development of vaccines.

The unfolding diplomatic crisis revealed a crucial, and previously unseen, problem for public health: bioweapons technology. As technological advances made in the 1980s allowed the possibility of formerly unthinkable forms of terrorism in the 1990s, governments had to distinguish natural microbial events from those that were man-made. This put the United States in a particularly dicey catch-22 situation, as its government employees were among the few scientists in the world capable of both making such horrible bioweapons and proving whether or not an outbreak was man-made. In the case of the Surat strain, Indian accusers charged that it was either manu-factured at the army's old Dugway Proving Grounds or in the Kazakh laboratory of Dr I. L. Martinevsky, a Russian biological warfare expert. His laboratory, the Indian press claimed, had been visited by US Secretary of Defense William Perry, and Martinevsky now worked for the US Defense Department making offensive biological warfare agents.

What was the motivation, and how did the alleged biological warfare weapon get to Surat? It was claimed that the United States used Suratis as guinea pigs, testing new biosensing devices in the city. That such devices were never seen in Surat, and are so enormous that they could hardly go unnoticed, was not mentioned. The release was allegedly conducted by none other than the CDC's David Dennis—the very individual who, two months after the epidemic began, led a team of investigations to Surat at the request of the Indian government.

Ambassador Wisner's role in the conspiracy was 'proven' because he had played a key role in treaty negotiations with China and India, trying to persuade the two massive nations to sign the 1972 Biological Weapons Convention. In other words, because he tried to broker peace, he must have actually been the kingpin in a horrible scheme to inflict plague on India.

The accusations proved embarrassing to the United States, and conveniently deflected anger away from the failed policies and negligence of Indian authorities. When plague first broke out in Surat the Indian press had loudly declaimed the lack of essential public health services, the filth, the squalor, the lack of plague surveillance, and the slow pace of government response. Now, with national elections approaching and Prime Minister Rao's leadership wildly unpopular even within his own Congress Party, it was convenient to point the finger at another nation.

But Indian public health authorities had much for which to answer.

'Let our nation learn the lesson: economic advancement requires adequate investment in human health,' said Dr Jacob John.[23] 'Second lesson: infectious diseases are the major causes of morbidity and mortality. Well-informed tourists coming to India take immunizations against Japanese encephalitis, hepatitis A, typhoid fever, and chemoprophylaxis against malaria; they carry with them drugs against giardiasis and cholera. Some even carry a few doses of rabies vaccine. And we want rich tourists to come and see India, risking their health? Third lesson: infectious diseases must be diagnosed by laboratory methods and not by government decree. Fourth lesson: microbiology laboratories and microbiologists should be available in all districts. . . . Fifth lesson: there should be continuous monitoring of causes of diseases and of death in order to detect epidemics of diseases.'

Indian expatriate researcher Dr Vikram Chand felt the most appalling event was the mass exodus of physicians away from Surat during the plague.

The gross disparity between the health status and care of India's poor versus her tiny elite of wealthy, upper-caste members formed the basis of the most sweeping critiques of the country's response to plague. In a nation where 53 per cent of all children under five are officially underweight and growth stunted, and 21 per cent are severely so, basic health needs were clearly unmet.[29] Perhaps the clearest illustration of the nation's public health weakness lay in its exploding *true* plague of HIV. Recognizing that India had all the social ingredients necessary for rapid spread of the almost 100 per cent lethal virus, the World Bank in 1992 awarded the country an $84 million grant for AIDS prevention efforts. Six years later Indian authorities were still trying to figure out how to spend that money, and the United Nations AIDS Programme (UNAIDS) was convinced that India's HIV population outnumbered that of Mexico, the United States, and Canada, combined. In 1998 the World Bank sadly estimated that India's failure to respond swiftly to the initial spread of HIV among prostitutes and intravenous drug users in the early 1990s would, by 2000, cost her $11 billion, or 5 per cent of her GDP, in direct medical care and lost worker productivity due to death and illness.[30] And by 1999 the UNAIDS Programme was convinced that more than 1.5 million Indians were infected. As with *Yersinia* plague, India's HIV epidemic spread primarily among its poorest citizens—a fact critics charged fully explained the country's inadequate public health response to both HIV and the plague.

'The chances of being rich and getting plague, in India or anywhere else in the world, are about as remote as the ability of the rat flea to jump from its slum habitat to the distant electronically protected environment of the rich,' wrote the *Lancet* in an editorial.[22] 'The distance between a slum environment and five-star comfort is rather more than an inch.'

The *British Medical Journal* labelled plague a disease of poverty, and concluded: 'Is it chance, or nemesis, that this revenge is taking place at a time when India, indeed the whole planet, is moving towards a "free market" economy that benefits some but not all. The epidemic of plague has meant that instead of being marginalised in their socially distant slums, the existence of the poor has abruptly impinged on the consciousness of the rich.'

Critics within India were less likely to beat the drum of international guilt, and more apt to aim their anger squarely at their nation's economic elite and inept leaders.

'If India can afford an aircraft carrier,' wrote Dr Eswar Krishnan, for example, 'she can very well afford more epidemiologists and the resources they need. It is merely a question of priorities.'[31]

In Bombay the press devoted November 1994 to dissecting blow by blow Maharashtra's response to the Beed and Surat outbreaks. It wasn't a pretty sight. By name, public health officials were accused of negligence, folly, and laziness. But the Indian media could hardly be considered guilt-free, as some of its less reputable members had wildly exaggerated the original threat of plague, whipped up national hysteria, and then, months later, joined in conspiracy fever.

Meanwhile, in Surat, poor women, one hand clutching their saris in place, spread white DDT powder with their bare hands along Ved Road. At an empty lot Kamlesh Patel supervised another crew of women who under orders plunged ungloved hands into piles of putrid waste, tossing animal carcasses and debris into a massive bonfire.

The poor were doing as they always had in India: taking care of themselves.

Four days before the first of November WHO finally recommended that all boycotts and travel restrictions against India be lifted. There had been no more deaths reported for twelve days. The epidemic had, officially, stopped.

WHO had by then allowed India to be treated as a global pariah for more than two months.

Shortly before WHOs declaration, but with the epidemic clearly under control, a weary reporter boarded a British Airways jet in Bombay, headed for London. The cabin was redolent with insecticides sprayed over every inch of the place. And more were then sprayed upon the seated passengers and their carry-on bags.

For hours the chemical stench reminded passengers that Britain feared they might be carrying *Yersinia*-infected fleas. It was, to say the least, an unpleasant thought.

Upon landing outside London the aircraft stopped just off the runway, not at a gate. Passengers were ordered to remain seated. A pair of public health service personnel in uniform boarded, flanking a robust, buxom blond physician in her sixties.

'Is anyone feeling unwell,' she called out as she slowly made her way down the aircraft aisles, studying each passenger closely. 'Anybody have a fever? Hmmm? Headache? Touch of delirium? Speak up, please. Fever?'

A smartly dressed Bombay businessman commented in the physician's wake, 'Only a bloody fool would answer yes,' and the passengers burst out in uproarious laughter.

Clearly nobody aboard the plane trusted such measures would stop plague, were it present.

In every possible way the essential public health trusts between authorities, science, medicine, and the global populace were violated during the 1994 plague outbreak in India. Indian citizens trusted that their governments—both local and federal—would respond swiftly to a disease crisis, reach sound scientific conclusions, and act rapidly in a manner that both staunched the outbreak and quelled panic. Indian authorities failed to reach timely and irrefutable diagnoses, to assist beleaguered plague respond-ers in Surat, to calm the public, or to offer accurate information as the epidemic unfolded. The plague tiger was well out of his cage, causing havoc across the country-side, before the hunters and trainers set out in search of the beast.

Global authorities also failed in their responses. The World Health Organization's only real power rests with its credibility as a voice of scientific reason that can rise above international politics to give timely guidance the global community can trust. But WHO's press releases and statements were weak, late, and politically influenced. Rather than decry all forms of international hysteria and punishment of India WHO fell under the influence of politically motivated rival nations. The agency dragged its feet, seemingly lending credibility to such inanity as Gulf State boycotts of such out-rageously misnamed plague-carrying items as Indian postage stamps, oranges, Madras bolts of silk, and Bangalore computer chips.

The very word *plague* still conjures fear decades after both its prevention and cure have been developed and globally distributed. No new technology is needed to conquer *Yersinia pestis*, just implementation of very basic public health measures. Nevertheless, WHO and health authorities worldwide failed to consider the historic, almost visceral, impact the word *plague* arouses. Perhaps in their offices chatting by telephone with colleagues around the world they dismissed word of *Yersinia* on the grounds that, well, it was a controllable, harmless agent. But in so doing they utterly failed to recognize that while the organism may be easily vanquished with modern tools of medicine, the panic it sparks cannot possibly be addressed in a technological or dismissive manner.

In the end it was that very panic which proved most costly during the plague outbreak. And in the months that followed, panic gave way to its close cousin, conspiratorial thinking. Cloak-and-dagger explanations for epidemics have always proven attractive in the absence of unambiguous, timely, scientifically validated public health pronounce-ments. And conspiracy thinking undermines the credibility of the very health authorities in whom the public ought to place its trust.

That trust would soon be tested again in one of the remotest locations on earth.

CHAPTER 2

Landa-landa

An Ebola virus epidemic in Zaire proves public health is imperilled by corruption.

One is always alert, protecting oneself against the objects that can steal your soul, the landa-landa *that can inflict all forms of ill fortune, illness, and, frequently, death. Death, in such cases, is the sober thief that comes.*
—Kibari N'sanga and Lungazi Mulala[1]

We are the ones who first bring life, but we never believed in such powerful disease. Now it is true: we have lost the brothers and sisters with whom we worked. In the name of our ancestors I say: remove this evil spirit from amongst us or we cannot work in peace.
—Twela Say Ntun, chief nurse of Kikwit Maternity Hospital No. 2[1]

The night air was, as always, redolent with the smells of burning cook fires fuelled by wood, wax, propane, or cheap petrol. The distorted sounds of over-modulated 1995 hit *ramba* music echoed from the few bars along Boulevard Mobutu that had electric generators or well-charged car batteries. Fully dilated pupils struggled to decipher shapes in the pitch darkness, spotting the pinpoint lights of millions of dancing fireflies. Gentle footsteps betrayed what the eye on a moonless night could not see; the constant movement of people, their dark skin hiding them in the unlit night.

From a distance a woman's voice rang sharply, calling out in KiCongo, '*Af-waka!* Someone has died! Someone has died! He was my husband! He was my husband.'

As she continued her call to heaven, detailing the virtues of the just-deceased, the woman's eerie cry was joined by a succession of her relatives' voices.

'Someone has died! Someone has died! He was my father!'

'Someone has died! Someone has died! He was my son!'

The padding of feet on Kikwit's mud paths paused as people turned their ears to catch the name of the latest *landa-landa* victim. In a city without newspapers, radio, television, telephones, or electricity, such cries in the night constituted local broadcast news. And no sooner had the flow of pedestrians resumed than another voice rang out from the opposite side of the emotionally electrified city-without-electricity.

'Someone has died!'

Landa-landa. Foreigners. Something called a virus. Something called Ebola. These things gripped the estimated 400 000 people of Kikwit with a terror unlike any they had ever felt. Fear was no stranger to them: hadn't they lived under the brutal Mobutu Sese Seko regime for more than thirty years? Wasn't death already a steady companion, fuelled by malaria, measles, HIV, TB, and malnutrition?

But this *landa-landa* was different, more terrifying than all the other diseases that had taken the lives of Kikwit's children and young adults. The victims died fast. But first, they bled, had long fits of hiccups, cried out in agonizing pain, even went mad, and screamed incoherent phrases of apparent devilish origin. They seemed possessed.

There were ancient ceremonies handed down by the ancestors that could purge evil spirits—they usually lifted the *landa-landa.* But not this time. The magic was too powerful. Surely it must be the work of an exceptionally evil one.[2] Who was the potent fount of Satanism?

The rumours were numerous, and were spread in hushed tones so as not to be overheard by the evil ones. Only the Christian leaders, imbued with the strength of Jesus, dared decry the evil out loud. Pentecostal preacher Eloi Mulengamungu declared it the work of Satan, himself, allowed to roam freely over doomed Kikwit by God, in punishment. Kikwit, the preacher declared, had become a modern Sodom replete with prostitutes, corruption, illegitimate children, abandoned elderly parents, and other wages of sin.

From the Baptist Community of West Africa (CBCO) the people also heard of Satan's mischief. As members of CBCO fell ill and died of the strange new malady their leader declared that Kikwit had lost sight of God. In the absence of a large core of true believers Satan could claim even a tiny pool of the pious. As his congregants also fell ill, Pastor Kutesa Mayele of the Assembly of God Church reached a similar conclusion: it was God's punishment for Kikwit's sins.

Only the Catholic church's Monseigneur Alexandre Mbuka Nzundu accepted the outsiders' verdict that there was no *landa-landa,* just a terrible virus that was passed by the loving touch one person gave another: a virus that exploited moments when a husband might daub the forehead of his ailing, feverish wife; a child might hand wash the bloodied sheets upon which his ailing brother slept; a mother might spoon-feed her delirious son; and a grieving family would reverentially wash down the body of their deceased relative, rinsing off the sweat and blood of his haemorrhagic demise.

It was not *landa-landa*; it was a mortal pestilence that passed from one human to another through acts of kindness and love.

The virus was named for the Ebola river in Northern Zaire, which passes near the site of the microbe's first known epidemic in Yambuku, in 1976.[3] Though the 1976 death toll in Yambuku was less than four hundred villagers and Catholic Belgian missionaries, those members of the international scientific team who were deployed to the region to conquer the mysterious outbreak still held Ebola in awe in 1995. In their meetings with other public health officials for years after the 1976 outbreak, surviving members of the Yambuku crew always placed the deadly filovirus in a special, particularly fearsome category: a small assemblage of haemorrhagic fever viruses that included Lassa, Yellow River, Marburg disease, and a handful of others, most of which were discovered only in the last three decades of the twentieth century.

The fear evoked by Ebola among Westerners was largely a matter of enigma: in classic European and American tradition, that which could be understood, even if still dangerous, was no longer fearsome. The act of explanation diminished Western terror. But nineteen years after the virus's last outbreak in Zaire Western science still could not answer the most basic questions about Ebola: where did it come from? In what animal or plant species did it normally reside, when not infecting the human species? Exactly how was it transmitted from person to person? Could it, under any circumstances, pass through the air, infecting people who had no physical contact with patients? Precisely how lethal was the virus? Was it treatable with any drugs or methods available to 1995 physicians?

At the close of the twentieth century these issues would remain largely enigmatic. And in the absence of clear understanding of the elusive Ebola virus public health responses would rely on classic measures, practiced by scientists, physicians, and nurses during epidemics for a hundred years.

For the Zairois Ebola's presence raised horror for very different reasons. The inexplicable nature of an event, or lack thereof, was rarely a primary cause for consternation among the people of Kikwit, as more than three decades of an increasingly brutal dictatorship had left few individuals with a sense of power over their own fates. The main shocks in their lives rarely involved circumstances of their own making or full comprehension, but might well result from an offhand remark made by the dictator the previous day in the faraway capital of Kinshasa. Besides, *landa-landa* served as the all-purpose explanation for otherwise mysterious horrors, deaths, pains, and traumas in life.

Nor could disease, alone, be the source of their collective trepidation. The United Nations Children's Fund (or UNICEF) ranked Zaire number twelve in child mortality, meaning only eleven nations in the world witnessed higher proportional death rates among their under-five-year-olds.[4] Every year the mothers of Zaire gave birth to just over two million babies. And 442 000 of them didn't live to see their fifth birthdays. Nearly half of the nation's children were, by strict medical definition, malnourished, 45 per cent of them growth-stunted as a result. The main causes of child death were malaria (increasing due to drug resistance among the parasites), malnutrition, measles, and HIV.

If a child survived to the age of five, there were good odds that he or she would reach adolescence. Then the youngster would face a new series of threats: AIDS, tuberculosis, murder, maternal death in childbirth.[5] Malarial episodes were frequent, as were the pains of syphilis, gonorrhoea, and chlamydia. The main road of Kikwit—Boulevard Mobutu, named after the dictator—was lined with mud hut pharmacies offering everything from, literally, snake oil to out-of-date antibiotics as remedies to the long list of ailments that formed an assumed, seemingly normal, part of life near the equator.

No, death and disease were not, in and of themselves, the causes of Kikwitians' grave fear in the face of Ebola.

The terror grew from the horror evoked by the illness itself and its rapid progression to death.

'I dare to say that anyone who has seen a case of Ebola will never forget it,' Dr Tamfum Muyembe said.[6] Recalling his first encounter with the virus in September 1976 Muyembe said that he'd worked barehanded on patients who were drenched in blood.

'I had never before seen blood continue to flow at the site of injection,' Muyembe recalled, describing Ebola as 'strange, a fever that responded neither to antibiotics or antimalarials.'

Muyembe spoke as a scientist and physician, finding concern in details similar to those that worried his Western counterparts. But in Kikwit's central marketplace, where all manner of rain forest meat and plants were sold, Ebola raised different fears.

'I pray most of the time now in order to get protection from God,' fishmonger Kieghilamga said, holding her palms upright beside her tattooed cheeks and raising her eyes to the clouded day. Those people who died, she insisted, 'were poisoned. I don't know who poisoned them. It makes me afraid.'

Brigitte Mwalanga sadly rearranged her display of smoked caterpillars, which because of their crunchy flavour usually sold quickly. But there were few buyers now, she said, because, 'everybody is afraid. I'm very afraid.'

The usually bustling market was oddly quiet and bereft of its typical mob of morning buyers. Sugar seller Pascaline waved at fellow traders, all of whom, like her, were having trouble moving the goods that they displayed upon makeshift wooden tables of crate boxes. Usually the plump woman drew crowds who admired her humourous banter and jolly mood. But Pascaline's outlook was cool now, and, 'Salutation is forbidden. I don't greet people and I don't like to eat with others or share food.'

Pascaline's usually gregarious behaviour was reined in by Ebola, which 'instantly,' she says, killed her good friend Willy Ndumba, a nurse at Kikwit General Hospital.

As Pascaline speaks, young peanut seller Brigitte nods sadly, then ticks off a list of those she knows who have died suddenly of the dreaded disease. When asked how she copes with her fears Catholic Brigitte looks down at her feet and whispers, 'I just pray.'

Far away from the quarantined Bandundu Province, accessible only by chartered plane or a drive of three and a half days over the potholed Mobutu Highway, a warlike state of siege reigned in the Zairois capital, Kinshasa. The rooftops of her few hotels are dotted with portable satellite dishes, impromptu news bureaux fill the hotels' suites, multilingual hustlers find ready employment as translators for the media, and cell phones beep in the hallways. A horde of journalists, most of them shell-shocked after previous weeks of bearing witness to the horrors of civil war in Rwanda, set up camp in Kinshasa. With the same aggressive verve that had kept them alive during one of Africa's most brutal conflicts, a media corps from all over the world clamoured and competed for news from the front of humanity's battle with a microbe. If the reporters feared the virus they did not show it, for missing deadlines or being trounced by their competitors were paramount concerns.

Not far from the media encampments another frenzied horde was gathered around Health Secretary Lonyangela Bompenda. Bureaucrats, generals, and the dictator's entourage struggled to guess Mobutu's whims while preventing panic in the capital. All too aware of the satellite dishes on the Hotel Intercontinental, the government leaders struggled to keep the nation's face while maintaining access to Zaire's oil and diamond reserves.

Reading the tea leaves to surmise the dictator's will was something of an art in Kinshasa. No one survived, either politically or in material reality, for long if Mobutu's ire was raised. But the sixty-five-year-old dictator offered little guidance. Indeed, he seldom set foot any longer in the capital, preferring the security and solitude of Gbadolite, some 750 miles to the north-east of Kinshasa. There he was surrounded by Mouvement Populaire de la Révolution cronies and leaders of the seventy-thousand-strong Zairois Army. The sycophants bowed to their 'democratically elected leader' who held court seated upon a throne, clutching the staff traditionally given to tribal chieftains and wearing the royal skins of leopards. With his eyes always invisible behind pitch dark glasses Mobutu had held sway since 1964.

Back then Zaire was called Belgian Congo and had suffered nearly four hundred years of brutal colonialism, slavery, and exploitation. Though it was seventy-seven times the size of tiny Belgium, the Congo was ruled from 1876 to 1908 by a white king enthroned in Brussels. Africa's largest nation was controlled by the Belgian Parliament from 1908 to 1960. A bold leader emerged named Patrice Lumumba who espoused African nationalism and vaguely socialist ideals. In 1960, after only months on the job, Lumumba threatened continued Western access to the vast natural resources of Congo, including cobalt and uranium, then in demand for nuclear weapons production.

Convinced Lumumba would open the African door to Soviet communism, CIA director Allen Dulles ordered Congo's head of state assassinated.[7] Driving Dulles's decision were a series of cables from Leopoldville (the colonial name of Kinshasa) sent by Congo CIA station chief Lawrence Devlin. In a key cable Devlin claimed that 'embassy and station believe the Congo experiencing classic communist effort take-over government. . . . Whether or not Lumumba actually Commie or just playing Commie game to assist his solidifying power, anti-West forces rapidly increasing power Congo, and there may be little time left in which take action to avoid another Cuba.'

Under direct orders from Dulles and President Eisenhower's National Security Council the CIA created violent riots in Kinshasa and selected thirty-one-year-old Colonel Joseph Mobutu as the heir apparent, pending assassination of Lumumba.

Two attempts to kill Lumumba using CIA-developed biological weapons failed. The CIA deliberately leaked word of Lumumba's pending murder, causing the legally elected head of state to flee the capital for distant Lumbumbashi. There, with CIA assistance, Mobutu's troops surrounded and murdered unarmed Lumumba on January 13, 1961, placing his body in the trunk of a car, much as a gang of Mafiosi might dispose of their enemies in a gangster hit.

Mobutu seized power but was immediately opposed in armed insurrections in the Katanga and Shaba provinces. To ensure the political survival of the Mobutu regime during the tempestuous years of 1961 to 1967 the CIA flew in Cuban anti-Communist mercenaries, trained an elite corps of 243 Zairois soldiers in Israel, and occasionally dropped top units of the US Special Forces into hotly contested areas. Belgium also bolstered Mobutu's climb to power, deploying commando units to lead his troops in combat in rebellious Katanga.

From the beginning Mobutu proved a wily leader. Outwardly he donned all the appearances of classic African nationalism. He wore the attire of traditional chiefs, mixed with his own version of business jackets—a stifling cross between Nehru jackets worn in India, Chinese Mao jackets, and thick European business suits. The nation's name was changed to Zaire, a wholly concocted amalgam of Bantu names. All Zairois were commanded in 1971 to change their names as well, dropping the Christian names that had been used for more than two centuries. The new leader changed his own name from Joseph to Sese Seko Kuku Ngbendu wa za Banga, or 'the all-conquering warrior who triumphs over all obstacles.'

The nationalistic veneer fooled many pan-Africanists, who thought Mobutu the equal of such contemporaries on the continent as Kwame Nkrumah in Ghana, Nelson Mandela in South Africa, and Tanzania's Julius Nyerere.

Prophetically, on his cancer deathbed in 1961, the Algerian intellectual Franz Fanon warned, 'Our mistake is to have believed that the [Western] enemy had lost his combativeness and his harmfulness. If Lumumba is in the way, Lumumba disappears. . . . Let us be sure never to forget it: the fate of all of us is at stake in the Congo.'

Throughout the 1970s and 1980s Mobutu proved a ready ally for Europe and the United States, offering his country as a staging and training ground for counterinsurgency forces bent on toppling governments and guerrilla fronts considered hostile to the apartheid state of South Africa: Angolan troops fighting in opposition to the MPLA (the Popular Movement for the Liberation of Angola); mercenaries and South African Special Forces troops battling Namibia's SWAPO (Southwest African People's Organization); Frelimo (Mozambique's anticolonial organization); and all presences of Cuban troops in Africa. That all of these organizations eventually attained power in their respective countries—and in some cases still retained that power at the close of the twentieth century—is indication of the failure of the West's Zaire strategy.

Nevertheless, the Zaire engagement stratagem remained in place throughout the Cold War and well into the 1980s. It was not until the arrival of the Clinton administration in the United States that Mobutu felt the slightest chill in his warm alliance with the West.

In exchange for Mobutu's willingness to act as Africa's proxy for Western anti-Soviet interests the dictator gained tremendous power and personal wealth. From 1963 to 1984 France, Belgium, South Africa, and the United States provided the dictator with astounding amounts of foreign aid—often in the form of zero-interest, no-strings-attached loans—and direct military assistance.[8]

Perhaps even more valuable to the dictator than the West's military support was its willingness to ignore Mobutu's obscene greed and corruption. As the Western governments poured cash into Zaire's coffers, everyone knew that the Mobutu regime couldn't provide legitimate receipts, for the funds rarely found their way to the programmes for which they were designated. A massive General Electric-built Congo river dam, sufficient to power the electrical needs of all sub-Saharan Africa, fell to ruin because US foreign aid funds for maintenance mysteriously never reached the electric power authority's bank account. Roads were never built. Hospitals and schools fell to ruin, most faring worse under Mobutu than they had when a Belgian colonial missionary system handled the bulk of Congo's health and education needs. Only 42 per cent of the nation had access to anything vaguely resembling safe drinking water, and sanitation and refuse services were available to just 15 per cent of the population. Nothing in the nation—from telephones to airports—functioned reliably. Agricultural production was poor, but distribution of foodstuffs even worse. The 42.3 million Zairois suffered in a country almost entirely lacking in infrastructure, their complaints met with brutal repression, torture, and military assault.

Meanwhile, North American and European companies routinely paid hefty 'fees' to Mobutu and his cronies in exchange for access to Zaire's genuine wealth: her cobalt (60 per cent of the world's reserves, and a strategic metal), copper, cadmium, gold, silver, uranium, tin, germanium, zinc, manganese, oil, diamonds, ivory, and rubber.[9] While per capita income stagnated for twenty years, never exceeding $180 per year, Mobutu became one of the world's wealthiest men, Belgium's biggest property owner, and a key property owner in France and Switzerland.

As early as 1977, after just twelve years of such graft and corruption, Mobutu is estimated to have amassed a personal fortune equal to Zaire's official foreign debt—$5 billion. To ensure the loyalty of his cronies, as well as his personal safety, Mobutu allowed graft to flow to a tiny coterie of fellow gangsters, most of whom lived near him in Gbadolite. His uncle, Litho, for example, died leaving assets in excess of $1 billion. His second wife was arrested in Belgium in 1977 trying to smuggle $6 million worth of diamonds into the country.

By the time Ebola struck Kikwit the dictator and his friends had stolen at least $11 billion from the Zairois people.[10] The national bank had been shut down since 1991, when soldiers looted Kinshasa having learned that the currency in which they were paid carried no value. There was no cash in the bank, and no legal exchange of currency. The black market was Zaire's only monetary system, and there a $100 bill could fetch two twenty-five-pound satchels full of 100- and 500-Zaire notes, each of which bore the portrait of the nation's greatest thief, Mobutu. Even at that exchange rate it was hard to see the worth of the Zaire note, given that a tankful of petrol required an inch-thick stack of the nation's highest denomination Z500 notes. For the seasoned traveller accustomed to the currency crises of developing countries the Zaire stood out as a 'funny money' challenge that defied space afforded by pockets, purses, wallets, and money belts. Zairois businessmen routinely carried foot-thick stacks of Z100 and Z500 notes, arranged in rubber-band-held bundles valued at Z5000 or Z20 000. Payments were usually negotiated by bundle, and only the most paltry of goods—such as Brigitte Mwalanga's smoked caterpillars—could be purchased with individual Z100 or Z500 notes.

It was in this national climate of corruption and currency fraud that the Ebola virus flourished in 1995. By the time it surfaced in Kikwit after a nineteen-year hiatus the nation's public health and medical infrastructure existed in name only. There were twenty-four thousand Zairois for every hospital bed in the nation. Most of the population was under eighteen years of age in a nation almost bereft of condoms and contraceptives. HIV was rampant, afflicting an estimated 10 per cent of the adult population. The multinational Project SIDA, once the most productive AIDS research centre in all of Africa, was shut down, its equipment looted during the 1991 soldiers' riots.

And, most importantly, the nation's civil servants, including more than 95 per cent of Zaire's physicians and nurses, had gone unpaid since the 1991 riots. The dictator, having grown smug in his old age, ceased even pretending to maintain national cash reserves to back civil service paychecks: Mobutu and his cronies were by 1995 overtly siphoning every penny of foreign exchange directly into their personal bank accounts.

When a Zairois became ill in 1995 his or her family had three choices: ignore the ailment and pray the individual muddled through somehow; carry or transport the ailing relative to a missionary hospital and there beg for free treatment; or, most often, get the relative to one of Zaire's government clinics or hospitals. In a foreign-funded mission facility Western-trained physicians offered good care, using reasonable equipment and drugs. But in the civil facilities the physician or nurse would make a diagnosis, usually without the use of such nonexistent or long-since-broken-down medicinal tools as X-rays, laboratory tests, CT scans, or blood pressure devices. Even thermometers were in short supply.

Once a diagnosis was reached, the government health-care worker would tell the family what was needed to ensure their relative's recovery, and the Zairois family would dutifully pool their resources and search their homes and local stores for the prescribed essentials: bedsheets, anaesthesia, sterile equipment, antibiotics, food, bandages, and the like. More often than not sterile equipment was the lowest priority and, frankly, unavailable. In contrast, the black market and private pharmacies were chock-full of medicines of all kinds, even state-of-the-art broad-spectrum antibiotics.

The market was well supplied because doctors and nurses, lacking paychecks or other means to support their own families, simply sold off whatever medical supplies reached their facilities, either doled out by the Ministry of Health or, more commonly, donated by foreign non-governmental charities and religious organizations. Everything that was saleable, from latex gloves to X-ray film, had disappeared from the nation's hospitals and clinics since 1991, and by 1995 the Zairois people had grown begrudgingly accustomed to bartering their worldly goods and services in exchange for medical supplies and the skills of local health-care workers.[11]

Two things are clear: Ebola spread in Kikwit because the most basic, essential elements of public health were non-existent. And those exigencies were lacking in Kikwit—indeed, throughout Zaire—because Mobutu Sese Seko and his cronies had for three decades looted the national treasuries. Ebola haunted Zaire because of corruption and political repression. The virus had no secret powers, nor was it unusually contagious. For centuries Ebola had lurked somewhere in the jungles of central Africa. Its emergence into human populations required the special assistance of humanity's greatest vices: greed, corruption, arrogance, tyranny, and callousness. What unfolded in Zaire in 1995 was not so much the rain forest terror widely depicted then in popular media worldwide as an inevitable outcome of disgraceful disconcern—even disdain—for the health of the Zairois public.

Gaspard Menga Kitambala was a forty-three-year-old charcoal maker, Jehovah's Witness, husband, and father of five small children. Those were his vital statistics, along with the fact that he resided near Ndala Avenue in a modest mud-and-brick house located along a precarious, steep, muddy pathway that was alternately engulfed by rain forest vegetation or transformed into a waterfall during equatorial monsoons. By all accounts Menga was a hard-working fellow, devout Jehovah's Witness Christian, and devoted father.

Menga's strong, muscular body bespoke the tough physicality of his profession. The making and transport of charcoal was arduous and phenomenally labour intensive, given the low cash return. Menga regularly bicycled or walked to the rain forest, which until the 1970s engulfed most of modern-day Kikwit, but each year retreated farther and farther away, yielding to the axes of firewood-hungry Kikwitians. After two decades of hacking at the forest the periphery was more than a full day's walk away. And reaching the denser regions where Menga toiled took up to three days.

Once there, Menga would make camp, dig large pits, and fill them with the wood of felled trees. Then he would set the wood afire, lightly bury it, and allow the smoldering heat to char the trees down to hefty chunks of charcoal. After two weeks of such labour Menga would haul his heavy cargo back to Kikwit, selling it to fuel-starved neighbours.

It was never difficult to sell charcoal at a comparatively decent price, for Kikwit had few other sources of cooking fuel. Propane and petrol were far more expensive, and in such short supply that idled vehicles awaiting petrol frequently lined the road. Most so-called petrol stations were little more than crates on top of which sat a haphazard selection of petrol-filled bottles and plastic jugs, thirty of which were usually needed to fill a car tank. Not surprisingly, there were few cars or trucks in Kikwit, and most people—Menga, included—walked everywhere, carrying their burdens on their heads.

In December 1994 Menga was camped deep in the forest, not far from the Lwemi River. It was a verdant place, redolent with well-mulched soil and fragrant flowers. Butterflies danced in the areas penetrated by the sun. Tall trees, laced with lianas, protruded from the dense undergrowth. In some spots a plant locally called 'quatre-vingt' or 'eighty' choked all rival growth, leaving patches where nothing but the local weed grew. No one knew from whence 'quatre-vingt' had come, but its name signified the year, 1980, when the alien vegetation suddenly sprung up all over Bandundu province. The tall weed crowded out all indigenous growth, much as kudzu had long ago taken over the untended areas of America's Deep South. In place of growth that was once diverse and filled with edible plants and animals, sprouted the poisonous 'quatre-vingt'.[12] Wherever stands of the tall weeds appeared the Bandundu wildlife was forced elsewhere, crowding into dwindling sites of indigenous growth.

In his own very small way Menga was contributing to the region's deforestation, knocking down trees and creating spaces into which the opportunistic 'quatre-vingt' could grow. The terrible weed, which choked manioc and corn crops as well as the forest, was just one of a long list of ecological changes Bandundu's forests had undergone since local human populations grew to their 1995 proportions. The so-called city of Kikwit with its 400 000 residents was little more than a gigantic village, as it lacked even a modicum of an urban infrastructure. A key missing item was employment: Kikwit had no industry or large businesses. If the people had stayed in their villages they might have lived off the land, growing cassava, manioc, and corn. But in Kikwit their village-style wattle huts were jammed one against the other, leaving no room for cultivation. In the absence of an urban employer Kikwitians had little choice but to arise with the dawn and trek to the forest in search of animals to sell as bushmeat, caterpillars, snakes, medicinal herbs, and other saleable items. Every year the people made their task more difficult as they chopped and pushed the forest's periphery, extending the distance of their periodic treks.

The fortunate, resourceful few laid claim to the newly timbered lands, planting small plots of corn, manioc, or cassava. They fought daily battles with encroaching 'quatre-vingt' weeds, but usually could eke out a subsistence from decent-size plots. Gaspard Menga had such a plot, located along his route to the rain forest. It was a source not of income but of food for the large, hungry Menga clan.

For Menga the long journeys to the forest signalled time away from his family, and hours of lonely work surrounded by enormous black and red ants, malarial mosquitoes, venomous snakes, spiders larger than a human hand, flying squirrels, mongoose, small antelopes, bats, and, rarely, monkeys. What he caught, Menga ate. And at night he slept in a makeshift hut, where he was undoubtedly tormented by insects.

Shortly after Christmas 1994 Menga loaded up another batch of charcoal and headed back to Kikwit. No one knows when the fever, sore throat, fatigue, and achy muscles first hit the hardworking man. No matter how sick he felt Menga had little choice but to push on for Kikwit, as there were no refuges nor medical aid along his route.

By the time he reached his humble home on Ndala Avenue Menga had a fever and was exhausted. His wife, Bébé Ando, tended to him and shooed away their youngest boys, seven-year-old Judo and Michael, age two. But by January 6, 1995, his fever had soared, and Menga had bloody diarrhoea. Alarmed, Bébé Ando took Menga to a local clinic where he began vomiting blood, becoming so weak he could not walk. The clinic transferred Menga to Kikwit General Hospital, where he was placed in Pavilion No. 3. The doctors who cared for Menga were understandably alarmed by their patient's rapid deterioration, and on the assumption he was suffering from Shigella-induced dysentery, filled him with locally available antibiotics.

On January 13 Gaspard Menga died, and the family brought his body home. There Bébé Ando and Gaspard's younger brothers, Pierre and Bilolo, lovingly washed down the dead man and dressed him in his church clothes. Menga family members from faraway villages came to the open-casket funeral and, as was customary among local Catholics, touched or kissed the body, bidding Gaspard speedy admittance into heaven. Photographs of the mourning depict a family deeply distraught by their loss, with some draping themselves in grief over Gaspard's body.

A few days later Gaspard's brother Bilolo fell ill, exhibiting symptoms the family knew were the same as those that had devastated Gaspard. On February 3 he died in the Kikwit General Hospital emergency room.

Sensing that she, too, was falling ill to some terrible *landa-landa*, Bébé Ando sent her children off with their aunt, Marie-José Nseke, to the care of their grandparents in the village of Ndobo. And then she, too, began to bleed uncontrollably from her anus and nose. At a local infirmary her condition was mistakenly diagnosed as malaria and, when she vomited blood, pneumonia. Like her brother-in-law before her, Bébé Ando died in the emergency room of Kikwit General Hospital.

Meanwhile, in the village of Ndobo, a day's drive away, Bébé Ando's youngest son, Michael Jackson Menga (named after the family's favourite pop star) became ill, suffering the now-familiar litany of Menga family symptoms: headache, fever, fatigue, depression, anorexia, muscle aches, sharp stomach pains, inability to swallow, bloody diarrhoea, bloody nose, bloody vomitus, hiccups, reddened eyes, and red urine. In short, he bled to death on February 11. His older brother, Judo, followed suit, five days later.

Ndobo was one of six villages affected by the tragedy unfurling for the Mengas. Located across the Kwilu River from Kikwit, the villages were connected by a spider's web of dirt roads barely traversable with a four-wheel-drive vehicle. In some stretches the roads were little more than metre-wide paths beaten out of stands of savannah grass by the steady treading of feet.

Every village had its own character, often dictated by its chief. Ndobo's chief, Santu, was a white-bearded, bald man who appeared to be elderly, though he was probably less than fifty years old. When visitors arrived Santu struggled to silence Ndobo's mobs of unruly children, which outnumbered the adults fifteen-to-one. Only by swinging his staff sharply, occasionally connecting with a youngster's backside, could Santu maintain a semblance of order.

In the centre of the village was a large, rectangular thatched building in which Michael Jackson, Judo, their Aunt Marie-José, and their three sisters Lenza, Asinta, and Gizelle stayed with their grandparents following Gaspard's funeral. By March 1, both grandparents had died of Ebola.[13]

Nobody in Ndobo understood the terrible *landa-landa* that struck the Menga relatives. It was months before explanations would come from distant Kikwit. For village chief Santu and the unruly herds of children that raced about the place the Menga clan's suffering was simply a more mysterious and frightening version of the death toll that haunted their lives. Some of the children were AIDS orphans, after all. But AIDS killed slowly—this *landa-landa* destroyed bodies and minds within a week. So the villagers ordered the family's bodies buried well outside of their tiny town, where the fearsome *landa-landa* could not reach them as they slept at night.

When the Menga death toll was counted, in Kikwit and the various villages, sixteen of the twenty-three who either had attended Gaspard's funeral or tended to those who contracted Ebola from Gaspard died of the disease. Amazingly, every Menga who developed symptoms eventually perished—an astounding 100 per cent kill rate. Perhaps equally amazing were the cases of Mengas who apparently never did get the disease. Twenty-six-year-old Pierre, for example, washed his brother's body which, unbeknown to him, was drenched in virus-rich blood and fluids. And he tended to his other dying brother, Bilolo, and sister-in-law, Bébé Ando. Yet Pierre said he never suffered as much as a headache. Neither did Pierre and Gaspard's father, Innocent, who participated in several Menga funerals. Most startling was elderly Innocent's survival. Having long suffered from tuberculosis, Innocent was a frail, weak man. He helped bury three of his sons, three daughters-in-law, and several grandchildren. Yet he never caught Ebola.

Similarly, Lenza, Asinta, and Gizelle touched their father's corpse and cared for their dying brothers, Judo and Michael Jackson. When the boys succumbed the sisters prepared the bodies for burial in Ndobo. And when their grandparents subsequently developed Ebola disease the three little girls were again exposed to the virus. Yet they never became ill. Nor did the members of the Mbelo family who helped the three little orphans and buried all of the Mengas who succumbed in Ndobo.

After the Menga grandparents died Ebola simply stopped in the village of Ndobo. Why? No one knows. But Ndobo's confrontation with the dreaded virus was long over before the people knew the cause of their tragedy or the world knew that Ebola had broken out in Zaire.

A similar pattern developed out in other villages where Menga relatives lived following Gaspard's funeral. In the neat, orderly village of Kimputu-Nseke, for example, thirty-five-year-old Romaine Mawita—wife of Gaspard's brother Nico Menga—and her two small children died in mid-February. And though the villagers helped to care for the ailing trio, and buried their bodies, no other residents of Kimputu-Nseke came down with the virus. By March the villages' struggles with the virus were over. When Ebola raged months later in Kikwit the people of Kimputu-Nseke remained untouched, both by the virus and by panic. While fear gripped most of the region, Kimputu-Nseke residents still greeted strangers with the palms-up gesture of friendship and salutations of *Mbote*.

By mid-March this cycle of death had passed, allowing the villages of Ndobo, Kimputu-Nseke, Nkara, Mukolo, Bulunga, and Ikubi to return to normal life—and death.

Such was not the case back in Kikwit. In the villages, where the only medical care available was the ministrations of friends and relatives, Ebola failed to pass beyond its initial chain of infections. But in Kikwit, where public health was a shambles, but medical clinics abounded, the virus found great opportunity.

Gaspard, Bilolo, and Bébé Ando all died in the decrepit emergency room of Kikwit General Hospital. So did Gaspard's aunt, Rosalie Sandrala, on February 14, 1995.

A wide dirt road, accessible from a back alleyway, met the ramp up to Kikwit's *Salle d'Urgence*. Rusted, heavy steel trolleys covered with thin, worn-out plastic pads, were strewn haphazardly about the area, some nestled among the weeds and mud of the hospital grounds, exposed to the equatorial heat and daily downpours, while others sat just at the top of the ramp under the cinder block turquoise veranda entryway to the emergency room. On any given day dozens of family members milled about the area, using the trolleys as benches and beds while they awaited word on the status of an ailing relative.

An officious ward clerk barred entry to the emergency room, using his table to create an obstacle that prevented the anxious families from mobbing the already crowded medical facility. Names and symptoms were dutifully entered into his logbook in a mix of KiCongo and French when one emergency room bed was vacated and another patient was allowed to come in. Protected from the tropical rain, usually lying on the concrete floor of the veranda, were the desperately ill waiting to see a doctor. Most were malnourished children—toddlers, really—whose eyes stared out vacantly from feverish heads. Malaria, measles, bacterial infections, and meningitis were among their predators.

The adult infirm were also largely victims of microbes, which caused them variously to spit up blood from tuberculosis-infested lungs; walk on stick-thin legs wasted by years of HIV infection; fight malarial fevers of more than 39.4 °C; or, most commonly, combat some mysterious *landa-landa* that produced sudden fatigue, fevers, head-aches, and malaise.

These patients could wait. That was what the clerk was taught. First priority was the comparatively rare case of trauma, a bleeding accident victim. Second priority were feverish babies, for everyone in Kikwit had seen how rapidly little ones could die: one day they seemed like normal babies, and the next day they were corpses.

Inside the dark emergency room only indirect sunlight could guide the physicians' and nurses' activities by day, kerosene lamps by night. Decades-old steel-framed beds lined two walls of the emergency room, leaving a narrow walkway between. So crowded was the place that health-care workers stumbled into one another as they moved among patients. Most patients stared out from pain or fever, an intravenous drip delivered through recycled needles silently passing into their bloodstreams saline, antibiotics, or antimalarial drugs, along with whatever microbes might be on the needle.

Next door in a tiny chamber was the transfusion table, set diagonally toward an east-ern window. When malarial parasites overwhelmed the oxygen-carrying red blood cells of an individual's body, minutes counted. Death could occur in the blink of an eye if the suffering one didn't immediately receive millions of healthy, oxygen-rich red blood cells. These, of course, had to come from a genetically matched relative or the victim's immune system would reject the transfusion, and death due to anaphylaxis would swiftly follow.

More often than not a child less than five years of age lay upon the transfusion table receiving blood drawn from a parent or older sibling. Encrusted with dried blood and rust, the transfusion table loomed like some medieval torture rack. And though it was a site for short-term cures, the old steel slab was also a daily source of infection where, through either nonsterile needles or directly from the contaminated donor's blood, the transfused received doses of HIV, hepatitis B, *Plasmodium falciparum* parasites, and assorted other microbes.

The health-care workers did the best they could, given their nearly complete lack of resources. There were syringes and surgical supplies which, when the electrical gener-ator worked, could be sterilized in an autoclave. A small supply of latex gloves were washed and recycled after a day's use. The hospital laboratory performed rapid tests to determine that transfusions involved matched blood types. But they lacked kits that could as rapidly test the blood for HIV, hepatitis, or other infections.

The surgical pavilions were similarly sparsely supplied. The sorts of massive, round overhead lights used in surgical theatres in Europe four or five decades previously loomed over the operating tables but were rarely powered, as electricity was a precious commodity. Sunlight pouring in through screenless windows typically guided the sur-geons' hands. The patients, nurses, anaesthesiologists, and surgeons were protected from one another's germs by a thin veneer of hygiene: cloth tie-up masks, recycled latex gloves, cotton surgical gowns. These items, as well as the surgical equipment, were washed every day in local water. The hospital had no tap water, nor any source of sterile liquid. Instead, physicians scrubbed in tubs of river water, often unable to obtain soap that might offer a modicum of hygiene. When electricity could not be generated, surgical instruments were boiled over a wood or charcoal fire—thus, the Bandundu forests offered both fuel for sterilization and refuge for the very microbes responsible for much of Kikwit's *landa-landa*.

Patients that were hospitalized ended up on designated one-story cinder block wards, lying upon bare steel-framed beds. Only a wafer-thin plastic pad shielded their bodies from jutting steel, and any amenities such as food, pillows, and sheets were provided by visiting relatives. The wards, or pavilions, were designated according to Kikwit's greatest health needs. The largest was paediatric, where mothers often slept with their ailing children. As those youngsters confronted death new babies were born in the hospital's most densely packed ward, maternity. There expectant mothers frequently had to share a twin hospital bed, lying diagonally head-to-foot alongside a stranger, their newborns jostling for space. Babies were delivered by gloveless mid-wives who toiled amidst maternal and neonatal blood, usually with only the faint flicker of a single kerosene lamp to guide their efforts as they slit episiotomies, cut umbilical cords, performed caesarean-sections, or corrected breech births.

Off to the side, disconnected from the rest of the hospital, was the *Salle du tuberculose et de la SIDA* where adult AIDS and TB patients languished.

And in two tiny chambers at the end of the long, blue open-air hallway that con-nected the pavilions were the hospital's laboratories and statistics office. There techni-cians hunched over one of two available light microscopes, usable only by sunlight. Their laboratory samples sat in unpowered refrigerators. Glass tubes, stoppered with rags or cotton balls, rested in racks awaiting analysis. And, as was the case with most of their hospital colleagues, the laboratory personnel lacked any protective gear to prevent their infection in the event contaminated samples spilled onto their hands, eyes, noses, or cut into their bloodstreams.

Even worse conditions reigned at Kikwit Maternity Hospital No. 2, where most of the city's babies were born. On March 2 Pauline Kabala, Rosalie Sandrala's best friend, checked into Kikwit Maternity Hospital No. 2 suffering bloody diarrhoea and vomit-ing blood. Eight nurses and several friends attended to Kabala, who was dying; within days all of them came down with the same bloody illness. Six of the eight hospital employees died of it in March. Before they died—indeed before they even realized that they were ill—these nurses and friends passed their infections on to still more hospital employees, family members, and patients, starting a chain of death that would in April spiral out of the maternity hospital and into the general community. Kikwit's mysteri-ous *landa-landa* was getting out of control.

Meanwhile at Kikwit General Hospital doctors had their hands full in March with cases of what looked like shigella bacterial infection, the leading cause of bloody diarrhoea. True, it was rare to see shigella patients also vomit blood, bleed from their noses and gums, and have bloodied eyes. Shigella didn't usually cause such things. But in 1995 a new type of shigella had emerged in the world, in the far east of the country in a rocky, volcanic place called Goma. There, tens of thousands of refugees had taken haven from the civil war slaughter in neighbouring Rwanda, living without viable shelter, food, or safe drinking water. Cholera and shigella broke out among the refugees, claiming thousands of lives.[14] And due to widespread misuse of antibiotics the strain of shigella rampant in the region became resistant to all available drugs. Only one drug in the entire world had any effect against the new superbug, and it was at least ten times more expensive than anything in use in the region. Ciprofloxacin, a German-made powerful, third-generation antibiotic was the last, completely unaffordable hope for Central African shigella sufferers.[15]

It seemed a logical conclusion, then, that the wave of bloody deaths in Kikwit General Hospital and Maternity Hospital No. 2 were caused by the new supershigella. Or so Dr Mungala Kipassa thought. To be certain, the young doctor, who had a master's in public health, ordered Maternity Hospital No. 2 laboratory technician Kakesa Kimfumu to take blood samples from several of the patients.[16] If shigella were in those samples Kipassa knew that steps would have to be taken to decontaminate Kikwit's water supplies lest a full-fledged dysentery epidemic might erupt.

Kimfumu, aged thirty-six, did his job in early April, drawing samples from several patients, including hospital administrator Kimbambu. Somehow Kimfumu became infected, probably through an accidental poke with the needle drawn from Kimbambu (who died on March 27), and Kimfumu went from being a hospital employee to patient.

On April 10 Kimfumu was transferred to Kikwit General Hospital where Kipassa's team struggled to understand what had happened to the laboratory worker. Kimfumu had some of the same symptoms seen in the other suspected shigella patients, with two key exceptions: he didn't have bloody diarrhoea, but he did have a hugely protruding, distended belly. In the eyes of his physicians it looked like Kimfumu was suffering from appendicitis.

That day he underwent an appendectomy, conducted by surgeon Nyembe. But the removal of his appendix failed to improve Kimfumu's status. Indeed, in subsequent hours he became delirious and the distension of his belly worsened. The physicians concluded that their first diagnosis had been incorrect: Kimfumu did not have appendicitis but an intestinal perforation caused by the bacterial infection typhoid fever.

So on April 12 Kimfumu underwent a second round of surgery intended to mend his perforated intestines. Present in the operating theatre were anaesthesiologist Willy Mubiala and nurses Mingweni Lakamoyo and Sister Floralba, a European nun with the Sisters of the Poor of Bengame. The surgeons were Doctors Nkuku and Bwaka, who were watched closely by local medical student Pila Puskas. As they prepared their patient for surgery the group was well aware that Kimfumu was one of their own—a fellow medical worker.

Things began to go wrong as soon as Nkuku made his incision, for Kimfumu's distension was full of blood, which spewed all over the unprotected surgical team.

As they tried frantically to comprehend what was happening and save their colleague, the team members became drenched by Kimfumu's blood. Unable to find a single source of Kimfumu's bleeding or distension the surgeons had no choice but to sew the laboratory technician back up and return him to the postoperative ward. There, on April 14, Kimfumu died.

On the same day as he performed Kimfumu's appendectomy surgeon Nyembe also operated on Géraldine Katadi, the wife of prominent Pentecostal Pastor Kabanga, a follower of the evangelical faith Nzambe Malamu, or God is God.[17] Katadi had suffered placenta praevia during a caesarean section of her baby and now required emergency surgery. Nyembe operated on Katadi immediately after completing Kimfumu's appendectomy. Nurses Anne Lusilu Manikasa and Jean Kingangi assisted Nyembe while Raymond Katima stood guard over the procedure.

And they would die: all but one person present during those three operations would perish, suffering the same litany of bloody symptoms as had tormented the Menga clan. But first they travelled, attended to other patients, and spent time with their families. The first to be taken ill was Dr Nyembe, who died on April 20, ten days after performing surgery on Kimfumu and Katadi. His cause of death was recorded as unknown aetiology.

Two days later in Kikwit medical student Puskas, too, succumbed, as did scrub nurse Lakamoyo.

So when seventy-year-old Sister Floralba was taken ill the members of her order placed the ailing nun in the care of people who were told to take her to Sister Daniella. A nurse, Sister Daniella worked in a Catholic-run hospital located 120 kilometres away in the town of Mosango. Funded by the US-based Catholic Relief Services, the Mosango 590-bed facility was larger, cleaner, and better supplied than Kikwit General.

The road to Mosango was in decent shape. Lined with jacarandas and palms the drive afforded a magnificent view, taking in verdant hillsides, tall monkeypod trees, red clay soil, and steady streams of colourfully dressed pedestrians toting on their heads baskets full of bananas, breadfruit, corn, and fish. The road crossed the Nko River to vast grasslands that reached up to open blue skies. The Mosango mission and hospital, perched on a hill at the end of the grasslands, offered solace from the tropical, sweltering heat.

It's doubtful that the sister noticed the view, as Floralba was deathly ill. By the time Belgian-born Dr Marie-Jo Bonnet saw the Italian nun the sister was suffering 'the worst haemorrhaging I've ever seen. She was elderly. And there was a huge amount of blood coming from her mouth. Her tongue was thick, covered with lesions and bleeding. Her gums, tongue, and lips . . . they all were bleeding,' Bonnet grimly recalled days later.

Upon her arrival in Monsango on April 23 Floralba could only speak in monosyllables, and her fever exceeded 39.4 °C. During the night, while Sister Daniella looked on, Sister Floralba's status worsened. Red, pinprick blood spots appeared all over her body, along with bruiselike splotches indicating uncontrolled bleeding under the skin. Wherever the doctors injected fluids and antibiotics bleeding started, and then never stopped.

By then Bonnet's group had tried five different antibiotic cocktails on Sister Floralba, with absolutely no effect.

The following day, on April 24, with Floralba's condition appearing hopeless and pressing matters awaiting her at another, distant clinic, Sister Daniella left. She'd only been in contact with Floralba for a few hours. After Daniella's departure, Bonnet tried desperately to stop Floralba's haemorrhaging, giving the nun high doses of vitamin K coagulant. 'It was incredible,' Bonnet recalled later. 'The blood simply would not coagulate. Anything we did, it just kept bleeding, . . . the haemorrhage was so profound.'

On April 25 Sister Floralba fell unconscious, her blood pressure plummeted, and at 10 a.m. she died.

Bonnet, who had worked in the Mosango hospital for a decade, was stunned. The sheer amount of the haemorrhaging, and no indications that Sister Floralba had contracted her illness from a patient in Kikwit General Hospital were both disturbing. Bonnet and physician colleagues Doctors Anicet Mazaya and Philippe Akamituna discussed the case, speculating as to whether Sister Floralba's death was caused by the same agent that had claimed four previous patients in Monsango.

Akamituna, a tall, young Zairois physician, noted the case of Pila Kikapindu, a male student nurse from Kikwit General Hospital. He'd arrived in Mosango on April 3, after being ill in Kikwit for four days.

'His brother-in-law said, "Oh, it's AIDS,"' Akamituna remembered. 'But his sister, who cared for him, came down with the same symptoms.'

As Sister Floralba lay dying, so did Kikapindu's sister. And his mother. Their only connection to the horrible disease was the care they gave to Pila, who, despite the hospital's best efforts, died on April 14. (The mother and sister also soon succumbed.) And the same day that Pila Kikapindu bled to death another diseased refugee from Kikwit had arrived: Sambubanda Wagona. He died, suffering similar symptoms, three days later.

The doctors debated every aspect of these cases: were they connected? What caused their deaths? Was there danger for the rest of the hospital, given Mosango had no more gloves, masks, or sterile gowns for the health-care workers?

Hours before Sister Floralba died another ailing nurse from Kikwit General Hospital arrived, seeking a cure that he knew could not be had in the far poorer government hospital. Twenty-five-year-old Ekara Mpolo had the now-classic set of haemorrhagic symptoms, and died a few hours after his arrival. His death sparked a chain of eight more cases, all among Mosango health-care workers. Sister Daniella died. So did nurse Nzaka Munsango, who had cared for Mpolo. A laboratory technician, more nurses, the wife of one of these men—all died in rapid succession between April 26 and May 11.

Watching Munsango's deterioration proved particularly difficult for the hospital staff, as the illness affected his brain. He became a wild man, shouting deranged thoughts, accusing his colleagues of all manner of evils, flailing his arms wildly. Panic started to set in among the hospital staff and rumours of strange goings-on spread to the nearby villages.

Then something truly fearful happened. The wife of one of the deceased laboratory technicians died of the mysterious disease. Her room was scrubbed down, the mattress cleansed, and no one entered the room for more than two weeks. Then twenty-year-old Mupangi, hospitalized for unrelated reasons, was placed in that room, on the dead woman's bed. When Mupangi developed the symptoms of the now-terrifying disease, Bonnet faced panicked insurrection among her staff.

Mupangi's situation was analysed thoroughly. It was clear the young woman had no other possible source of infection, Bonnet insisted. She could only have caught the disease from the plastic-and-foam padding that was her mattress. And the agent of death had somehow survived on that surface for fifteen days.

Bonnet's staff threatened to abandon the hospital, but top doctors staved off desertion by creating true isolation rooms for the remaining patients, and personally caring for Munsango and the rest. One, thirty-nine-year-old nurse Jean-Pierre Sabkuti, was caring for Munsango. When, at the end of April, he died, 'no one here agreed to deal with the body,' Bonnet said. 'I did it, wearing a mask and gown and so on that I had. I, and Akamituna and Mazaya. We took the body for burial.'

As the trio of physicians carried the body of their nurse down the hill to the cemetery, terrified Mosango villagers grabbed up their children and fled into their homes, hiding from the *landa-landa*. When the grieving doctors returned to the hospital the staff announced they would not enter Sabkuti's room to clean it. One nurse, when directly ordered to do so, quit. The three doctors thereafter had to perform all the saddest tasks themselves: placing the dead in coffins, hauling the bodies to the cemetery, burial, and the cleansing of the deceased's rooms.

On May 11 Nzaka Munsango died. And that afternoon shortwave radio reports broadcast from France informed the doctors that the culprit responsible for so many deaths in their hospital was a virus called Ebola.

That conclusion had not been reached swiftly. Indeed, the cause of the Bandundu *landa-landa* crisis was not determined until May, five months after the first Ebola death, that of Gaspard Menga. And the diagnosis was reached as much by luck and fate as by science.

In April other regional hospitals, like Mosango, experienced outbreaks of the bizarre, frightening disease, always commencing with a visitor from Kikwit. And nearly all the deaths in these facilities were among health-care workers.

One such case turned out to be crucial. In the Yasa-Bonga hospital, located about 180 kilometres away from Kikwit, nurse Jean Kingangi underwent treatment, and there died of massive haemorrhaging sixteen days after becoming infected during

Géraldine Katadi's surgery at Kikwit General Hospital. The doctors of Yasa-Bonga had tried every imaginable treatment on Kingangi, including attempts to clot his blood and antibiotic therapy to halt his presumed bacterial dysentery. Numerous blood and urine tests were done on Kingangi: his was the most extensively documented case.

And it would prove fortunate that a Zairois military surgeon, Dr Kongolo, who specialized in tropical medicine, happened to pass through and personally see Kingangi's death. Kongolo speculated that the cause could be Ebola virus, about which he had read a great deal. Kongolo was the first person to reach that hypothesis, which he voiced shortly after Kingangi's death on April 26.

There were no telephones in Yasa-Bonga and therefore it was at first impossible for Kongolo to notify authorities or scientists who might confirm his dire suspicions. His only choice was to make the arduous 420-kilometre journey to Kinshasa and search for Professor Tamfum Muyembe, the famed veteran of the Yambuku outbreak of 1976.

Meanwhile, in Kikwit Dr Kipassa was worried sick. His hospital seemed full of this bizarre, bloody disease, and most of the ill were members of his own staff. He was desperate. Convinced the supershigella had arrived in Kikwit, Kipassa sent pleas for better antibiotics to UNICEF and Muyembe, both in Kinshasa.

By the end of April Muyembe was, as a result, well aware that something terrible was afoot in Zaire. Zaire's leading scientist, Muyembe was a thoughtful, multilingual University of Kinshasa virologist whose serious nature was nicely counterbalanced by his warmth and strong sense of humour. One minute Muyembe would wrinkle his brow in deep thought over a dangerous conundrum, and the next his eyes would sparkle mischievously and he'd let loose with a loud guffaw.

His first action upon receiving Kipassa's desperate plea was to fire off a cable to Sister Agnes, a Catholic nun who had once served as a regional pharmacist in Bandundu. She had long since retired and now lived in a convent outside Antwerp, Belgium.

After hearing the military surgeon's conclusion that the Yasa-Banga case could have been caused by his old nemesis, Ebola, Muyembe packed his bags and grabbed the first charter plane to Kikwit.[18]

Meanwhile, in Belgium Sister Agnes was in a quandary. Muyembe's cable asked for thousands of doses of ciprofloxacin, an antishigella drug far more expensive than anything her poor order could handle. She estimated that she would need more than one million Belgian francs (or $37 000) to fill Muyembe's request: an impossible sum. Uncertain where or how to rapidly obtain the life-saving drugs, eighty-year-old Sister Agnes visited Dr Simon van Nieuwenhove, showed him Muyembe's missive, and asked for advice.

Van Nieuwenhove worked in the tropical research institute in Antwerp, Belgium, and had done work in Zaire. What disturbed the middle-aged Flemish scientist was not the almost prohibitively expensive drug request, but a postscript Muyembe had hastily tagged onto the message: this might not be shigella, but Ebola. Muyembe had added that postscript after speaking to Kongolo, though the Zairois virologist hadn't yet tested blood samples from Kikwit patients. The word *Ebola* gave van Nieuwenhove a shudder, for his entire life had been influenced by that virus. While still a young scientist he had been part of the international team that investigated the Yambuku Ebola outbreak in 1976. He knew Muyembe, and respected the Zairois scientist's hunches.

So van Nieuwenhove told Sister Agnes to delay her search for ciprofloxacin. And he called up another veteran of the 1976 epidemic, American Dr David Heymann. On loan from the CDC to the World Health Organization Heymann was working in Geneva at the WHO Global Programme on AIDS. His colleague had barely whispered the word *Ebola* when Heymann mentally packed his bags, considered which WHO and CDC people he'd like on his team, and visualized what needed to be done.

But first, he said, they needed laboratory samples for analysis. Nobody at WHO wanted to utter out loud the word *Ebola* unless they were certain that the virus had, indeed, reappeared after its nineteen-year hiatus. Having watched the global panic a few months earlier over India's plague outbreak, Heymann realized that a new era had dawned for public health. Back in 1976 when genuine fear had gripped the scientific team in Yambuku their terror had not been reflected in media coverage: fewer than ten newspaper stories had reported on the events, and there was no broadcast coverage. The scientists back then had toiled only under the watchful eyes of the Zairois soldiers and the terrified people of Yambuku. Frankly, at that time nobody outside of Zaire seemed to take note of the event.

But times had changed. The avalanche of global media attention that greeted India's epidemic signalled a warning to Heymann. And there was more: the number one best-selling book in the English language at the time was *The Hot Zone*, by Richard Preston. A gripping account of an Ebola outbreak inside a monkey colony in Reston, Virginia, *The Hot Zone* had captured international attention, focusing a vague sense of public phobia on a virus of which few had previously heard. The book caught Hollywood's interest, and as Heymann pondered the Kikwit situation from his vantage point in Switzerland cinema audiences from Rio de Janeiro to Tokyo were queuing up to see *Outbreak*, a Dustin Hoffman thriller about an imaginary Ebola epidemic.

So Heymann was discreet. He packed his bags, bought tickets to Kinshasa, and quietly informed only a handful of colleagues of Muyembe's suspicion.

Meanwhile, on May 1 Muyembe and his technical staff arrived in Kikwit, examined the patients, and collected blood samples. They were immediately able, based on laboratory analysis, to rule out shigella. And by the time he left Kikwit that day Muyembe was convinced that the Ebola virus had resurfaced. On May 6 Muyembe sent samples to Antwerp, which were rerouted immediately to the CDCs Biohazard Level 4 laboratory in Atlanta, Georgia.

On May 9 C. J. Peters, director of the Special Pathogens Laboratory, received the samples and within less than ten hours his team was able to say that the disease was, indeed, Ebola. Within two days the laboratory confirmed not only that it was Ebola, but also that the viral strain in Kikwit was almost identical genetically to that seen nineteen years earlier in faraway Yambuku.

A skeleton crew of just six scientists toiled round-the-clock in rotating shifts throughout the Ebola crisis inside the CDCs Biohazard Level-4 (BL-4) laboratory. The agency was overwhelmed by the deluge of human and animal blood and tissue samples that arrived from Kikwit and neighbouring villages. Though many—perhaps most—of the samples came up negative for Ebola infection, all had to be handled with the same level of care and caution a scientist might exercise while working with a container of weapons-grade plutonium. Because nobody knew precisely how the virus was transmitted, but did know that Ebola infection was incurable, all laboratory work was performed by scientists who wore full-body space suits that were attached to respiratory umbilical cords that pumped fresh air into their protective gear. The people living outside the Atlanta laboratory were protected by a system similar to nesting Russian dolls: the BL-4 laboratory was inside another, larger building which, in turn, was inside yet another. Each of these structures was airtight, maintained under tight security and accessible to fewer than a hundred people. The innermost, highest security chambers were forbidden to all but a dozen human beings and a host of research animals.

Inside their respiratory suits C. J. Peters's team worked with great care. Each one knew that any slip-up could be immediately lethal to the scientist, and pose a significant risk to society as a whole should the organism have escaped its BL-4 containment.

Shortly after the CDCs Special Pathogens Laboratory confirmed on May 9 that blood samples from Kikwit General Hospital contained the Ebola haemorrhagic fever virus, laboratory director Peters issued memos to higher-ups at CDC warning that there was a distinct possibility that exhaustion, due to overwork among his reduced scientific team, could result in a serious accident.

Because of the extremely highly skilled nature of BL-4 work it was not possible for the agency to simply draft personnel from other sections of the CDC to temporarily fill in gaps left by the budget cuts and congressionally mandated downsizing that had rendered the lab's seven scientists short of its former staffing level. His staff was too small, and the scientists were exhausted. Twenty years previously the CDC had been able to respond to such crises by shifting some laboratory work in two directions: non-BL-4 samples could go to its next security tiered Biohazard Level-3 facility and some of the extremely dangerous BL-4 load could be shared with one of the four other maximum security laboratories in the world.

But in the spring of 1995 some of the other BL-4 options simply were no longer reasonable. For example, there was a BL-4 laboratory in Siberia—a holdover from the heydays of Soviet science—but its security and safety had deteriorated considerably along with every other aspect of Russian public health and scientific research. Britain's Porton Down biological warfare facility was once considered suitable, and had played a role in the 1976 Ebola crisis. But due to changing political considerations vis-à-vis biowarfare and several rounds of budget cuts, Porton Down did not meet 1995 BL-4 standards.

For decades the leading backup to the CDC was France's Institut Pasteur in Paris. But WHO officials were reluctant to direct 'hot' samples to the French laboratory because a scientist studying Ebola-contaminated blood there in the fall of 1994 had come down with the disease, indicating a security breach.

That left only one alternative BL-4 facility: the US Army's Fort Detrick laboratory in Maryland. There, too, cutbacks had taken a toll, as the Department of Defense sought to reduce its share of the national debt. However, the CDC's C. J. Peters, who had once worked at the Fort Detrick laboratory and maintained close contact with colleagues there, was unable to convince the army facility to help the CDC with analysis of Ebola samples.

Meanwhile, the CDC was reluctant to pass non-Ebola work down the security tier to its two BL-3 facilities because the forty-year-old laboratory buildings had so deteriorated that a team of inspectors from outside the federal government had urged their condemnation more than five years previously.

So serious was the decay that air ducts meant to draw biological hazards away from laboratory benches and into safety filtres actually did the reverse: they blew microbes right into scientists' faces. On at least three occasions in the previous eighteen months scientists had, as a result, caught the very diseases they were studying.

In 1993, the US Public Health Service had requested funds from Congress to construct a new BL-3 laboratory, and in the interim Congress had appropriated $88 million of the more than $110 million that was needed to build the facility. All but $1 million of this had been accumulating in an earmarked federal account, awaiting a time when sufficient additional funds were available to purchase land in the Atlanta area and construct the laboratory.

Shortly after the world learned of the Kikwit Ebola outbreak Congress voted to rescind $40 million of that accumulated fund, and apply it toward retirement of the national debt. The Senate voted to rescind all $87 million remaining in the fund. President Clinton vetoed the two budget proposals, hoping to salvage at least $47 million of the BL-3 funds.

Republican staffers for the committees on Capitol Hill that oversaw the Department of Health and Human Services (HHS) and CDC budgets said that the funding situation for all aspects of public health was 'very fluid'. As one staffer put it, 'It's all a moving target—difficult to predict.'

Perhaps the strangest twist in funding events concerned WHO. Long reliant upon largesse from the United States, WHO initially faced the Ebola crisis with a budget of less than $10 000. But on May 19 a handful of private European corporations and foundations came up with $2 million in special aid to support Ebola control efforts. For most Americans and Europeans an outbreak of an exotic disease in a far-off African country seemed none of their business—particularly during post-Cold War national budget crises. Thus, the governments that traditionally underwrote such public health efforts initially demurred in the face of resurgent Ebola.

'The CDC is the only ball game in town,' Dr James LeDuc, head of WHO's special virus division, insisted, emphasizing the world's complete, utter dependence on the American facility.

On May 10 Heymann's tiny WHO team of three Ebola-fighters left Geneva, bound for Zaire. That same day the US government officially declared the Kikwit epidemic a disaster. Over the following five days additional epidemic-fighters streamed in from France, Belgium, the Netherlands, the United States, Sweden, Ghana, Zimbabwe, and South Africa. Laying the groundwork for all these foreigners were Muyembe, Kipassa, and a team of Zairois health-care workers that included local medical school students and the Kikwit Red Cross. Together these people, speaking more than ten different languages and representing the cultures and worldviews of three different continents, faced the toughest challenge of public health: stopping an epidemic firestorm and the panic it produces. In the following six weeks, 2793 English-language media reports on Ebola were stored in the LEXIS/NEXIS computer system, and media in every one of the world's major languages filed daily reports on the unfolding epidemic. Heymann's media hunch almost immediately proved correct: things indeed had changed for public health.

But that wasn't obvious when Muyembe and Heymann first sat down on May 10 on battered vinyl chairs in an abandoned Kikwit VD clinic to assess the city's situation and map out a public health strategy.

Cries of 'Afwaka! Afwaka!' or 'They died!' filled the air in Kikwit. At Kikwit General Hospital those staff members who hadn't caught Ebola or died were hysterical: terrified and grief-stricken. Rumours of deadly landa-landa at the hospital had nearly closed the facility, Kikwitians, perhaps rightly, had begun to prefer remaining ill at home rather than dying in Kikwit General Hospital. Only twenty patients, most suffering from Ebola, remained in the hospital.

In town the people concluded that the facts spoke for themselves: everybody who'd died had been in one of the local hospitals. In each outbreak surgery was directly or indirectly involved. Doctors are corrupt, the townspeople said. Therefore, the doctors were killing people. The dominant explanation for this apparent raft of hospital-caused murders was diamonds.

Much of the world's diamond reservoir is located in northern Angola and Zaire. To prevent theft diamond workers were routinely strip-searched at the end of their shifts. The only way a worker might smuggle a promising gem out of the mines was by swallowing the diamond. Some physicians earned handsome sums of cash by performing surgical removals of diamonds that became lodged somewhere in the individual's gastrointestinal tract rather than finding their way 'naturally' out of the smuggler's body.

The rumour that was all over Kikwit during the second week of May was that Kikwit General Hospital physicians, no longer satisfied with their customary payments for such smuggler surgery, were now killing the patients, and taking the diamonds for themselves. There was no *landa-landa* in the hospital, people said, just greed.

The diamond story didn't carry any currency with those who had actually seen the agonized, bleeding Ebola patients. But it was a hugely popular myth in Kikwit that terribly undermined the credibility not only of Kipassa's staff but also of physicians in general.

Faced with demoralized, even hysterical local health-care workers, a public rife with panic and suspicion, a virtual absence of all essential public health and medical resources, and, at that point, no cash from outside the country, Muyembe and Heymann confronted a daunting challenge.

Exhausted from their long journeys, Heymann and WHO's Mark Szczeniowski were shell-shocked by what they saw. The usually open-faced Heymann wore a strained, emotionless mask, overwhelmed as he was by the horror. It was Heymann's practiced way of confronting chaotic disasters: with stony calm. Szczeniowski, who had for years in the 1970s lived in Zaire working on WHO monkeypox surveys, was no less ashen. Even the ever-gregarious Muyembe was at an emotional loss.

'There was blood everywhere,' Heymann later recalled. 'Blood on the mattresses, on the floors, on the walls. Vomit, diarrhoea . . . When we got here it was really awful. Apocalyptic. There were people dying everywhere. And the women were wailing. It was surreal. They were filling up the graves and we realized that this was not like Yambuku.'

Heymann and Muyembe, the Yambuku veterans, knew that by the time an international team of scientists had arrived in Zaire in 1976 the original Ebola epidemic was already winding down. Some of the international team members back in 1976 never saw an Ebola case, and even Muyembe—first on the scene in Yambuku—came after that outbreak's zenith. In Yambuku, it turned out, nearly every case was spread by one of three syringes that Belgian nuns used over and over again in a tiny mission hospital. Once the nuns succumbed and the hospital closed, the Yambuku epidemic wound down. All this was determined retrospectively by the international scientific team in 1976, which reached Yambuku after the nuns had self-imposed a quarantine on their mission and clinic.

But this time, in Kikwit, Heymann recalled, 'I said to Muyembe, "We're right in the middle of it." The women sat here, family after family, wailing, facing the mortuary. And the Red Cross truck was right here,' he continued, just days later, pointing at locals on the grounds of Kikwit General Hospital, 'taking the bodies straight to the cemetery. The volunteers were doing it with only surgical masks on.'

The stunned trio watched as Ebola-contaminated blood dripped from corpses onto the brave Red Cross volunteers. Heymann then turned to Muyembe and said, 'Our number one priority is to stop the epidemic. Number two is everything else.'

Heymann, Szczeniowski, and Muyembe sat down immediately to map out their plan. Szczeniowski's role was the most obvious, for it was one he had played brilliantly in countless previous epidemics: logistics. The athletic forty-something American moved swiftly in the sweltering, 90 per cent humidity torpidity, rarely seeming to break a sweat or smudge his spotless wire-rimmed glasses. A walking polyglot, Szczeniowski was an American-born man of Polish descent who grew up in an itinerant family and was multilingual before even setting foot in school. His facility with languages—which included Zaire-dialect French and KiCongo—was a valuable asset, especially when coupled with his easygoing manner and efficient ease with complex logistic concerns. It was Szczeniowski's job to ensure that all the material necessities were in place: satellite telephones and fax machines, four-wheel-drive vehicles, gallon upon gallon of safe drinking water, housing, local maps, translators, paper, pens, food—each and every item scarce or unavailable in Kikwit. It was a testament to Szczeniowski's past performances in epidemics all over the world that Heymann and Muyembe simply assumed the resourceful WHO point man could handle his end of things, and after Szczeniowski took charge they had no concerns about dwindling petrol supplies, choleral water, or lack of bedding for the large crew of scientists that was *en route*. If lack of sleep and the tremendous pressure ever got to Szczeniowski he never showed it.

Muyembe, the noted Zarois scientist, of course, would be the leader. He would set the priorities, deal with the Zairois government, and act as the team's general.

Heymann, who for nearly all of his adult life had worked for the CDC, had recently had a spell of bad luck. Assigned by CDC to work at WHO in Geneva, Heymann had for the last two years been ensconced in a tiny, windowless office inside the AIDS programme. There he had fallen out of favour, finding himself on the losing side of too many political arguments. So completely had his star fallen that there was talk in Atlanta of terminating Heymann's employment before he could qualify for significant government retirement funds. Just weeks before he learned of the Kikwit epidemic Heymann had felt desperate about his career future.

Yet there could be no doubt, even among his detractors in Geneva, that Heymann was the right man—the *only* man—for the Ebola problem. Though American, he spoke perfect French. The slim, boyish-looking scientist had a reputation for being cool under fire and not cracking under pressure. Heymann had faced Ebola before and spent time in Zaire, as well as other central African nations. Finally, he was trained in epidemic control and surveillance. That the forty-nine-year-old Heymann hadn't been compelled to resign his WHO post was a stroke of luck for the people of Kikwit.

Under the leadership of Director-General Hiroshi Nakajima many once-vital WHO capacities fell into ruin amid changing budget priorities, staff purges, and the generally poor morale that marked the mood in the Geneva headquarters. Heymann was hardly the only scientist whose status was precarious. By 1995 WHO had no emergency response office and only one employee—funded entirely by the CDC—who monitored typically tropical epidemics. The CDC's Dr James LeDuc held that position in 1995, primarily overseeing the laboratory capacities of WHO's far-flung string of affiliated surveillance sites. LeDuc's research career had focused on animal- and insect-carried microbes such as yellow fever and hantaviral diseases, and he had never supervised response to an emergency epidemic.

Nearly all of the disease cowboys who had tackled epidemics during the 1960s, 1970s, and early 1980s had long gone, disillusioned and dispirited by the Nakajima regime. Donors were also giving up on the World Health Organization, no longer convinced that the once-vital agency had the vision, will, or resources to fulfil its mission. Nakajima, who had recently claimed diplomatic immunity when arrested trying to smuggle religious icons out of Russia, was the object of much disdain.

So it fell to a disgruntled employee to wave the WHO flag in the crisis. Heymann's role was to function as a combination diplomat, attaché, colonel, and chief epidemiologist. Keeping all the various physicians and scientists, as well as the institutions for which they worked, functioning as a unit would be a monumental challenge. Initially limited to a handful, the team grew to more than a hundred scientists and volunteers. Egos, language differences, institutional power struggles, and legitimate cultural and scientific variations in how individuals pursued their respective jobs all had to be carefully smoothed over. Egos had to be massaged.

Heymann told Muyembe that it was preferable to have a small but well-coordinated team in place. Large numbers of loose-cannon scientists would surely spell disaster. Muyembe agreed, and the pair set about mapping the most crucial tasks ahead. Muyembe proved deft at mobilizing local volunteers and abating potential rivalries among African scientists. Together, Heymann and Muyembe formed a strong leadership team.

The fourth key player in the team's leadership arrived the following day from Amsterdam: Dr Barbara Kiersteins of Médecins Sans Frontières (MSF), or Doctors Without Borders. The humanitarian, European-based organization had offered crucial support in hundreds of crises all over the world, with a track record dating back more than twenty-five years. Formed in response to another African crisis—the famine of civil war–torn Nigeria in 1968—MSFs doctors and volunteers were deployed all over the world to health crises spawned by war, famine, tyranny, or epidemics. From its outset MSF was committed to principles atypical for international relief organizations: its staff did not seek governments' permission to assist in civilian crises; doctors were encouraged to denounce publicly political or economic conditions they felt contributed to such catastrophes; and nobody in MSF was expected to make a lifelong career of such work. The organization strongly believed that career relief workers tended to make too many compromises with corrupt governments or use local disasters as rungs on their personal ladders of prestige ascendancy.

Though only in her early thirties, Kiersteins had already seen more of humanity's horrors than most people glimpse in a lifetime. Just two weeks before arriving in Kikwit MSFs Kiersteins had wrapped up her extensive tenure battling cholera and shigella in the refugee camps of Goma. Like most educated Europeans, Kiersteins spoke several languages, including Dutch, French, and English. If she appeared humourless under pressure, she also stayed emotionally cool and focused. Kiersteins was indefatigable: even the rivers of tropical sweat that seemed perpetually dripping from her body failed to slow her down.

Kiersteins's arrival on May 11 was a welcome sight for the Heymann/Muyembe/ Szczeniowski trio. They all respected the organization she worked for and were in desperate need of the supplies, vehicles, and volunteer MSF logicians that Kiersteins brought with her on a chartered plane from Kinshasa. Wasting no time, Kiersteins drove straight to Kikwit General Hospital to assess the situation and determine how best MSF might help.

'The hospital was in a sorry state,' she said a few days later when, for the first time, she allowed herself a moment of reflective relaxation. 'The patients were in a sorrier state. The staff had no protection and they hadn't been paid for risking their lives. So we decided to focus on hospital sanitation and establishment of an isolation ward.'

The MSF crew began by trying to repair the hospital's ancient, long-unused water system but gave up after a few futile hours. The pipes were choked with weeds, eroded, rusty, and irreparable. So they switched to plan B, erecting a plastic rainwater collector attached to a filtration unit.

Across the central courtyard of Kikwit General Hospital the MSF team stretched bright yellow plastic tape, demarking a *cordon sanitaire* line that only authorized medical personnel could cross.

Muyembe ordered all non-Ebola patients sent away from Kikwit General Hospital, and he decreed that all suspected Ebola cases in any other clinic, or in people's homes, be collected by the local Red Cross and brought immediately to Pavilion No. 3, the hastily designated isolation ward.

Barely had the *cordons sanitaires* been stretched around the pillars of the hospital's arcaded central hallway than dozens of family members gathered at its edge, anxiously staring at Pavilion No. 3. To one side of the line was the mortuary, and for days to come a ghastly ritual would repeat itself: as nurses carried a deceased patient to the mortuary all of the family members would strain to see who had died, often calling out, 'Who is it?' Once the identity was known, that individual's family would commence their wailing to heaven, crying, 'Someone has died! Someone has died,' often in a loud huddle beside another family still mourning their own recently deceased kin. This wailing would persist for hours. And it could be heard by the staff and ailing Ebola victims in Pavilion No. 3. Kiersteins realized immediately that the deaths, wailing, and stress had taken a terrible toll on the medical staff, most of whom continued to toil away in the hospital despite their lack of pay and tremendous dismay over the demise of their colleagues. The staff was scared, sleep deprived, and grieving. A steady stream of local Red Cross volunteers carried in ailing patients and hauled away the dead for burial. None of these brave Kikwitians possessed protective gear, and all were terrified and exhausted. At least three had become infected performing their heroic deeds. Remarkably, as volunteers died others eagerly took their places, displaying levels of courage that Kiersteins and Heymann found truly awe-inspiring.

But none of them need have died. Muyembe ordered that all of the staff and volunteers brought under MSF's wings receive immediate training in infection control, and Kiersteins ensured that every one of them was fitted out with scrub gowns, rubber galoshes, long rubber aprons, latex gloves, goggles, masks, and hair coverings. Though the team didn't know whether or not Ebola could be transmitted through the air, it was obvious to them that contact with the blood or bodily fluids of the sick or dead was extremely dangerous. Heymann and Muyembe reasoned that any measures that placed barriers—such as latex gloves—between infected patients and health providers would block transmission.

Kiersteins also knew from experience that exhausted, frightened health-care workers make mistakes: needles slip, bottles break, hands tremble, all creating opportunities for spread of the virus. When she spoke to the Kikwit crew she could see that they had all long since exceeded reasonable levels of sleep deprivation and exhaustion. A first priority had to be the professionalization of the volunteers' work routines.

Making matters worse, the physicians and nurses had to pass a small cemetery every day on their way to the hospital, which by now was full of their colleagues' bodies. Nestled among weeds and monkeypod trees were rows of wooden crosses, marked with the names of Kikwit's Ebola victims.

'I have seen many African countries, and this is, by comparison, shocking,' Kiersteins told Heymann. Strong words from a woman who had just been in the deadly Rwandan refugee camps. But Kiersteins could plainly see that infection control practices in Kikwit were even worse than those executed in emergency medical tents in Goma. Supplies were non-existent, and the medical facilities of Kikwit were in states of fatigued chaos.

Kipassa chastised Kiersteins, urging her to look at the poverty of the hospital, the lack of resources: 'The only thing we have to work with is our brains,' he complained.

'And your brains,' Kiersteins responded, 'can't think properly. You all need a rest.'

MSF erected a series of tents on a small lawn space in the interior of the *cordons sanitaires*, positioning beds and chairs for the staff inside. She set up work schedules, making sure that all hospital personnel had breaks, naps, and far shorter shifts. No more all-nighters were allowed. Meals and safe water were provided to the staff for the first time. And, perhaps oddly crucial, paychecks. In order to improve the situation Kiersteins used MSF resources and made every person on the Pavilion No. 3 and mortuary staff employees of her organization, clocking hours for which they were paid. With the imposition of a routine came a sense of calm. As a result the hospital spread of Ebola came to an immediate and grinding halt.

Similarly, MSF put the Red Cross burial crews on modest salaries and helped their leaders create manageable schedules for their grim tasks. Trucks and a bulldozer were found, applied to the horrible job of creating enormous mass graves on the edge of town, in which the plastic-wrapped bodies of the dead were stacked.

But MSF's supplies were limited: enough protective gear and sterile equipment to match Kikwit's needs did not arrive until May 27. In the meantime, everyone simply made do. On Friday, May 12, Kiersteins spent the morning on her satellite telephone talking to MSF headquarters in Brussels: 'Send respirator masks, latex gloves, protective gowns, disinfectant, hospital linens and plastic mattress covers, plastic aprons, basic cleaning supplies and cleansers, water pumps and filtres, galoshes, tents . . .'

It was not the high-tech equipment popularized in science fiction movies that would halt Ebola's spread, Kiersteins knew. What Kikwit needed were the basics: soap, gear, and safe water.

Between Friday afternoon and Monday, May 15, the vital members of Heymann's crew arrived. Dr Philipe Calain, a Swiss physician attached to the US CDC, was given command of Pavilion No. 3 and put in charge of the Ebola isolation ward. Belgian Dr Bob Colebunders took over the hospital's emergency room and screened incoming patients, sending all new Ebola cases to Calain and the rest to alternative hospitals. The CDC's Drs Pierre Rollin and Ali Khan worked with WHO's Dr Güenal Rodier to track down all of the region's Ebola cases and figure out how the virus was spreading. South Africa's Robert Swanepoel of the National Virology Institute, located outside Johannesburg, set up an on-site Ebola laboratory, carved out of the hospital's tuberculosis centre. From WHO's Zimbabwe office came veterinarian Oyewale Tomori, whose task was to investigate whether any animals within Kikwit were carrying—and possibly spreading—the virus. His samples were hastily analysed by Swanepoel. Their efforts were supplemented by dozens of volunteers drafted from a local medical school, as well as a host of research institutes in the United States, Europe, and Africa.

Heymann and Muyembe had made rough counts of the Ebola toll, and realized that the numbers of dead were quadrupling daily. In his conversations with Kipassa, Muyembe learned of the Ebola-spreading operations performed on Kimfumu and Katadi, and subsequent illnesses in the medical staff. When he tallied it all up on Friday Muyembe estimated that 73 per cent of the dead were health-care workers.

More alarming, Muyembe told Heymann, 'This epidemic has been going on since March,'—for three full months—and clearly had spread well beyond Kikwit General Hospital. He didn't yet know about Mosango and all of the nearby villages—that would be learned over the next week—but Muyembe already realized that Kikwit's epidemic was more explosive than what he had seen nineteen years earlier in Yambuku. Though many pieces of the Kikwit puzzle were yet to fall in to place, Muyembe could see that unlike in Yambuku (where most cases traced back to those reused missionary syringes) this epidemic was spreading out from many different sources. In Yambuku the epidemic chain of transmission from one person to another had flowed from a single stem, with only tiny branches extending along the way. But in Kikwit in May there seemed to be several apparently unrelated sprouting outbreaks.

The links among them—and the Menga family roots of the epidemic—had yet to be unearthed.

Heymann immediately set to work with Rollin and Khan, training a group of medical students in basic epidemiology and planning a schedule of surveillance. Teams were dispatched on Sunday and Monday to every neighbourhood in Kikwit, where they went door to door in search of Ebola cases. As they returned to headquarters the team members brought news of active cases, sending the Red Cross to pick up the ailing. The mounting data they amassed helped to fill in a rapidly expanding tree of infections Muyembe was sketching out, depicting who transmitted Ebola to whom. It all seemed to trace back to those March operating procedures in Kikwit General and the maternity hospital, particularly the operations performed on laboratory technician Kimfumu. At Heymann's request the sketch was faxed to WHO and the Ministry of Health offices in Kinshasa.

Trusting to Kinshasa's discretion would later prove to have been a mistake.

As the team interacted they were careful not to embrace, shake hands, share food or water. A novel form of greeting was invented to prevent passage of Ebola: in salutation friends tapped the backs of their forearms against one another, carefully keeping their hands pointed toward their own chests, palms away from the friend. Team members worked closely without wearing masks or protective gear, but avoided touching one another. Blood and tissue samples were drawn and handled with well-gloved hands. And all of the team members exclusively imbibed bottled water that Szczeniowski had flown into the city from Kinshasa.

Based on their first, cursory examination of the city the team relayed their primary field report via satellite telephone to Geneva on May 11, and daily thereafter. The Zairois government placed Kikwit under quarantine, halting all trade and transport to and from the city, except for airlifts of medical supplies and personnel. Almost immediately the canned foods, sacks of rice, batteries, tools, and other goods usually sold in Kikwit markets disappeared and store shelves became barren.

By that time Kikwit authorities had identified twenty laboratory-confirmed Ebola deaths and sixty-one haemorrhagic cases assumed to be caused by the virus. Many more suspected cases awaited laboratory confirmation.

On May 13, team members returned from Mosango and a sweep of the villages, unfortunately confirming that Muyembe's fears were well founded: the virus had spread well beyond the confines of Kikwit. Heymann decided that the surveillance net needed to be widened, and team members embarked on long journeys over bumpy dirt roads in search of Ebola cases.

Meanwhile, cases continued to pour into Kikwit General Hospital's emergency room, usually carried in by Red Cross volunteers, wailing relatives in tow. Belgian physician Colebunders saw immediately that conditions in the chaotic emergency room were outrageous.

'People were moving in and out, Ebola cases and other emergencies were all mixed together and six ER nurses had died of Ebola,' Colebunders explained a few days later. 'I said, "I can't keep aseptic conditions here if people are just wandering about," and the Red Cross had walked off with all the protective gear. So we went around with the protection leftovers. All of the best equipment went to Pavilion No. 3.'

Colebunders, who wasn't able to reach Kikwit until Tuesday, May 16, discovered that all of the supplies had already been claimed by Calain for Pavilion No. 3 or by MSF. And the emergency room staff were examining bleeding, delirious patients without even the basics—masks and gloves—to protect themselves. The tall, nervous Belgian pleaded for supplies, but it was ten days before more protective equipment would arrive.

Nevertheless, the emergency room served as the screening and triage site for every case of diarrhoea and fever found in Kikwit. Colebunders tried to minimize the risks for himself and the hospital staff, but he knew that they were all in considerable danger. And he struggled to hide a terror that continued to build within him over subsequent days.

Colebunders was perhaps ill-suited to the task. The very day that the CDC laboratory confirmed that Ebola was the cause of Kikwit's crisis Colebunders had attended the funeral in Antwerp of a longtime friend and colleague. This death had come close on the heels of his father-in-law's demise. Despite his grief, when Colebunders learned of the CDC's laboratory results he rushed to volunteer. He had never before worked under such desperate third world conditions. But having devoted his career to AIDS research at Antwerp's Institute of Tropical Medicine, Colebunders seized upon the opportunity to participate in a great adventure, and, in the process, advance his status within the claustrophobic Belgian scientific community.

Now he was doing his best to hold down a fear that was welling up from his insides, threatening to push him over the brink into hysteria. As patients arrived in the emergency room Colebunders anxiously examined their bleeding noses, bloody diarrhoea, fever-ridden faces—always careful to minimize how much he actually touched them. He developed a case definition of Ebola—a way to diagnose patients in the absence of confirmatory laboratory findings. He tried desperately to stay focused on his tasks, to not let the horror of the situation overcome him.

Nevertheless, after six nearly sleepless days of the greatest stress he had ever experienced the forty-seven-year-old doctor suddenly collapsed on a trolley. His body felt leaden. His mind was spinning. He struggled to gather his thoughts, reaching the diagnosis that he was having a nervous breakdown.

Each of the team members had come to do battle with the notorious virus for their own reasons and fought internal battles with competing emotions of duty, fear, compassion, ambition, and scientific curiosity. Though Colebunders was the only team member who completely broke down under the pressure, each of the scientists had moments of high temper, sharp words, exhausted malaise, or self-doubt.

On Sunday, May 14, a group of twenty-three reporters pooled their resources, chartering a hulking old airplane for a flight from Kinshasa to Kikwit. Upon landing on the cracked tarmac at the tiny Kikwit airport the reporters immediately fanned out across the city in search of Ebola cases and scientists. With the skilled guile and instincts of seasoned Africa-based journalists the horde, though unfamiliar with Kikwit, soon found Heymann's team and the hospital's Pavilion No. 3.

The scientific team was caught completely off guard. No one among them had given a thought to the media, largely because Africa's many epidemics and health crises rarely rated more than a few minutes per year of broadcast news time in North America, Western Europe, or any of the non-African world. Only a handful of foreign reporters had travelled to Surat during India's plague epidemic: media coverage had largely come from government sources in far-off Delhi. And Ebola was certainly more dangerous than plague, the scientists reasoned. Therefore, it seemed unlikely that more than an easily ignored number of reporters would turn up in Kikwit, or so they had reasoned.

They were, of course, forgetting that since *The Hot Zone, Outbreak*, and other TV films and documentaries Ebola now carried a certain cachet among diseases. The public had become fascinated by the haemorrhagic fever virus and the special fearsome status Ebola had among microbe fighters. Every large news organization in the world either dispatched a reporter to the site or bought stories and film from freelancers who had made their way to Kinshasa. The Italian media, in particular, were well represented because of the deaths of their countrywomen, the Sisters.

On May 14 the scientists, physicians, and people of Kikwit got a small taste of what important political candidates and celebrities went through in the West at that time, when confronted by camera crews, photographers, and reporters.

Three other reporters had already been in Kikwit for two days, filing their stories overseas and causing little consternation within the Ebola control team. Heymann had added the role of press secretary onto his long list of tasks, showing the three the lay of the land and ensuring that they got the tape, stories, and photos that were needed to document the unfolding epidemic.

But even Heymann was taken aback by the additional twenty-three reporters and photographers who arrived on May 14. His agitation grew as cameras shot the new cemetery plots, Red Cross teams gathering bodies, the hospital, and the epidemic command post.

Brooklyn-born Ali Khan stood to the side and watched, aghast, as camera crews filmed a chart he had made, listing the names of the dead and dying.

'Outrageous!' Khan cried. 'We posted those lists for the team so we could keep track. They're never supposed to be public. What about patient confidentiality? These people have the same rights to privacy as Americans.'

Khan, the son of Pakistani immigrants, took propriety so seriously that despite the stifling Kikwit heat he always wore a smart shirt and tie: 'a sign of respect,' Khan said, for the people of Kikwit. If such attire had been appropriate in New Mexico in 1993 when he investigated the hantavirus epidemic, Khan reasoned, then it should also be correct in Kikwit. He expected similar ethics and propriety from everyone else, including journalists.

So it was with outrage that he helplessly stood by watching the photographers and TV camera people shoot his precious chart of death, and hours later saw patients and weeping funeral participants filmed without their consent. These things, he shouted, were not right.

And then and there Khan started to hate the media. As did Pierre Rollin, a French scientist on loan from the Pasteur Institute to the CDC.

'I detest reporters!' Rollin hissed. 'I will never again give another interview. You are a member of the lowest, most vile profession on earth.'

The most demonstrative expression of antipathy toward the pack of reporters came from Switzerland's Calain. The photographers, not surprisingly, wanted to take pictures of the patients inside Pavilion No. 3. Given that the ward was intended as an isolation area and most of the patients were too ill to grant consent, Calain objected. Tempers rose, shouts were heard, and Calain threw a punch at a female photographer on assignment for Reuters. Witnesses later insisted that both parties were out of line. Regardless, the photographer apparently scraped her knee on the possibly contaminated floor during the fracas. At the very least this constituted a break in infection protocols, and the photographer, who would soon return to Kinshasa, could have been an unwitting vehicle for spread of the virus. (Fortunately, the photographer was not infected, though nobody knew that when she departed Kikwit.)

Some member of the enraged medical team radioed word of the reporters to Kinshasa, and when the group of twenty-three landed at dusk back in the capital later that day Zairois soldiers surrounded the plane. Held inside the aircraft in the blistering equatorial heat, the reporters were first informed that they would be confined indefinitely under quarantine. After an hour's standoff diplomats from several embassies intervened, convincing Zairois officials that the reporters could safely be released.[19]

The incident prompted greater attention to accreditation details on the part of Zaire's Ministry of Information. The agency, which might better have been termed the Ministry of Bribery and Disinformation, welcomed money in exchange for accreditations for foreigners and rarely provided anyone—foreigner or citizen—with accurate news about anything, especially public health. Located in one of several decrepit, thirty-year-old government buildings at considerable distance from Kinshasa's hub, the Ministry was on the nineteenth floor of a decaying structure with only one remaining, marginally functional lift.

Though the Ministry officials emphasized the grand panoramas afforded from their windows of Kinshasa and the Congo River, it was the offices, themselves, that offered the clearest views of the Mobutu regime. Water stains and creeping fungi on the walls and ceilings betrayed the building's inability to withstand Zaire's equatorial downpours. Exposed, rusted pipes explained why no water ran from the nineteenth-floor taps. A collapsed ceiling spoke to the generally shoddy workmanship and poor maintenance of the building. And looking down from every wall was the dictator, scowling from photographs shot during his youth, postured arrogantly, attired in his trademark mix of Pierre Cardin glasses, Rolex watch, leopard skin hat, and Western-style jacket. Without meaning to the Ministry of Information staff thus presented a perfectly realistic image of modern Zaire.

The information officers were at a loss when it came to providing an accounting of Zaire's epidemic. Genuine information was not their forte; concealment was. But while hiding the truth might ward off the dictator's domestic critics, such action only further provoked foreign journalists.

So epidemic information control fell to the Ministry of Health. On May 15, with Minister of Health Mbumb Musong oddly out of the country during his nation's most significant international medical fiasco, the Ministry staff muddled through. Secretary-General Lonyangela Bompenda derided the large foreign press corps in a briefing in Kinshasa, saying that they 'are putting people in danger' by their movements.

'If the quarantine cannot be held the country will be closed. *Voici la verité!* You—if you go to Kikwit, you break the quarantine,' Bompenda said, adding ominously, 'so I will repeat: if we have to detain some people it will be the police that will detain them.'

Meanwhile, a virtual industry sprang up in Kinshasa, focused on obtaining as much of the foreign journalists' currency as possible. Taxis raised their rates, phone calls out of local hotels suddenly required $20 and even $50 bribes to switchboard operators, room rates skyrocketed, and the price of meals at the local cafés soared. As competition among the journalists escalated—particularly among rival television networks—basic bribery rates jumped to astonishing levels. Airport officials and local charter companies were negotiating prices in excess of $25 000 to cover transport and bribery fees for flights to Kikwit in violation of the quarantine. With the government obfuscating, even threatening, and rumours of deaths and disease rife in the capital both the international media and local Zarois were at pains to separate fact from fiction.

Mobutu, who flew into Kinshasa to meet visiting American televangelist Pat Robertson and later returned to his distant retreat in northern Zaire, far from the Kikwit crisis, thanked Robertson 'from the bottom of my heart.'

Addressing his country's Ebola epidemic, Mobutu said, 'I would have liked to go [to Kikwit] but my doctors have forbidden me to go to this area. The first responsibility of a chief is to show solidarity with his people and be strong for his people. My purpose is to help the people and cooperate with all international groups.'

With that the dictator thanked the international team then working in Kikwit, expressed gushing gratitude to his political supporter Robertson, and disappeared. For the remainder of the epidemic the Zarois leader would stay secluded, never issuing another word of concern or condolence for his people.

In Kinshasa's enormous slum La Cité the dictator's brief appearance was greeted with open derision. One of the popular local newspapers, *Salongo*, brazenly asked in a bold headline, 'EBOLA VIRUS. BLOODY DIARRHOEA. WHO IS AT FAULT?' The rhetorical headline's answer: MOBUTU. The paper noted that the epidemic 'is without a doubt' the result of widespread social and environmental 'degradation' brought about by 'demagogues' in the government who were clinging 'to the old order' and blocking democracy. As the epidemic unfolded even the scientists toiling in Kikwit would be compelled to conclude that the aetiology of Zaire's epidemic was at least as much political and economic as it was biological. Authoritarianism and corruption may not have spawned the Ebola virus, but they certainly created formidably fertile ground for its spread.

One week after the CDC had confirmed that Ebola had returned to Zaire, unfounded rumours of cases loose in Kinshasa had finally been quashed with the apprehension of two suspected patients, both of whom proved to be well, and tested negative for the virus. On the streets of the capital vendors complained that they could not obtain fruits and vegetables from Bandundu Province, thanks to the quarantine. People along the boulevards and alleyways stopped white-skinned journalists, begging for news of the epidemic and asking their assessments of the regime's efforts to control Ebola.

'Are there enough scientists in Kikwit?' they asked.

'Is the government telling the truth—are there really no cases in Kinshasa?'

'Don't believe the government—it only lies!'

'Will the world save us?'

It was clear that the government hadn't a shred of credibility in La Cité, or perhaps anywhere else in the troubled nation. The populace was counting upon WHO and the foreigners, whose presence offered them the only consolation they could see in the unfolding crisis.

By then eighty-six people had died of laboratory-confirmed Ebola—numerous other suspected cases had surfaced or died. And in Kikwit a new wave of cases, results of spread not in the hospitals but within households, was sweeping through the community. The growing international team was watching what had begun primarily as a health-care worker epidemic turn into a more generalized phenomenon.

Heymann's teams of local medical students and foreign scientists were finding what he dubbed 'hot houses' in which whole families had contracted Ebola and most died.

For example, in one of Kikwit's barely accessible neighbourhoods where no vehicles could manage the muddy, rutted roads, a young woman slowly rocked back and forth on her tiny porch, her baby nursing at her breast. She stared straight ahead, shell-shocked. She suddenly had found herself the sole support and caretaker of her baby, her teenage sister, and sixteen other children.

The horror started, she said, when in April her niece had a caesarean-section at Kikwit General Hospital. Nine days later the new mother died of Ebola. Her newborn followed suit two days later. Then their mother, who had cared for the dying mother and child, suddenly developed a piercing headache at her daughter's funeral. The family rushed her to a local dispensary where a nurse diagnosed the problem as a tipped uterus and reached in, barehanded, to adjust the bereaved woman's womb.

A week later both she and the nurse were dead, victims of Ebola. And soon thereafter relatives at that funeral died: the shell-shocked woman's father and two more sisters.

'They hiccuped,' the survivor said, seemingly stunned by the curiosity of it. As they neared death, the Ebola victims each had fallen into fits of uncontrollable hiccuping.

An international team member asked if he could take blood samples from the surviving woman and the pack of orphans that she now had in her charge. She leapt to her feet in horror, crying, 'My sisters got needles in their arms! *Afwaka*—they died. My mother got needles. *Afwaka!* My father—*Afwaka!* No! I will not!'

The fear of Kikwit's hospitals, particularly their needles and surgical equipment, was, of course, quite rational, even wise. It was obvious to the international team that several of the Bandundu Provinces medical facilities had served as Ebola amplifiers: turning isolated cases that entered the facility into outbreaks, multiplied several times over as a result of poor hospital hygiene. Thus, the local health establishments performed roles in precise opposition to their mission: rather than preventing an epidemic, they had created one out of what previously had been a problem isolated within the Menga family.

But, thanks largely to the efforts of MSF, by mid-May hospital transmission had stopped and the team knew that Ebola was primarily continuing to spread within so-called hot houses. Though everyone agreed that Ebola was exploiting human altruism, spreading via acts of compassion among Kikwitians, the precise biology of that transmission wasn't clear.

In the evenings, exhausted and emotionally drained from their day's work, members of the international team gathered in one of Kikwit's few restaurants, located inside her only hotel, Kwilu—named after the river that bisected the city and until less than a decade earlier was the rain forest's border. Like soldiers at war the scientists tended to be boisterous and drink plenty of Primus beer on such occasions. And often they would speculate about what they had seen during their investigations that day. Inevitably they were drawn to one key question: are we sure that we are taking correct preventive precautions in this epidemic?

Over several meals of local fish, bananas, rice, and tough goat meat spiced with hot peppers, the men—and nearly all were men—ruminated over the vagaries of the deadly, haemorrhagic fever virus. The Mosango case, in particular, troubled them because it indicated that the virus could survive on open-air surfaces in the tropical climate for days on end. But was Dr Bonnet's observation correct? Was it the hospital room itself that was the source of that ill-fated patient's infection, or might there have been other possibilities? Perhaps, they agreed, the virus was on the hands of a health-care worker who tended to the woman. Or on her dishes. Or in the drinking water.

WHOs Rodier voiced a shared concern: if the virus is in a well or on a glass of water is it safe to use that water? He reflected on lessons from Yambuku. Recalling the original laboratory work done in 1976 Rodier felt that there were grounds for such a suspicion because the original Yambuku samples were improperly packaged and arrived at the Institut Pasteur in Paris in a condition that, with most organisms, proved useless for analysis. The liquid nitrogen that was supposed to keep test tubes full of virally contaminated blood cold had long since melted and the viruses had been at room temperature for days. Nevertheless, Dr Pierre Sureau had had no trouble isolating living Ebola viruses from those containers.

That, Rodier concluded, dictated that scientists take a conservative course in Kikwit, assuming that the virus thrived in tropical heat and could live in food and water. Muyembe didn't like that idea one bit: it might be all right for the foreigners to take such precautions as drinking and washing in bottled water hauled at considerable expense from Kinshasa, but such measures were impossible for Kikwitians. Any talk of virally contaminated food or water would only exacerbate the already near-hysterical public panic.[20]

Back in America Fort Detrick researchers at the US Army Medical Research Institute for Infectious Diseases, or USAMRID, and at the CDC were studying the Ebola transmission question closely. Perhaps fortunately, for the sake of limiting panic, their findings would not be known until the Kikwit epidemic was over. Dr Nancy Jaax of USAMRID, for example, would demonstrate using monkeys that inhalation of aerosolized Ebola viruses could cause infection and death.[21] And the BL-4 group at the CDC would discover evidence of secreted Ebola viruses in cells of human skin, indicating that mere touch might lead to infection.[22] Taken together, these two discoveries might have raised fears in the international team about casual inhalation or skin contact and transmission of the terrifying virus.

Based on what they did know at the time, however, the team felt American provisions for universal precautions, modified to include goggles and rubber boots, were probably adequate for the Red Cross and health-care workers. For Swanepoel and his tiny group of on-site laboratory workers full-body space suits were, despite the stifling heat and humidity, deemed wise.

And for the people of Kikwit door-to-door education efforts advised two modes of protection: do not care for people suffering from high fevers or diarrhoea, and do not perform mortuary procedures, washing down the dead and having open-casket funeral rites. Rather, they advised, send a runner to the Red Cross as soon as a family member falls ill. In a city bereft of mortuaries and funeral parlours this meant that the families should abandon ailing loved ones and allow their bodies to be buried unclean and without Catholic ritual. Though such measures were emotionally wrenching for family members, they were, Muyembe insisted, the precautions most likely to stop the epidemic successfully.

'Someone has died! He was my papa!' screamed a teenage girl. Surrounded by her six younger, grieving siblings the girl's face and blouse were drenched in tears. 'He was my papa,' she cried again, pushing a photograph of the deceased into the hands of a passing stranger. While her brothers and sisters wailed, sometimes jerking in spasmodic death dances, the distraught girl told a foreigner what tragedy had befallen her family.

'Mama got the Ebola,' she explained, foisting a photo of a plump woman in her thirties at the visitor. 'They took her from us. They took her to the hospital. Then Papa took ill, and they took him away. And today he died there! He died in the hospital. *Afwaka!*'

On hearing the fatal *Afwaka* the other children escalated their wailing, one boy, appearing to be about five years old, collapsed facedown on their small earth garden, lost in his screams.

'Mama had a headache. And she had a high fever,' the eldest child continued. 'She is still at the hospital. Oh, Mama! Oh, Papa! Who will care for us?'

For days the children had fended for themselves and watched the steady flow of Red Cross trucks that lumbered past their tidy home, *en route* to the mass graves at the top of the hill. With each passing truck they had worried: is this one carrying Mama? Papa? And just now the eerie caravan had, indeed, passed by, its cargo including the white plastic wrapped body of their father, they were told.

The children's tragic cries faded and were eventually drowned out by the grinding noise of a large Red Cross truck stuck in a muddy rut on the hilltop. A cluster of men and women, dressed in their colourful protective attire, held a row of body bags laid out on the truck bed, lest the lurches of the vehicle send one shooting out onto the roadside. Such a thing would be ghastly and undignified—certain to provoke anxiety among the crowds of people who stared from a safe distance at the sorry sight. At last freed from the rut, the truck manoeuvred to the edge of a deep trench some thirty feet wide, and already layered with dirt-covered bodies. Two Red Cross volunteers adjusted their big, knee-high, European rubber boots and jumped off the truck bed, into the pit. The others handed down the heavy, ominous white body bags: one tall one here, a baby-size one there, a medium-size adult shape . . . the corpse of the father of the wailing children down the road.

Carefully, the two volunteers in the pit received the bodies, some of which still bled Ebola-rich fluids, and placed them side by side along the pit floor. Then a third man, wearing a large metal backpack tank, leaped into the pit, pointed a nozzle at the bodies, and doused them with a veneer of DDT. Their job nearly complete, the DDT was sprayed on all of the volunteers, a second layer of dirt was added to the pit, and the crew headed back to the hospital in search of another grim cargo.

Each team included seven volunteers and there were fourteen teams toiling around the clock in Kikwit, finding the ill and taking them to the hospital and hauling the dead in trucks for burial. Three of the volunteers had died of Ebola before Kiersteins doled out protective gear, and two were fighting for their lives in Pavilion No. 3.

'They are volunteers who are doing this of their own free will,' Red Cross Secretary-General Kadiata Vunga said. 'No one from government has told them to. They are willing to die for others. They will do what God says to relieve suffering.'

Neither the International Committees of Red Cross and Red Crescent, nor any wealthy nation's sister organizations (such as the American Red Cross) offered assistance to the heroic Kikwit group. Indeed, volunteers canvassed local businesses for stacks of nearly worthless Zaires currency with which to buy petrol and spare tyres for their trucks and bulldozers. When donations ran out, the volunteers reached into their own near-empty pockets.

'There is no help from anyone,' Vunga said, barely hiding his anger. 'We do it all ourselves. . . . If the American Red Cross can see our situation here—we are suffering a lot! We need money and resources. They should see the conditions we are working under here in Zaire.'

Perhaps equally vital to their grim task of shuttling bodies was mass education, as it was the Red Cross volunteers who canvassed the community, warning of the deadly disease. Their protective gear, Vunga said, frightened people. So volunteers also travelled about in their normal clothing, telling Kikwitians, 'See? We are just like you! Don't be afraid.'

But suspicions, superstitions, and fears persisted. The crowds that witnessed the by now regular burials spread word of the DDT sprayings, suggesting that the Red Cross was keeping a magic potion from them. Ten days after Heymann, Muyembe, and their team arrived a runner came to the hospital, announcing that his neighbour had just died of Ebola. Because the name was not on any surveillance list Khan and Heymann followed the Red Cross to the site.

A funeral was in progress. An older, thin man stared, bewildered, beside the open casket of his deceased wife. He had, unfortunately, cared for her himself, never sending her to the hospital for treatment. Like most Kikwitians the widower feared the hospitals. He had also prepared his wife's body for burial. She was the second family member to die of Ebola, the first having been their adult son.

The old man appeared dazed, uncomprehending when Red Cross volunteers, dressed in protective gear, asked if they could remove the body. He silently nodded, and the horde of wailers screeched and cried when the casket was covered and Red Cross volunteers carried it to their truck. As the truck slowly departed the old man beseeched Heymann for an explanation. Dutifully, in perfect French, the angular American explained how the virus spread from one person to another, in the loving ministrations the well gave to the sick. He then asked the old man if he would provide a sample of his blood. As medical student Norbert Lafulu inserted a needle in the old man's arm he did not wince nor take his eyes off Heymann's deliberately emotionless, calm face.

'Can you give me a drug now?' the old man asked as the realization that he might be infected dawned. Heymann shook his head sadly. The man—who though only fifty looked quite old—turned plaintively to the more than one hundred mourners gathered around him, and one shouted, 'Look at the Red Cross—Le Croix Rouge! Regardez!'

Those volunteers who hadn't followed the truck were busily scrubbing the site in the house where the coffin had lain, and spraying the area with DDT pesticides.

'Why did you spray the house?' the old man asked. And then, raising his arms and preparing for a mist he pleaded, 'Spray me, too! Spray me! Why not me, too?'

Heymann patiently explained that the DDT was a precaution, in case insects could carry the virus. Nobody knew, Heymann added, whether or not insects played a role in the spread of Ebola. But such sprays could not protect him if the virus was already in the old man's body.

An American photographer, without asking his permission, shot the old man's stunned face. Ali Khan quietly cursed the photographer. Heymann thanked the old man for his blood. And the outsiders departed, leaving the widower agape, amid a throng of tear-soaked friends and family.

In another misunderstanding between the populace and epidemic control efforts an entire neighbourhood rose up in a near riot. It began when a man and woman drove up to a house located on a street near the University of Bandundu. The exhausted, frail woman waited in the car while the man called out for her brother. No one responded, so the man returned to the vehicle and ordered the woman out. She stood silently, clutching her cloth-tied parcels, as the man sped off. With great difficulty she hobbled toward the house, collapsing on the road. Neighbours ran to her aid, finding her to be feverish, weak, and semilucid. She explained that her husband had died of the new disease at their home in Mosango village, and now she was searching for help from her brother.

But no one in the swelling neighbourhood crowd had ever heard of her brother. She was delirious. She had come to the wrong address. Hearing the word *Ebola* a local teenager took off on a full sprint for the Red Cross. And when the Red Cross volunteers loaded the woman onto a stretcher shouts and fights broke out.

'Why are you taking her away,' cried a woman, demanding that, instead, the Red Cross bring the ailing stranger into her home. 'I must take care of her! They will kill her because of this disease! Everybody who suffers from this Ebola, they [the Red Cross] destroy him forever!'

A robust, authoritative man—the neighbourhood political chief—went up to his neighbour, shouting at the top of his lungs, 'If someone wants to debate this thing I will accuse him!'

'You are crying with your politics here in order to destroy people,' countered another large woman of the neighbourhood. 'You know this town is dangerous! You are the chief of the area, it's your duty to protect people. Why don't you?'

'I'm not sure she will ever come back alive,' screamed the first woman, brandishing her fist at the chief. 'Most of the time when someone is taken from here, he dies! Maybe he gets the disease at the hospital.'

The chief waved at the Red Cross to depart swiftly, and turned on his accuser, asking the woman, 'Are you afraid to go to the hospital?'

'Everybody is running away,' she retorted. 'How can you ask me such a question?'

As dusk darkened the neighbours shouted and threatened one another, each convinced of one of two positions: either the sick and dead were the sources of contamination and therefore had to be removed for the sake of the community, or malevolent doctors were gathering up sick people and murdering them—intentionally or accidentally—with the virus.

The first woman continued: 'As I'm not a doctor, I haven't heard anything about this virus. But I have heard that it is a virus that kills. And so I am afraid to go to the hospital because we have seen the source is there.'

While the shouting escalated and fists flew in that neighbourhood Heymann and Muyembe burned the midnight oil at their impromptu offices, discussing what to do about other communities that were overreaching, going too far, putting virtually every ailing person out on the road for Red Cross pickup, regardless of the nature or cause of their illnesses. And Vunga was outraged because some Kikwitians were using the Red Cross as a way to get free burials for relatives they knew had died of AIDS, malaria, or other non-Ebola causes.

Outside of Kikwit even greater difficulties were arising. In the village of Kimbinga, for example, Chief Justin Muntunu ruled with an iron fist and was determined to use his own brand of public health to stop Ebola. There had been cases in Kimbinga, the lanky chief told a visitor, 'of the disease which in Kikwit is called Ebola.'

In Kimbinga it seemed to have begun when a village woman went to Kikwit to care for her ailing brother. After he died of Ebola, Muntunu said, this woman returned to her home in Kimbinga. Muntunu visited the woman in her thatched hut and, upon discovering that she was ailing, commanded her to depart immediately to her family's nearby village of Insomi, which she did. Under local tradition women can always be ordered to return to the village of their birth if they in any way displease their chiefs, husbands, mothers-in-law, or eldest sons. Two days later she died in Insomi.

And for the last four days, by order of Chief Muntunu, the two young men who had carried the ailing woman to her parents' village had been incarcerated in a sort of makeshift village quarantine.

'I have heard that the virus can take twenty-one days to cause disease,' said the chief accurately, 'so they will remain there for seventeen more days.'

Pointing to a thatched building some hundred yards away, Muntunu gestured with authority. A young girl busy pounding manioc near the quarantine site started to giggle, as did other children near the building. Angrily Muntunu strode to the building, finding it empty.

'They went into the forest,' a village woman defiantly told the chief.

'You should not have let them go,' Muntunu cried. 'If they die it's your problem, not mine!'

A fight ensued among the villagers, fists flew, and in the scuffle a huge cloud of dust arose, enveloping the participants. The chief's son, a tall, strapping young man, raced into the dust storm shouting, 'My father is the chief of the village! When he tells you to take care of these boys you must do it! People are dying in Kikwit. You have to respect the chief and pay attention to the lives of all of the people!'

Back in Kikwit the international team doggedly pursued information about Ebola cases, their surveillance net now firmly in place. By May 19—ten days after the first members of the team had arrived—Heymann had begun to feel confident that the epidemic control effort was working well. His troops were deployed, all known Ebola cases were in Pavilion No. 3, and investigators were scouring nearby villages. So, he said, the epidemiologists could return to 'hot houses', gather blood samples from survivors, and pursue larger scientific issues. For example, he pointed out, nothing was really known about healthy Ebola carriers: did such people exist? Could they spread the virus to others? And it was clear some people survived Ebola—why? How had they outwitted the virus, given there was no treatment for the disease?

Heymann and Khan decided to go back to what appeared to be the epidemic's origin in the hospitals: the case of technician Kimfumu. Walking through hills not accessible by vehicles or bicycles, the duo reached Kimfumu's pretty, young widow. Seated outside a wattle house next to her sister the widow calmly answered the scientists' questions. No one in her family had acquired the disease, even though they'd attended to Kimfumu during the first days of his illness.

Suddenly the widow's brother-in-law stormed in, angrily demanding to know what Khan and Heymann were up to.

'We are all well,' he insisted, 'why are you here?'

Heymann calmly began to respond, but the brother-in-law interrupted, shouting, 'Why is all of the world saying Kimfumu started this epidemic? I heard it on the radio—on Radio France and VOA!'

Heymann knew that it was true—that poor Kimfumu's name was broadcast world-wide. And Heymann knew he was helpless to stop it. He shook his head sadly, trying to gain the brother-in-law's confidence. But it was useless. Heymann and Khan learned nothing from the visit except that their patient's confidentiality had been betrayed.

The betrayal originated in Kinshasa, where government officials were still trying to fight off panic.

The capital city, with its run-down, tawdry buildings and pot-holed roads, was abuzz with rumours. District Governor Bernadin Mungul Diaka declared that what-ever was necessary should be done to protect the population, estimated at six million: 'If the disease penetrates to Kinshasa, that will be a catastrophe,' he cried, noting grimly that the city's mortuary only had room for 150 corpses.

Secretary-general of the Ministry of Health Loyangela Bonkuma Bompenda, acknowledging rumours on Tuesday, May 16, that at least two Ebola-infected individ-uals were 'on the loose in Kinshasa,' decreed that the army would protect the city—at all costs.

Muyembe's hastily drafted chart, depicting Kimfumu at the centre of Kikwit's epidemic, was mysteriously, anonymously distributed all over Kinshasa. No one ever took credit for its release, but obviously somebody had violated a basic tenet of public health: patient confidentiality. Muyembe's chart noted all of the patients involved in the original hospital outbreak, and had arrows pointing from 'Kimfumu' to several names. Within hours poor Kimfumu was the Typhoid Mary of Kikwit, named in media accounts from Hong Kong to Buenos Aires as the source of Africa's latest disaster.

That boomeranged on his grieving family. Neighbours attacked the widow, accusing her of spreading disease, and she had been forced to flee with her children to her sister's family home in a remote part of Kikwit. In his blind rage the brother-in-law accused Heymann and Khan not only of libelling Kimfumu, but of misdiagnosis. The technician did not die of Ebola, he claimed, but of a sliced artery, cut by a murderous doctor at Kikwit General Hospital.

There would be no further discourse and certainly no blood samples from Kimfumu's survivors. Heymann and Khan trudged back to their vehicle, enraged at authorities in Kinshasa, who they assumed had released Muyembe's chart to the media. Khan sneered and cursed in the car. Heymann, who was equally angry but less demonstrative by nature, simply shook his head and quietly said, 'We didn't have that problem in Yambuku. No press came. Now they bring their satellite links and set up shop. And we can't control it.'

It was dawning on Heymann that public health had entered a new era in which at times of crisis scientists' every move would be scrutinized. Live television coverage of unfolding epidemics was now, and in the future, inevitable. He pondered what this could mean for the future of public health: it worried him deeply.

Meanwhile Nigerian veterinarian Oyewale Tomori, a veteran of Lassa fever epidemics in his home country, wanted to be sure that animals within Kikwit weren't spreading the virus. He began by combing the city for monkeys, chimps, and gorillas, which were kept in homes all over the town, as pets or possible sources of future revenue. Many of the animals—particularly the gorillas and chimps—were in alarming shape, clearly suffering from a variety of bacterial infections. But none appeared to have Ebola symptoms.

At considerable personal risk Tomori, assisted by the pets' owners and the CDC's Scott Dowell, held the strong animals down and drew blood samples. This was not, of course, a procedure the cousins of Homo sapiens enjoy; teeth were bared and struggles ensued. Clearly, Tomori's latex gloves would have proved useless if one of the animals had managed to sink its teeth into the veterinarian. Fortunately, Tomori escaped unscathed, loaded with monkey and ape blood samples.

Analysis fell to Swanepoel, who worked in just ten-minute shifts, the brevity necessitated by the sweat and torpor produced by working inside a space suit in the tropics. He swiftly ruled out Ebola infection in the primates, and set about searching for other possible Ebola-carrying animals. The amiable South African managed to recruit local volunteers who helped snare bats from Kikwit's trees and church belfries. In following days he captured dozens of species of birds, bats, rodents, and insects in the Forêt Pont Mwembe, or Mwembe Forest.

By May 20, with the epidemic slowing but still under way, Kikwit's mayor, Ignace Gata Mavita, felt thoroughly overwhelmed. The problems and petitioners just kept piling up at the *Hôtel du Ville*, the one-story cinder block town hall, nestled in a weedy, run-down former park. Deeply grateful for the international assistance, Mavita felt that, at long last, the epidemic was coming under control, but now new problems were proving invulnerable to his best efforts.

'The town is in isolation,' the handsome young politician explained. 'It is difficult for people to get goods at decent prices. Those traders in other regions are afraid to come here. And those who have goods are increasing their prices. And you can imagine how the people are suffering, because they are so poor. It's good to issue a quarantine, but they have to find a solution or we will have dire economic consequences. If not, the world may have its solution, but we will starve . . . and they will create another crisis here in Kikwit.'

Mavita noted sadly that Ebola was creating hundreds of orphans, and Kikwit had no orphanages.

'This is the greatest challenge that Kikwit has ever faced,' he concluded.

While Mavita exerted pressure on officials in Kinshasa to lift Kikwit's crippling quarantine Heymann and Muyembe felt that they were soon going to complete their primary mission: stop the epidemic. Heymann sent word to CDC and WHO that relief crews should come soon, allowing the crisis team to head home after two gruelling weeks for well-deserved rests. As the numbers of new cases slowed to a daily trickle the team concentrated on setting in place two key scientific efforts. The first, using the far-flung surveillance system they'd created, would focus on mapping out the epidemic's history, from Gaspard Menga to the end, noting who had caught the virus from whom and how it had been transmitted. Further, that mission would search for evidence of uninfected Ebola carriers.

The second mission, already begun by Tomori, Swanepoel, and Dowell, would hunt for whatever animal, plant, or insect normally carries the mysterious virus. To accomplish that, they reasoned, a large team of ecology experts would have to comb Mwembe Forest, gather thousands of samples, and ship the carefully catalogued material back to the CDC for BL-4 laboratory analysis.

But before any such activities could be undertaken in earnest Kikwit desperately needed more supplies, particularly protective gear for use in the hospitals and by the Red Cross. For seemingly the millionth time, on May 23 Szczeniowski telephoned via satellite requests to Geneva. WHO, short on cash and lacking any genuine emergency response capability, simply passed the request along to various North American and Western European governments.

On May 26, with a fresh scientific team on its way and no new Ebola cases in the previous forty-eight hours, Heymann decided to head home. His one concern was that vital supplies *still* had not arrived, and if doctors performed procedures without infection protection the epidemic could start all over again. And then, of course, all of their heroic efforts would come to nothing.

The next morning Heymann stood in the blistering heat on Kikwit's tiny runway, awaiting a chartered plane to Kinshasa. In vain he scoured the skies for signs of his oft-requested supplies. But the only plane he saw was that which flew him to Kinshasa.

Several hours after Heymann departed, however, a huge Hercules transport plane lumbered down the Kikwit runway, loaded with supplies and scientists from Sweden. Among the much-needed syringes, gloves, masks, and such were a few supersuits, designed with built-in air-conditioning units. These were the suits Hollywood expected to see. And they arrived after the epidemic was nearly over.

At the Hotel Intercontinental in Kinshasa later that evening Heymann savoured his first shower in sixteen days, as well as news of the Swedish supplies, which he celebrated with an ice cold Primus beer.

'We did it!' he cried jubilantly. 'We beat the virus!'

A month later the CDC and WHO reported that 296 people had died of Ebola during the Kikwit epidemic, and 79 per cent of all identified infections had proved lethal. A third of the dead were health-care workers. The epidemic had waxed and waned several times between February and June; it had peaked exactly when Heymann first arrived. In August, with all possible incubation periods—the hypothesized lengthiest being twenty-one days—long past since the last Ebola case had been seen, WHO officially declared the epidemic over.

Barely had the world issued a sigh of relief when the virus resurfaced, hundreds of miles away in the West African nation of Côte d'Ivoire. Twenty-five-year-old Jaster Chea travelled from nearby Liberia to the Ivory Coast, was taken ill on December 8, 1995. A WHO team led by Dr Deo Barakanfitiye—who had been part of Muyembe's group in Kikwit—discovered within a few hours that Chea was from the Liberian village of Plibo, where three other men were suffering from the disease. In short order a fifth case—a woman, also from Plibo—was found in Abidjan, the capital of Ivory Coast.[23]

The government of Ivory Coast immediately shut down its border with Liberia, suspending all trade between the two nations. And the WHO investigators found themselves entangled in ongoing civil war disputes, as Plibo was located in a region controlled by the guerrilla National Patriotic Front of Liberia, led by rebel warlord Charles Taylor. The rebels cooperated with WHO, allowing an investigation. The team concluded that the outbreak was limited to the Chea family.

But that incident prompted a review of two previous Ebola incidents in the same rain forest region. In November 1994 a mini-epidemic broke out in gold mining camps that were deep in the forests of Gabon.[24] Accessible only by canoe, the camps were particularly remote, located in a region called Makokou. The suspected Ebola cases were transferred by canoe to a Gabonese military hospital where they were immediately placed under quarantine and treated exclusively by physicians and nurses attired in basic protective gear. Blood samples were analysed in Paris, at the Institut Pasteur, where four of the first eight cases were confirmed as Ebola.

After three years of analysis French researchers concluded that forty-four people had contracted Ebola in the camps, twenty-eight of whom died of the disease. And the military hospital, thanks to appropriate infection control efforts, prevented any further spread of the virus.

The outbreak caught the interest of local chimpanzee researchers who had noted die-offs among the animals in the 4200-square-kilometre Tai rain forest that spans parts of Liberia, Gabon, Ivory Coast, and Cameroon. A few months before the mining camp outbreak a team led by Swiss Institute of Zoology scientist Cristophe Boesch had collected twelve dead chimps (out of forty in a colony) and discovered on autopsy that the animals' blood wasn't coagulating, and there was evidence of internal bleeding. The scientists feared that a terrible new disease had surfaced.

Eight days after those chimp autopsies were performed one of the Swiss scientists fell ill and was evacuated to Institut Pasteur. Though diagnosed with Ebola, she survived, and standard infection control procedures prevented any further spread. No one was able to determine how the veterinarian had become infected in the first place, however, as she'd worn protective gear throughout the autopsies.

The two Tai Forest outbreaks sparked widespread speculation among scientists that whatever creature normally harboured the Ebola virus was located in abundance in the area and had close contact with human beings. That, they said, was exciting news, as it might mean they were close to finding the source, the Ebola reservoir.

Eight weeks after the Liberian Chea incident, Ebola surfaced again, this time in Gabon, in villages located in the same Makokou region in which the prior mining camp incidents had occurred.[25] At least nineteen villagers from the remote Mayibout settlement were infected; all were immediately placed under quarantine in the Makokou Hospital, where infection control standards were elevated to minimize spread. The diagnosis of Ebola was made at the Centre International de Recherches Médicales de Franceville, a local state-of-the-art laboratory built by the French government.

Teams of internationally known scientists poured into Gabon, taking the arduous ninety-three-mile canoe journey to remote Mayibout, population 150 people. By late February it appeared that one-fifth of the village's population was infected with the terrifying virus.

The Gabonese government swiftly rounded up everybody who might have had contact with the initial Mayibout cases, placing them under observation.

In the village, researchers discovered that children had found a dead chimpanzee on January 26, and all of the original ten deaths were among people who had feasted that night on the chimp. The Gabonese government, on learning of the chimp connection, issued radio bulletins nationwide warning citizens not to touch or eat dead chimps or monkeys.

By February 19 twenty cases had been confirmed: thirteen were dead. WHO intervened successfully to prevent international airlines and bordering nations from placing sanctions on Gabon, and the military imposed a strict quarantine on Makokou district. Given the area's inaccessibility such a quarantine was easily enforced, even when it came to keeping the media out. WHO officially praised the Gabonese efforts, saying that the government had taken 'all appropriate measures...to limit the outbreak.'

By the end of February, 20 per cent of the Mayibout populace had fallen ill: 9 per cent had died. But the rapid control measures taken by the Gabonese government and local hospitals prevented any further spread. Twelve of the dead had helped butcher and consume the chimpanzee. The remainder were relatives who had cared for the original group of Ebola sufferers.

And then Ebola broke out again in Gabon, nine months later in an area called Boué.

The WHO team, which included Kikwit veteran Rodier and the CDCs Mike Ryan, identified some fifty possible cases and eight Ebola deaths in Boué during October 1996. And though Boué was relatively close to Makokou district, Ryan and Rodier felt certain that the new epidemic was unconnected to the earlier Mayibout outbreak.

Reviews of local medical records revealed that for at least a decade the villagers living around the periphery of the Tai Forest in Gabon suffered three to nine apparent Ebola deaths every year.

Suspicions mounted that the notorious virus's natural habitat was in that rain forest. Heymann, who had been in the process of creating a new emerging diseases unit inside WHO ever since his triumphant return from Kikwit, started hunting for funds for construction of an Ebola station in the Tai Forest.

A year after the 1996 Boué outbreak an ailing Gabonese doctor flew to Johannesburg, South Africa, for treatment at the exclusive Morningside Clinic in the smart Sandton suburb of the city. The patient found himself, said Dr Adrian Dusé, 'in a town setting in a first-class hospital.'

Physicians did not diagnose Ebola immediately but imposed isolation care on the Gabonese, who recovered fully within two weeks. On November 11 his case was still officially undiagnosed, and the doctor was released from the hospital.

But on November 2, 1997, Morningside Clinic nurse Marilyn Lehana, age forty-six, came down with a sharp headache, spiking fever, and elevated white blood cell count. Initially, no one suspected a link between Lehana's case and that of the Gabonese doctor. And it would only be in retrospect that Dusé and infection control nurse Gerry Sharpe would recall that Lehana had been poked with a needle while trying to insert a blood line into the Gabonese.

As Lehana steadily deteriorated her medical colleagues struggled to understand: What was ailing her? How should it be treated? The hospital laboratory tested for every organism ever previously seen in South Africa, finding Lehana negative for all. Then on November 11 Lehana developed petechia, or pinhole bleeding spots all over her body, which appeared something like a measles rash. And the laboratory reported seeing microscopically the classic question mark form of the Ebola virus in Lehana's blood.

As word of her diagnosis spread within the hospital one doctor cried out, 'We are all going to die!' Sharpe recalled emotionally. Panic set in, and soon local radio stations were spreading the news. The following day hundreds of parents kept their children home from schools, while others put masks on their youngsters, instructing them to keep the coverings on in class. Attendance at Johannesburg sporting and cultural events plummeted, and even the enormously popular rugby games were sparsely attended.

Lehana's illness drew particular attention because her husband was a celebrated lawn bowler, a popular sport in South Africa. Her illness became a national obsession, updated live from Morningside Clinic every morning on Johannesburg's top station, Radio 702. Throughout her illness local newspapers carried detailed accounts of her progress along with letters and prayers penned by Lehana's thousands of supporters.

Meanwhile, Dusé and Sharpe set to work tracking down every hospital worker who had had contact with the Gabonese doctor, Lehana, or their blood and tissue samples. 'The number was mind-boggling,' Sharpe said: 360. Every one of them was tested for antibodies to Ebola and counselled.

Meanwhile, despite their Ebola fears, Lehana's colleagues found it hard to constantly wear gloves and masks while tending to the popular nurse. Many admitted removing their gear and spending time chatting at Lehana's bedside, trying to cheer up their ailing colleague. Similarly, Dusé and Sharpe discovered countless cases of lax infection control in the hospital: laboratory accidents, people eating or smoking in the laboratory, nurses tending to patients ungloved, inappropriate waste disposal. Even in the obviously dangerous crisis health-care workers found it difficult to adhere to strict infection control guidelines.

Fortunately, none of Lehana's 360 contacts tested positive for Ebola infection. But on November 24 Lehana died, her brain filled with Ebola-saturated blood.

'So even in a top-of-the-line modern hospital you can get spread of Ebola,' Dr Neil Cameron, secretary-general of communicable diseases for the South African Ministry of Health, said. 'Morningside is the best private hospital in Africa. It is better than many of your American hospitals—certainly better than your urban, public hospitals.'[26]

The South African incident hadn't yet occurred when most of the world's Ebola virus experts gathered in Antwerp, Belgium, to compare notes, in September 1996. It had been thirteen months since WHO officially declared the Kikwit epidemic over, and at least three small outbreaks had occurred in West Africa's Tai Forest region. Enough time had elapsed to allow the scientists to assemble laboratory and field data, in the hope of making sense of the haemorrhagic filovirus. Yambuku outbreak veteran Guido van der Groen organized the International Colloquium on Ebola Virus Research, convened at his Institute of Tropical Medicine.

Nearly all of the Ebola veterans were there—the elder statesmen who'd witnessed Yambuku, the Kikwit team, and a host of young Turks who were working on advanced molecular biology or blanketing the Tai Forest in search of Ebola's reservoir. One excited participant pronounced it 'The Ebola Woodstock.' Missing, however, were most of Africa's Ebola experts, with the exception of Muyembe. The Zairois virologist bitterly explained that the Belgian government had refused visas for his colleagues because it feared the Africans would not return to their home countries. It was, Muyembe explained, typical of how Belgium prevented African immigration to its little piece of the European continent.[27]

Heymann set the meeting's tone, telling the scientists that there was little about which they could gloat. Ebola broke out in January 1995 in Kikwit: the world didn't hear of it until May 9. He ticked off a long list of public health catastrophes of the 1990s, noting a consistent trend. The crises occurred in poor countries, largely because of essential public health failures.[28] The outside world didn't learn of the problems until things had spread beyond easy control. And resources from the wealthy world were scarce. All told, he said, $3.5 million was spent on Kikwit's epidemic efforts, more than $2 million of which came from European companies and humanitarian aid groups. Only $1 million had come from the US CDC. To prepare the world for the twenty-first century, Heymann insisted, 'We need a whole new vision of the function of the World Health Organization.'

In the absence of genuine infrastructures of public health, separate from but in tandem to medical treatment systems, episodes such as the Kikwit Ebola epidemic would repeat, and repeat, and repeat—well into the twenty-first century. Few of the world's poor nations at the close of the twentieth century had a genuine public health infrastructure. Instead, they had a poorly funded medical care system and small offices located in large cities, inside which bureaucrats tallied up the nation's annual death counts.

But numbers alone could not make a public health infrastructure. Indeed, they could offer little more than false reflections used to justify bad policies.

At the time of the Antwerp meeting 92 of 193 nations surveyed by UNICEF spent less than 10 per cent of their budgets on health-related services.[29] That's 48 per cent of the countries, providing services to well over four billion human beings. In contrast 12 per cent of the budget of industrialized nations—19 per cent of the US budget—were directed to health spending.

At the bottom of the bottom was the Democratic Republic of the Congo, formerly Zaire, which spent less than 1 per cent of its budget on health. Globally, 16 per cent of all governments devoted less than 5 per cent of their budgets to protecting and improving the health of their citizens.

The Ebola virus and innumerable other less exotic organisms would always be part of the global ecology, Heymann warned. And they would always have opportunities to infect *Homo sapiens.*

It was a sentiment echoed by the CDC's Dr Reva Khabbaz, who noted that haemorrhagic fever viruses had broken out at least thirteen times in Africa since 1986, in almost every case noted only after epidemics were well under way. Better disease surveillance was essential, she declared.

'Ah, but you cannot establish a surveillance system if there is no public health system at all,' Michel Pletschette of the European Commission countered, noting that the fifteen nations of the European Union reacted poorly to Kikwit's outbreak. Lack of public health infrastructure created Zaire's crisis, Pletschette insisted, but the inability of Europe to respond wisely was indicative of those wealthy nations' public health inadequacies, as well. For example, during the epidemic some European governments banned all African primate imports—a measure Pletschette labelled 'dumb'. After all, there was no evidence Ebola was transmitted from monkeys to humans except, per-haps, when people ate chimps which, of course, was a practice Europeans condemned. Four countries stopped all flights from Zaire—also a move he considered 'dumb'. No European nation had a laboratory any longer that WHO would certify BL-4. And nearly all Europeans who took part in epidemic control in Kikwit did so under the aegis of the American CDC, Medécins Sans Frontières, or WHO—not under their own country's sponsorship. In general, he concluded, European governments did not want to spend money on an African problem and lacked clear, scientifically based public health leadership to guide their domestic Ebola-prevention policies.

Veterinary researcher Frederick Murphy of the University of California, Davis, was even blunter; funding to date in North America and Western Europe was merely 'tokenism; token funds to get us scientists out of [politicians'] offices. . . . Who is to pay? Today for lack of funds the infrastructure of tropical diseases is a mere skeleton of what it was twenty years ago. That says something about the political acumen of those involved.'

'So who is to be the world's public health doctor?' he asked. Who, indeed, was the leader? As colonial interests in Africa had waned after World War II, so had all North American and European commitment to tropical diseases research and control. Eng-land, France, and the United States, once the clear leaders in the arena, had stepped back, leaving no nation or institution in charge. Funding had all but disappeared for most 'tropical diseases'—better termed 'diseases of poor nations'. Murphy bemoaned the absence of a powerful leadership voice.

The list of unknowns regarding Kikwit's epidemic remained enormous, despite hundreds of hours of research and collection of more than fifty thousand samples of human blood, and animals, plants, and insects of the Mwembe Rain Forest. South Africa's Swanepoel said that transmission was still an open question, as the CDC team was unable to explain how 5 per cent of Kikwit's sufferers were exposed to Ebola: could it have been airborne contagion? Or, perhaps, utensils and food? In support of the lat-ter hypothesis Swanepoel revealed that he had analysed a set of contaminated syringes he'd collected at Kikwit General Hospital. More than a month after he'd collected them, and left them sitting on a desktop at 90 °F (32.2 °C) the whole time, Swanepoel harvested living Ebola viruses off the needles.

The South African criticized the international team's medical efforts, noting that very little data existed on the immunological responses of Ebola survivors, 'so we have *no* idea what is an effective immune response,' the bombastic South African insisted. Further, he had found upon return to Kikwit after the epidemic that patient samples were mislabelled, virtually all were collected only between May 14 to 29 of the epidemic, and nothing of substance could be conjured regarding the Menga cases or any of the other pre-May 14 infections.

Murphy also bemoaned the lack of reliable immunological data, noting that the 'level of destruction by this virus, the speed, begs the question why did 12 per cent of the infected people of Yambuku survive? And 21 per cent in Kikwit? It's one of the most overwhelming pathological images of any acute disease you can imagine.'

After the international team had left, doctors in Kikwit transfused blood from Ebola survivors into eight still-ailing patients in hopes that it would prove curative. One of the patients died, seven survived. Did the experiment work? Muyembe argued no, noting that all of an additional five acute Ebola cases who were later given similar transfusions died. It was possible, therefore, that the seven transfused survivors, all of whom were less acute cases to begin with, would have survived regardless. But in the absence of reliable antibody and immune system data on any of the Kikwit cases it was impossible to judge.

Animal studies done by Peter Jahrling at USAMRIID suggested that such antibody transfusion can't succeed once monkeys or guinea pigs have developed Ebola-like symptoms.

Science similarly remained in the dark regarding the elusive source of Ebola. Researchers throughout the summer of 1995 combed Mwembe Forest, searching for anything that might have infected Gaspard Menga. Around Menga's campsite, 'everything that crawled, we collected,' a British expert said. Scientists from Belgium, France, the United States, England, and Zaire combed the area. And CDC and USAMRIID dedicated tremendous human resources to analysing those samples.

'It was a lot of work,' the CDC's BL-4 laboratory analyst Tom Ksiazcek said. 'But so far the Holy Grail is still out there and up for grabs.'

Privately several scientists complained of turf battles among the Institut Pasteur, CDC, and USAMRIID, each of which hoped to find that Holy Grail. One researcher complained that each of these three institutes were hoarding their samples and reagents, forbidding access to other scientists. Another griped that discoveries, when made, were never shared with African scientists who reside in Ebola-endemic areas.

And then Dr Karl Johnson, the retired CDC officer who led the international response in Yambuku, rose and took the microphone. Renowned for decades of ground-breaking haemorrhagic fever research, Johnson was a sort of senior statesman of the field. Now living outside Bozeman, Montana, Johnson felt no need to pull his punches. He ran down the list of scientific failures in the Kikwit investigation, concluding with a sharp attack on the searches in Mwembe Forest: 'I would like to ask you, number one, whether you were working under *any* kind of hypothesis at all. And number two, do you think you can even eliminate any species, as possible reservoirs, based on your investigation?'

The CDCs Paul Reiter was chagrined. 'I felt the same way as Karl. The fact is we went out there to do the best we could. I'm afraid that it was just a fishing expedition.'

Further, the teams had tramped all over Mwembe a full six months after Menga's original infection. It was a different season, Reiter said, and probably unrealistic to think any reservoir could be found at that late date.

'There wasn't a lot of good planning,' the CDC's C. J. Peters conceded.

The most tantalizing revelation came not from the heart of Africa, but via a little-known plant researcher in the Danish Royal Veterinary and Agriculture University in Copenhagen. Dr Thorben Lundsgaard had spent years studying the festuca leaf streak virus, which attacks grasses used to feed livestock in Europe and North America. He had a hunch that the virus was carried to grasses by tiny flying insects called leaf-hoppers. So he grew a batch of leafhoppers, mashed them up, and scoured cell samples, using a powerful electron microscope. He never found his leaf streak virus.

'But I did find something else,' the shy Danish scientist recalled. 'And it was by chance. I see something and then I go, of course, in more detail. I look and it looks like a filovirus. And I was very excited, in fact.'

Old Ebola hands at the colloquium were stunned by Lundsgaard's photographs, and most agreed that the microbe looked remarkably similar—but not identical—to Ebola. Still, it caught the CDC's Jim LeDuc's excited attention, because he had taken part in a 1981 US Army search for Ebola's sources in northern Zaire.

'Everybody in the villages was raising guinea pigs to eat,' LeDuc recalled. 'And they feed the animals these grasses that are loaded with leafhoppers.'

In 1981, Dr Joseph McCormick ran the top-security Special Pathogens Laboratory at the US Centers for Disease Control, where he conducted tests on guinea pig blood and tissue samples LeDuc sent from Zaire.

'Those animals did test positive for Ebola,' said McCormick. But the test methods used to verify Ebola infection fifteen years ago often provided false positives, so the reliability of such findings was questionable.

Dr Elena Ryabchikova of the State Research Centre of Virology (or VECTOR) in Novosibirsk, Russia, infected laboratory guinea pigs with Ebola. First, she said, they seemed resistant. But when she passed the virus through eight generations of guinea pigs, a strain of Ebola surfaced that was 100 per cent lethal to them. This probably meant, Ryabchikova said, that guinea pigs rarely got sick with Ebola in nature, though they might carry the virus.

The leafhopper/guinea pig connection was pure speculation, of course. And no one was suggesting that Euro-American leafhoppers carried the virus. Only a handful of tests had been performed on African leafhoppers, all by Robert Swanepoel of the National Institute of Virology in South Africa. Swanepoel was unable to infect the insects, but he was able to infect three species of bats found only in the so-called Ebola Belt of

Central Africa.[30] The virus quickly replicated in the bats, with no deleterious effects on them. Most disturbing, Swanepoel said, was the discovery of large amounts of Ebola in the salivary glands and lungs of the bats, pointing at a possible respiratory route of Ebola transmission from the winged rodents to other animals or human beings.

An entirely different line of observation was offered by French researchers working in the Tai Forest. WHO's Dr Pierre Formenty was studying wild chimpanzees, which had experienced die-offs due to Ebola. Most of the chimp deaths seemed to have occurred during the rainy season, when male apes hunt for Colobus monkeys. Chimpanzees who ate the Colobus, Formenty said, were five times more likely to develop Ebola than were those who avoided monkey meat.

Dr Tom Monath of Oravax in Boston said that he had discovered that another deadly haemorrhagic virus, Lassa, was carried by the brown *Mastomys* rats in West Africa and passed to humans via inhalation of dust contaminated with rat urine. Monath told the Antwerp gathering that the Ebola puzzle was likely to be complex, possibly involving insects that were eaten by animals. Those animals were, in turn, eaten by people. Or Ebola was passed via a bite to another animal species, which were eaten by yet another animal or by people.

'I'd be very surprised if this doesn't turn out to be a complicated story,' Monath concluded.

'Ah, yes,' Swanepoel said with considerable gusto, 'but a damned fascinating one!'

Throughout 1997 and 1998 researchers continued their efforts in the Tai Forest, erecting elaborate networks of observation stations high in the jungle canopy from where they could observe chimpanzee activities. It was, perhaps, a long shot, but the scientists thought they might witness something that could finally solve not only the Ebola mystery but also the larger question of how viruses jump from one target species to another, and eventually to human beings.

In five Tai Forest countries (Central African Republic, Cameroon, Congo, Gabon, and Equatorial Guinea) a Pasteur Institute team led by Jean-Paul Gonzalez ran blood tests on a variety of animals, as well as local Pygmy tribes people, looking for the presence of antibodies against Ebola. Nearly 8 per cent of the *Mastomys* rats tested positive, meaning that they had at some time been infected with the virus. More striking were antibody-positive rates in wild pigs, guinea pigs, and dogs in the 16 to 18 per cent range.

The human results were particularly intriguing and clearly demonstrated that the Ebola virus frequently infected *Homo sapiens* who lived their lives in the Tai/Congolese rain forest. Further, it appeared that infection rates varied year by year, indicating that exposure to the virus was, for people, erratic. In Pygmy blood samples taken in 1979, for example, about 5 per cent proved positive. In 1985 it peaked at 35 per cent seropositive blood samples.

It seemed, then, that Ebola epidemics were a rarity among the human and animal denizens of the Congo Basin and Tai Forest, but individuals were frequently exposed to the virus, perhaps infected, and probably more commonly than anyone realized, killed by the virus.

Ebola was hardly the only relatively recently discovered virus toward which the region's animals and peoples had antibodies. HTLV types I and II, Marburg virus, and HIV types 1 and 2 were also present and infected several species besides human beings. In the early 1990s several research groups showed that the less pathogenic AIDS virus, HIV-2, was a monkey microbe. So closely did HIV-2 strains resemble those found in monkey populations in any given West African area that scientists concluded the two primate populations were being exposed over and over again. That meant that people in the region were in contact with monkey blood—probably while butchering animals for consumption—so often that the monkey SIV-2 viruses were reintroduced over and over again into the human population, becoming HIV-2.[31]

In 1999 two separate teams of scientists, led by Beatrice Hahn of the University of Alabama in Birmingham and Francoise Barré-Sinoussi of the Institut Pasteur, discovered that the same might be true for the far more dangerous HIV-1. The virus was exclusively seen in one of four subspecies of chimpanzees, the *Pan troglodytes troglodytes*, which live in the Tai and Congo Basin rain forest area. Based on observations of only a handful of the infected animals it appeared that the virus was harmless for the chimps, though lethal to more than 95 per cent of all infected *Homo sapiens*.

Given that chimpanzees and *Homo sapiens* differ genetically in only 1.5 per cent of their total genetic makeup this seemed startling. It suggested to Hahn that study of wild *Pan troglodytes troglodytes* might reveal immunological secrets vital to finding effective treatments or a vaccine for AIDS.[32]

But since 1991, Hahn learned, chimpanzees in the region have grown scarce, their ecologies and very existence thrown upside down. It was a turn of events with implications for not only the future of HIV-1 but also of all Central African animal viruses.

Prior to 1991 the government of France had subsidized the currency of all of its former West African colonies, artificially bolstering its value. But in 1991 France dropped the subsidy, allowing the African currencies to plummet to their 'natural' values. Overnight the resources of those countries—which included Central African Republic, Equatorial Guinea, Côte d'Ivoire, Cameroon, and Gabon—became highly desirous for European investors. The costs of resource development and transport, labour, and goods fell so far that even comparatively low value items, such as scrub trees, were profitably exploited. By 1992 dozens of European companies were logging the region's rain forests at a feverish pace.[33]

In their zeal the loggers were slicing roads deep into previously inaccessible rain forest regions. And a new industry arose across the region: bushmeat hunting. In its new incarnation the exploits varied, both in quantity and form, from the traditional hunter-gatherer search for subsistence. The new hunters came from cities in the region, wielded rifles and automatic weapons, and sold the meat in urban marketplaces for tidy profits. The actual rate of bushmeat kill, its impact on the local ecology, and the numbers of primates hunted were all matters of considerable controversy, due largely to their powerful political repercussions.[34]

While controversy and the bushmeat trade swelled in tandem, so silently did the risk of transmission of monkey and ape diseases to human beings, as the slaughter and butchering of these animals exposed hunters and cooks to tremendous amounts of primate blood.

It only took exposure to one dead chimp to spark Mayibout's 1996 Ebola outbreak. Escalating the primate hunt obviously increased the odds that such viruses as simian forms of HIV, HTLV, Ebola, Marburg, and monkeypox—as well as microbes not previously known to human beings—would make the cross-species jump, infecting *Homo sapiens*.

In Zaire the bushmeat trade was driven not so much by foreign logging operations as starvation. Without the animal meat of Mwembe Forest, for example, the children of Kikwit would no doubt have suffered even worse kwashiorkor, malnutrition. The dictator's greed was their burden, and the tax upon their ecology. It was also the focus of their collective rage, which had risen steadily as Mobutu's reign wore on.

Not long after the Kikwit epidemic ended, old, simmering civil war activities in Zaire heated up. Sensing that ageing Mobutu was losing his grip upon the Zairois Army, and having formed an advantageous pact with the neighbouring Rwandan government, rebels took bold steps. For years rival rebel groups had waged tiny battles from isolated parts of Shaba, Katanga, and the Mitumba regions, sparring with Zairois troops. But from the Mitumba Mountains that border Lakes Kivu and Tanganyika, and Rwanda and Burundi, arose a new organization, the alliance of Democratic Forces for the Liberation of Congo-Zaire. It was an amalgam, made up of a host of different anti-Mobutu forces and tough, seasoned killers drawn from the Tutsi population that had been living in exile in Zaire since conflicts heated up in their home countries of Burundi and Rwanda.[35]

At an extraordinary pace the new movement, led by long-obscure rebel Laurent Kabila, captured Zaire's towns and cities in its drive from the country's eastern-most border to the Atlantic Ocean. So great was the populace's hatred of the dictator that rebels barely had to engage in genuine conflict as Zairois troops fled, steadily westward, looting everything in sight in their hasty retreats. Hailed by jubilant, cheering throngs, Kabila's army entered towns from Lumbumbashi to Mbuji-Mayi. As Kabila's forces closed on the capital in May 1997 the dictator was fighting his own battle in France with malignant cancer. Realizing that Mobutu could, after thirty-one years in power, no longer command fear and respect in his army and general Zairois populace, the exclusive circle of his cronies who had so benefited from the dictator's greed-fest fled Kinshasa, and took anything of value that they could grab with them to European hideaways.

Kabila's march into Kinshasa was greeted by enormous, cheering crowds from La Cité ghetto, and hailed by Western officials and businesses that had long before grown weary of the Mobutu regime. The dictator's corruption had made business dealings and investment nearly suicidal.

Kabila took control of a capital that bore little resemblance to beautiful Leopoldville, the colonial name of Kinshasa. Gone were the lazy palms and bougainvillaeas, the well-swept boulevards and quiet bistros. Gone, too, were the promising commercial buildings that during the first years of Mobutu's reign had housed representatives of foreign banks, businesses, and diplomatic corps. In their place were stench, decay, rot, refuse heaps, potholes big enough to destroy a chassis, street beggars, barefoot gangs of starving children, and rain-soaked buildings covered in fungus.

The jungle was reclaiming the capital, as lianas, mildew, weeds, and rain forest shrubs overgrew the streets and buildings. Like a postapocalyptic vision from 1950s science fiction, pavements were splintered by aggressive roots and weeds, trees sprouted through rooftops, turning whole buildings into seeming multistory flowerpots, waves of mud rolled with the afternoon rains through the dirt roads, and human waste visible in open sewer lines filled the tropical air with an eye-stinging redolence.

The day Laurent Kabila took power Zaire's external debt was $14 billion. The national bank vaults were, literally, empty. And the World Bank estimated that repairing the country's essential infrastructure—key roads, telephone system, power generators, and the like—would cost $4.5 billion. Overall, Africa's gross domestic product grew a promising 4.6 per cent in 1996, and 3.3 per cent in 1997. But Zaire's *shrank*, went backward, by 8 per cent from 1990 to 1995 and 6 per cent in 1997 alone.[36]

In June Mobutu was on his French deathbed and Kabila was surrounded in Kinshasa by petitioners, foreign advisers, and businessmen eager to cut deals for access to Zaire's vast oil, mineral, and gem wealth. It was a moment of optimism. Western leaders, the World Bank, and the International Monetary Fund paid homage to Kabila but cautiously avoided offers of cash until the new leader's intentions were clear. At the close of 1997 US Secretary of State Madeleine Albright paid Kabila a visit, calling the new leader 'a friend of democracy.'

But if it was democracy Kabila intended his approach was unusual. The robust, bald leader who, ominously, dressed in the famous Mobutu suits declined to name a date for national elections. Much-needed funds for repairing Zaire's decay—including her clinics, hospitals, and public health infrastructure—weren't forthcoming from United Nations agencies because Kabila, amid reports of genocide in eastern Congo, refused their access to the country's eastern regions for human rights investigations.

When the New Year of 1998 dawned euphoria had vanished from Zaire, replaced by disquiet amid fears that one dictator had simply been replaced by another. Worse yet, the new one seemed more beholden to African foreigners than to his own people.

Amid the military and political chaos another monkey disease made the leap from rain forest animals to human beings: monkeypox. Though the first human cases of the disease surfaced in the Katako-Kombe region in February 1996—almost exactly one year after Ebola had made its way out of the Mwembe Forest—notification of WHO and field investigations were severely hampered by the war. It was a year before WHO scientists got a look at the problem firsthand, and that investigation was aborted because of guerrilla military operations in the region. In October 1998 WHO returned to the area, discovering that the epidemic was still under way and could well constitute the largest known human monkeypox outbreak.[37]

The single biggest killer of the twentieth century was the smallpox virus which, before its 1977 eradication, claimed more lives than all of the century's wars, combined. The smallpox virus only infected *Homo sapiens*, and was spread through casual contact and in the air.

The monkey form of the virus was similar enough to smallpox that many scientists had protested WHOs declaration of eradicating smallpox, insisting that as long as monkeypox existed in the jungles of Africa the threat of reemergent smallpox remained.[38]

The new monkeypox epidemic worried WHO because it seemed that the virus was spreading among people, rather than merely from monkey-to-person. During seventeen years of prior investigation in the entire Central African rain forest region only 476 human monkeypox cases were found, and few were more than two rounds of transmission away from a monkey source.

But in this new epidemic at least 511 human cases of the disease had occurred between February 1996 and October 1998, and some appeared to be more than twelve generations of transmission away from the original monkey source.

Though the connection to smallpox made monkeypox worrisome, it was not a terribly dangerous disease to humans, and only eight people had died in the latest epidemic. However, it illustrated to WHO that the political and ecological crises in the region were increasing the probability of epidemics that could have implications well beyond the country Kabila had renamed the Democratic Republic of the Congo, or DROC. Local WHO representative Dr Abdou Moudi warned that there were an 'alarming' number of epidemics in the country, and information systems were rapidly breaking down.

The story wasn't over.

By March 1998 the already abominable conditions in Kikwit under which its 400 000 residents survived had, amazingly, worsened. The Hotel Kwilu's kitchen and power generator had been looted by soldiers, as had its water pump, doorknobs, curtains, mosquito nets, bedsheets, and even pencils and paper. That paucity of valuables was echoed in every sector of Kikwit society, rendering cast-off beer cans and shipping crates treasured replacements for stolen pots, pans, baskets, and totes. Even fewer cars crawled the streets, as spare parts for the ageing vehicles no longer could be found, and soldiers had stolen everything from steering wheels to spark plugs.

In 1995 the largest denomination bill had been the 500-Zaire note, large stacks of which were needed to purchase even one banana. In 1998 the largest currencies were the 500 000- and one-million-Zaire notes, which still carried the profile of Mobutu Sese Seko. The size of the stacks needed for rudimentary purchases were thinner, but it remained Monopoly money, so worthless as to be laughable. A 100 000-Zaire note was worth $1.10. A bottle of Primus beer cost 600 000 Zaires.

As was the case in most of DROC, roads connecting Kikwit to other major cities were destroyed during the war. Trade never had a chance to recover from the Ebola-required quarantine of 1995. For most of the now-dubbed 'Congolese' traders, over-heads had become almost prohibitively high, as all goods had to be transmitted either by boat or air. In the case of Kikwit, river transport didn't carry goods in profitable directions. Only chartered aeroplanes carried goods in 1998, along with paying pas-sengers who sat on the cargo, sipping colas that flight attendants distributed as they carefully manoeuvred among packing crates inside old Soviet cargo planes.

Though the configuration of the army and the flag under which it served had changed, soldiers holding M-16 rifles still stood guard in the same positions in 1998 as in 1995. More than two hundred pharmacies still lined Boulevard Mobutu, and no one had got around to changing the name of Kikwit's only surfaced road. In Kikwit's markets the usual paltry display of smuggled plastic goods and packed foods was presented, along with the plants and animals gathered from Mwembe Forest.

But among government officials only Makarios Manikasa, chief of the National Security Services' Bandundu office, retained his job. The rest of the Mobutu-era officials were swept away, replaced by those loyal to Laurent Kabila.

'There is little peace in the country now,' Manikasa said sadly, seated behind his large wooden desk in a small office bathed in sun, sweltering heat, and mosquitoes. The security chief never removed his black sunglasses, nor would he permit photographs, because, he explained, 'I don't want the CIA to know what I look like. As you know I am an agent and must remain under cover.'

Manikasa took his area's safety seriously, seeing his role as one that extended well beyond the usual security concerns of intrigue, rebels, smuggling, and insurgency. That was because, he explained, 'As I am responsible for security, I don't see security just in terms of weapons but in all things.'

Including disease.

In 1995 Manikasa's wife, Lusilu, was a nurse at Kikwit General Hospital. She was in the operating room when hapless Kimfumu's abdomen was cut open releasing Ebola-rich blood that spattered over everyone, herself included.

'She got it in that first surgical case in that cluster after the orderly took ill,' Manikasa said, still stiffening when he recalled those events three years later. 'She was sick for three weeks. Nobody could touch her. Everybody was afraid. Even myself, in the hos-pital, could not touch her. Especially when we learned it was a deadly virus.'

It took Lusilu Manikasa many more weeks to recover all of her physical health. But after three years the pretty thirty-year-old nurse still had not bounced back emotion-ally. For reasons she could not fathom, but troubled her deeply, Manikasa alone survived that first cluster of cases. As she had lain in Pavilion No. 3 during April and May of 1995 Manikasa watched each of her colleagues die around her, listened to the seemingly non-stop wailing of grieving families standing in front of the nearby mortuary, and felt certain that at any moment the virus would claim her life, too.

'For four days I didn't eat anything,' Lusilu Manikasa recalled, relaxing under a shade tree on a steamy, equatorial afternoon. 'My throat burned and my gums hurt. I had bloody spots on my thighs. And bloody diarrhoea. I felt weak.'

Manikasa patted her multicoloured full-length cotton skirt, touching her thighs, and said, 'One more thing. I don't understand. Every now and then those bloody spots on my thighs return. They're like . . . you know, when you hit something. Like big bruises. What could that be?'

Manikasa's relatives gathered around the corner of their cinder block ramshackle home, peering at the white woman who had come to speak to their cousin. Nervous about her life in Kikwit, Manikasa was spending most of her days far from her husband and two children, living with relatives in Kinshasa. Though she missed her family, Manikasa explained, it was frightening to return to Kikwit and her nursing job.

'It takes courage to go to work,' she insisted. 'The conditions are not good!'

A forty-minute aeroplane flight away in Kikwit Manikasa's security chief husband said that his wife had 'beaucoups de courage.' Every time she returned to the Kikwit General Hospital he worried. By mutual agreement she rarely came to Kikwit any more.

'It is certain that we will have another epidemic because conditions are unchanged,' Manikasa insisted.

'And when the international response came we were happy. We knew WHO came here to save our lives. A good part of Zaire at that time, now the Congo, could have been decimated,' Manikasa continued. 'In that time the entire world community was organized to come here to Kikwit, and Kikwit became the centre of the world. The population believed that because of the terrible disease a health infrastructure would be developed. Some even believed the hospital here would become the reference facility for the whole country. The hospital believed that from then on Kikwit would develop a genuine health infrastructure.'

Manikasa lowered his voice and spat out his words bitterly as he concluded, 'But everything has returned to square one, where people are suffering to find medicine and medical support. Everything is forgotten. Could it happen again? For sure! There are no changes!'

Well, that wasn't exactly true. There had been changes: for the worse.

In 1997 Kabila appointed Marc Katshunga to be the Bandundu Province's governor, which, among other things, meant that the plump politician and his wife, Cornelie, could move into the sprawling two-story governor's mansion in Kikwit and maintain a staff of servants and gardeners who kept the lace table-cloths well ironed and the colourful, tropical garden well weeded. A similar well-staffed mansion was at his disposal in Bandundu City. And among his entourage were several advisers and a video cameraman who documented the governor's every move. Puffing up for the camera the politician explained that, in the long run, the Ebola epidemic had little—if any—

lasting impact on Kikwit and its neighbouring villages. He credited 'aggressive polit-ical mobilization,' engineered by himself, with 'almost annihilating the fear.'

Apparently confident that Kikwit no longer needed to be prepared for such emer-gencies Governor Katshunga confiscated the region's only ambulance, had it painted and fitted with sofas, and pressed it into the service of his office. In 1998 the ambulance that had previously carried Ebola patients to Kikwit General Hospital functioned as Katshunga's chauffeur-driven limousine.

For Kikwitians poverty had become a constant. A local Catholic nun put it in perspective by noting that her order found the resources to supply one pen to each family every school term. When siblings took exams in school, they shared their fam-ily's sole writing implement.

It was, of course, the utter lack of infection control and hygiene in Kikwit's hospitals that the Ebola virus had exploited, turning an isolated chain of cases occurring in the community into a profound epidemic. Once the virus had entered a hospital that lacked even the most minimal elements of infection control—soap and clear water—it raced through the patients and medical staff like fire burning its way up a hillside of dry grass.

WHO's David Heymann said that 'this epidemic was driven by hospital workers who did not respect the most minimal health standards.'

It was a 'lack of respect' driven largely by the paucity of options.

But in 1998 conditions in Kikwit's frail health infrastructure were, remarkably, even worse.

What few medical supplies reached cut-off Kikwit in 1998 cost far more than they had in 1995 because the only remaining form of transport was a network of private aircraft. Flying post-World War II Russian cargo planes, three newly created com-panies carried passengers and shipments daily to and from Kikwit. Every now and then a plane bore X-ray film for tuberculosis diagnosis, antibiotics to treat bacterial infections, chloroquine for malaria, surgical gloves, or other life-and-death supplies.

In 1997 Dr Pius Kongolo had moved from Bomba some two hundred kilometres away to become the new chief of Kikwit General Hospital. Though his colleagues warned him against moving for fear he would encounter Ebola in Kikwit, Kongolo, a handsome Kinshasa-trained internist, decided the job 'represented a certain amount of risk, but it was a calculated risk.'

A big part of Kongolo's thinking that led him to accept the Kikwit job was word that the international response to the Ebola epidemic brought 'a lot of equipment here. But my surprise was huge when I discovered it was not here.'

Every microscope, water purifier, specialized protective gear, laboratory instru-ment, test kit, and piece of laboratory equipment that scientists from the CDC, WHO, Institut Pasteur, and Medécins Sans Frontières had brought in May 1995 were gone by September of that year.

Kikwit's primary medical facility by 1998 had only the same two microscopes that were there before the Ebola epidemic, both of which could only be used with the aid of sunlight. It had one ageing X-ray machine. One of the diagnostic labs had a forty-year-old centrifuge—a device essential for preparing blood samples for analysis. The hospital's ancient, rusted generator provided only sporadic electricity, so there were no freezers to hold blood and tissue samples, or refrigerators for safe storage of transfusion blood or temperature-sensitive drugs and vaccines. Unless boiled on coal fires, the hospital's water was unsafe for human consumption. Night-time labours and deliveries—including emergency caesarean-sections—were performed with the aid of one of the three kerosene lamps on the obstetrics and gynaecology ward.

In the surgical theatre—the same operating room in which Lusilu Manikasa had been infected with Ebola three years before—every piece of equipment was recycled, from gloves to masks, scalpels to haemostats. And the equipment that was inserted in one body after another was usually not sterile, Kongolo said, 'because we lack the fuel to run our generator and therefore have no power for the autoclaves,' which would heat-sterilize surgical instruments.

For the previous fifteen months—since the civil war—the medical staff of Kikwit's hospital had not yet been paid. And Hospital Director Baudouin Ndulu had to lay off 30 per cent of the staff, leaving 265 doctors, nurses, maintenance workers, and other essential personnel. It had been more than ten years since he had received federal funds for equipment, Ndulu said, and the hospital was so deeply in debt to medical suppliers that it technically was insolvent.

'Apart from the human factor, the infrastructure is demeaning,' Kongolo insisted. 'We always have to do makeshift things in order to achieve the minimum. There are times when we feel as if we've been sacrificed.'

Ndulu—as well as every other Kikwit health-care worker—insisted that were Ebola to hit the hospital then, 'It would be worse! Because no preventative measures have been taken and nothing has come to this hospital.'

Ndulu claimed promises were made by all the international agencies that responded to the 1995 epidemic, but none of the pledged supplies ever materialized.

'That's the usual behaviour of international people,' DROC's Health Minister Dr Jean-Baptiste Sondji said dismissively. 'They came when there is a lot of coverage in the media, then they leave as if nothing happened.'[39]

But it was not just international health agencies that forgot poor Kikwit's plight. Her own officials, citizens, and health providers appeared to have shoved Ebola out of their minds, forgetting all the lessons of prevention they were taught three years earlier by the international team.

'I haven't noticed any change in Kikwit because people in Kikwit did not believe really that it was a virus that attacked,' University of Bandundu history professor N'sanga Kibari explained. Kibari, whose twenty-seven-year-old brother, Mombolo, perished in the epidemic, wrote a detailed history of the crisis entitled, *The Ebola Virus in Kikwit: Myth, Mystery or Reality?* He concluded that despite all the obvious scientific evidence that the Ebola virus caused Kikwit's calamity, most of the populace, still in 1998, believed something else had been responsible for the 296 deaths.

'First people believed it was an experiment conducted by the Americans,' Kibari recalled. Then the concept of *landa-landa* swept Kikwit. In nearby Vanga it was rumoured that a local American missionary physician who had run a hospital in the village since 1960 was capable of transforming himself into a hippopotamus that trawled the Kwilu River, performing ominous spiritual acts. And because the first person to contract Ebola in January 1995 was Gaspard Menga, a Jehovah's Witness, it was widely suggested among the majority Catholic population that the epidemic constituted God's revenge for deviant beliefs and behaviours.

All these beliefs, coupled with the poverty of the health-care system, conspired to create a profound level of post-epidemic denial. The people returned to practices that spread Ebola in 1995, including cleansing bodies of dead family members and thus exposing themselves to infected fluids. At the hospitals all the infection control practices followed during the epidemic were swiftly abandoned.

At Kikwit Hospital statistician Ebwala Dambwala saw that fear ruled nearly all behaviours during the epidemic, particularly among health-care workers. Nearly 22 per cent of the deaths were hospital employees, he noted, pointing to stacks of charts and tables he had painstakingly hand-drawn, depicting the epidemic's toll. But by 1998 Dambwala asserted, 'They don't think of it anymore. They have forgotten.'

Most had put Ebola out of their minds, except the survivors. Like Lusilu Manikasa, most of the eighty-eight Ebola survivors now saw life through prisms of apprehension. In Kikwit they formed a club that met monthly to discuss their fears about future returns of the deadly virus.

Enery-Raphael Mikolo had a pile of photographs of his bout with Ebola in a drawer in the hospital's leprosy and tuberculosis laboratory. He had been taken ill on April 29, three days after burying a friend who had died of the disease. And when he recovered doctors at the hospital used his blood as an antiserum for other Ebola patients.

Three years later Mikolo was still haunted by his battle with the virus. He ate constantly to stay strong and had a nervous manner. Despite his fears, Mikolo continued to work at the hospital, taking sputum and blood samples from TB and leprosy patients.

'We test saliva with no protection. We don't have the necessary gloves and equipment,' Mikolo said, his voice high-strung. 'We do all we can not to position ourselves in front of patients who are coughing. But for lepers there is no means of protection. You see, here washing hands is difficult because I don't have any soap.'

When a visitor offered Mikolo a small container of antiseptic hand-wash liquid he grabbed it in an instant, immediately hiding it from the view of colleagues. For the next ten minutes Mikolo hovered around the soap's hiding place, eyeing his colleagues. Once certain they were unaware of his treasure Mikolo grinned broadly.

Pierre Menga still vividly recalled the January 1995 funeral of his brother Gaspard. He had photos of the funeral depicting the Menga family gathered around Gaspard's open casket.

Of all his siblings only Pierre was alive in 1998. He was saddled with a number of small children—his, Gaspard's, and those of other deceased relatives. And he cared for his ageing, tubercular father, Innocent. In all, Pierre cared for twelve people.

'We look and search every day,' for food and money, Pierre, who was unemployed, said. 'But everyone is kind to us in Kikwit.'

Innocent glared through rheumy eyes at his son and retorted, 'Don't sound as if we're all right—we're suffering!'

And indeed, they were. The Menga clan of thirteen people lived in a two-room wattle home located in an almost inaccessible gully well off Ndala Road. The densely crowded neighbourhood resonated with the laughter and cries of small children. During heavy rains the clay grounds flooded. And after each downpour the humid, steamy air filled with malarial mosquitoes. The children were all barefoot, their clothes tattered and ill-fitting.

Pierre, who was unmarried, had his hands full caring for all of the children and hustling for work and money. During the Ebola epidemic Pierre set aside grief over the deaths in his family to assist WHO and the CDC in their investigations. For his services Menga received no money or compensation.

'Between that time and now there's no change at all,' Menga said of Kikwit and of his family. 'We've gone back to our old ways. We are suffering. Of course, now many of us are missing. We just wish that the international community would be aware of our suffering here.'

The thirty-four-year-old man looked overwhelmed as he introduced the many children in his care.

'We have kept one child in school all along, but [because of the fees] we cannot afford to put the others, with all our losses, through school. And we are wondering what will be the future of our family.'

Every morning Pierre awakened from a dream. Someone had given him enough money to start a business, and he had built a house large enough for all of the surviving Mengas to live in comfort, dry during storms and free of disease-carrying insects.

That, he said, 'Would stop the pain and anguish.'

In Kinshasa, meanwhile, it was hard to detect any action and effort to improve matters. 'The problem is they're overwhelmed,' a Western gold developer said. 'Mobutu left such a massive disaster that they just don't know where to start.'

Congo's Health Minister Sondji added that the crisis in Kikwit's health-care infrastructure was no better or worse than what was the current state of affairs 'in hundreds of towns all over the nation. We estimate that minimally $530 million will be needed to address the problem. We are battling very hard to find those funds. But look, $700 million is just the entire national budget!'

Obviously, the tall, middle-aged Sondji said grimly, health must compete for every one of those $700 million against every other sector of the society. And Congo, just two years before the millennium, had few of the necessities of the twentieth century. Most Congolese had no electricity, running water, telephones, surfaced roads, or other essentials of life.

For Professor Muyembe the sorry state of affairs in his country was deeply painful. He grew up in Bandundu Province, not far from Kikwit, during colonial days when strict nuns sharply doled out lessons in Latin, classical Greek, French, and the Western humanities. A worldly father of five, Muyembe remained in Kinshasa despite invitations for appointments in Europe. But he used his European connections to fund research and clinical work in Kinshasa, and to keep a back door open should escape from his beloved Congo be necessary. Few, if any, of his colleagues were so fortunate.

The situation, even in April of 1998, was ominous enough. It soon worsened.

By May counterrevolutions were breaking out all over DROC as disenchantment with the seemingly paralysed Kabila government grew. Political activists in Kinshasa who had courageously tolerated beatings and imprisonment under Mobutu found little improvement in the democratic climate. Opposition political parties, though officially legal, were harassed to such a degree that local newspapers called the era the Time of Darkness.

Rebel counterforces surrounded key Congolese cities, including the capital, by August 1998. An exodus of foreigners followed, bringing all mining, oil, and general large business operations to a halt. Even within his own ranks Kabila was finding dissent, as breakaway factions of his army seized aeroplanes, airports, and whole towns.

By the end of August Kabila's alliance had collapsed, and for all intents and purposes his rule extended only a few miles beyond Kinshasa. The already beleaguered economy went into a tailspin. All foreign investors disappeared. The Zaire/DROC war was threatening to expand, drawing in adversaries from all over Africa. Angola now backed Kabila. Uganda and Rwanda had switched their allegiances, supporting Tutsi dissidents that formerly were part of the Kabila alliance. Zimbabwe sent military 'advisers' to Kinshasa. Namibia flew in twenty-one tons of military equipment, also backing Kabila. Water and electricity for Kinshasa were cut off by rebels.

From South Africa President Nelson Mandela pleaded for a peaceful resolution. He was ignored.

By September 1998 troops from at least five African countries were on the ground in DROC, fighting alongside either the Kabila government's soldiers or rebel forces. The entire east of the country was under rebel/Rwanda/Uganda control.

By October it seemed that, thanks to foreign troops, Kabila had driven the rebels back to the far east and maintained control. It had cost the government $5 billion, sinking the nation toward the $20 billion debt mark.[40] To the victors went the spoils: each of Kabila's supporting nations laid claim to various Congolese oil, mineral, and gem reserves.

As the last year of the twentieth century dawned the armies of Africa were mobilizing to decide the fate of the continent's massive equatorial nation.

And on November 13, 1998, armed soldiers, by order of Laurent Kabila, marched into Health Minister Sondji's office. He was removed from his office for 'insufficient display of solidarity,' having voiced concern that the new dictator had no intention of holding elections or creating a democracy. Sondji was arrested, leaving the nation—and the people of Kikwit—without any health leadership.

The public health implications of Ebola extended well beyond the dismissive notes that were usually struck by Westerners when discussing seemingly intractable African problems. Failure to take action guaranteed that such public health crises would recur, not only in the Congo Basin but also wherever there is a confluence of similar social and biological factors.

Clearly the Kikwit outbreak was nosocomial. The local hospitals functioned as amplification systems: a pianissimo stream of individual cases went in; a loud fortissimo din of epidemic proportions came out.

At the peak of the Ebola outbreak nothing more exotic than latex gloves and basic protective gear was needed, along with clearheaded planning, to bring the epidemic under control. The sorts of high-technology tools favoured in North America and Europe not only would have been useless in Kikwit, but they might even, in the long run, have proved deleterious. If Kikwit's demoralized doctors toiled in fear in 1998 because they couldn't afford latex gloves, their paranoia could only have been compounded further if the control of Ebola had necessitated even costlier items, such as the air-conditioned space suits brought—too late to be used—by Swedish volunteers.

High-tech solutions are also unlikely to hasten diagnosis and notification of such crises in Kikwit or any other isolated, impoverished pocket of the earth. If Kikwit General Hospital had been left a $10 000 satellite telephone with which to call David Heymann in Geneva in the event of another epidemic, it would not now possess the device. More than likely the exotic phone would long since have been 'liberated' for the use of a general in one or another of the armies now fighting over the future of DROC/Zaire. Or perhaps it would be used by Bandundu Province's governor, making phone calls from inside the ambulance he 'liberated' from Kikwit General Hospital.

CHAPTER 3

Bourgeois physiology

The collapse of all semblances of public health in the former Soviet Socialist Republics.

Moscow meanwhile was empty. There were still people in the city; a fiftieth part of all the former inhabitants still remained in it, but it was empty.
    It was deserted as a dying, queenless hive is deserted. . . .
    Almost all have died, unconscious of their coming end, sitting in the holy place, which they had watched—now no more. They reek of death and corruption. But a few of them stir still, rise up, fly languidly and settle on the hand of the foe, without the spirit to die stinging him; the rest are dead and easily brushed aside as fishes' scales. The beekeeper closes the partition, chalks a mark on the hive, and choosing his own time, breaks it up and burns it.
—Leo Tolstoy, War and Peace

Either socialists defeat lice or lice will defeat Socialism!
—Joseph Stalin

The public health situation worsened so much that at first it seemed unbelievable. No country has ever exhibited such an abrupt change in peacetime.
—Vladimir Shkolnikov, Moscow epidemiologist, 1994

What we face is unprecedented, colossal!
—Dr Gerasimenko of the Russian Academy of Medical Sciences in a May 1997 address to the Duma

By the time Leonid Brezhnev died in the autumn of 1982 there wasn't much left of his seventy-five-year-old cardiovascular system. The ironfisted dictator who had served as Soviet premier and then president for eighteen years had blood veins and arteries that were so clogged with atherosclerotic plaque that blood cells could barely pass. In his abdomen the aorta had ballooned into a massive aneurysm. His heart, scarred after innumerable heart attacks—the exact number was a state secret—fluttered irregularly, struggling for years before finally giving up, felling the leader of the Union of Soviet Socialist Republics. The all-powerful leader died as a result of decades of overeating, overdrinking, and chain-smoking.

Less than two years later his successor, Yuri Andropov, also succumbed. The once-feared leader of the KGB secret police, famed for always wearing sinister darkened glasses, was buried in the winter of 1984 alongside the KGB's notorious founder, Feliks E. Dzerzhinsky. Officially Andropov died of kidney failure. But like Brezhnev, it was a lousy diet, smoking, and alcohol that brought down the man once considered the most fearsome Soviet of his day.

And thirteen months later seventy-three-year-old Konstantin Chernenko was also buried in Red Square, having served as the last of the Soviet Union's Stalinist-style premiers. Years of smoking cigarettes and drinking massive quantities of vodka felled him as well, turning his lungs into emphysema-besieged, wheezing apparati and his liver into cirrhotic jelly.

In March 1985 the Politburo finally gave up on placing men who had served in Stalin's shadow in power, turning to Mikhail Gorbachev, comparatively youthful at the age of fifty-four.

It was the beginning of the great change.

Gorbachev was the first leader of the Soviet Union—indeed, in Russian history dating back to AD 913—to survive his political tenure, not either dying in office or forced out, having been crippled by fatal physical or mental illness.

If Gorbachev's physical health signalled improvement for Soviet leadership it did not augur commensurate enhancement in the health of the Soviet masses. Indeed, it marked the beginning of the most astounding collapse in public health ever witnessed in peacetime in the industrialized world. For the Euro-Slavic world it would be the most radical reversal, in the absence of war, since the Black Death of the fourteenth century.

I

Then that frightening word demography appears, and it is clear that Russia today is on the eve of a demographic catastrophe: the death rate is exceeding the birth rate, life expectancy is declining sharply, the number of suicides is rising, and there are 240 abortions per 100 live births.
—Andrei Sinyavsky, 1997[1]

If there was one thing the Soviet Union seemed justified in bragging about it was their health-care system.

In a series of bold five-year plans executed from Moscow, the Soviets, and their counterparts in Eastern Europe, claimed one victory after another over disease and illness in the Communist world. By 1970, Russia had raised life expectancies from 1917 pre-Bolshevik Revolution levels of thirty-eight years of age for men and forty-three for women to sixty-five and seventy-four, respectively. And infant mortality plummeted from 250 deaths per 1000 babies born in 1917 to about 20 per 1000 in 1970.

Trumpeted globally as evidence of the human, caring face of communism, the successes were buttressed by a public health infrastructure so massive that the Soviets could honestly claim to have more doctors, nurses, and hospital beds per capita than anyone else in the world. So it came as something of a shock to the global health establishment when a series of epidemics suddenly exploded across twelve time zones of the Communist world less than a year after the Soviet Union collapsed in 1991.

Diphtheria infected 200 000 people regionally over this time period, killing 5000; polio rolled into Azerbaijan in 1991, Uzbekistan in 1993, and Chechnya in 1995; and hepatitis was suddenly so commonplace as to be considered endemic, rather than epidemic. Flu hit so hard in 1995 that the Ukrainian government closed for more than a week; typhoid infected 20 000 in Tajikistan in 1996 and then stayed endemic; St Petersburg coped with dual epidemics of cholera and dysentery four times from 1993 to 1998. AIDS grew exponentially, with 20 000 full-blown cases projected in Ukraine alone by the year 2001; TB, syphilis, and gonorrhoea followed suit. And alcoholism, drug abuse, and suicide were by 1995 considered epidemic, according to international health standards.

Even childhood mumps became a serious problem, rising 30 per cent from 1992 to 1994 alone.

Life expectancy nose-dived—men's, for instance, dropped three years between 1992 and 1993. Suddenly, just eight years after the Soviet state ceased to exist, the grandest health-care system known to man was spiralling into chaos.

What had functioned as the 'human, caring face' of communism became, instead, a vision of despair and disease.

In Moscow, that vision was personified by Konstantin, an emaciated, former Soviet soldier who was dying from drug-resistant TB, developed in a Russian prison, that had invaded his lungs, liver, kidneys, and heart. And in Tblisi by frail, tiny Irakli Sherodzle, fifteen, huddled with his mother around an orange hot electric coil, suffering from the drug-resistant flesh-eating streptococci that was inexorably destroying his body.

In the Ukraine, it was most obvious in the killing field surrounding a neighbourhood where drugs were sold openly, then injected by hundreds of teenagers and young adults who shared their needles while squatting on the ice-cold parkland. And on the streets of Odessa, where a pretty, fourteen-year-old prostitute said that she always used condoms, then laughed derisively and winked knowingly at a nearby friend.

The new face of health-care in the former USSR could be seen at an AIDS clinic in Kiev, where a nurse took blood from an HIV-positive man without wearing protective latex gloves, using her bare forefinger to apply pressure to the site of injection. It could be seen in Georgia, at the Deserter's Bazaar in Tblisi, where Goga, an economics student with no medical training, sold antibiotics from an open-air booth, advising customers how to use the drugs, and which to take.

It was in Tskhinvali, Georgia, on the empty paediatric wing of Republican Hospital. Asked about the patients, a nurse—holding a log in her hand, as if it were a baby—was contemptuous: 'Can't you feel the cold?' she asked. 'We sent them home. It's safer for them, no matter how sick they are, to be home than to be here where we have no heat.' And it was on the hospital's top floor, where a hernia operation was being conducted. The patient's respiratory ventilator was hand-pumped by a nurse, his anaesthesia was dripped onto a cloth over his face. The surgeon was working quickly because the generator only provided fifteen minutes of electricity for the lights.

The depth of this public health catastrophe varied among the former Soviet and Eastern Bloc nations as the twentieth century reached its close. But it was undeniably grave regionwide.

'No country in peacetime has ever exhibited such an abrupt change,' said epidemiologists Vladimir Shkolnikov and France Meslé, of Russia's Centre for Demography and Human Ecology and France's Institut National D'etudes Demographique, respectively, in a 1997 report to the Russian nation.[2]

In 1970 Soviet scientists were so impressed with their nation's health achievements that they forecast a population of 160 million people in Russia alone by the year 2000. But Russia's population was shrinking so rapidly during the 1990s that it was expected to dip to between 126 million and 140 million by 2010—its lowest level since the eve of the 1917 Bolshevik Revolution.[3]

But the prognosticators were fooled. In 1999 Russian murder rates declined, yet premature death rates continued to soar. Sombre forecasters predicted in revised 2000 projections that by 2050 Russia's population might be a mere 80–90 million, or the smallest number of people in more than two centuries. If such an abysmal forecast proved correct, in sixty years Russia's population would shrink by more than any Northern Hemisphere society had in known human history, including during wartime. Even by 2016, American demographer Murray Feshbach predicted, Russia's population would decrease by up to 17 million people.

The average male born somewhere between Vladivostock and St Petersburg in 1917 could have expected to live to the age of thirty-eight years. His most likely cause of death would have been any of a number of infectious diseases that raged across the region with terrifying regularity. In the hot summers mosquitoes carried malaria, yellow fever, and encephalitis. Ticks passed local haemorrhagic fever viruses. Rats carried bubonic plague. In the winters influenza, bacterial pneumonias, scarlet fever, typhus, tuberculosis, and a host of other diseases swept through hovels high in the Caucasus, mansions in St Petersburg, and cabins in the steppes.

However, thanks to the creation of a vast public health infrastructure, provision of housing, and improved nutrition during the Communist years, the grandsons of those boys that had been born in the year of the October Revolution could expect to live almost twice as long: Russian boys born in 1970 faced an average life expectancy of sixty-five years.

But by 1993 when the first post-Communist generation of Russian boys was born, life expectancy had plummeted to a grim fifty-eight years. And it kept declining, reaching fifty-seven in the autumn of 1998, and fifty-six by that Christmas.

Such a thing would have been utterly inconceivable to Soviet public health planners. With crusading zeal they had pursued the dream of a disease-free workers' state.

'There were huge, fantastic epidemics,' recalled Dr Sergei Pozorovskii, in 1997 the director of the Gamaleya Institute, considered Russia's most prestigious medical research centre. 'Then came World War I, the civil war, and by the end of the 1920s millions were dying of infectious diseases, especially typhus. So The Ruler [Stalin] came out with an eloquent slogan: either lice conquer socialism or socialists conquer lice.'

With a chuckle Pozorovskii admitted that Stalin's command was followed vigorously, but 'not quite democratic ways were used to accomplish this.' The vaccine for typhus hadn't yet been invented, nor were effective antilice pesticides that could kill the insects that carried the deadly bacteria. So, by order of Stalin, every man, woman, and child in the Soviet Union was ordered to a bathhouse, their clothing and bedsheets deloused, and infested homes were often burnt to the ground.

What this first sweeping Soviet public health campaign lacked in scientific finesse it made up for in zeal and, where that failed, authoritarian action. The result was an astounding success that became an international propaganda bonanza. While typhus continued to rage in many capitalist nations the Communists could claim a victory for the proletariat.

Stalin, who had terrible scars all over his face that attested to his childhood battle with smallpox, embraced the battle against infectious diseases. It was wholeheartedly enjoined by the new public health establishment—Stalin-style.

A vast network of sanitation and epidemiology was created, eventually reaching into nearly every village in the nation. Medical schools and sanitation training centres were constructed all over the Soviet Union during the 1920s, churning out specialists for the powerful Sanitation and Epidemiology Service, or SanEp. SanEp had powers akin to those of the KGB. It spied on doctors, looking for deviant behaviour, both medical and political. SanEp agents rounded up infectious disease carriers and removed them from greater society until they either recovered or died. Those who suffered so-called social diseases—such as tuberculosis, syphilis, gonorrhoea, and alcoholism—were publicly named, denounced in their factories and schools, and made to list all other people with whom they might have had intimate contact.

As preventive treatments and vaccines were developed the masses were compelled to undergo immunizations and such at the hands of SanEp. The leaders of SanEp were always loyal Communist Party members, and eager Komsomol (Communist Youth League) volunteers were typically put to the task of rounding up the proletariat for its latest public health intervention.

With time the system of both SanEp and hospitals and clinics became so enormous that it was one of the three biggest lines of employment in the state.

At laboratories such as Gamaleya work focused on inventing and mass-producing antitoxins, vaccines, and eventually antibiotics. After World War II that role shifted to huge so-called biodefence factories—the Soviet equivalent of pharmaceutical plants in the capitalist world—which mass-produced materials for use by SanEp.

During the Khrushchev years of the 1950s the most prestigious biomedical laboratories, such as Gamaleya, became basic research centres, much as they had been before the revolution. The scientists functioned within an elaborate hierarchy, with academics—equivalent to senior PhDs—at the top. For them life was grand. Their offices were often plushly decorated with details taken from bourgeois homes and palaces; they had meals and tea services brought to them by a staff of state-employed servants, and chauffeurs drove their free cars.

In addition SanEp built five plague laboratories, dedicated to the control and eventual eradication of *Yersinia pestis* and its rat and flea carriers.

And by 1970 the goal set officially by the Politburo was nothing less than the complete eradication of all infectious disease in the Soviet Union.

'When we started working we realized that these tasks were hard, if not impossible, to fulfil,' Pozorovskii admitted. 'But for a time that goal was inspiring.'

One by one diseases that had until quite recently devastated Soviet people were, indeed, nearly vanquished: diphtheria, smallpox, cholera, malaria, tuberculosis, typhus, polio, typhoid fever, whooping cough, measles, tick-borne encephalitis, tetanus—all brought under control by SanEp. And if the methods they used were a bit repressive, even cruel, to some people, well, Pozorovskii said, they worked—'and wasn't that what mattered?'

'Then came 1991,' Pozorovskii said, his body visibly slumping, facial muscles sagging. 'The change caused not only political crumbling, but also a crumbling of public health, medical care, and medical science.'

First the Warsaw Pact nations and Baltic states broke away from Soviet influence and ousted their old Communist rulers. Then the Soviet nation ceased to exist, each of the former Socialist Republics splitting off to become fifteen separate nations. Thousands of scientists left the laboratories of Moscow and Siberia for their home countries.

'And starting from 1993 the [Russian] state stopped funding all research subsidies,' Pozorovskii said. 'Starting from 1994 the state stopped funding the overhead of the Institute. But salaries were still paid. It's a laughable salary—the head of a laboratory here receives less than $100 a month.... But then in 1996 we saw more change—no salaries, at all.'

Pozorovskii sighed, nearly breaking down as he concluded, 'The Gamaleya Institute is dying. I feel like I'm a watchman at a cemetery.'

But the real graveyard sentries were those who counted the region's demographic numbers, tallying the grim reversals witnessed after the collapse of the Soviet Union. Among their numbers was Pozorovskii, who died a few weeks after welcoming his American visitor, suffering from, a colleague insisted, 'a broken heart.'

There was no category for broken hearts in the statistical tables of Russian, Ukrainian, Moldavian, and other ex-Soviet epidemiologists. But there were categories for cardiovascular diseases deaths, all of which soared after 1991, in populations from the shipyards of Poland's Gdansk to the ports of Vladivostock. The shift in the body politic was, it seemed, breaking the hearts of the masses.

In a May speech before the Russian Duma Dr N. F. Gerasimenko of the Academy of Medical Sciences summarized the situation in exceptionally strong language. 'We want to make it clear to everybody... that the national security of the country is threatened.'

Gerasimenko then listed a dramatic series of statistics: the Russian mortality rate, he said, was 1.6 times the birth rate in 1992, with about three million young men dying as a direct result of the health-care crisis, or about ten times the number killed in the Afghan and Chechnyan wars, combined. And he said that every third recruit for the army could not be accepted into the armed forces for health reasons in the last few years, as opposed to one in twenty in 1985.

'In other words, the situation is catastrophic,' he said. 'If it doesn't change, only 54 per cent of the sixteen-year-olds [males] will live to pension age. It's even worse than it was in Russia a hundred years ago.'

Gerasimenko turned on the Russian medical system, placing at least part of the blame on state-supported care: 'Article 41 of the Russian Constitution guarantees 'health protection and medical aid to the population,' he continued. 'But, in federal medical centres patients have to pay up to fifty million roubles for surgery—and if they don't have the surgery they die! But where can millions of our citizens get such money, especially when their salaries are delayed?... Further, federal centres in 1996 only received 46 per cent of allocated funds. This is something between financial isch-aemia and fiscal infarction!'

In a report to President Boris Yeltsin from his Committee on Issues of Females, Family and Democracy in 1997, public health experts stated that between 1991 and 1996 the premature death rate for Russians grew by a ghastly 126 per cent, with the most striking increases seen in alcohol-related mortality, accidents, suicides, trauma deaths, respiratory tract infections, infectious disease deaths generally, poisonings, murder, and road traffic accidents.

Between 1990 and 1994 Russian men lost, on average, six years of their life expect-ancies; women lost three years according to a 1998 joint US/Russian study. And death rates in that period soared 100 per cent for men.

Russian epidemiologist Vladimir Shkolnikov and French scientists France Meslé and Jacques Vallin collaborated on a series of studies aimed at appreciating the enor-mity of Russia's gruesome statistics and when, exactly, the great decline commenced. They discovered that the disintegration of Russian public health actually had begun in Soviet days, as early as 1966, and was partially covered up through a series of neat accounting tricks used by the statisticians of that time. For example the statisticians moved the goalposts of the health field by adjusting data for the age of the subjects in ways considered completely unorthodox in the West.

Nevertheless, the Russian/French team asserted that the dramatic escalation in the pace of public health collapse after 1991 was genuine and 'express[es] unambiguously the failure of the health-care system to make any headway in cardiovascular mortality and to contain the upsurge in "man-made disease,"' such as alcoholism, drug abuse, and tuberculosis.

This failure to control heart disease, either through prevention or treatment, appeared even more significant when the researchers compared death trends in Russia to those in France, England, and Wales. During a period when those European areas witnessed fivefold decreases in heart disease death rates, Russia's rose threefold to five-fold from 1970 to 1995. And most of that death rate magnification had never appeared in Soviet official data tables.

Murray Feshbach had spotted it, though. Indeed Feshbach, who was approaching his seventh decade of life as the world neared its millennium, had devoted most of his life and career to finding truth amid Soviet—and after 1991, Russian—obfuscation and 'damnable lies', as some labelled all statistics. Since 1956, working first for the US Census Bureau and then as a professor at Georgetown University in Washington, DC, Feshbach had successively uncovered one horrendous canard, prevarication, or deceit hidden in Soviet data after another. He was obsessed with the pursuit, driven by the same desire to command a field of information as guided his endless searches for rare postage stamps and obscure rocks. A fluent speaker of Russian, Feshbach had been making data-hunting trips to the USSR since 1973. And make no mistake about it: Feshbach was relentless, if not ruthless, in his pursuit of numbers.

Long before the collapse of the Soviet Union occurred Feshbach uncovered evidence of public health failure hidden by the creative accountants in the Kremlin. For example, adult premature death rates started climbing in 1964 right across the USSR, jumping from 6.9 per 1000 adults annually to 10.3 per 1000 in 1980. And by 1980, he discovered, the life expectancy gap between Soviet men and women was more than eleven years—already the widest gender chasm in the world. Buried in 1979 data he found the measles rate in Soviet children was fifteen times that for American young-sters, and the typhoid fever rate was twenty-nine times America's.

In 1980 Feshbach discovered that the Soviets used two creative statistics methods to cover up soaring infant mortality rates. Beginning in 1975 they simply stopped pub-lishing any infant mortality numbers at all, burying the toll of dead babies inside the broader category of deceased children. And then, sometime around 1976, the Soviets redefined 'infant' to be a baby born maturely (after twenty-eight weeks gestation), weighing more than a thousand grams, being of more than thirty-five centimetres in length, and surviving at least seven days after birth. Thus, all premature births were neatly wiped out of the records, eliminating the very group of babies that accounted for the bulk of all American and Western European infant mortality.

The Bronx-born son of Ukrainian immigrant Jews discovered mountains more evidence of public health deterioration throughout the Brezhnev years, including extreme nutritional deficits in the region's children, tremendous shortages in medical equipment and supplies at state hospitals, an adult alcohol-associated death rate that by 1978 was one hundred times that of the United States, and hints of mounting cardiovascular disease problems in the population.

With the Gorbachev era came *glasnost*, or openness, a gold mine for Feshbach. Although *pravda*—truth—didn't immediately surface, *glasnost* gave access to Russian colleagues and tantalizing clues, which in turn led to *pravda*.

What he then saw in the trail of tallies, noted in lengthy, boring columns of fudged data, prompted Feshbach to ask: 'If it's so bad why isn't everybody dead?'

And in answer to his own question Feshbach answered, 'My feeling is they are dead.'

While most Westerners, including the US government employees who had for decades relied on Feshbach's findings, celebrated the end of communism the plump, bespectacled Georgetown University professor declared that calamity had struck. His office reflected the deluge of data suddenly available, stacked in precarious piles that nearly reached the ceiling. Miraculously, when prompted by an incredulous visitor, Feshbach could immediately locate and pull evidence from a seemingly random pile, without toppling the entire mass. As with everything else, Feshbach saw order in what to mere mortals seemed utter chaos. And the order he saw in the ruins of the Soviet Union was calamitous.

'You can look at these figures. See?' he demanded, punching a stubby digit at a Cyrillic column. 'What can you make of these figures? I don't care how exaggerated they are, you have a disaster!'

Feshbach confronted stacks of grim data. 'Look at this one. In the US roughly two hundred to four hundred people in any given year die of alcohol poisoning, okay? Okay, so look. In 1994 fifty thousand Russians died of it. Okay? Okay, now this, syphilis. Incredible! A thirtyfold increase in ten-to-fourteen-year-old Russian girls between 1990 and 1994. See that? How about this. Look. It says—and this is an official document, you see. It says, "38 per cent of babies are born normal." Well what does that mean? It means 62 per cent of all Russian babies born in 1991 were *abnormal!*'

According to Feshbach's crunching of Russia's population data 1992 marked a telltale turning point, from which few civilizations have ever historically recovered. That was the year more people died in the Russian Federation than were born. Every year since then the gap has widened. By January 2000, the Russian death rate was two and a half times its birth rate, and in some regions of the country the death rate was a staggering four times the birth rate.

Of particular concern for the future, Feshbach predicted, was the observation that most premature deaths were in men, aged fifteen to fifty. These were the productive workforce and would-be fathers of the region's future generation. These men were dying in the 1990s at four times the rate of their female peers, and Feshbach asked, 'Where are the men?' He predicted that the 1996 life-expectancy gap of 13.1 years between men and women in Russia would widen by 2010 to 17 years. Given that most of those deaths were among marriageable men, Feshbach predicted a second great crisis loomed as women, unable to find mates, all but stopped bearing children. In such a scenario even the grimmest of population forecasts for 2010—namely, that Russia's population will have fallen back to 1917 levels—would fall short of the eventual reality.

In 1994 UNICEF decried the regional situation as 'a societal crisis of unexpected proportions, unknown implications and uncertain solutions. . . . The "excess mortality" accumulated between 1989–93 is far greater than that wrought by the Great Depression of 1929–33 in North America. The "excess mortality" over the entire 1989–93 period amounts to approximately 800 000 people, a figure that reveals all too clearly the severity of the current crisis.'

Why was this nightmare occurring? Why had the world's largest public health safety net completely failed?

II

Around forty-three thousand people have died in Russia this year from drinking low-quality vodka, the Interior Ministry said today.
—Agence-France Presse, November 28, 1997

The recent upsurge in criminality, in synergy with alcoholism, is above all the after-math of the sweeping economic reforms and accompanying lower standards of living and of the dismantling of the former political and administrative system.
—Shkolnikov, Meslé, and Vallin, 1996[2]

Drinking is the joy of the Rus. We cannot live without it.
—Vladimir of Kiev, founder of the Russian state, tenth century

On a frigid, dank night in Moscow, beefy bodyguards, armed with automatic weapons, served as sentinels, eyeing the entrance to the posh eighteenth-century building that until recently housed the Writers' Union, and had been occupied at one time by famed Soviet author Maxim Gorky.

Known to Muscovites as the Griboyedov House, named after its original aristocratic owner, the mansion was a crucial location for all Soviet-era writers. It was here that judgements were passed: this writer deserves a free trip to the Crimea to give a lecture; this enemy-of-the-people author merits a trip to the gulag! And it was here that the proletariats' scribes—voices of the supposedly classless society—dined on meals available to precious few other Soviet citizens.

With the fall of the Soviet Union and Communist Party the state no longer subsidized the grand, palatial writers' restaurant, so a private company took over its management. By the late 1990s the former hall of politically correct purveyors of prose was

Moscow's most elegant restaurant, complete with waiters attired in formal tuxedos, sparkling crystal chandeliers, concert pianists, ample supplies of beluga caviar, and the best reserve supplies of Russian vodka, Georgian wines, and Armenian cognacs to be found anywhere in the world.

While the French embassy staff enjoyed a private party in the upstairs room that once had housed Gorky, diners quietly feasted in the main hall, sipping vodka while listening to the lilting tones of Chopin produced by a talented concert pianist.

One group of diners deviated. Dressed in black turtleneck sweaters and leather Gucci coats, signifying that the four men were gangsters, the quartet was accompanied by a younger, spandex-attired woman. The men drank heavily, growing collectively louder with each round of fiery Russian vodka and peppery Georgian wine, their language becoming increasingly vulgar. The plump leader of the group in a grandiose gesture withdrew a two-inch-thick wad of US $100 notes from his pocket, waved it in the air for all to see, and called out for the bill. An obedient waiter brought the bill, noting that it was illegal to accept payment in foreign money.

After glancing at the bill the head gangster sneered and in a movement so rapid that its details could not be discerned the gangsters had the waiter on the floor and were pummelling the poor man with clenched fists and stabbing forks. Little noise was produced, as the drunken mobsters were professionals and the waiter quickly went into shock. The pianist never missed a note, and most of the posh restaurant's clientele seemed unaware of what was transpiring.

A team of waiters, apparently accustomed to such drunken outbursts, formed a human wedge, plowing into the fray, rescuing their unconscious colleague and repairing to the kitchen. The gangsters gave chase; the kitchen door was bolted.

'So much for our dessert,' muttered one of the few diners who had paid heed to the bout. Seamlessly the pianist switched to a Cole Porter tune, and the gangsters, puffed with victory, poured themselves another round of cognac and laughed loudly. The maître d' quietly approached the robust chief mobster, whispering a negotiation stance on behalf of the restaurant. And in an instance—*pow!*—he, too, was on the floor, showered with sharp jabs and fisted blows. As he crawled out in retreat, the pianist—who had yet to miss a note—began to sweat, her eyes widening in fear. The clientele, however, remained largely oblivious.

A triumphant gangster rolled the spirit trolley to their table, and the criminal quintet happily served themselves vintage French cognac. The staff remained safely behind locked doors. The pianist moved to Gershwin's *Rhapsody in Blue*.

One of the security guards that had been on post outside the restaurant entered, moving his hulking, muscular frame with deliberate nonchalance. He wore a suit that seemed to be bursting at the seams under the stress of his impressive musculature: a Russian Arnold Schwarzenegger. Recognizing a fellow-professional the gangsters stiffened and, after exchanging words, rose and headed toward the restaurant's exit. Peace, it seemed, was at hand.

But suddenly, standing at the pianist's back in the restaurant's threshold, the head gangster spun on his heels and swiftly slapped the security guard back and forth across his cheeks. In a microsecond the guard had an automatic magnum lodged against the chief mobster's left temple. And instantly a gang lieutenant had his arm stretched over his boss's shoulder, a pistol pointed back at the guard.

The pianist ceased playing Gershwin and crawled out of crossfire range. Some diners, finally taking notice of the escalating stand off, quietly moved their chairs out of the presumed line of fire and watched. Seconds passed, neither man lowering his weapon. Waiters, peering out of the kitchen, collectively held their breaths.

Suddenly a balalaika player performing for the upstairs French Embassy crowd shouted, 'Hey! Hey! Hey!' and was greeted with a rousing stomping and cheering from his French audience. The performance was a classic tourist treat, the sort of thing Westerners who had seen *Dr Zhivago* more than once savoured. The guard and gangsters stifled a shared laugh and, having found a mutually face-saving way to stand down, lowered their weapons. Negotiations ensued, the chief mobster dismissed his sidekicks, grabbed his girlfriend, and returned to savour yet another round of cognac.

When the waiters returned, attending to their tables, the cause of what was nearly at least two murders was clarified. The mobsters, it seemed, didn't like the exchange rate the restaurant was using to compute dollar-to-rouble values. They were willing to kill, in front of scores of witnesses, over what amounted to less than a ten-dollar dispute.

All over the former Communist region murders, suicides, car accidents, and outright alcohol poisonings were occurring in record numbers, fuelled by elegant cognac, run-of-the-mill vodka, and, more often, cheap rotgut moonshine.

Outside the Siberian city of Ulan Ude, a village has been created downwind of the municipal rubbish dump. Fifty-two adults and eight children live in a pine grove that is covered in an artificial forest floor made of refuse that blows off the ten-story-high, redolent waste heaps. The loose group of otherwise homeless Siberians had dug holes in the earth, some twelve feet deep and ten feet wide, in which they live, even during the harsh, snowbound winters.

Wooden beams stabilize their underground homes, which are lined with items scavenged off the nearby rubbish heaps. The group lives without running water, electricity, heat, or fresh food, says Nikolai Constantinovich, the encampment's unofficial leader. Most of them were cheated out of their housing in the city, talked into selling when property was privatized but too naive—and eager for quick cash—to realize their apartments' true values. Unable, with the paltry sums they obtained, to buy new homes the three score Ulan Udeans had ended up homeless, Constantinovich explains.

Seventy-year-old Alexander pops his head above ground, sees strangers, and ducks back into his hovel. Constantinovich allays Alexander's fear that the police have arrived, and the ageing pensioner, his breath thick with the smell of moonshine, emerges, greeting his visitors.

'We never, never could imagine that we would end up here,' says Alexander. 'We were supposedly living in a worker's paradise. Well, I was a worker—where is my paradise?'

During the day, the children's job is to search through the stinking dump for saleable items that can be rescued from the vicious rats that live there and can be converted into cash. It's a disgusting task, which, Alexander tearfully says, 'breaks my heart,' but the children obediently return each day with their sacks full of items.

Then, the adults take turns riding a bus into the city for supplies—including bread, to survive on, and alcohol.

'Don't think badly of us,' cries Alexander's neighbour, middle-aged Lena, her face reddened by years of alcoholism. 'We live underground, but we are not murderers. The drink has just got us.'

At nine on a dreary Moscow morning homeless Nikolai Yelizarov, a thirty-four-year-old ex-convict, is in line, as he has been every weekday for twelve months, trying to get a work permit. He was robbed one day as he lay unconscious somewhere in Moscow, lost in an alcoholic stupor. The thief got Yelizarov's most valuable possessions—Moscow residency and work permits. Without these, Yelizarov says, his blue eyes tearing, 'I cannot have a home, and I cannot have a job. Ever since [the robbery] I've been dealing with this damned bureaucracy.'

Yelizarov 'deals with the bureaucracy' by arising from whatever hovel he's shivered in the night before, downing a high-proof rotgut, and queuing up to beg, again, for new papers.

In Moscow's Pushkin Square metro station a middle-aged drunkard tries to enter an exit-only turnstile and bounces off the machinery, landing headfirst on the tiled floor. Stunned, he lies semi-conscious for several minutes while a gang of fourteen-year-old boys, high on heroin-and-speed cocktails, loudly mock, 'the filthy old drunk,' kicking at the downed man. Unable to comprehend what has happened, the drunk pulls himself up onto his feet. The boys stand aside, laughing and shouting, 'Come on, Old Man, you can do it. Walk!' Once again the man tries to enter the wrong way, is rebuffed, and lands on his head. The boys surround him, ready for another round of mockery, but lose interest when they realize that this time the drunk is truly unconscious.

By the mid-1990s public drunkenness was so common as to leave the visitor uncertain what was reality: the steady view seen by the sober eye, or the wavering, blurred perspective of the throngs of swaying fellow pedestrians. In devastated old industrial cities, from Bohemia to Vladivostock, unemployed men, no longer able to imagine the future, simply pulled daily alcohol curtains over the present.

Alcohol-inspired violence and self-destruction were not new to the Eastern European world. No. But after 1991 it was far more extreme and dangerous. As was the case with abortions and other basic public health indicators the rise of alcoholism and its associated catastrophes was the result of a trend dating to Soviet years that spiked dramatically after 1991.

In 1999 just over 1.2 million babies were born in Russia, for example, while more than 2.1 million people died. Any nation with such a profoundly greater death, versus birth, rate was bound to shrink dramatically. Some of the contraction was due to a plummeting birth rate, which, in turn, was driven regionally by astonishing abortion rates.

The trend began during the late 1970s in large part because of the very poor quality of Soviet-made contraceptives. Condoms, diaphragms, and other safe forms of contraception were virtually unavailable, and Soviet-made birth control pills contained higher levels of hormones than were found in Western-made products—and, therefore, induced more horrendous side-effects, including cardiac failure.

So women in the Soviet Union and Eastern Europe accepted abortion as their primary form of birth control. The numbers of abortions performed every year in Soviet state-run clinics rose steadily, reaching 7 228 000 in 1988, or 1.2 officially registered abortions for every one live birth.

A survey conducted by the Zhordania Institute of Human Reproduction in Tblisi in 1995 revealed that the average Georgian woman, by the age of twenty-six, had undergone ten to twelve abortions, with dangerous illegal procedures outnumbering officially registered hospital ones by two-to-one. And though slight improvements in the Georgian economy subsequently lowered the abortion rate, in 1996 the country of 5.5 million people witnessed 25 000 legal abortions and at least 50 000 illegal ones, the institute found.

'I have met women who have had more than thirty abortions. The highest number I ever saw was a sixty-nine-year-old woman who told me she had sixty abortions,' Institute director Dr Archil Khomassuridze asserted. As the leading expert on family planning for Georgia and the Soviet Union, Khomassuridze was responsible for filing fertility and abortion data with the World Health Organization in Geneva. In the late 1980s the WHO computer rejected his reports because it wasn't programmed to believe data claiming any woman underwent more than twenty lifetime abortions.

As shocking as these figures may seem, Khomassuridze explained that he understood, and sympathized, with the women, for two reasons. First, 'I am surprised how they can exist. How they can work. How they can have sexual lives. Why they don't hate their sexual partners. I still don't understand—not only for Georgian women but Russian women, too. I have deep sympathy.'

Their lives were not only filled with financial difficulty, Khomassuridze explained, but with abusive, often drunken, men. Not only was sex often involuntary for the women, they told Khomassuridze, it was rarely pleasurable even when mutually consenting. When asked how they abided the brutality of their lives as prostitutes, hookers in Russia, Estonia, and Ukraine typically said, 'It's no worse than marriage.'

Although some women were heavy drinkers, alcoholism regionally was an overwhelmingly male phenomenon. And vodka, when consumed at Russian levels, drove men to astounding heights of violence and brutality committed against their wives, girlfriends, children, even suicidally against themselves.

In the six years Mikhail Gorbachev led the Soviet Union, he had saved, conservatively, more than a half million lives in the region—but not because of any military or political decision he made.

Startled to learn that in 1983 Soviets were consuming, on average, three litres a year of pure ethanol equivalent, Gorbachev waged an all-out war on alcoholism, using the classically repressive apparatus of the Soviet state. Warehouses were destroyed; illegal sellers were jailed; vodka prices were artificially raised; and police were given free rein to arrest public drinkers.

But in 1988, the campaign collapsed, a surprise victim of Gorbachev's own political reforms, *perestroika* and *glasnost*. Overnight, alcohol so regained its high stature that Vladimir Zhirinovsky, an ultra-nationalist presidential hopeful, raised campaign funds selling his own brand of vodka, picturing himself on the label attired as Vladimir Lenin.

It is estimated that Gorbachev saved 600 000 lives over three years, dropping the combined incidence of alcohol poisoning, cirrhosis of the liver, and alcohol-induced violence and accidents to 179 deaths per 100 000 in 1988, a level not seen since 1965.

But after the fall of the USSR per capita consumption jumped by 600 per cent and incidence of alcohol-related deaths followed suit. Government figures from 1995 showed a rate approaching 500 per 100 000, in contrast to an American alcohol-associated death rate in 1995 of just 77. Russia witnessed a 550 per cent increase in alcohol psychosis cases between 1989 and 1993.

Regionally violence, particularly against women, rose in tandem with soaring male alcoholism. Up to ten per cent of women in the region, according to UNICEF in 1999, reported experiencing at least one beating from a spouse that was severe enough to require hospitalization, and about a fifth of married women complained of regular beating.

Some estimates were that eighty per cent of all Russian men were alcoholics, consuming in 1999—*on average*—600 grams of drink a day, or roughly three litres of vodka every week. The male alcohol poisoning death rate in Russia was about 200 times that of the United States.

Murray Feshbach argued that Russians were not only drinking more than they had in the past, they were also drinking more dangerously. What was marketed as vodka or whisky in Moscow could be anything from 100 proof genuine vodka to 'rotgut moonshine,' aftershave, or even—commonly—jet fuel. And much of the alcohol was sold in pop-top, non-resealable bottles that prompted the drinker to consume the entire contents in a single sitting.

'It's not just that consumption is high, although it is,' Feshbach said. 'It's the way they consume. It's chug-a-lug vodka drinking that starts at the office during the morning coffee break and goes right into the night-time.'

Drinking on the job was a practice that went across all levels of society in the region, even among health-care workers.

At a Moscow hospital a visitor was invited to join a cognac party among doctors, held on a weekday at 10 a.m. In the Arctic city of Talnakh a group of four cardiac physicians downed a bottle of champagne and a couple of rounds of cognac over lunch—a routine break, they said. And in the physicians' lounge at a Kiev hospital, surgeons relaxed between operations by sharing a bottle of vodka. A private doctor in Bohemia proudly displayed a large and diverse alcohol selection, spread out all over his office, most bottles having been given to the physician in lieu of monetary payment for medical services.

This form of abusive binge drinking was historic in the region, although not at the levels being evidenced in the post-USSR era. 'Russians drink, essentially, to obliterate themselves, to blot out the tedium of life, to warm themselves from the winters,' Hedrick Smith wrote in 1976 during the Brezhnev years 'and they eagerly embrace the escapism it offers.'

Two Russian customs added to the problem: one, that a vodka bottle once opened must be finished, never recorked; and two, that a shot glass of vodka must be downed in one gulp. Violation of either custom within the male community in particular was roundly considered rude and insulting to one's host, and prima-facie evidence of a lack of manhood.

Dr Boris Logna had watched this alcohol trend closely over the years from his vantage point as chief of the largest poison control centre in Estonia, located in the capital city of Tallinn. During the Gorbachev campaign, Logna said, the country had about 120 alcohol poisoning deaths per year. In 1995, there were 400 such deaths in Tallinn alone.

'There is no national alcohol policy here,' Logna says, echoing complaints from his counterparts throughout the former Communist bloc. 'As you see, everywhere alcohol is for sale—even in petrol stations at night. More people go late to petrol stations for a drink than to fill their tanks.'

The problem also started early: teenage arrests for alcohol-related crimes more than tripled from 1991 to 1997, and suicide rates—which many health experts link directly to drinking—were also on the rise.

For teens and adults alike, alcohol was a way of life that was easily available, legal, and remarkably cheap.

Because export-quality vodka, such as Stolichnaya Cristall, sold for about thirty dollars a litre in Moscow or Kiev, few local people would dream of wasting their money on such a product. Most vodka was sold for less than eight dollars a litre, and some was available in street kiosks for a dollar.

'Between December 1990 and December 1994, consumer prices [in Russia] increased by 2020 times for all goods and services, by 2154 times for food products, but only 653 times for alcoholic beverages,' stated a report issued jointly by the California-based Rand Corporation and Moscow's Centre for Demography and Human Ecology. 'This means that over this period, in relative terms, alcohol became over three times cheaper than these other products.'

Adult alcohol consumption in 1996 was 18 litres a year of pure alcohol, or the rough equivalent of 38 litres of 100-proof vodka, according to the Russian Ministry of Health. That's equivalent to consuming one and a half bottles of high-proof vodka weekly. The rate for other countries in the region was as high: in Estonia, for instance, it was 16.5 litres annually; in Ukraine, 17 litres.

Bad as that was, it soon got much worse in Russia, Belarus, Ukraine, and other parts of the region. In the fall of 1998 Russia's President Yeltsin announced that Russia's populationwide average had reached more than 25 litres of pure ethanol equivalent a year. Adjusting for age, that implied that Russian adults were—*on average*—consuming an astonishing three bottles of high-proof vodka a week.

Another terrible trend emerged from the adult alcoholism upswing: child abuse and abandonment.

At Father Alexander's crisis centre for children in Odessa, Ukraine, dozens of rag-clothed youngsters live together, abandoned by their parents or escapees from homes of poverty and alcoholism. Young Misha, for example, has lived in the sparsely deco-rated quarters of Father Alexander's haven—a converted nursery school—for two months. He sports a hip pierced ear and scratches his head absentmindedly while making conversation, probably because of the lice that infect his scalp. Admired by the younger children for his tough-guy swagger, the blue-eyed blond fourteen-year-old loses his cool when he tries to explain why he is now homeless.

'My parents drink a lot. And then they humiliate me and beat me. The problem is they don't like me,' Misha says, tears drenching his pink cheeks, his voice cracking. 'Even my grandmother doesn't like me. I often went to school hungry,' Misha concludes.

Misha's story is echoed a thousand times over by the sorrowful tales of the ultimate victims of the alcoholism and drug abuse sweeping from Prague to Vladivostock: the children. Pyotor, for example, left his three sisters and brother when he was ten, moving into Alexander's haven because his parents drank themselves—and their children—into homelessness and, he concluded, 'There is nothing to eat.'

Eleven-year-old Andrei ended up in the centre after his stepfather in a drunken rage poisoned Andrei's mother. Now his stepfather is on the run from the police and Andrei is alone in the world.

Since 1988, Catholic priest Father Alexander says, the number of abandoned chil-dren in Odessa has increased twentyfold. And for those who still have parents and homes, alcohol and poverty often makes abandonment seem preferable.

'Nowadays we have children living at home whose malnutrition is even worse than the street kids,' Father Alexander says. 'I know boys who weren't allowed to go to school in winter because they had no shoes. So one wrapped his feet in plastic bags. They eat once a day and work as cleaning boys.'

When he was eighteen years old Father Alexander took the unusual step of getting baptized as a Catholic and undergoing training for the priesthood—political suicide during Communist days. He studied in Poland, Brussels, and Rome, ultimately returning to establish this ramshackle home for wayward and abandoned children. Plump, bearded, and bombastic Father Alexander has few friends in the Odessa power structure and is openly hated by the police, who suspect most Catholic clerics.

But, he claims, without him children like Misha, Pyotor, and Andrei would have nowhere to go.

In 1997 the Moscow Human Rights Research Centre estimated that there were a million homeless children in Russia; the government said 700 000. No one knew how many more children had parents in homes but were left largely to survive on their own because of their parents' alcoholism. In Russia a term was coined to describe these children: the Lost Generation.

In Moscow, Sapar Kulyanov runs a small charitably funded shelter for children, some 92 per cent of whom come from families of drug or alcohol abuse. Kulyanov, a gentle forty-five-year-old man, has witnessed 'an avalanche', he says, of abandoned and abused children since the fall of communism.

'It's true that there was less openness in Soviet days and the problem existed before,' Kulyanov says. 'But I am absolutely sure the bulk of this is new, because of social change.... When *perestroika* started all the old links and ties broke. Families had to confront their problems. Some families started to drown their problems in drink, and children had to learn to live their own lives.'

Most of the children in Kulyanov's centre suffer classic symptoms of parental abuse: bed-wetting, crying out in their sleep, nightmares, inability to respond to direct questions. Eight-year-old Katia, for example, boldly approaches a stranger and responds to a smile with heartbreaking warmth, crawling into the adult's arms. But she cannot answer when asked about her parents' names or whereabouts. When asked, Katia's face, framed in a blue Russian scarf, takes on the innocent look of an angel, but all she can recall of her past is that 'at home I was in school and I graduated from first grade.'

She remembers nothing more, and stares blankly into the eyes of a stranger when asked, 'And where was your home?'

Asked to tell his story eleven-year-old Vanya reluctantly jumps from a high perch to the floor and collects himself into a ball, sitting on his heels, his striped shirt-covered arms wrapped tightly around his knees. Vanya can't control the involuntary nervous tics in his face that make him blink and give his cheeks sudden ripples. But the tics are his only animation: he is otherwise almost without affect, seemingly emotionless.

When Vanya was just nine years old, he explains with utter lack of emotion, his parents' drinking escalated. His father—whom Vanya says he detests—beat the boy and his mother repeatedly. And his mother drowned her sorrows in moonshine purchased at local kiosks. The bad drink drove her insane, and escalated the violence in the household.

One day, after his father had committed a night of household bloodletting, Vanya's mother gathered the child's belongings into a small bag, hers in a larger one, and said, 'We're leaving.' She dragged little Vanya to the massive Belarus train station, located on the western end of Moscow. He had never been there before, and Vanya stared at all of the strange immigrants who seemed to be living in the station. There were the so-called Blacks from the Caucasus, the Orientals from southern Siberia and Central Asia, the White Siberians...packed so densely that the child and his mother could barely squeeze by.

And then it happened. As a train was about to leave the station Vanya's mother let go of his hand and jumped into the departing train, never looking back.

'I lost her at the railway station,' Vanya says, taking blame for what Kulyanov says was a classic case of abandonment. For a full year—his tenth year of life—Vanya survived on the streets of Moscow, begging for food and sleeping in a telephone booth. He discovered hundreds of other similarly abandoned children, and they formed a gang to protect one another against the older bullies of the streets.

Now Vanya's only emotional moment comes when he thinks of the other street waifs: 'I wish they would come here,' to the shelter, he says.

Kulyanov's centre was one of only five in all of Moscow—and that's five more than existed in virtually every other city in the region. There were, instead, old Soviet orphanages, famed for the abusive way in which they warehoused abandoned and 'defective' children—those born with disabilities of one kind or another. Kulyanov was trying to build a Western-style network of halfway houses for children, focused on rehabilitating and reuniting Russian families. Until 1993 such activities, even shelters, were illegal in Russia, and it was illegal until 1996 to remove—under *any* circumstances— a child from his parents. Even when a child was hospitalized prior to 1996 with evidence of life-threatening beatings the youngsters would, if they survived, simply be returned to the home of their tormenters.

Seated in his office before a table coated with the photos of abused and neglected children, Kulyanov points out the stacks of stuffed animals and toys that clutter every other surface in the room. Such things, he said, were not found in the homes of these abused children. When they reached the shelter most of these children received the very first playthings they ever had.

'In the past we had many expenses covered by the state, greater egalitarianism in income without such extremes,' forty-five-year-old Kulyanov softly continues. 'I grew up in a safe society. After school we went to Young Pioneers clubs and lessons and sports, all available for free....But now there are no children's clubs, no Young Pioneers, no puppet shows....'

'So now kids get their fun from criminals. From motley crews of thieves and drug dealers,' Kulyanov said.

In Novosibirsk, Siberia, the Club 888 was a hip oasis filled with ironic Communist memorabilia displayed as kitsch, complete with an empty but bona fide nuclear bomb shell painted with a bright red star and CCCP, which is Cyrillic for USSR. Adolescent artists and college intellectuals huddled in niches throughout the labyrinthine nightclub, drinking, smoking, and debating their futures.

'I'm just a human, rolling through life,' boasts twenty-year-old diskjockey Sevi. 'I'm totally against drugs. My choice is vodka. I'm an alcoholic!'

Fyodor adjusts his black leather motorcycle jacket, denounces Moscow (as Siberians are frequently wont to do), and declares, 'Heroin is an American drug! Our drugs are different. We take drugs as camouflage—we are only pretending to give up.'

That said, he hoists his vodka and murmurs to twenty-two-year-old Sergei that perennial presidential candidate Zhirinovsky is trying to win over the youth with vodka—and may succeed.

Sergei shakes his head, reminding Fyodor that they have all experimented with shooting opium extracts and amphetamines. The group of young men grows momentarily quiet, the only sounds the background rock 'n' roll and the gentle sucking noises they make as they all simultaneously drag on their American cigarettes.

'What is a Russian?' they are asked.

'Drinking,' eighteen-year-old Alex answers. 'And loneliness. No one is lonelier than a Russian.'

Later, when the discussion turns to alcohol's effects on their future, Sergei blurts out a bit of his past. 'I tried to commit suicide,' he says, pulling up his black leather sleeve to reveal the scars of slit wrists.

'Me too!' Alex says, displaying a similar set of scars, and quickly, all five of the young men in the group roll up their sleeves to the astonishment of a reporter, excitedly comparing suicide methods and scarred reminders.

Sergei then speaks up again, silencing the group when he takes a visitor's hand and raises it to his temple. 'Here, feel this,' he says as the visitor traces the outline of a bullet still lodged in his skull, left over from a failed attempt to blow out his brains. 'I thought suicide was the best drug.'

Psychologist Anna Terentjeva said that the feelings expressed by the young men of Novosibirsk were typical of what she's heard throughout the region. On the staff of the Moscow-based drug group NAN, which stands for 'No to Alcoholism and Drug Addiction,' she said she saw a steady daily stream of young men and women similar to those at Club 888.

The issues for many of these young men and women 'has to do with recognizing oneself, one's identity,' she says, adding, 'they think they have nothing else' other than alcohol.

'What is self?' she asks. 'Where are the borders of me versus us? This is all new. The [Soviet] state used to decide such things. The value of one's self was not supported. Individualism and personal reflection were discouraged, even penalized.'

Terentjeva's staff had just completed surveys in Moscow colleges that revealed a startling 100 per cent of the students have tried drugs; all drank hard liquor, and half of them said that they use heroin, other narcotics, or amphetamines regularly. In their survey responses most of the young Muscovites said that they saw no other alternative—no other way to face each day—except inebriated or stoned.

At Club 888 Sergei changed tables, plopping down under a speaker that blasted rock 'n' roll. For the first time since meeting the visiting foreigner Sergei smiles, content to hear his favorite tune: *Revolution in Paradise.*

III

There are no conditions to which a man cannot become used, especially if he sees that all around him are living the same way.
—Leo Tolstoy, *Anna Karenina*

Beside a white concrete bandshell that protrudes into the Angara River, dozens of teenagers are dancing, dressed in outfits that imitate the looks of American rock videos. The lyrics to a techno-pop tune are blaring in the background: 'Here we go, here we play! It's revolution in paradise!'

It is May Day, the traditional Communist day for celebrating the triumphs of the proletariat. But today, the teens celebrate nothing more, or less, than the end of winter. They couldn't care less about politics. The Siberian teens of Irkutsk flirt, frolic, and strut, as do adolescents the world over. One draws admiring throngs of girls as he strolls nonchalantly into the bandshell, dressed in a genuine Nike jacket and trousers made from an American flag, one leg the stars, the other red and white stripes.

The first generation to come of age absent the social restrictions of the Soviet state, these teens seem healthy enough. But to hear their parents talk, there is a generational time bomb of cancer, genetic mutation, immune deficiency, and disease hidden beneath their youthful glow. These youngsters are damaged goods, they say, weakened to the genetic level by a dual legacy of environmental devastation and misanthropic social engineering.

'The Russian gene pool has been destroyed,' Dr Askold Maiboroda, dean of the Federal Medical University in Irkutsk, explained. 'First there were Stalin's slaughters of millions of people, especially the Jews and the most creative and intelligent people. Then the Nazis slaughtered more of the strongest people in the Great Patriotic War. Then more perished in the gulags—our best minds: artists, writers, poets. And now we suffer this environmental assault.'

'We have been weakened. Our genes are damaged,' he said. 'You cannot expect much from the Russian people—do not ask much of us.'

It was a jarring view, to say the least. But it was a perspective widely shared by physicians and parents from Warsaw to Sakhalin—labelled Chernobyl Syndrome by those who believed it to be an example of mass psychosis. And no one—from the doctors working in the small cities throughout the former Soviet Union to the medical experts located in the region's grandest cities—knew whether this view was based on fact or fear fuelled by regionwide feelings of helplessness.

Certainly there was strong anecdotal evidence of a link between cancer and the Chernobyl nuclear power plant explosion. And there was equally strong anecdotal evidence that the rape of the land in places like Noril'sk and Murmansk, key mining and industrial centres, contributed to rising incidence of cancer, cardiovascular disease, and the like.

But there were very few focused, well-planned general population studies that allowed these links to be viewed in either a historical or scientific context. Indeed, during Soviet days most key industrial centres, nuclear power plants, and military installations weren't even on official maps, and some seventy entire cities were classified as state secrets, their very names protected by a veil of KGB surveillance. In another sixty or so cities, where chemical weapons were manufactured, it was illegal during Soviet days to publish any scientific information regarding local pollution. Similarly, it was illegal to study the environmental impacts of the Soviet nuclear power or weapons industries, or even ask where the nuclear waste was dumped.

Prior to 1991, therefore, no legitimate academic departments of toxicology, environmental sciences, human environmental epidemiology, or epidemiological oncology existed in the Soviet Union. There was no trained pool of scientists who could sift through the evidence, separating fact from fiction.

The first time the Soviet government tried to confront the pollution issue came in 1988. In a startling address to the nation, then-Soviet leader Mikhail Gorbachev said that fifty million Soviet citizens were living in 102 cities in which air pollution exceeded the USSR health standards by more than tenfold.

In the following years the Yeltsin government determined that, minimally, two hundred cities in Russia alone posed 'ecological danger to human health' due to toxic pollution of the air and/or water.

And the facts—the horrible ecological truths—didn't really begin to be revealed until 1994 when Article 7 of the Russian State Secrets Act was enacted, requiring publication of long-clandestine environmental data.

The result was a regional collective gasp of horror and a tendency among caregivers simply to throw up their hands in defeat, blaming all public health crises—even the staggering regional demographics—on pollution and radiation.

The Chernobyl incident was a good case in point. Precise figures on the number of people exposed to fallout from the Chernobyl meltdown don't exist. Most Moscow authorities have said it was fewer than ten thousand, whereas the Ukrainians say more than thirty-four million of their countrymen were exposed. Not a single aspect of the Chernobyl incident—from details of what occurred on April 26, 1986, to how many Ukrainians, Belarusans, Russians, and Moldavians were subsequently taken ill—is settled.

'For years after the explosion, physicians would just tell parents that every ailment in their children is related to Chernobyl,' psychiatrist Semyon Gluzman, a member of the Joint Ukrainian/American Project to Study Post-Chernobyl Children, explained. 'But this is not so. It's just an outsized reaction to all the lies we were told when Chernobyl occurred.'

The April 25, 1986 Chernobyl nuclear power plant disaster ranked as the largest civilian nuclear contamination event in history. Radioactive fallout blanketed 17 million acres of Ukraine and then moved north-west to cover Belarus, St Petersburg and western Russia, eastern Poland, eastern Germany, the Baltic States, and Scandinavia.

Hardest hit, of course, was a circular area of 30 kilometres around the Chernobyl complex. It is still officially dubbed the Alienation Zone.

Encircled by a security perimeter, the Alienation Zone was at the dawn of the twenty-first century closed to all but Chernobyl employees and government approved visitors. Ghost towns dotted the zone. More than 135 000 former residents fled for their lives in April 1986, never returning to pull the sheets off their clotheslines: eleven years later shreds of fabric flapped in the wind, offering anthropological clues to the lives once lived here. Once-cultivated fields had gone fallow. Baby pine trees sprouted like weeds out of former potato fields.

Closer to the Chernobyl site, 100-foot-tall steel structures that looked like the Imperial Army's megatanks in *The Empire Strikes Back* stood rusted into rigid positions. Weeds surrounded their footings; the cables and pulleys that once were functional components of the hulking steel cranes dangled and creaked in the wind. The ground was brown, trees few and far between.

Eleven years after the explosion, Prypat City, which once housed most of the Chernobyl workforce, was empty save for a few black crows and three Ukrainian army guards who lazily smoked cigarettes. The only sound in Prypat City, except for crows, was a vague hum from one of the still functioning reactors at the power plant, located more than a mile away.

The risk of protest actions by alienated workers is rising, claims Chernobyl information officer Mikhail Bogdonov. 'The [Ukrainian] legislature now forbids the personnel to go on strike. I wouldn't talk of sabotage—it's practically impossible. The person who is normal, sane, it's unimaginable that he would do something harmful. But of course it's natural one who works at the controls and he's anxious about money for his family, his children, you can say his attitude is not what it should be,' Bogdonov said, shrugging his shoulders.

Every day the 6252 Chernobyl workers pass by a large silver bust of Lenin as they enter the building, then show their security passes and walk through metal detectors. There is little chatter or animation among the grim-faced nuclear workers. A visitor was not permitted to speak to workers inside the Chernobyl facility or to people spotted in the Alienation Zone.

The workers know that Ukranian president Leonid Kuchma, eager to please future NATO allies, had agreed to shut down all the Chernobyl reactors by 2000, reinforce the concrete sarcophgus that currently enshrouds the damaged reactor,[4] and remove the nuclear cores from the other reactors. But by mid-2000, decommissioning had yet to commence, and Ukrainian president Leonid Kuchma claimed that there wasn't adequate evidence of cancer in Chernobyl workers to warrant an immediate shutdown.

'My friend worked here since before the accident and he's still healthy,' biologist Boris Oskolkov, chief of the Chernobyl Ecology Service, says dismissively, speaking broken English. 'What concerns cancer and other long-term effects of radiation, weakened immunity, and increased morbidity—there are no reliable data to prove such increases.... The main factor affecting morbidity is the psychological effect of the stress of the accident. That psychological effect is in place. Definitely. But it doesn't have any physical foundation.'

The blond, goateed Oskolkov discounts the infirmity and disability claims filed by hundreds of Chernobyl workers since 1986 as mere ploys to obtain early pensions and sick pay. Though it is illegal to eat wild boar or mushrooms from the Alienation Zone, Oskolkov insists the food, water, soil, and air of the area are now completely safe. And due to reports from his staff the Ukrainian government has loosened up regulation of the Alienation Zone, allowing about one thousand people to move back into the outer perimeter area.

But scientists from Russia's Severtsov Institute of Ecological and Evolutionary Problems measured topsoil samples in villages both inside the Alienation Zone and up to one hundred kilometres north-east in Russia and Belarus. They found gamma radiation levels of 100 to 320 micro-Roentgens per hour.[5] That is, according to sources at Brookhaven National Laboratory, fourteen to forty-six times the amount of background radiation emanating from the soils of Long Island, New York, even in close proximity to that US nuclear research facility.

In 1996 the Centre for Russian Environment Policy, an independent scientific group based in Moscow, published strong evidence of radioactive contamination and cellular mutations in plants and wild animals collected from the Bryansk oblast and eastern Belarus.

And Ukrainian physicist Valery Kukhar readily conceded that the Chernobyl ecology would never be the same. Extensive research indicated that the overall extent of biodiversity in plants and animals was unchanged after the 1986 radioactive catastrophe. But the comparative sizes of animal and plant populations, and therefore the overall balance of the ecology, changed radically. Concentrations of plutonium isotopes found in soil samples up to ten years after the accident exceeded those produced by *all* nuclear weapons tests that were conducted in 1960, combined—in some cases by a factor of 89.

Invertebrate insects were decimated by the radiation, some species of spiders and worms nearing the local level of extinction.

Among small mammals, such as voles, rats, and mice, populations initially fell, then restored to pre-1986 levels. But the nuts and plant seeds these animals were consuming were radioactive, and there was evidence of declining photosynthesis rates in trees and other large flora, resulting in growth stunting.

Local fish were highly contaminated with Cs^{137} radionuclides, and several species showed signs of abnormal development. Frogs and other amphibians showed similar evidence of radiation-induced abnormality, and their immune systems—levels of functional lymphocytes and neutrophils—appeared to be weakened.

Mutation rates escalated, based on study of animal and plant chromosomes. And the mutation rates correlated perfectly with the amount of radiation that had fallen on any specific site, indicating what toxicologists referred to as a dose/response curve.

But Chernobyl's Oskolkov insists, 'Everything, all of this fallout, now lies at the bottom of the water and doesn't make a problem. And there radiation is now measured in 10^{-11} cu/litre level, so it is not a problem, I tell you.'

Psychiatrist Semyon Gluzman, an intense Ukrainian Jew who has studied regional psychosocial reactions to Chernobyl, says that the nuclear authorities are entirely to blame for the degree to which people suffer some post-Chernobyl hypochondria.

'The former [Soviet] Ministry of Health said, "A certain amount of radiation is good for you." It's natural that the absence of precise information, accurate information, gives rise to anxiety.'

For years after the accident the Gorbachev Soviet regime refused to extend *perestroika* and *glasnost* to Chernobyl, instead denying any possibility of a widespread deleterious health impact, Gluzman recalled. And people who expressed fear that Chernobyl's deadly isotopes were hurting them were labelled 'radiophobic', meaning they suffered a psychiatric state of hysterical fear of radiation brought on by the traumatic event.

But since the fall of the USSR, Gluzman continued, 'the same medical *nomenklatura* are shouting that "everything is *so terrible*! People are just dying walking down the streets." They can get Western grants and trips out of this, of course.'

Radiophobia, or Chernobyl Syndrome—whatever name it is given—swept the former Soviet Union and Eastern Bloc nations in the wake of the 1986 Chernobyl accident. And with each passing year it grew, affecting every aspect of how the region's adults viewed their health, and that of their children.

For example, at Novosibirsk Paediatric Infectious Disease Hospital No. 3, located a thirty-minute drive outside the Siberian city, Natalia Nikiforova, the chief physician, is convinced that the Siberian children under her care suffer from immunological disorders caused by environmental pollution. Though she has absolutely no white blood cell data to prove the need, Nikiforova has ordered her staff to care for ailing children differently in 1997 from how their counterparts in 1987 were treated. Antibiotics are shunned in favour of Siberian herbs made from reindeer horns and rhododendron plants. Animal thymuses are mashed up and injected into the children. And in some cases vaccinations are avoided because, she says, the Siberian children are too weak to tolerate preparations made for stronger Western youngsters. Though there is little scientific evidence to support these beliefs, the notion is so widespread that doctors and parents living more than four thousand miles apart spout nearly identical claims. The only thing that varies from place to place is the culprit charged with the crime of generational devastation: in Belarus and Ukraine the finger is pointed at the Chernobyl nuclear power plant accident in 1986; in Siberia the horrendous industrial pollution is blamed; in Eastern Europe it is the old Communist mining and manufacturing centres and in Moscow they accuse the air and water of violating their children's vitality.

The pollution was undeniable. It assaulted the senses, both physically and aesthetically. Seen through Western eyes the Soviet style of industry was reminiscent of a Hollywood science fiction version of a postapocalyptic society replete with pollution-darkened skies, greyness, and hulking concrete-and-steel structures. Perhaps with more relevance it brought to mind America's Pittsburgh in the 1880s, London during the Industrial Revolution, or Germany's Ruhr Valley during World War II military production—all periods of capitalist development during which human health, aesthetics, and the environment were sacrificed in favour of enormous scales of productivity and profit. Soviet planners clearly believed in two principles: bigness and utilitarianism. The niceties of human health and aesthetics were ignored. Having grown up amidst industrial filth dissident Russian poet Irina Ratushinskaya wrote: 'Do we have to know why/ the river turns black?'

There was no denying that the environmental devastation was an affront to the senses. But was it killing people? What chemical and radioactive threat was actually present, and was it at least partly to blame for the observed deterioration of the health of the people of the former USSR and Eastern Bloc?

'At issue is not only the scope and coverage but also the quality of environmental and health information,' wrote Feshbach. 'Many experts concluded that available statistics on air pollution, for example, are 30 to 50 per cent lower than the real figures.... Communism may be dead, but Lenin's dictum that "statistics are not scholarly but practical" lives on. The normal bureaucratic response to requests for information is often to conceal what might be embarrassing or costly.'

Had Chernobyl radiation exposure caused widespread illness in people who lived more than twenty miles away from the nuclear power plant in 1986? Could it be blamed for perceived health deficiencies of the children living a decade later in the western parts of the former Soviet Union?

Cancer is genuinely a problem. Though national cancer rates are generally below those seen in the West, cancer hot spots exist all over the former Eastern Bloc and Soviet Union. In the industrial regions of Siberia, for example, the incidence of adult leukaemia is nearly twice that seen in Western Europe (15 cases per 100 000 Siberians annually versus 8 per 100 000 Europeans).[6] Hodgkin's disease incidence is about double that seen in Europe.

'We see oncological heamatological problems—leukaemias and lymphomas. There is a real upward trend among children, especially,' Dr Tatyana Boyko, deputy president of the Public Health Committee of Irkutsk, said. Diagnoses of cancer in adults increased 130 per cent between 1992 and 1996, she said. And for children under fourteen years of age cancer was diagnosed 145 per cent more frequently in 1996 versus 1992.[7] In 1996 the diagnosed child cancer rate in Irkutsk was 247.5 per 100 000 children—nearly fifteen times the US paediatric cancer rate.

As far as Boyko was concerned the culprit was clearly 'the ecological disaster—after all, the real concentrations [of pollutants] exceed allowed ones by many-fold in this region.'

Official Ministry of Health data indicated that there had been a slow but steady increase during the last two decades of the twentieth century in the numbers of Russian children and adults diagnosed with cancer. The child incidence rose 14 per cent from 1993 to 1995; adult cancer incidence rose by 6 per cent.

Overall adult and child cancer rates also rose in Ukraine, jumping from 300 per 100 000 in 1988 to 410 per 100 000 in 1994, according to physicist Valery Kukhar.

'But the problem is that since 1990 the health status—all markers of health—have shown a worsening situation in Ukraine,' Kukhar said. Infectious diseases were increasing, as were heart disease, traumas, poisoning, accidents . . . everything.

'All these figures—including the rise in cancer—may be the result of the deterioration of the environment, but also of psychological stress, economics, political instability—all of it,' Kukhar insisted. And he gave the example of an ulcer to illustrate his point. If a man developed a peptic ulcer in Kiev in 1999 was it because of the stress of his unemployment, a lowering in the quality of his diet, a newly acquired bacterial infection, or ingestion of radioactive food grown in the Chernobyl zone?

'One thing we can be absolutely sure of is that the thyroid cancer is the result of Chernobyl,' Kukhar said.

Even the most conservative officials in Moscow, and the current operators of Chernobyl, agreed that there had been a striking radiation-induced increase in thyroid cancer, particularly in children, since the accident. In Ukraine the incidence of thyroid cancer in children by 1998 was 52 times higher than it was before the accident; the incidence in Belarus, which bore the brunt of the fallout, was 113 times above its 1986 level.[8] As the century closed, the Chernobyl district led the world in thyroid cancer, with a rate of one diagnosed case in every 3700 local residents, or 500 times the pre-1986 rate.[9] The incidence of thyroid diseases of all kinds in children was far above normal. By the end of 1997 fifteen thousand paediatric thyroid disease cases had been diagnosed in Belarus and fifty thousand in Ukraine. And eight years after the accident 19.5 per cent of Belarusan children who were exposed to the fallout were making antibodies against their own thyroids—only 3.8 per cent of children in Belarus who lived in unradiated areas made such antibodies.

The Ukrainian authorities estimated that 700 000 children under fourteen years of age at the time of the accident were exposed to Chernobyl radiation and that 336 107 children lived in 1998 in radiation-contaminated areas. Dr Daniel Gluzman—brother of psychiatrist Semyon—and his team of molecular biologists at the R. E. Kavetsky Institute of Experimental Pathology in Kiev used advanced immunological methods to study some of these children, looking for signs of developing leukaemias, lymphomas, and other types of blood cancers that were seen in victims of the Hiroshima nuclear bomb. In one such study Gluzman's group found a variety of blood disorders—such as leukcopenia and thrombocytopenia—in 1275 of 7250 Chernobyl-exposed children. And in half of those children there were clear changes in their white blood cells, particularly T-cell lymphocytes. The sorts of alterations Gluzman saw in the T cells of these children were not found in any of the cells of control children from other parts of Ukraine that weren't affected by the accident. But they did correspond to some of the lymphocyte changes seen in cancer patients.

Perhaps more disturbing were Gluzman's studies of children who were born within nine months after the accident to mothers who were definitely exposed to Chernobyl radiation. More than half of these children had abnormal lymphocytes.

'We have also seen forty cases of leukaemia in clean-up workers' who entered Chernobyl shortly after the meltdown, the white-haired elderly Gluzman explained, chatting in his chilly Kiev laboratory. 'So probably we will expect to see an increase in breast cancer, lung cancer, central nervous system neoplasms,' over coming years.

But in 1996 the Ukraine Institute of Biophysics convened a meeting of so-called radiobiologists, most of whom were from Moscow. The forum released a statement concluding that beyond the observed thyroid cancer cases, there was no long-term deleterious effect from Chernobyl at all, which, they argued, wasn't surprising given human beings could tolerate 70 rems of radiation. Based on average US annual radiation exposure, however, it would take 19 000 years for a typical American to receive that dose of radiation.

A large-scale study carried out by researchers at Harvard University concluded that the incidence of childhood leukaemias in the radiated areas was 50 per cent higher than that seen in parts of Ukraine not exposed to Chernobyl fallout: 37.7 cases per 100 000 in the radiated zones versus 25.4 cases per 100 000 in control areas.

Perhaps remarkably there was no evidence of birth defects, other types of cancer, elevated numbers of miscarriages, or heightened sterility among residents of the radiated area. Nor was there evidence of widespread damage to human immune systems.

But there was plenty of fear. Surveys showed that ten years after the accident up to half of the adults who had lived in radiated areas were still taking sedatives.[10] They were caught between information extremes, between polarizing views of their futures. At one extreme was the Ukrainian government, telling them that 125 000 citizens had already died in the first decade following the near meltdown, victims of unspecified forms of radiation damage. And at the other extreme were researchers who argued that only a handful of verified deaths had, or would, occur, all of them among the men who died in the accident itself, or children downwind who developed thyroid cancers.

The Chernobyl radiation debate was mirrored all across the region as residents of the former Soviet states learned that nuclear waste had simply been dumped in local lakes, seas, and refuse heaps; ugly 'factories' were actually secret nuclear facilities;

nuclear submarines lay decommissioned upon the floor of the Baltic Sea; and within dense cities Soviet engineers had conducted dangerous radioactive experiments, leaving residue behind that would still emit radiation for thousands of years.

All of these sites, charged physicist Alesey Yablokov, contributed to an overwhelming burden of radioactive contamination across the region, especially in his beloved Russia. Having served as President Yeltsin's environmental advisor, Yablokov was privy to long-secret documents that delineated the horrors. In 1992 Yablokov lost a tooth and, out of curiosity, ran radiation tests on it. He was astonished to discover that it was highly radioactive, containing traces of several different isotopes. Determined to learn where the radiation had come from, Yablokov urged his colleagues in a Moscow laboratory to be tested: all returned with similarly disturbing results. Eventually, Yablokov found documents, he said, that proved his laboratory building, and many other Moscow structures, were built of concrete made in part from waste products produced by Soviet nuclear facilities.

He resigned after three years in Yeltsin's service, despairing of the obstacles against change. After 1995 the bombastic Yablokov worked from outside the government, acting as chair of the independent Centre for Russian Environmental Policy: 'Your society wants to be protected,' he said, 'but ours is not mature. . . . My government has no money to combat pollution. And every new fact showing disaster demands more money. So the government doesn't want to have good information.'

The Russian government created a 'dirty cities' programme—a rough equivalent of the US Superfund for toxic waste clean-up. About thirty cities were officially designated 'dirtiest' in Russia, giving them highest priority for the paltry reserve of funds Moscow could muster for ecological research and clean-up. In addition the Russian government during the 1990s designated two hundred cities as ones that posed 'ecological danger to human health' due to toxic pollution of the air and/or water.

Dr Boris Revich, of the Centre for Demography and Human Ecology in Moscow, sits on the panel that decided which cities should receive the dubious 'dirty' accolade, and what sorts of scientific interventions should be executed. As documents were declassified and data mounted the extent of Soviet pollution proved so overwhelming that Revich and his fellow scientists couldn't begin to decipher the impact it was all having on human health.

'So the first task we want to solve is to make a short list of the most dangerous contaminants for Russia. Where are the pollution/environment problems most acute? What are the problems? We have no sense of priorities,' Revich lamented.

Efforts were hampered not only by money, Revich said, but also by horrible Soviet-era statistics and a dearth of skilled epidemiologists. The old database on such things as birth defects, child asthma rates, child deformities, and even child cancers was, Revich insisted, 'almost useless.'

'When they try to link [anything] to the environment they say, "The level of unborn deformities has gone up." We say, "You didn't have any statistics before! They weren't calculated properly ten years ago,'" Revich said. And because all aspects of the study of environmental damage to health stepped on the toes of Soviet military and industrial planners scientists weren't foolish enough to wade into such research waters prior to 1991.

The Lake Baikal region of Siberia offered a perfect illustration of the problem. The lake itself is a national treasure of rare size and beauty. More than a mile deep and 636 kilometres long, Lake Baikal is the crystal clear source of one-fifth of the world's fresh water supply. During the winter the lake—which is larger than the nation of Belgium—freezes on top with an ice crust more than a metre thick. So solid is this winter ice mass that the Japanese Army drove over it and into Siberia during World War II, surprising Soviet forces. Called the Pearl of Siberia, Lake Baikal holds a special, precious position in Russian culture.

In 1988 Soviet leader Mikhail Gorbachev gave his startling address to the USSR nation, disclosing for the first time the extent of the great Soviet pollution cover-up. He deliberately opened by referring to Russia's natural treasure, Lake Baikal. But he went on to tell the stunned Soviet masses that damage to their beloved lake was minimal compared to what had been done elsewhere in the nation, including in seven industrial cities located along the Angara River, the only body of water that flows out of Lake Baikal. Angara meanders first to the metropolis of Irkutsk and then northwest past the industrial cities of Angarsk, Usol'ye Sibirskoye, Cheremukhovo, Zima, and several smaller cities. As the Angara flowed farther from Lake Baikal its pollution levels increased significantly, particularly with dioxins, lead, and PCBs—all substances closely regulated in Western Europe and the United States.

At the Federal Medical University in Irkutsk Larisa Ignatyeva used mass spectrometres and gas chromatographs to measure dioxins in the region. Such dioxin compounds as 2,4-D, 2,4,5-T, and TCDD were used as pesticides and produced as waste by-products of pulp and paper processing. They were considered highly carcinogenic, teratogenic, and mutagenic, making these chemicals prime suspects for any observed increases in cancer or birth defects.

Ignatyeva found dioxins everywhere she looked: in local food, water, soil, sewage. The highest levels were in locally produced butter, milk, riverbank soil, and sewage water pouring into the Angara and Irkutsk drinking water.

The TCDD levels Ignatyeva found were low—in some cases within safe US standards. But Ignatyeva, who had been nicknamed the Dioxin Lady by her colleagues, was convinced that dioxins were causing a marked 'effect on the human body, the immune systems,' she said.

Toxicologist Nina Ivanova Motorova of the Siberian Academy of Science's research station in Angarsk wasn't convinced. While she was quite sure that the health of people living in the Angara River industrial cities had been severely damaged she did not think exotic compounds like dioxins were the key problem. It was the overall burden of pollution, compounded by social stress, that was killing people, she said.

The Taiga forests around Angarsk were denuded by acid rain. No floor of scrub and greenery formed a protective bed for dying trees, their trunks encrusted with black filth. Nearing the city the amount of blackness on struggling trees increased, covering not only their trunks but their limbs and leaf buds as well. Weighed down by their pollution burden trees leaned at sad angles, eventually collapsing.

The sky, too, changed as one neared the city, its blueness fading. In place of azure appeared greyness, haze, and, at sunset, a vermillion glow.

The city was ringed with oil refineries and energy production plants. The landscape was criss-crossed with enormous rusting steel ducts that carried petroleum products from one plant to another.

The city centre of Angarsk, population 280 000, was bisected by streets that, as was the case in every city in the Soviet Union, were named after Karl Marx and Vladimir Lenin. Next to the requisite stern statue of Lenin was a sign: 'Angarsk City—Born by Victory!' From behind the sign American disco music blared. Rows of concrete apartment buildings, each exactly the same as the last, lined the streets of Angarsk, creating a visually numbing landscape. It was hard to fathom in the 1990s, but thirty years earlier when Komsomol volunteers built the apartments and factories of Angarsk it was considered a great Soviet honour to live and work in the city.

All around the city stood gargantuan steel factories and plants, most built during or soon after World War II. Everywhere the ground literally smoked, smouldered, and flamed as some buried pipes leaked, their contents spontaneously combusting in the chilly Siberian air. The area was densely littered with abandoned hunks of machinery, oil drums, chemical containers, and rubbish. The air routinely exceeded all Russian air pollution standards, Motorova said, and the soil was severely contaminated with heavy metals and lead.

Everyone in the city was in some way connected to the chemical or oil industries. And all of the factories and plants dumped their wastes into the ice- cold swift Angara River, carrying the pollutants all over Siberia, Motorova explained.

When Nina Motorova moved to Angarsk in 1973 she found the city horribly polluted and was kept busy scurrying among factories and sites of contamination in her capacity as an environmental health scientist.

'I got enough of a pollution dose in the seventies to influence my body,' Motorova says. Though only in her forties, blue-eyed Motorova manoeuvres with difficulty, leaning heavily on a cane and any fellow pedestrian willing to assist. 'I have a rare disease because I have visited so many polluted sites. So I have a disease of my central nervous system.'

Motorova has reticulohistiocytosis, a profound, rare immune system disorder that is always crippling and may prove fatal. The cause of the syndrome, which is usually found in older women, isn't known. But she insists, 'I got this syndrome from all the bad places I've visited.'

As Motorova guides her visitors about the unsightly Angarsk mess, she nervously avoids eye contact with passing pedestrians and car passengers. Unemployment in all the old Soviet industrial cities was rising as these outmoded old plants went bankrupt. The people were angry, and they resented any outside inquiry that might further worsen their economic situation—even if it was intended to improve the health of the populace.

Once the stars of the proletariat state, Angarsk and dozens of other industrial cities in Siberia were, by the late 1990s, foci of mass public health fear. At the top of the phobia list, garnering the popular distinction of 'most polluted place on Earth,' was Noril'sk.

From the air, northern Siberia's mountainous, white frozen landscape, spotted with pockets of heavy pine forests, offers a breathtaking panorama. Until the plane nears Noril'sk.

A plume of chocolate brown air hovers over the city and a diameter area about fifty miles surrounding it. The white landscape takes on a dark, greyish-green tone from the air, though there are places where the snow is jet black. It is a devastated region— its chimneys belching out 2 041 000 metric tons of 'atmospheric particulate' each year.

On landing, three alarming sensations took hold: a metallic taste in the mouth reminiscent of sucking on a penny; a painful burning in the back of the throat that caused a reflexive tightening of the larynx and oesophagus; and an almost constant tearing from eyes unused to the grit that quickly collected on eyelashes, crusting on the lids.

Welcome to the most polluted place on Earth, Noril'sk. Located 200 kilometres north of the Arctic Circle. No sunlight four months out of the year. Population 280 000.

Once the cash cow for the Soviet Union, Noril'sk sits on more than a third of the planet's nickel reserves, a fifth of the platinum, half the palladium, and 10 per cent each of copper and cobalt. It is rich in high-grade coal, is the world's second largest producer of diamonds behind South Africa, and contains significant quantities of gold and amethyst.

But along with the sweet cream of these natural riches came curd: in addition to the airborne particulates, the area's mining and processing operation produced 28 million tons of solid waste, at least 10 million of which was toxic by Russian government standards. Every year some 5500 tons of black particulate crud fell on each square kilometre of Noril'sk, giving each inch of surface a charcoal veneer. It was estimated that Noril'sk's industrial effluent routinely blanketed more than two thousand hectares of the Arctic.

And the pollution didn't stop there. Noril'sk annually pumped an astonishing burden of filth into the earth's atmosphere, including: 2.1 million metric tons of sulphur dioxide, 1.8 million tons of copper oxides, 1.2 thousand tons of nickel, 10.1 million metric tons of carbon monoxide, 19 million tons of nitrogen oxides, 43.7 million tons of lead, 30 million tons of hydrogen sulphide, a tenth of a million tons of sulphuric acid, and 0.3 million tons of chlorinated hydrocarbons.

The wind blew toxic dust filled with heavy metals—30 per cent of it iron oxide— swirling down in visible clouds off the black slag mountains dotted around the city.

And when the wind didn't blow, in midwinter for instance, the pollutants hung heavily over the sunless city like a dirty, wet, wool coat.

Along Leninski Prospect, the city's main boulevard, the populace is taking its Sunday evening stroll. Dressed in mink and sable coats and hats the people parade down the boulevard, walking its seventeen-block length and then turning around. They wear their finest clothing on this popular promenade and many women stroll behind baby prams, taking care in their high-heeled boots lest they fall on the icy pavements. The men tug thoroughbred dogs by their leads. Children toss soccer balls to one another as they play in parallel progress to their slowly meandering parents. Clusters of friends greet one another, remarking on the weather, their children's grades, one another's attire, maybe sports.

Remarkably—perhaps astonishingly—these Noril'sk paraders seem unaware that with each step they are pushing their feet into several inches of black metallic filth. The marching masses produce a *crunch crunch crunch* cacophony, treading upon industrial waste. Their fur coats and pets blacken as they go, accruing layers of carbon, iron, copper, lead, nickel, and other pollutants. To either side of the pavements, also seemingly unnoticed by the citizens of Noril'sk, stand banks of black snow. The only thing that appears to irritate those out for their constitutionals are the metal kiosks that have recently sprung up along the pavements, forcing occasional detours and bottlenecks. The kiosks, from which all manner of goods are vended, indicated that capitalism has come to Noril'sk.

And there was no mistaking the imprint of the old Soviet *nomenklatura* upon Noril'sk, which they dubbed 'The Pearl Set in Snow.' Though hints of Noril'sk's astonishing mineral wealth were known to Czar Peter the Great in the 1750s, the city was not built until 1935, when Stalin ordered its construction. Prior to that time the region was inhabited by nomadic Shamanistic tribes—the Evenkis, Tungus, Nganasan, Dolgan, and Nenets—who herded reindeer and hunted fish and animals along the Taimyr Peninsula. Stalin ordered them shoved into gulags, outlawed their languages, and did his best to obliterate their cultures.

Between 1939 and 1953 slave labourers, most of whom were interned for alleged acts or thoughts contrary to Communist ideology, toiled in the Arctic wasteland, building the 'Pearl' of which the Moscow *nomenklatura* dreamed. It is estimated that at the gulag's peak 100 000 political slaves toiled in Noril'sk, a quarter of them dying every year, quickly replaced by new shipments of dissident poets, intellectuals, nationalists, and labour organizers.

To lure otherwise rational, highly skilled human beings to lives of darkness, ice, and dismal pollution the Moscow *nomenklatura* created a second class within the 'classless society' composed of privileged scientists, engineers, miners, and industrial personnel who enjoyed certain opportunities not afforded to the rest of the proletariat. Certain cities, such as Noril'sk, were designated 'A Class' meaning that their stores had top priority for all goods. Residents of Noril'sk took satisfaction in being able to fly—at state expense—all over the USSR on holidays, and see barren shelves in markets elsewhere, bereft of the same toys, tomatoes, and television sets that they could readily obtain back home. Workers in 'A Class' cities were among the highest paid Soviet citizens.

No matter how bad things got in the icy darkness of a Noril'sk January the workers could always be consoled in knowing that they were superior to the slaves who toiled, and died, all around them. Russian poet Galich neatly summarized the caste system of Noril'sk, and other gulag/cities:

> We dug and we toiled,
> And we bit the iron,
> We offered our chests
> To the muzzles of submachine guns.
> And you, driving past
> On your Victory motorcars,
> Shouted to us:
> 'Achieve your norm.'
> And we forgot
> about sleep and food,
> And you led us
> From victory to victory.
> Meanwhile you
> Exchanged your Victories for Volgas,
> And later
> You exchanged your Volgas for Zims,
> And later
> You exchanged your Zims for chaikas,
> And later
> You exchanged your chaikas for ZILs.
> And we wore ourselves to the bone,
> We dug and we loaded,
> And you led us
> From victory to victory
> And shouted toasts
> To victory.

By the 1990s the ugly history of Noril'sk, including the enormity of the Schmidt Mountain gulag cemetery, was known. Nearly every resident was desperately trying to get off of what they called their 'island', a place escapable only by air. But they were trapped. Pay was down—if it arrived at all. The airlines were no longer state enterprises that provided free tickets to Noril'sk's workers. To decamp Noril'sk in the late 1990s one needed money—more of it than anyone was now earning.

'It's an economic gulag now,' Komsomolsky Mine director Hamby Kozhijev said. Paranoia forced denial: fear of job loss, of freezing in an unheated Arctic hovel, helped keep complaints unsaid.

But denial was getting harder every day, as the populace learned long-secret public health truths.

Though precise, analysed statistics were hard to come by, it was clear that the pervasive pollution was linked to internationally high rates of miscarriage, lung cancers, various forms of chronic respiratory diseases, cardiovascular disease, allergies, and skin disease. At one hospital in neighbouring Talnakh, for example, 90 per cent of patients admitted from 1993 to 1998 suffered from lung diseases and 'practically 100 per cent of the children hospitalized in the area have allergies and skin problems,' said Vladimir Koshubarov, deputy chairman of Noril'sk's Committee on Environmental Protection.

'Lung cancer is the number one killer in Noril'sk. Cardiovascular disease is number two. Without any doubt we know Noril'sk has the lowest life expectancy in all of Russia,' Koshubarov continued.

An average infant in Noril'sk suffered 1.7 bouts of respiratory illness per year. Mothers in Noril'sk were three times more likely to give birth to a child with congenital birth defects than were women living elsewhere on Taimyr Peninsula, and ten times more likely than was the average Russian mother.

Outside Noril'sk, along the roadsides that connected the city to neighbouring mines, smelters, foundries, and workers' settlements, the permafrost was disappearing under the heat of mile upon mile of leaking pipelines of pollution. In places hundred-foot-tall geysers of steam spewed from leaking conduits. Slag heaps, discarded cars and steel machinery, and sacks of mysterious rubbish covered the imperiled permafrost. In places the permafrost had completely disappeared, all of its ice having long since melted and been replaced by lakes of red, putrid liquid that, like some organic mass, spontaneously belched, burped, and spewed forth fountains of nausea-inducing, putrid steam.

St Petersburg-born Boris started life in Noril'sk as foreman of a metal furnace, rising through the ranks to reach one of the Kombinat's top positions. As a Jew Boris couldn't hope to attain such stature without having become a devout Communist Party member during Soviet times. With the KGB long gone, USSR dead, and the old *nomenklatura* vanished, Boris was still frightened—perhaps more so. He was afraid of the Kombinat.

In 1992–94 the Yeltsin government sold off most of the old state-run industries. A consortium of banking and investment firms, working with Russia's second largest bank, Oneximbank, bought 51 per cent of the Kombinat Noril'sk Nikel and in its first year shared an estimated $2.4 billion worth of mined metals sales with the Russian government, which retained 49 per cent ownership of the Kombinat. But at the end of 1994 Noril'sk's largest turbine engine blew up, killing several workers and plunging most of the citizens into a long, horrible, heatless winter.

Among the citizens of Noril'sk rumours spread of gangsters who had bought out several original partners and sent thugs to force greater productivity. For men like Boris this meant that where once they feared KGB spies in their midst, now it was the company thugs, famed for their brutality, who gave them daily cause for concern.

No wonder, then, that Noril'sk had become an island of paranoia. Parents pulled their children away from strangers, passengers on buses hastily moved to the far end of the vehicle when foreigners boarded, workers and the mayor declined to speak of their situation....

Though Noril'sk is often cited for a dramatically lower than normal life expectancy for the region, it was difficult to confirm because of the Kombinat's retirement policy. Life in the mines and plants was so hard that men could retire at forty-five, women at forty, receiving full life pensions.

'A man works his shift, spends some time at home. He does this for years. Then he goes to the "Continent" and dies. Who cares? Who blames Noril'sk?' Koshubarov says with a shrug.

'So data are hard to come by because usually when workers retire they leave Noril'sk and die elsewhere,' Komsomolsky Mine chief engineer Alexander Borodai said. That could explain why there were few graves in Noril'sk's cemetery for people who died after the age of forty-five. And why he was considered 'elderly' in Noril'sk, fifty-five-year-old Borodai said.

'For us Noril'sk is an information black hole,' said Russian government scientist Boris Revich. Moscow had repeatedly offered to designate Noril'sk a 'dirty city' which would qualify the region for special cleanup and scientific research funds. But the Kombinat refused both the designation and Moscow's offer of scientific inquiry.

Or it may be true that *average* life expectancy for men was below forty. That wouldn't surprise Dr Nikolai Pavlov, chief physician of Medical Sanitary Unit No. 2, located thirty-five kilometres from Noril'sk in the satellite city of Talnakh. Two of the Noril'sk Kombinat mines and seventy thousand people reside in Talnakh.

The incidence of lung disease in Talnakh adults is, Pavlov says, 'three times the average in Russia.' His 310-bed hospital over the last six years admitted 1207 lung disease patients, accounting for 90 per cent of its in-patients. Malignant lung cancer killed 231 of them. Emphysema, tuberculosis, pneumonia, chronic bronchitis, and acute asthma claimed the rest.

The six-foot six-inch white-haired Pavlov strolled the noisy, crowded hallways of his hospital inured to the sounds of harsh coughs and raspy breathing. No longer subsidized by the state and ignored by the Kombinat, the hospital's unpaid staff survives by directly billing patients for each procedure and compelling the ill to purchase their own drugs, meals, linens, syringes—'the whole lot,' Pavlov says.

Pavlov had recently logged a stupendous increase in drug-resistant tuberculosis cases, more than doubling in number in just two years. He had no resources to support scientific research, but he had a hypothesis: the pollution had so devastasted the lungs of the seventy thousand residents of Talnakh that any cases of TB brought by visitors from outside the area swiftly spread. Nearly 2 per cent of the population had active pulmonary tuberculosis in 1997, Pavlov said. And his hospital 'had no TB drugs.'

'In the winter there is a waiting list here when we see outbreaks of upper respiratory infections,' Pavlov points out. 'And it keeps our surgeons busy, breaking up lung cavities of tuberculosis, removing cancerous lungs, cutting [tracheal] bypasses,' so patients can breathe.

The future of Talnakh, suggests Pavlov, could be one of 'slow, slow death.'

One thing was certain. Working conditions in the mines and plants were incredibly dangerous.

Down the road from Noril'sk is the huge Nadezhda ore processing plant, where 10-story-tall furnaces heat copper, nickel, and cobalt to temperatures of 1100 to 1400 degrees centigrade. Thousands of workers toil with the vermillion, molten ore in front of them radiating searing heat, and winter's minus 40 degree centigrade chill at their backs.

'You'll never know what that feels like,' manager Boris says, noting that it 'confuses your heart,' because half the worker's body is exposed to frigid, sub-zero air, signalling a need for fast-pumping blood. And the other half is boiling hot, telling the heart to slow down.

A suppressed study by the Medical School of Sverdlovsk, provided to a visitor, showed that workers in the mines were far more likely to suffer cardiovascular disease and lung cancer, even when compared to other residents of Noril'sk. Measurements of their work space air revealed that they were inhaling 19.2 micrograms per metre squared of nickel and up to 134 micrograms of cobalt—levels 20 and 135 times more, respectively, than considered normal by Russian standards.

The study, which was completed in 1990, was never published, by order of the Kombinat. Nor were the results of a recent Kombinat-financed environmental survey of a 53 000 square kilometre Arctic area around Noril'sk. Geologists Yuri Melnikov and Sergei Snisar, both aged thirty, led a seven-man team that collected ten thousand samples in the vast region, braving all Arctic weather conditions. By pulling core samples out of the permafrost, drawn from appropriate depths, Snisar and Melnikov could compare contemporary pollution levels with those of two hundred years ago.

In the areas farthest from Noril'sk, Melnikov said, 'contemporary snow samples contain 18 times the amount of cobalt, 6 times the copper, 11 times the nickel, 14.5 times the barium, and 3.2 times the zinc,' than were present two hundred years ago. Acid rain from the Kombinat's smokestacks has destroyed up to 90 per cent of the original tree population.

Moss and lichen had become saturated with heavy metals at levels up to twelve times what they were before the Russian Revolution of 1917, killing off half the plants.

And, 'we see a dangerous potential for avalanches due to degradation of surface plant life that protects the permafrost,' Melnikov concluded.

Three days after Melnikov and Snisar shared their unpublished findings with their visitor, the Kombinat cut off all their funds and ordered the young scientists not to speak. The Kombinat representatives declined to discuss any health or environment-related matters.

According to the Russian Ministry of Health the relative hazard of dying prematurely in Noril'sk in 1994 was 85. In Angarsk, which ranked fourth worst, it was 15. No city ranked above a 22—except Noril'sk.

Noril'sk was at the extreme end of a Soviet ecological legacy that could be felt from East Berlin all the way to the Pacific Ocean. In Bohemia, the Czech Republic, fifty years of strip mining and coal smelting had devastated what had once been the preferred holiday location of the Hapsburgs and aristocracy all over Central Europe. The fall of the Berlin Wall gave West Germans a shocking look at the industrial filth and putrid air of their eastern countrymen. The Central Asian nations of Uzbekistan and Kazakhstan were suffering from an insane irrigation scheme begun by Lenin, draining the vast, landlocked Aral Sea to provide water for cotton fields, resulting in increased incidence of throat cancer due to environmental dust. The visual and physical filth was pervasive. It assaulted the senses.

But was it the cause of the region's radical demographic shift?

On that experts stridently disagreed.

Former Yeltsin advisor Yablokov became visibly agitated when the question was posed. The grey-haired, bearded Russian dismissively said that despite a lack of reliable data the illnesses and deaths seen in Noril'sk 'are obviously due to pollution.'

'Look,' he says, stabbing his points home with pokes in the air. 'Fourteen per cent of our young children in Russia meet primary school healthy child standards. Why?'

'I have personally had a high level of radiation exposure—why? No one knows how. It may be possible that a pipe somewhere comes free, releasing radiation. All over Moscow every year an average of seventy places are discovered with dangerous levels of radiation. It's amazing,' Yablokov, a physicist, says, gesticulating wildly. 'Nobody can feel safety even inside Moscow.'

Zoologist Maria Cherkasova shares Yablokov's views. As head of the Moscow-based Centre for Independent Ecological Programs Cherkasova cites the same figures as Yablokov. Her chief concerns are rocket and missile launches, and the d-methylhydrazine fuel used as a propellant.

'The whole world should work on safe fuel for rockets,' Cherkasova says, insisting that children all over Russia and Central Asia were dying due to exposure to missile fuel. Other key contributors to the region's rising death rates, the fifty-five-year-old ornithologist says, are dioxins, lead, DDT, and a generalized dampening of people's immune systems prompted by environmental assaults.

The key problems with the environmental argument were that the epidemiology, if it existed at all, was poorly done. And pollution had actually declined dramatically after 1991 all across the region due to the economic collapse of local industries.

Thus, during the very time in which the region experienced its most dramatic increase in deaths and health crises the amount of pollution in people's environments decreased.

Boris Revich had no doubt that the ecological tragedy was playing a role in human illness, and he had personally documented pollution-induced asthma, lead-associated child health problems, and dioxin impacts in Russia. But he found most assertions that the pollution was directly responsible for the region's demographic shift 'nonsense— complete crap!'

Beldrich Moldan was the first minister of the environment in the Czech Republic following the fall of communism. His country underwent the same debate, perhaps starting three years earlier in the nations to his east. The focus of the Czech public's fears was industrial Bohemia.

'In 1990 when I was minister I went there. And to my amazement there was a slogan: "The first three words our children learn are *Mummy, Daddy*, and *inversion*,"' a reference to air inversions that held smog and pollution inside the Bohemian valleys. When just two months after the Czech revolution the populace was accusing Moldan of not doing enough to clean up their environment, he realized the depth of their collective panic. After decades of lies and cover-ups by the former Soviet-aligned government the Bohemians suddenly realized what was in their air, water, and food.

He poured over all available data, Moldan recalled, and found it was 'mostly shit! Really! So bad you cannot believe it.'

In the end blue-eyed, silver-haired Moldan concluded that 'life expectancy in Bohemia is about five years behind the Czech average,' for a number of reasons, including—but not limited to—the environment.

Six years after the Czech revolution that country's demographics shifted back, even in Bohemia, in favour of longer life expectancies and better public health, 'and nobody can say our environment has improved that much.'

Moldan, dressed casually but seated in a meticulous office lined from floor to ceiling with books and scientific journals, saw the issue philosophically. After decades of communism, he explained, people had no sense of personal responsibility. Because they had little control over their personal fates during totalitarianism the new societies found individuals unable to imagine that their own behaviour—drinking, smoking, driving while inebriated—were key to their health.

'I told those people in Bohemia, "Look, you have done nothing to clean this up. You just wait for the government to do everything. But if you don't take some responsibility, too, this place will look like Russia."'

'And I remembered that in 1987—maybe it was 1988—I met a young Russian colleague. We discussed political evolution, a favourite topic of mine. He said, "I see you have hope—forty years of Communist rule is bad, but you can recover. But seventy years of Communists—we will never recover!" And that man's remarks will always live with me.'

IV

What are the present Russian authorities offering the people? 'Support Yeltsin and you'll live the way people do in America!'. . . How is it possible not to see that everything in Russia is being done not 'like in America' (or in France or Sweden), but the way things were done in Uganda under President Idi Amin?
—Andrei Sinyavsky, 1997[1]

From the point of view of the United Nations Children's Fund the public health crisis of the nations of the former Soviet Union and Eastern Bloc boiled down to one thing: history.

'Hopes that, with the elimination of authoritarianism and the introduction of a demand-led market economy, the needs of children would be better met in the short-term have been largely betrayed,' read UNICEF's 1997 report.[11] 'Systematic changes have for the most part been too large and sudden, with negative effects to the economy; and the bursting out of national pride and ethnic intolerance has led to heightened tensions and, in a few cases, warfare. Child welfare has once again become the victim of dramatic historic changes.'

'The transition has been accompanied by a severe region-wide economic crisis, the effects of which have hit even the most successful countries. Moreover, the transition is also based on market forces, which can free powerful human energies, but which also need support from societal values and social institutions for a balanced development. As social norms and institutions collapsed, values eroded—it will take time for new values to take root, which will also require support from laws, law enforcement and the recognition of a common interest.'

As the demographic nightmare unfolded in the region UNICEF, viewing matters through the prism of children, felt that public health had collapsed because the societies themselves had lost their social fabrics. It was more than just economic peril that drove individuals to the brink, UNICEF argued, it was economic peril coupled with the cessation of all social cohesion.

In other words, change was killing people.

The World Bank, on the other hand, argued in its 1996 World Development Report that the problem wasn't too much change: it was that not enough change had occurred. Those societies that made the transition to market economies most rapidly, such as the Czech Republic and Poland, suffered the briefest demographic disaster. Public health catastrophes persisted, according to the Bank, where governments kept one foot in the old Soviet system and another in capitalism.

'What has happened to health during transition?' the Bank's analysts asked. 'Two conclusions emerge: rapid reform is not necessarily detrimental to health indicators, but slow reform or the absence of reform does little to impede a long-run deterioration.'

In 1993 the entire region appeared to be in public health hell. But by 1996 demo-graphic disasters in Poland, the Czech Republic, Slovakia, and Hungary appeared to have reached their nadir and were heading toward recovery. This, the Bank's analysts felt, offered proof that populations could, indeed, tolerate 'shock therapy' economic reform and, in the long run, would benefit from such drastic measures.

From its inception the Soviet Union's economy was dictated by Communist Party planners in Moscow who seemingly cavalierly moved entire ethnic populations from one place to another, started industries in the middle of unpopulated tundra, demanded that corn be grown in icy climes, and placed the means of production for different segments of the same industry thousands of gruelling, wintry miles apart. Inefficiency was the rule of the game.

When the USSR collapsed, industries fell with it, as the various segments of its typically long outmoded production were now located in different countries. Over-night millions of workers lost their jobs, and most of the people residing in the Eastern Bloc and former Soviet Union fell into poverty—perhaps 25 per cent of them were, according to UNICEF, living in acute poverty within eighteen months of the break-up of the Soviet Union.

In Russia 45 million people, or a third of the population, had incomes *below* sub-sistence level in 1995, meaning they were surviving off their wits and dacha gar-dens—or weren't surviving at all. Those who actually had paying jobs were earning a paltry average wage in 1996 of $153 a month, which was 10 per cent less than they earned in 1992. The World Bank and International Monetary Fund broke all historic lending records in a scramble to save Russia, and, of course, bring it into the capitalist fold. By 1996 the IMF had loaned the Russian Federation more than $12 billion, a good deal of which the Yeltsin government used to cover the cost of its war in Chechnya and, it would later be revealed, to line the pockets of the Yeltsin family and cronies.[12]

In 1997, however, there was talk of economic recovery. For a few financial moments Russia looked promising, as its trade balance and industrial production levels were both firmly in the asset columns at the dawn of 1997.

Yet these positive indicators glossed over a distressing picture that would have profound regional implications for public health: the concentration of wealth in the hands of an elite oligarchy. Rising out of the post-1991 chaos came the phoenixes of the supposedly free markets. The 'New Rockefellers', as they were dubbed, snapped up de-nationalized industries, built regional banking systems, created vast energy and tele-communications monopolies, and without a second's concern for the once-dominant proletariat, shut down inefficient industries and created economic ghost towns that dotted the lands across twelve time zones. In some cases their cosy relations with gov-ernment regulators and mobsters were so obvious as to recall Al Capone and Chicago in the 1920s. Indeed, many may have aspired to be John D. Rockefeller, but in practice appeared more reminiscent of the Familia Corleone.

For ordinary Ukrainians, Georgians, and Siberians, this concentration of wealth in corrupt hands spelled disaster. As the greedy took over industries, they not only laid off more than a third of the workforce, but also stopped paying those who theoretically still had jobs. Tens of millions of workers continued for years on end to tromp to work every day, toiling in increasingly unsafe, antiquated factories, in the hope that one day a miracle would occur and months of back wages would be paid. Rarely, this occurred and supplied the necessary carrot that kept the old proletariat trudging its way to the means of production throughout the dismal 1990s.

Despair and gloom set in on a mass basis as the people came to appreciate that their futures were in the hands of gangsters. In Russia, for example, the Ministry of the Interior estimated that by mid-1997 forty thousand former state enterprises and five hundred banks were controlled by mobsters, and the gap between rich and poor had reached levels not seen since the days of the czars.

One by one government services collapsed as these gangster businesses evaded taxes, denying Moscow, Kiev, Baku, and Tblisi billions of dollars' worth of revenue that might—ought—to have been used to run hospitals, pay schoolteachers, repair highways, and take care of the public health needs of the regional populace.

As the plight of the majority worsened, average, normally sane people in the region resorted to acts of madness. On a spring day in 1997 Muscovite Irina Smirnova threw her six-year-old daughter, Dina, out of a fourth-floor apartment window and then followed, plunging to her death. *Komsomolskaya Pravda* noted on May 23 that Smirnova was the third Moscow mother that week to commit suicide, taking her starving children with her. Weeks later Colonel Aleksandr Terekhov sat down in a Moscow subway station and set himself on fire. The same week, three thousand miles away, Private Sergei Polyansky stuck a pistol in his mouth and blew his brains out while on duty. Everywhere groups of unpaid workers staged hunger strikes, hoping—in vain—that protests would promote government action.

Reactions took many forms, including the region's ancient bottom line, anti-Semitism. Average citizens and politicians blamed 'the Jews' for the region's nightmares, sure, as they were, that behind every corrupt gangster and banker stood a vast Zionist conspiracy.

Bad as all of this was, it soon grew far, far worse. After months of haggling amid concerns about corruption the IMF on April 13, 1998, finally approved a $22.6 billion loan package for Russia, offering $4.8 billion of it immediately to bolster the precarious rouble.

But by August 1, 1998, the Russian Central Bank was putting out half a billion dollars a day in a scramble to keep the rouble from collapsing. Though the government claimed that these efforts were keeping the currency stable, black market trade in roubles went wild, with the number of roubles needed to purchase one US dollar inflating by more than 30 per cent a week. Anticipating disaster, smart players moved their capital out of the country—at a rate of more than $2 billion a month. For several tense days the

Yeltsin government continued the bailout until Western billionaire currency speculator George Soros said on August 13 that the rouble wasn't worth a fig.

The Russian stock market collapsed, and the value of the rouble plummeted. An instant inflation backlash resulted, pushing the prices of food to levels never before seen in Russia. Beef soared in cost by 85 per cent in a single day, milk by 60 per cent. An already desperate populace fell into a mad scramble for the basics: food.

By the end of 1998 Russia's political and economic situations were in a tailspin, the nation owed $17 billion but only had $12.3 billion in its Central Bank, hyper-inflation set in at local food markets, the Moscow stock market had lost more than 100 per cent of its value compared to the dollar, and capital haemorrhaged out of the country at an estimated rate of $3 billion each month.

'Each day without a government is a day closer to the abyss,' a member of the Duma said. Briefly in early 1997 it had looked like Russia might follow Poland and the Czech Republic down the road toward stability and free market success. Now it was clear that, instead, she was on a highway to hell. And she was dragging her neighbours down with her.

No nation owed the world's investors and IMF as much money in 1999 as Russia did, and the government wanted still more. The Russian bear was panhandling, offering the prospect of political instability in the nuclear weapons nations of Russia, Ukraine, and Belarus as ample incentive for continued Western spare change.

By 1999 many leading Western economists and politicians openly argued that it would be in the best interests of the Russians, Ukrainians, Moldovans, Belarusans, and others in the region if the flow of loans from the West simply stopped, cold.

The threat of instability, however, seemed all too real, as terrorist bombings killed some three hundred Muscovites in the summer of 1999, prompting a resurrection of warfare in the province of Chechnya. Billions of foreign aid dollars were drained, blood was shed, yet the war proved immensely popular among Russians, who favoured strong, patriotic action to prevent further erosion in the nation's geographic and military influence. Riding the crest of that newfound national pride was Yeltsin's designated heir, former KGB operative Vladimir Putin, who was elected president of Russia in March 2000.

By then Russia's economy, along with that of its allied neighbours Ukraine and Belarus, was generating only 1 per cent of global merchandise trade, and domestic inflation was running ahead of the nation's GDP growth rate. One man, Boris Berezovsky, controlled the bulk of the region's wealth and assets. And the once-feared Russian superpower was ranked by the influential Swiss International Institute for Management Development in 2000 as the least competitive large economy in the world, well behind such troubled economies as the Czech Republic, South Africa, Slovenia, Mexico, and India.[13]

Possibilities for the near future regionally included civil war, widespread anarchy, painfully slow stabilization of market economies, the splintering of Russia into as many as ten different nations, military coups, a regionwide return of Stalin-style Sovietism, and a sort of endless period of 'muddling through'.

All of this boded agony for public health. By the end of 1998 at least forty-four million Russians were living on *less* than $32 a month: that's one out of every three Russians. In Ukraine matters were so bad that the government couldn't even provide such statistics. In Belarus the Communist government may have had the grim numbers but refused to provide them.

Russian children bore the brunt of it all, turning into a massive, orphaned subpopulation that lived by its wits on the streets of the snowy nation. The Russian Association of Child Psychologists and Psychiatrists estimated in November 1998 that the number of abandoned and orphaned children suddenly doubled, to two million children—up from essentially zero in 1990. And the annual suicide rate among these cast-off youngsters was an astonishing 10 per cent. UNICEF estimated that since 1989 the region had experienced a 33 per cent increase in the rate of child abandonment, suicide rates in under-nineteen-year-olds had more than doubled, and child school enrollment had fallen by more than 10 per cent.

In late 1998 the University of North Carolina conducted a survey that revealed that *all*—100 per cent—of Russian children suffered iron deficiencies, most having only 3 to 4 per cent of minimum daily requirement needs met in their terrible diets.[14] As Russians prepared for the bleak winter of 1998, a Moscow-based polling service queried them, asking how they expected to survive. Forty-four per cent said that they hoped to live off the vegetables they had grown over the summer in their dacha gardens; 12 per cent intended to live on game they planned to hunt in the Siberian tundra and taiga. By 1999, the fastest-growing occupation in Russia was 'dacha thievery', or stealing vegetables from strangers' gardens.

Starvation was not common in the region's pregnant women and children, but malnutrition was. According to UNICEF, in Georgia, the average mother and child daily calorie consumption fell from 2790 calories in 1980 to 1940 in 1995: a 30 per cent decrease. Russians were consuming an average of 21 per cent fewer calories in 1996; Ukrainians 23 per cent. Following the 1998 crash of the rouble caloric consumption fell still further.

Nothing weakens an immune system and overall health as efficiently as malnutrition, especially if families are, for economic reasons, substituting cheap fat and starch for more expensive proteins and fresh vegetables.

Georgian families in 1997 consumed only a third as much dairy products and almost four times less meat, poultry, and fish as they had in 1980, UNICEF figures showed. And Ukrainian, Russian, Estonian, and Armenian protein consumption declined by nearly as much.

The US Centers for Disease Control and Prevention and World Health Organization considered the shocking deficiencies in micronutrients, such as iodine, potassium, calcium, and iron, to be so severe in much of the former Soviet Union that the agencies were blaming it for declining IQs, anaemia, stunted growth, and other developmental deficiencies seen on a mass scale in the region. And some of these micronutrient deficiencies could also have rendered the children more vulnerable to pollution and radiation.

A joint 1996 US-Russian health study conducted by top government scientists from each country concluded that 60 per cent of Russia's territory was deficient in fluoride, accounting for the 85 per cent tooth cavity rate in the nation's children.

When these nations were all part of the USSR and Soviet Bloc such things as iodine and iron supplements were universally available, shipped from one part of the vast region to another. After 1991, however, impoverished Georgia struggled to find cash reserves with which to purchase iodized salt, and the Ukrainian people had to do without fluoride entirely.

In the end, Russian analyst Revich said, it was clear that the children of modern Russia and the rest of the former USSR were, indeed, less healthy than their counterparts a decade previously. But the causes of their infirmities were certainly more complex than the public believed. Pollution and radiation played roles. But so did stress, economics, and diet.

'Any epidemiological research that uses immune system measurements sees changes in the status of Russian children,' Revich concluded.

'But as far as the quality and quantity of analysis and the reasons it has happened—all of that we must say is unclear.'

It might never be possible to state empirically how much regionwide malnutrition contributed to the 1990s demographic and public health catastrophe. It certainly didn't help. During Soviet days the masses had money, but grocery store shelves were empty.

But after the collapse of the Soviet Union the situation inverted. Suddenly fruit, vegetable, and meat markets sprang up in even the remotest parts of Siberia, where such exotica as Nicaraguan bananas, Dutch tomatoes, and Florida oranges could be seen. But that was all most people could afford to do: look. Food markets became something like museums through which the masses strolled, their pockets bereft of *hryvnyas, laris,* or roubles.

And evidence of deprivation of even basic foodstuffs was starkly outlined by visits to the marketplaces of the region.

In Zhitniy Market in Kiev, Ukraine, gold-toothed peasant Galina sold an average of two hundred kilos of potatoes a day in 1992—now she feels lucky if she sells ninety. Tatyana says she can still afford to buy chicken once a week for her five-year-old son, Dima, 'because I deny it for myself.'

The elderly babushkas who for years have made cheese in their village homes and sold it in Zhitniy Market tell a visitor that the current sales are 'tragic.'

'No customers! You stay here all day and then you take all the cheese home because you cannot sell it,' toothless, elderly Katya cries.

Gori was Joseph Stalin's birthplace: a mountainous city of 160 000 residents, dominated by a three-storey-tall, imperious statue of the 'Father' as he was called, and a marble enshrined cabin in which Stalin was said to have been born.

About a mile from the Stalin shrine is a complex of rundown buildings, strafed with bullet holes during the mid-1990s civil war, that serves as the region's key hospital.

Paediatrician Tamriko Iluridze fights back tears as she speaks. 'In comparison to ten to fifteen years ago we see that the quality of children's health is decreasing. We can't do neurological examinations, but we see involuntary shivering, inabilities to hold their heads. The children's neurological status is impaired.'

Behind her ten newborn babies, swaddled tightly in wool against the icy room temperature, lie two to a bassinet.

All too often Iluridze's boss, Dr Nori Jorhadze, says babies here are born 'hypoxic, the central nervous system is ill-prepared for external conditions.... The mothers say they are okay, but really they are not okay because the food isn't good enough for them. Nine out of ten women say they are eating, but what are they eating? Fat and bread.'

Inside the central hospital's unheated corridors, lit dimly by clouded sunlight, the hospital director wrings his hands in despair, saying, 'God save us from such conditions here! We are witnessing the ecological genocide of the nation.'

V

The word progress was always one of the key words in political speeches of my youth: look what progress we have made for a poor, peasant country; how many asphalt roads we have built, how many factories! Look how your life has improved! You're not starving any longer, your children go to school and have proper shoes, and everyone has electricity nowadays. No more tuberculosis or epidemics of other terrible diseases! Isn't that progress? And communism has brought you all that.
—Slavenka Drakulić, 1997[15]

When the ancient scourge of diphtheria swept across the former Soviet Union beginning in 1990 the international health officials were stunned by its speed and frightened by its make-up. After all, diphtheria was a fully vaccine-preventable disease the occurrence of which in North America, Western Europe, and Japan was limited in the 1990s to one or two isolated cases per year.

When the *Corynebacterium diphtheriae* infected a human being the course of illness depended crucially on two factors: the site of bacterial colonization and which genetic subtype of bacteriophage was lodged inside the larger bacteria. The former determined the likelihood that an individual's immune system might bring the disease swiftly under control, with or without treatment. The latter was the key to diphtheria's virulence, as it was the viral corynebacteriophage lurking inside diphtheria bacteria that emitted lethal poisons. If the most toxic of bacteriophage were in an epidemic's bacteria, antibiotics would not prove effective in treatment and acute diphtheria cases would require antitoxin therapy.

In most cases *Corynebacterium diphtheriae* infected the mucous linings of the nose, mouth, and throat, forming a classic white membrane mass across the back of the victim's throat that prompted gagging and laboured swallowing and breathing. In more severe cases the bacteria made their way into the victim's heart, brain, or nervous system, killing 10 per cent of those so infected.

In 1994 diphtheria rates in the former Soviet region ranged from one case per 100 000 people to Tajikistan's abysmal 31.8 per 100 000—the highest seen anywhere in the world since the 1950s. Russia's was the second highest rate at 26.6 per 100 000, which was nearly thirty times the US diphtheria rate and rose to more than forty thousand cases in a single year. Cases were reported in every former Soviet and Eastern Bloc state, as well as Finland and Germany.

'This is the biggest public health threat in Europe since World War II,' declared WHO's Dr Jo Asvall. And it was one that 'presents a danger and a risk for the population of a good many parts of the world that might have thought they were safe from such a disease as diphtheria,' UNICEF's Richard Reid added.

World Health Organization researchers, working with colleagues in Moscow, traced the epidemic back, concluding that it was rooted in the long Soviet/Afghanistan war. During the 1980s Afghanistan had experienced a diphtheria epidemic involving nearly 14 000 cases of the disease. Beginning in 1988 some 100 000 Soviet soldiers left Afghanistan, returning to their respective homes or regimental bases. Unconfirmed anecdotes placed the first adult diphtheria cases in Russia in an army barracks located in Moscow, sometime in early 1990.

Most cases, they found, involved previously vaccinated adults, sparking fear that the epidemic that infected 200 000 people in the former Soviet Union, killing 5000, could infect immunized adults worldwide. The last time that the USSR had experienced such a profound diphtheria epidemic was 1955, when 104 000 cases occurred. That was three years *before* the USSR began mass immunization. Was the world facing a new, resistant form of the disease, or was something else at play?

In fact, experts discovered, something else was at play.

A 1995 study by the American Centres for Disease Control and Prevention found that nearly all of these cases occurred in a narrow group of people immunized either by natural exposure or with Soviet-made vaccines from the 1950s that didn't have enough diphtheria toxoid. The report went on to say that even though this group wasn't properly protected, they probably wouldn't have contracted diphtheria unless the level of disease in unvaccinated children during the late 1980s and 1990s was high enough to pose a threat.

Even though mistakes were made in the 1950s, it was the collapse of immunization in the 1980s and 1990s that put these adults at risk.

This collapse was fuelled by two key factors: first, a surprising lack of expertise among immunologists trained during a Soviet era dominated by ideology, when access to Western medical journals—indeed, to any Western-based science—was banned; second, a mystifying theory of immunology that evolved in the region, suggesting that there were hundreds of good reasons *not* to vaccinate.

The theory—which ran counter to all Western scientific experience—held that vaccines sparked reactions that could be dangerous to 'weak' children. Thus, any child who was ill for any reason (including a simple cold), who had a white blood cell count 5 per cent below normal, or who had a family history of illness, would be harmed rather than helped.

'Vaccine coverage was very low in the 1980s. In Moscow in 1983, for example, only 40 per cent of the children were fully immunized,' according to Dr Alexi Savinykh of the Russian Ministry of Health's MEDSOCECONOMINFORM, the government's main health think tank. And by 1992 the Moscow vaccination rate had dropped to an abysmal 34 per cent, according to Dr Eugene Tikhomirov of the emerging diseases division in the World Health Organization in Geneva. 'It makes no sense to say Russian [or former Soviet] children are immunosuppressed and can't tolerate vaccines— none! But there it was.'

Although by 1997 the diphtheria epidemic appeared to have been brought largely under control in Russia, at least, with the help of health agencies from the United States and Europe, the attitudes and conditions that spawned it remained in place, driving other formidable diseases.

And vaccine expert Robert Steinglass, who was technical officer of the US Agency for International Development-funded campaign to control the diphtheria epidemic, warned that it was only a matter of time before pertussis—or whooping cough— swept the region. This was because, he said, Soviets did not combine pertussis and diphtheria vaccines into DPT, as was done in the West. Rather, pertussis was given separately and rates of successful immunization varied wildly across the region.

When Steinglass and his American colleagues first assessed the vaccination situation in 1992 they were stunned. In some areas, they found childhood immunization rates had fallen during the 1980s below levels seen in many sub-Saharan African countries. And basic requirements of vaccine delivery, such as consistent refrigeration of supplies—or maintaining a cold chain—were routinely ignored.

'They don't know how to manage stocks and inventories of vaccines,' Steinglass explained. 'They don't know how to manage a cold chain, which by now every African country understands.'

It wasn't always so. Not at the height of the Soviet Sanitation and Epidemiology Service's (SanEp) power when upward of 280 million citizens could be lined up and immunized in a single month.

'It was a point of ideology,' Steinglass explained. 'People were pretty much told, "You will report to this station on this date for a vaccination."'

'Russian paediatricians were kind enough to try to save the Soviet children from vaccines,' Dr V. K. Tatochenko, chief paediatrician for the Russian Ministry of Health, said sarcastically. In 1978 and 1979, he said, Soviet officials introduced a long list of 'contraindications' that told doctors to avoid vaccinating children with *any* condition—real or imagined—that could cause a child's white blood count to fall marginally. This, despite the fact that paediatricians in Western Europe and the United States found no need for such precautions.

Part of the problem, Tatochenko and others said, was that Western medical journals had been banned in the Soviet Union for more than fifty years. So the 'science' of immunology, as well as principles of paediatric practice, evolved despite controlled studies or serious data.

By the mid-1980s paediatricians all over the Soviet Union had been trained to believe, Tatochenko said, 'that Russian children are weak, perishable. It doesn't mean [the child] has a pathology, but he's just not what he should be.' And this belief eventually led to the 'weak child' theory of immunology that at the dawn of the twenty-first century remained an important contributor to rates of death and disease that rivalled the third world.

Furthermore, in the absence of a sound, scientifically based concept of vaccination theory and practice during the 1980s doors opened for crackpots and pseudo-scientists, such as eighty-two-year-old Boris Nikitin, a bearded, bespectacled engineer and self-declared expert on child rearing who was often referred to as the Russian equivalent of America's Dr Benjamin Spock. However, there was a key difference between the two highly read and influential authors: Nikitin lacked medical training and was proudly antiscience.

In the Moscow suburb of Bolshevo Nikitin lived in a three-storey blue wooden home with his wife, seven adult children, and fifteen grandchildren. All of them went barefoot, even during the notorious Russian winter, and the grandchildren scampered about on a chilly, cloudy day in little more than their underwear.

This was all part of the Nikitin Doctrine, which held that most clothing, food, or water treatment and medical interventions weakened children.

'Nature,' he tells visitors one spring afternoon, 'has designed a certain stage in child development when natural immunity is formed. This natural mechanism is called children's infections.'

'So this immunization of society is a great medical mistake.'

As he plays with his naked granddaughter outdoors during the dusk chill, Nikitin explains his rationale: 'Animals go barefoot. They don't have influenza or respiratory diseases.'

Actually animals do have flu and respiratory diseases. But facts don't seem to stand in the way of Nikitin's philosophy: 'You can decrease immunity,' he says. 'I don't know how, but I see the relationship. We must train our muscles. . . . Even medical people see that! But they don't see that you can train your immune system, as well.'

Training, under the Nikitin Doctrine, is illness or exposure to pathogens. Indeed, Nikitin was thrilled that SanEp had lost its legal power to force immunization after 1991, allowing him to 'save' two of his grandchildren from 'the clutches of the vaccinologists.'

But asked repeatedly about the diphtheria epidemic, he declines to comment, changing the subject.

Journalist Boris Umnov—another key figure in the history of this sad doctrine—also refused to discuss the diphtheria epidemic. In 1988 Umnov wrote a much-cited article in *Komsomolskaya Pravda* declaring adamant opposition to vaccinations, based on a claim by a single Russian scientist—Dr Galena Petrovna Chervonskaya, then a virologist in the Tereseeva State Research Institution of Medical Preparation in Moscow—that existing Russian-made diphtheria and pertussis vaccines contained dangerous poisons.

Since this publication was read by young adults throughout the USSR, the impact was profound: parents began avoiding vaccinations for their children whenever possible, and paediatricians, fearing Chervonskaya could be right, did not aggressively push the vaccine on fretful parents.

Chervonskaya claimed the levels of Merthiolate (which she referred to as a pesticide, though it is not) and mercury salts found in the vaccine were toxic. And despite a study by the World Health Organization that disputed this, she and the influential Umnov continued a campaign into the mid-1990s—in most of Russia's leading newspapers and magazines—that suggested that use of the vaccine should be ended.

Similar voices were heard in other former Soviet countries.

In 1996 in Kazakhstan, for example, Dr Raisa Sadykovna Amandzholova was given the nation's highest meritorious award for her medical efforts. During the award ceremony, she argued that vaccination programmes were killing children with 'AIDS, tumours or blood cancer. The whole of children's oncology is overfilled. And that is the consequence of vaccination.'

Amandzholova, who was seventy-six years old in 1996, said on the occasion of receipt of the 'Honorary Degree for the honorary title of Peace and Culture' that vaccines were responsible for disintegration of the human gene pool.

'I want to pose a question as a scientist: what goal is harder? To protect children against infectious diseases but creating for them the risk of getting diseases and the plague of the twentieth century [AIDS and cancer]? As a result children are delivered unhealthy and this is passed from one generation to another. But it is time to think that perhaps natural selection is better than to spoil the genome of our people and cause mutations, the consequences of which are unpredictable.'

While voices such as Nikitin's, Chervonskaya's, and Amandzholova's got widespread play in the post-Communist media, vaccination supporters such as Tatochenko received virtually none. Tatochenko insisted that he argued constantly with Russian reporters, but realized they were looking for sensational angles. Steinglass and Tatochenko teamed up to spread a counterinformation campaign to the region's paediatricians and medical schools. But it was tough going. Old ideas died hard.

For example, in the former Soviet state of Estonia, Dr Toomas Trei explained, 'The reason why the immunization rate in children is low is simple: 95 per cent of the nation's doctors were trained at Tartu University. And the [Soviet] professor in charge of paediatrics taught that vaccines are dangerous. He said babies needed to grow without vaccines.'

By 1991, according to the World Health Organization, only 60 per cent of Russia's children under five years of age had received the three doses of diphtheria, pertussis, and tetanus vaccines necessary to ensure immunity—even though WHO experts contended a 95 per cent rate was needed to prevent epidemics. The anti-vaccine sentiment had even reached Germany, on both sides of the Berlin Wall, where diphtheria vaccination was incomplete or absent altogether for nearly a quarter of the adult population in 1997.

And that was only one part of the story, statistics showed. Russian measles vaccine coverage was only 78 per cent in 1991; its polio coverage a mere 71 per cent; and virtually *no* girls were vaccinated against rubella.

The diphtheria epidemic first surfaced in the USSR in 1987, when the number of confirmed cases reached 2000. Then in 1990 soldiers returning from Afghanistan apparently introduced the particular strain of the bacteria that would spread. That diphtheria toll then grew to more than 12 000 in 1991, when Moscow asked for help from the World Health Organization and the United States. The Bush administration agreed to provide assistance, sending scientific teams to Russia, Ukraine, Georgia, and other former Soviet states throughout 1992 and '93.

What the Western researchers found was shocking. First, their own stocks of vaccine—indeed, global supplies—were desperately low.

And in the former Soviet nations, the Westerners learned, millions of children had received inappropriate adult-dosed vaccinations and these children had five times the diphtheria rate seen in children immunized with appropriate doses. And they found that, as Steinglass had noted, their Soviet counterparts knew nothing of one of the most essential principles of vaccinology, the so-called Cold Chain or necessity to maintain refrigeration of vaccines throughout transport and storage.

Even more astounding were the regional death rates. By 1994 diphtheria had made its way into every single one of the former Soviet states, prompting an only marginally above-normal death rate in Russia of 2.8 per cent of all active cases. But in Lithuania and Turkmenistan an astonishing 23 per cent of all diphtheria cases proved fatal.

After two years of intense effort and distribution of more than 30 million vaccine doses the international team had, by mid-1996, vaccinated 70 per cent of all Ukrainians, pushing diphtheria incidence down by 30 per cent. But as nearly a third of all children and adults in the country remain unvaccinated, the situation was still critical.

Dr Alla Shcherbynska of the L. V. Gromashevski Epidemiology and Infectious Diseases Research Institute in Kiev said that during the 1970s, before all of the anti-vaccine sentiment arose among Soviet paediatricians, Ukraine's fifty-two million people experienced an average of seven diphtheria cases a year. By 1990, she said, that number had risen to two hundred and in 1992 one out of every 100 000 Ukrainians (or nearly 50 000 people) suffered a case of diphtheria—a level of disease not witnessed since Czarist days.

The incentive to 'smash' the anti-vaccine movement might ironically not be diphtheria but polio, which also resurged in the region. The paralytic effect of the polio virus upon children and the microbe's highly contagious nature rendered this disease especially worrying. Further, the World Health Organization, backed strongly by the USSR, had long ago set a goal of complete global eradication of polio by 2000. Any return of polio to the former Soviet Socialist Republics was, then, a genuine slap in the faces of SanEp and its antecedents.

Between 1959 and 1991 all supplies of polio vaccine used in the Eastern Bloc and Soviet Union were manufactured by the Institute of Poliomyelitis and Viral Encephalitis, located in Moscow. Like the iodine to prevent goitres, chlorine for water purification, and fluoride for dental care, supplies of polio vaccines suddenly disappeared with the collapse of the Soviet Union. By mid-1992 every single one of the former Soviet republics—except the Russian Federation—was using up the last of their polio vaccine inventories.

In late 1991 a strain of the most virulent form of polio—poliovirus type 1—surfaced in Tajikistan. And it continued for four years, as Tajik public health leaders proved incapable of mounting an effective national polio vaccine campaign until late 1995.

The Tajik polio strain spread to Ukraine in 1992, infecting thousands more people and causing a small number of paralytic cases.

The following year a different, thankfully less virulent, type 3 strain of poliovirus emerged in Uzbekistan, where all supplies of vaccine had long since dried up and thousands of youngsters were not immunized. An estimated 146 000 children were infected between 1993 and 1994, equalling more than a third of the affected area's under-four-year-old children.

These polio outbreaks, like the larger diphtheria epidemic, were brought under control through massive vaccination campaigns, underwritten by European and North American governments.

In war-torn Chechnya, however, all child immunization efforts ground to a complete halt in 1992. And in 1995 the Tajik type 3 virus found its way into Chechnya, resulting in an epidemic that infected most under-five-year-olds in the breakaway area, causing paralytic disease in 154 of them.

Fearing that the Chechnyan polio epidemic could quickly spread across Russia, Dr Gennady Onyschenko, the Ministry of Health's top infectious disease official, loaded up vaccine supplies and flew to the Chechnyan capital, Grozny. A tall, charismatic man with piercing blue eyes, Onyschenko was accustomed to holding sway during Soviet health crises. In post-Soviet Russia, however, he said he had a 'revelation— a rather unpleasant shock to us—to discover even the medical specialists were not aware how important immunization is.'

Having spent considerable time arguing with Russian doctors in order to raise diphtheria immunization rates and halt that bacterial epidemic, Onyschenko was in no mood for debate about polio. Despite a bloody civil war, he planned to simply march into Grozny and start vaccinating every single young child he saw.

But the Chechnyan leaders had other ideas. One of the several gangs vying for control of Chechnya kidnaped Onyschenko and held him—and the precious polio vaccines—hostage for several months. Eventually freed, Onyschenko was physically and mentally exhausted by his captivity, and the polio vaccines he'd brought had long since deteriorated into a useless liquid.

At the war's end Chechnyan vaccination resumed, bringing an end to the polio outbreak during the final weeks of 1996.

A key set of lessons for public health were revealed. First, immunization levels could not be permitted to fall below the 95 per cent level in any corner of the world without creating pockets of vulnerability into which lurking microbes rapidly emerged. Vaccine supply shortages, local wars, and cash flow problems could not be considered adequate excuses, as microbial surges were spectacularly swift and, ultimately, far more costly than continued immunization campaigns. Happily, the diphtheria and polio events also demonstrated that mass scale immunization works, halting outbreaks and swiftly slowing epidemics to manageable proportions. In short, vaccines remained marvellously effective elements in the public health toolbox.

Sadly, the same could not be said for antibiotics.

It came as a sad shock to anyone who met him to learn that Irakli Sherodzle was fifteen years old. Frail and tiny, Sherodzle looked like a primary school child of ten or eleven years.

Sherodzle and his mother, Rovena, are civil war refugees who live in a one-room apartment with no light, because they can't afford a light bulb. Their tiny apartment is inside an enormous hotel converted by the Georgian government to emergency shelter for civil war refugees. Ice-cold, lacking light bulbs in its halls, and with stair-cases ringing with sounds of arguments and political debates, it is a grim setting. On a day made colder by bone-chilling rain, mother and son huddle around an orange hot steel electronic coil on the floor—their only source of heat—and talk in gentle voices that whisper out of the room's darkness.

Weakened by illness, Irakli speaks with effort and deliberation. His mother, an unemployed widow, talks quickly. Irakli is dying from streptococcus, a type of microbe an American might pause to consider only for about as long as it takes to say the word *penicillin*.

'He has no father,' Rovena tells a visitor. 'Maybe America can help him.'

Similar cries for help echoed all across the former Soviet Union where rampant misuse of antibiotics and archaic hospital hygiene practices were promoting the emergence of more and more deadly, drug-resistant strains of common bacteria.

Though the ingredients for antibiotic disaster were in place before the 1991 collapse of communism, the ensuing economic chaos dramatically worsened matters. As the pace of bacterial mutation and spread quickened in this region, neighbouring nations in Western Europe and immigration destinations such as the United States and Canada were becoming concerned about the spread of bacterial superbugs.

In Georgia, Irakli pulls up his pant legs and with great difficulty stands, supported by Rovena's firm grip. Both legs have a large gash up the front, revealing fetid flesh-eating infection and the boy's shin bones. Irakli can only stand long enough to give visitors a quick glimpse of his osteomyelitis—a condition in which the streptococci eat both flesh and bone. Since January, when Irakli developed a high fever, heart flutters, and severe weakness, streptococcus has invaded his heart, blood, flesh, and bones.

Back in January mother and child had gone to Republican Hospital—a huge, deteriorating medical complex in downtown Tblisi—where Irakli was hospitalized for what was then a routine infection: he was given penicillin. After several days of treatment, however, the boy's situation nose-dived.

'That's because every microbe in the nation of Georgia is now resistant to penicillin,' said paediatric surgeon Irakli Gogorishvili, who did not treat the young patient. 'People took it for everything—even for a bad mood. So for sepsis [blood poisoning], meningitis, and so on we now assume penicillin won't work. So we start with cephalosporins.'

Expensive and more complicated to use properly, cephalosporins are a class of newer antibiotics. In February, the doctors told Rovena she would have to supply Irakli with cephalosporins, which in Georgia cost ten times more than penicillin. To buy the drugs—even at bargained down black-market prices—Rovena sold all but two outfits of her clothing, leaving her one set for winter, one for summer. She sold the emergency relief food she received as a refugee, and every memento except her dead husband's portrait. She even sold the wedding ring she had removed from his finger before he was buried.

After a week, though, Irakli's fever rose again. And doctors said Irakli's streptococcus was probably resistant to that treatment as well—though they weren't sure, since the hospital had no way to test the bacteria.

Laboratory capacity was largely absent throughout the former Soviet Union, both for fiscal reasons and because physicians in the former Communist regime were never trained to work with their microbiology counterparts. Laboratories existed in hospitals not so much to help with diagnosis and treatment, but to police SanEp hygienic practices that, in the end, contributed little to patient well-being.

Because no laboratory work was done, no one will know whether the bacteria that originally made Irakli mildly ill was the same strain that, after three weeks of hospitalization, was threatening his life. But given conditions in Soviet-era hospitals, it is quite possible that Irakli's deadly streptococcus was a microbe acquired in the very place he sought refuge from infection: Republican Hospital.

In Georgia's hospitals, Gogorishvili said, 'Ciprofloxacin you can forget about. People use it like tea in the morning. Doxycycline—people buy it on the black market and use it for STDs [sexually transmitted diseases], so it's useless now.' Amoxicillin is following the same route, he said, though tetracycline remains effective.

The doctors treating Irakli told Rovena to find more money, to buy third-generation cephalosporins. When she discovered that a week's worth of those drugs, plus syringes to inject them and vitamins to help rebuild his body, would cost more than $300, Rovena was horrified.

Many stepped forward to help. 'The head of the committee of refugees...here raised the money for his antibiotics,' Rovena said; the surgeon who dressed Irakli's infection wounds waived his fees; the hospital charged nothing for three weeks' stay; friends brought donated meals to the bedside.

But it was not enough. Though the boy improved briefly from the initial treatment, returning home in March, Rovena couldn't afford to keep the treatment up indefinitely and, in April, mother and son huddled together in their icy room, without options, watching the streptococcus resurge.

In the Deserters Bazaar—so named because hundreds of Georgian draft dodgers congregated there during the Soviet war in Afghanistan—Goga sells antibiotics to customers like Rovena. An economics student with no medical training, Goga advises customers on how to use the drugs and which to take for their ailments—which he is also happy to diagnose, if asked. Goga's stand offers everything from Ukrainian transfusion kits, Turkish syringes and intravenous saline, and Indian-manufactured condoms, to Bulgarian-made kanomycin and expired antituberculosis drugs bearing insignias of Western humanitarian organizations.

'The official pharmacies have to pay taxes, rent, and so on,' Goga explains. 'So their prices are two times higher. I also have a much greater supply of drugs here and no drug lies on a table for more than two days. We have a huge turnover.'

The Deserters Bazaar, and hundreds of markets like it all over the former Soviet Union, was full of such impromptu, illegal pharmacies. At a similar stand in Kiev, Ukraine, a former schoolteacher diagnosed an elderly woman's arthritis and sold her ampules of steroids that the bewildered woman was told to self-inject. In the Siberian city of Irkutsk, a woman who described herself as a housewife diagnosed ailments in an open market and freely prescribed antibiotics.

While quacks and marketeers dispensed admonishments against vaccination and bolstered the widespread misuse of antibiotics, infectious disease tolls rose dramatically.

Rheumatic fever raged across western Ukraine, for example, in the rural Lviv area. Caused by type A streptococcus bacterial infection, rheumatic fever was an infection of the heart that commonly led to growth stunting and severe, lifelong cardiac disease.

'The problem is very severe,' elderly Dr Miraslava Strouck, chief statistician for the Lviv Institute, explained in an insistent, throaty voice. 'About 19 per cent of the patients become invalids.'

In 1994 Strouck began to realize that doctors were filing too many heart disease reports on teenagers. When she added up the numbers it looked like nearly one out of every one hundred youngsters aged fifteen to seventeen years was suffering major cardiac disease, which on the face of it made no sense. Then, in 1995, she received reports on 710 'heart defects' in teenagers—a figure far too high to be due to any normal event.

Working backwards with her painstaking attention to detail Strouck realized that western Ukraine was in the midst of a largely unrecognized streptococcus A epidemic, prompting astonishing rheumatic fever rates. In 1996, she found, the teenage rheumatic fever rate was 7.1 per 1000 and the adult rate was 9.3 per 1000.

The US rheumatic fever rate in 1995 was about one case in every 2.6 million Americans, for a total nationwide of 112 cases.

'By the end of 1996 we had about 20 000 cases in Lviv Oblast,' Strouck said. 'There were 1500 paediatric, 800 teenager, and 18 000 adults.'

Donated American antibiotics proved far more effective in treating the streptococcus A infections than the locally available drugs, Strouck said, causing her to conclude that the Lviv strain was resistant to first-line, affordable drugs. But she wasn't certain.

'In the former USSR there was only one laboratory, in St Petersburg, which could identify streptococcus A. That's why there are no labs in all of Ukraine which could identify this streptococcus and give us data about its virulence. . . . To start such a laboratory we need supplies, reagents, and, unfortunately, the economic conditions right now prevent us.'

So rheumatic fever continued its spread in rural Lviv Oblast.

At the World Health Organization's Geneva headquarters Dr Maria Neira was wringing her hands over an even more basic public health crisis in the East: water. Everywhere that she cast her surveillance net Neira found more outbreaks in the formerly Communist world of cholera, typhoid fever, shigella—all diseases that were entirely preventable with proper water and sewage treatment facilities. There need not be epidemics in the modern world of any of these diseases, Neira argued, as treatment was cheap and highly effective.

So Neira was stunned, she said, by the East's inability to control such outbreaks. Beginning in 1992 she and other WHO technical experts made frequent trips eastward, hoping to decipher the causes of both the outbreaks and treatment failures.

'We did a seminar in Kiev, Ukraine [in 1995], and it was *very* hard to convince the old [public health] leadership,' Neira recalled. 'They wanted to call the army in, encircle the entire place where cholera broke out, go out to the frontiers and round people up, forcing them into hospitals. And then they wanted to keep them in those hospitals until they had three successive stools negative for cholera vibrio,' after, typically, fifteen to eighteen days of hospitalization.

That was the old Soviet, SanEp, model: bring in the military and police, compel obedience from the masses, and enforce a treatment protocol that was both phenomenally expensive to the state and personally offensive to the affected population.

Meanwhile, simpler, cheaper solutions were ignored. For example, when a cholera epidemic exploded in Romania in 1994, lasting two years and felling thousands of Romanians with severe diarrhoeal disease, Neira's office was dumbfounded by the country's public health response:

'In Romania they injected all sorts of high-dose antibiotics to treat cholera. They don't understand that cholera vibrio do not respond to antibiotics,' Neira said, her face expressing frank astonishment. 'They want electrophoresis and amyloid analysing equipment,' all expensive and entirely unnecessary. When Neira's team carefully explained that worldwide cholera was best treated simply with oral rehydration therapy—a mixture of clean water and salts that stop the deadly dehydration induced by cholera—the Romanian public health officials snapped at WHO experts: 'Don't come here with your guidelines for African poor people—cholera guidelines are for Africans. We are Europeans!'

But WHO concluded that some former Soviet-dominated countries—particularly Ukraine—had 'sanitation that is worse than in Africa,' Neira said.

WHO water engineers discovered that all over the region Soviet urban planners had bundled drinking water and sewage pipes together, burying them one on top of the other under the region's densely populated cities. The pipes, which typically were of iron or steel, had been subjected to decades of freezing winters during which they were encased in ice, followed by summer thaws when rust claimed the conduits. There had been little attention to maintenance over the years, and by the 1990s sewer pipes commonly leaked directly into drinking water carriers.

The result was that the people of places such as St Petersburg, Tblisi, Bucharest, Dushanbe, Kiev, and Moscow were—literally—drinking and washing in their own waste. That obvious disaster was compounded by acute chlorine shortages that were the result of the same production and distribution problems that rendered the region deficient in micronutrients, such as iron and iodine.

A long litany of diarrhoeal epidemics ensued, and due to leaking stagnant water supplies, so did mosquito-carried diseases such as malaria and encephalitis.

At the close of 1995 the Russian Environment Ministry concluded that half of the nation's drinking water supply was unsafe, either due to severe industrial pollution or biological contamination. Without funds to improve the situation the water remains at the close of the twentieth century only marginally better in most of Russia than it was at the century's beginning.

'How can a nation feel safe if her air and water are polluted . . . and half of the population drinks water that doesn't meet basic standards?' asked the Russian Academy of Medical Science's Gerasimenko in 1997.

The typhoid fever epidemic was a particularly critical example of the water crisis. Spread through contaminated water supplies, the *Salmonella typhi* bacterium readily exploited any disaster situation that led to reduced water safety. In January 1996 in Tajikistan's capital city of Dushanbe a handful of typhoid fever cases were diagnosed. By mid-1997 hospitals in the capital were diagnosing 200 new cases *per day*, 10 per cent of the city's 600 000 residents had active cases of the disease, and no one could even count the typhoid rates outside the city—in part because of the nation's ongoing civil war.

In addition to eroded water and sewer systems, massively scaled, badly conceived Soviet water projects also ended up increasing the incidences of human waterborne diseases.

Taking a visitor to stand before a map-covered wall in his small office Ivan Rusiev, ecosystems expert for the Soviet Plague Laboratory in Odessa, pointed to the Dnieper River: 'The main idea in the Soviet Union was that they planned to transfer fresh water from north rivers—here—to the south—down here. They planned to pump the Danube River into the Dnieper. And the first stage of the master plan was here—Saslyk Lake.'

All of southern Ukraine was, Rusiev explained, a swampy delta estuary, right up to the Black Sea. The Soviets wanted to bring fresh river water down to the delta region for irrigation. The fresh water was dumped into salty Saslyk Lake, which actually was a Black Sea estuary.

The plan was a disaster. Misguided Soviet engineers ended up miscalculating the ratios of salty and fresh water in Saslyk Lake, flooding the delta fields with overly salty water that left sixty thousand devastated hectares upon which no crops would grow. And they turned Saslyk into a gigantic blue/green algae pond in which all sorts of mosquitoes and disease-causing microbes thrived. For two decades—well into the Brezhnev era—Soviet planners ignored the rising incidence of diseases, refusing to acknowledge their profound environmental plumbing fiasco. Finally in 1985 they erected a dam across the Dniester River, hoping to improve matters. But this completely eliminated fresh water supplies to the delta, turning the area into a salted moonscape.

Meanwhile, Saslyk and other similarly altered lakes in Ukraine bred cholera vibrio, which thrived in the new algae colonies. And the dams slowed water-flow rates so badly that there was little mixing. The lakes became bacterial stew pots, especially in the summer, when the water was sixteen degrees centigrade, emitting classic organic stenches. They also bred mosquitoes that carried malaria, West Nile Virus, and Sindbis virus. And the slowed rivers no longer flushed out the tons of unprocessed human waste dumped into them by upstream municipalities.

By the time all of this water reached Odessa and the Crimean Sea ports it was so microbially contaminated that local water, if consumed unboiled, was guaranteed to cause dysentery.

'Our authorities do their best, but everything stumbles over finances,' Rusiev says with a shrug. But then he amends his statement: 'But I tell them we have not only problems with finances, but also problems with our brains. When problems arise you need to think of the river. It's the source of water for ten million people!'

What could be more basic an element of public health than water? Or immunization? Or safe and adequate food supplies? Or elimination of antibiotic-resistant microbes?

Yet in each of these cases the Soviet leadership failed, blundering its way through one poorly designed and executed scheme after another. What happened in these arenas after 1991 constituted collapse of houses of Communist cards, not decimation of once-solid systems of public health.

VI

When a prolonged, stubborn, and heated struggle is in progress, there usually begins to emerge after a time the central and fundamental points at issue, upon the decision of which the ultimate outcome of the campaign depends, and in comparison with which all the minor and petty episodes of the struggle recede more and more into the background.
—V. I. Lenin, 'One step forward, two steps back', 1904

Konstantin, an emaciated, bedridden thirty-nine-year-old former Soviet soldier, lies dying at the Moscow Tuberculosis Research Centre. Drug-resistant TB has invaded his lungs, liver, kidneys, and heart.

Still, he says with a smirk that he appreciates the irony of the situation. 'It's like a joke,' he notes, his soft, ruined voice interrupted frequently by fits of coughing, 'a particularly Russian joke.'

It's hard to see the humour in Konstantin's situation. An intravenous drip pumps cocktails of antibiotics into his body twenty-four hours a day. Despite a bath of warm sunlight spread across his hospital bed Konstantin wears a wool knit cap and two sweaters, lies under layers of blankets, and still shivers. His colourless face and sunken eyes betray Konstantin's peril, and a doctor whispers that there is little hope for the man, as every vital organ of Konstantin's body is overwhelmed with tuberculosis bacteria.

Still, Konstantin sees irony in his plight, he says between bouts of coughs that seem to shake his lungs right out of their protective rib cage. And for a Russian, he continues, irony equals a joke. A Russian joke.

'I did it all,' Konstantin begins. 'Komsomol, Communist Party, fighting in Afghanistan...'

A decorated intelligence officer in the Afghanistan War, Konstantin returned to Moscow suffering from post-traumatic stress and was discharged in 1991, just before the Soviet dissolution. When Moscow radio announced in 1993 that fellow-Communists and a hotchpotch of other anti-Yeltsin forces had seized the Russian White House, Konstantin grabbed the Afghani rifle he had brought home with him and dutifully reinforced the barricades.

'In 1993 I took an active part in the political turmoil. I supported the coup,' Konstantin recalled.

But the rebellion failed, and a year later Konstantin was arrested for high treason. He was sent to Butirka prison without a trial, or formal sentencing, where, he recalls, 'I got TB in 1995.'

For months after that, his health deteriorated as he was transferred from one prison facility to another, his medications constantly interrupted and changed. Finally, in January 1997, a judge reviewed his case for the first time, ruling that since he wasn't in the army when the coup occurred, he couldn't have committed high treason. And for the first time in nearly three years, Konstantin was free.

But the exoneration was cold comfort. 'In principle,' Konstantin says with Russian stoicism, 'I was given a death sentence. The paradox is that most people are in there like me, waiting for court action, not even sentenced. I remember several people in prison who died of TB and never had a day in court.'

Mirian wanders the halls of the Moscow TB sanatorium, bored but exhausted. The skinny, pale Georgian also caught tuberculosis in jail—in his case at the notorious Matrosskaya Tishina prison—in 1993 and four years later is still struggling with the now multidrug-resistant microbes that have overrun his lungs. Arrested for robbery, Mirian served three years in a thirty-square-metre jail cell inhabited by more than a hundred prisoners, he softly says. Each prisoner, then, had less than a half a square metre of space, or about a chunk of personal turf measuring one foot by one foot. To sit or sleep the men rotated, Mirian said, taking turns alternately packing like sardines to stand for eight hours while other men lay down and slept.

The crowding in Russian jails and prisons was a post-1991 crisis born of the new nation's need to create a judicial system. Where once a mere KGB whisper backed by no evidence had been enough to land someone in a life-time of imprisonment now judges were required impartially to oversee trials in which prosecutors and defence attorneys argued over the merits of available evidence. But few such judges and attorneys existed in Russia, as the very concept of legal defence in the face of prosecution had long been anathema. While the nation struggled to invent a system of jurisprudence men piled up in the nation's jails, most having never formally been indicted. As Russia's crime rate escalated after 1991, so did the size of her unindicted prison population, reaching 500 000 in 1996. And Russia was hardly alone: the entire region was struggling to create judicial systems while untried prisoner populations piled up.

Released in October 1996 Mirian transferred to the Moscow sanatorium. And there he remained nearly a year later, held captive by tubercular microbes.

Asked why his TB has proven incurable, twenty-five-year-old Mirian shrugs: 'I can remember that at Butirka there were different tablets we got once a day. Different ones, changing all of the time.'

According to TB experts, staying just three years in the Russian jail system—home to an amazing 1 in 148 Russian residents in 1997—was tantamount to a death sentence from tuberculosis. And world health experts argued that unless Russia stopped the rampant spread of TB there, it hadn't a prayer of controlling it in the society at large.

'The easiest way to bring the Russian TB epidemic under control is with a focus on prisoners,' said Belgian physician Tine Demeulenaere of Médecins Sans Frontières (MSF). 'Cure them. Stop the recycling of TB.'

With up to one million people jamming the jails, overcrowding had become acute. At Moscow's Matrosskaya Tishina pre-trial detention centre, for example, there were 140 prisoners per 35-bed cell, with a per-prisoner 'space' rate of 0.1 square metres, according to photo documentation provided by the independent Centre for Prison Reform. By the summer of 1995 people were actually dying of lack of oxygen, as there were simply too many men packed in each cell.

'We now know that some 50 per cent of [Russian] prisoners are estimated to have TB,' says Murray Feshbach. 'And we also are now told that some 850 000 to one million persons are in prison.'

So it seems logical, he said, to conclude that there were up to 500 000 Russian prisoners with TB—a rate forty times higher than in the general population. Indeed, an unpublished Ministry memo supported that claim, noting that prisoners in Siberian jails, alone, were contracting more than 6500 new cases per year per 100 000 prisoners—the highest infection rate recorded in the latter half of the twentieth century in any risk group in the world, according to the World Health Organization.

Nestled in the Caucasus Mountains in the southern region of the former Soviet Union, the little nation of Georgia was trying to tackle its tuberculosis epidemic in the late 1990s with a strategy that met Western approval. And key to stopping its TB epidemic was elimination of the disease in Georgian prisons.

Dr George Nashievili, director of the nation's TB services, was waging a two-pronged attack on the problem, focusing on Georgia's urban centres. Following a World Health Organization approach called DOTS (Directly Observed Therapy System), Nashievili was trying to rebuild Georgia's demolished network of TB outpatient clinics and from them dispense appropriate antibiotics to identified tuberculosis cases and carriers. But he knew that it would be impossible to stop the spread of TB in the general population unless it was first eliminated from the nation's jails and prisons.

Though the numbers of prisoners dying each year of TB in Georgia paled when compared to neighbouring Russia, tuberculosis was the leading cause of death in prison, surpassing violence and heart disease, according to Givi Kvarelashvili, head of the National Committee of Incarceration.

To conquer the TB problem in prisons, Kvarelashvili's medical staff regularly scours the prison population in search of visibly ill men, who are then given chest X-rays. Those who are confirmed TB cases are separated: acute cases go to one special holding area, chronic tuberculosis sufferers to another. All patients are given DOTS antibiotic therapy, involving four drugs, daily. In addition, TB prisoners are put on special, highly nutritious diets and issued wool blankets.

As a result of this programme TB death rates fell by 50 per cent over the two years of the new prison programme according to Nashievili.

Normally that would be cause for joy, but Nashievili was cautious about interpreting TB trends either in the jails or on the outside—due to unreliable Soviet-era records and non-existent records during the post-1991 chaos and civil war. Still he was convinced that Georgia's TB situation had begun to improve.

Dr Maya Sharashidze wasn't so sure. Her privately funded Georgia Foundation surveyed and treated TB in the remote Sagarejo region of the country. In every village the medical team had found hidden cases—individuals who for one reason or another never sought medical attention for the TB that they knew was responsible for their weakness and coughing.

'Georgians feel ashamed of TB,' Sharashidze explained over tea and *khachapuri* cheese bread in her Tblisi home. 'They try to keep it confidential. They do not tell neighbours, and do not go to doctors.'

Though no one in Georgia had the necessary laboratory equipment to conduct drug resistance tests, Sharashidze said, it was also clear that most TB in the country was resistant to at least one of the five antibiotics used in the primary treatment cocktail.

So even if Georgia one day managed to get its prison outbreaks and Tblisi epidemics under control, Sharashidze said, the rural epidemic would persist and increase in drug resistance. Furthermore, in the wake of the civil war Georgia faced newer TB problems among refugees and civilians living in the contested areas.

In Southern Ossetia, for example, four tuberculosis patients huddle in a bombed-out hospital, trying to absorb heat from a log that smouldered on the concrete floor. They are the only patients in what had been the City Hospital of Tskhinvali, population 42 000. Volunteers from Médecins Sans Frontières built a toilet at the site, and puttied glass into the windows of the TB ward. But the patients use the former operating room to chop wood and furniture for their tiny fires. They are, in essence, camping out inside the rubble hull left by war.

MSF nurse Jean-Luc Seugy says the people of devastated Ossetia approach TB with 'aggressive denial,' taking whatever antibiotics they can buy on the black market until their money runs out. And never seeking medical attention. In the process they are breeding drug-resistant strains of tuberculosis. Even when family members die of TB the relatives refuse to be tested.

Amid the chaos that had become the norm in Ukraine's health system, children were suffering the highest levels of TB seen in that country since the 1950s, when antibiotic-based public health approaches to the disease were initiated.

'The situation is just dreadful. It is dreadful,' exclaimed Dr Victoria Kostromira, director of paediatric services for the Kiev Institute of Pulmonology. 'There are not only many more children with TB than we've seen in the past, they are getting forms of the disease we've never seen before.'

The number of diagnosed tuberculosis cases in Ukrainian children under the age of fifteen doubled between 1990 and 1996, Kostromira said, and with diagnostic capacity down to near-zero levels for mild cases, it had become almost impossible to estimate the disease's true rate.

And more of the Ukrainian paediatric tuberculosis cases were proving fatal. Prior to 1992, for instance, Ukraine had no TB-related meningitis cases. In 1996 there were thirty such cases, and twenty-four children died.

Kostromira's institute had a supply of just four first-line antibiotics, she said, and every day their usefulness diminished. That was because the front line TB dispensaries in the former Soviet state of 52 million people had run out of money.

When the Soviet Union was intact, Moscow created single production centres for specific items and shipped the products all over the vast nation: chlorine, vaccines, iodine. In the past, raw materials for antibiotics were made in one area, and packaged as useful drugs in another. Almost immediately after the 1991 breakup of the Soviet Union the chain of production collapsed. The result, in terms of TB treatment, was that Ukraine had to import all of its antibiotics; nothing was manufactured inside the country. And that meant that the essential drugs were anywhere from ten to one hundred times more expensive for Kostromira and her patients in 1997 than they were in 1987.

Once the frail tubercular children reached the institute, their care—including meals—was free. The trick for anxious families spread out over the large nation was getting diagnosed at a local TB clinic and finding the resources to travel to Kiev.

'We used to be full,' Kostromira said of her institute, built under the Soviet regime to serve patients diagnosed at local TB clinics throughout the large republic. 'Now patients can't afford to get here.' Galina managed to bring her grandson, Janya, to the institute in August 1996. They lived only fifteen kilometres outside Kiev, so it wasn't a difficult journey, Galina says.

On a cold, overcast day, she and her grandson lie quietly on his hospital bed in a room that is also home to three other children. The lights are turned off to save hospital electricity costs, and there is no heat. In the late afternoon shadows, Galina reads slowly to the tiny five-year-old boy, whose growth has been visibly stunted by his bout with tuberculosis. She hesitates while he coughs, which is frequently, since he suffers from a bronchial infection.

But it was Russia's out-of-control tuberculosis epidemic that most worried WHO and Western public health experts. By the close of the 1990s, the multidrug-resistant tuberculosis epidemic, spawned in packed prison populations, spanned the entire nation, often at incidence rates unseen anywhere else in the world at that time.

Prison treatment options were limited. Although the Russian Interior Ministry made TB treatment available to prisoners at its own medical facilities, health officials throughout Russia complained that the treatment could do more harm than good. That was because it remained standard practice to give prisoners only one or two antibiotics at a time, rather than the four or five recommended by the World Health Organization. And the drugs were often 'take what you are offered', since ministry officials allocated little money to the effort. Further, prisoners were subject to frequent transfers among jails, which meant they often underwent the type of treatment changes that promote the emergence of drug resistance. And once released, 95 per cent fell out of the public health system entirely.

The result: Dr Alexey Priymak, then director of TB services for the Ministry of Health, said that about 80 per cent of all infected ex-prisoners in Russia carried drug-resistant strains of bacteria, and half would die of TB-related symptoms within twelve months of their release from prison.

In Soviet times TB care was simple and straightforward. Every single man, woman, and child in the USSR was required by law to undergo an annual chest X-ray. Any suspicious X-ray films were sent to SanEp, which rounded up the possible TB carriers and compelled sputum tests. If proved to be infected, the individual was placed in a sanatorium for months, often years, isolated from contact with friends or family until several repeated sputum tests came up negative for TB. This was policy for infants, as well as older children and adults. During their sanatorium stay the Soviet TB patients received, typically, one or two antibiotics in high doses.

But with the collapse of the Communist state no one had the power to impose TB incarceration upon Russian or Georgian citizens. As a result all public health TB control measures had fallen to pieces because during Soviet days they relied upon the power of the state to impose screening and treatment upon its citizens.

By 1997, officials said, Russia's primary drug resistance rate was 23.4 per cent; 21 per cent to two drugs; 19.4 per cent to three drugs; 6.4 per cent to more than four antibiotics.

In the jails incidence of TB, and resistant tuberculosis, continued to rise. At the Tomsk central prison, for example, the TB incidence was 7000 per 100 000—ten times the general Siberian TB rate. Estimated rates in other Russian prisons ranged from 2481 per 100 000 to more than 7000 per 100 000.

And every day the prison system was feeding costly, multidrug-resistant, TB-infected patients into the beleaguered state public health network. A 1997 Ministry of Interior memo leaked to a visiting foreigner contained these disturbing lines:

'By the year 2000 the incidence [of tuberculosis] will increase fifty times compared with now; mortality will increase seventyfold; and deaths in children are expected to rise ninetyfold.'

Murray Feshbach interpreted that statement as follows: 'In 2000, according to these numbers, tuberculosis deaths in Russia will reach approximately 1.75 million, whereas I estimate that heart disease and cancer deaths will number about 1.5 million. This says something extraordinary about the state of public health.'

Meanwhile, Russia's prisons only worsened with time. With the 1998 collapse of the rouble came a government services crunch that, among other things, signalled food shortages and reported starvation in some Russian prisons. By late 1998 the Yeltsin government, realizing that imprisonment, even in the absence of indictment, had become a death sentence, enacted waves of amnesties, releasing inmates who hadn't been convicted of serious violent crimes. Tens of thousands of TB-ailing former inmates were released into the arms of a grossly overwhelmed health-care system.

Every TB hospital and sanatorium in Russia was full: some had waiting lists. Staff were either unpaid or, if they were lucky, underpaid. Less than half of the public health system's TB-related equipment, such as laparoscopes and X-ray devices, worked. The number of doctors and nurses willing to endanger their own health, working without protective gear in such facilities, steadily declined: by 1997 nearly half nationwide had quit. Who could blame them: mortality rates among health-care workers employed by the tuberculosis system was ten times higher than that of the general population.

Of greatest concern was Russia's eastern Siberian region, where TB traditionally ran at rates higher than were seen in Moscow and west of the Ural mountains.

When nature calls for Dr Galina Dugarova, the sixty-two-year-old head of tuberculosis control for Russia's Southern Buryatia state has to hike down a flight of dilapidated wooden stairs and step outside to an outhouse. The chief TB dispensary, which contains all the administrative offices and laboratories for the state of 1 150 000 people, has no running water, no sewage system, no heat, no laboratory supplies, scarce supplies of antibiotics, no modern chest X-ray devices, no protective masks and gloves for the staff and physicians, and no money to pay said staff. It is housed inside a 150-year-old wooden building that leans sharply to one side, has gaping holes in its roof, and is sinking.

The semiautonomous Buryatia Republic, located in Siberia just 150 miles north of the Mongolian border, hasn't a spare rouble to deal with tuberculosis. But it has plenty of TB.

'It's like a genocide,' declares Dugarova. 'A holocaust. We're dying.'

Though she was until recently a prominent member of the Soviet Communist Party, Dugarova concedes that the dramatic tuberculosis epidemic sweeping over her people began during the USSR days and has steadily worsened since 1991.

She is one of 260 000 ethnic Buryatis living in the mountainous republic—high cheekboned Buddhists (or in the case of devout Communists, atheists) who proudly declare their heritage to include Genghis Khan. Probably for genetic reasons, though no one was sure, ethnic Buryatis and other indigenous peoples of Siberia are especially vulnerable to the tuberculosis mycobacteria. In 1996 some 211 of every 100 000 Buryatis suffered active, symptomatic tuberculosis. That's twice the TB rate seen in their ethnic Russian neighbours.

For Buryati Minister of Health Blair Balzhirov the particular susceptibility of his Mongolian people to TB was a focus of great sorrow. He hoped that a blend of seventeenth-century Tibetan medical practices and Soviet-style TB control approaches would soon obliterate the tuberculosis crisis. But he had few health-care workers at his disposal trained in either tradition—who could travel the 354 000-square-kilometre republic in search of TB cases.

Patriot Day in Ulan Ude—May Day in the West—the city's population pours into Ploshehad Sovietov, a central square accessed via Ulitsa Lenina, a broad, tree-lined boulevard. Though it is still chilly, the sun bathes the celebrants as they parade past the two-storey-tall, black head of Lenin, which nestles atop a marble pedestal like the decapitated, neckless face of John the Baptist sitting upon Salome's platter. Russian Army soldiers and sailors stand to attention in dress uniforms while units of protofacist Cossacks, red flag-waving Communist Party members, and World War II medal-bedecked veterans march past.

So it comes as no surprise to discover Buryati's TB officer, Dugarova, and her political leaders favour a return to the old Soviet methods in their search for a way to staunch the area's rapidly expanding tuberculosis catastrophe. Every individual found to have tuberculosis in Ulan Ude is, by Dugarova's command, brought to the log cabins that currently constitute her TB sanatorium. One is entirely paediatric, housing children—forcibly separated from their parents—aged twelve months to fourteen years. Tiny Misha, fifteen months old, has languished on the ward for three months, separated from his loving parents during key weeks of infant development. He has pulmonary TB.

Pretty, blond Tatyana, her hair wound in tight braids, plays with her 'doll', a baby named Dulma. For more than a year Tatyana has lived in this tiny cabin, alongside a horde of other children, playing with the babies that at an increasing rate are dying in Dugarova's sanatorium.

Dugarova has no resistance laboratory test kits, no medical microbiology capacity, and—worse yet—no drug options. She just keeps giving the patients what antibiotics she can find, generally one or two drugs daily, and hopes the babies and adults muddle through. It's less than satisfactory, she admits.

But things will be better, Dugarova insists, when the giant 200-bed concrete sanatorium that has been under construction for six years is completed. The TB director takes her visitors to the edifice, which must be guarded twenty-four hours a day by armed men who shoot at would-be thieves. The nine-square-metre, six-storey building is Dugarova's pride, though all its windows are broken, its stair banisters are rusted, and the entire structure seems about to collapse.

Yet, Dugarova insisted repeatedly, this shell will one day be a sanatorium. And a sanatorium will stop the Buryatian epidemic.

Though the Buryatia Republic's situation may have ranked as the worst in the world—especially for ethnic Buryatis—there were hot spots within the former Soviet Union that, remarkably, had even higher incidences of tuberculosis in specific risk groups. Officials at WHO described the situation as 'eighteenth century,' and were doing all they could to pressure the governments in the region not only to pour more money on the problem but to change the way they tackled tuberculosis control.

Some of the governments, particularly those of Georgia, Armenia, Azerbaijan, and the Kyrgyz Republic, were listening and had radically altered their TB control efforts to follow WHO guidelines. But the huge nations of Ukraine, Belarus, and Russia, as well as much of the Baltics and Central Asia, remained stubbornly locked into old Soviet approaches to TB.

New York City learned its lesson in 1991 when TB erupted in the city, driven by neglectful treatment, inappropriate antibiotic use, emergence of multidrug-resistant strains of the bacteria, and the presence of a uniquely vulnerable population—hospitalized AIDS patients who lacked immunological capacity to fight off infection. After a few months of bumbling and fumbling the city adopted the Czech model developed by Dr. Karyl Stiblo, instituting a Directly Observed Therapy System—DOTS—to monitor medicine compliance every day in the city's identified TB patients. It worked.

WHO had promoted the DOTS approach vigorously worldwide. Wherever it had been properly implemented, officials said, TB rates fell dramatically.

But the approach adhered to—stubbornly and rigidly—in Russia, Ukraine, Belarus, and most of the rest of the former USSR was diametrically opposite. Tuberculosis was handled in the 1990s as it was in the 1950s when Nikita Khrushchev ran the far-flung nation with a Communist iron hand.

A massive system of sanatoriums staffed by doctors, nurses, and phthisiologists (a TB specialty that no longer existed in the West), coupled with an even more sizeable network of out-patient screening clinics, monitored the population, testing every citizen annually with chest X-rays. Anyone who came up positive was given skin and culture tests—laboratory assays. If either of those also proved positive, the individual was removed from employment for two years, placed in mandatory sanatorium confinement for a minimum of one year, and treated with huge injections of one or two types of antibiotics. All of the patient's family members and co-workers were also tested, ensuring that the patient's TB was publicly known. If any of them proved positive, they, too, were pulled out of school or stripped of employment for two years. If after one year treatment appeared to be successful, the patient would be given a temporary job involving no contact with food products or the public. If unsuccessful, infected parts of the patient's body were surgically removed. Twenty to 25 per cent of all TB patients underwent lung surgeries in which some or all of the lung was removed.

To the degree that dwindling finances permitted this highly labour-intensive, repressive approach to TB control, it was still practiced. But few TB officials could afford routine X-rays, tracing to find all of the familial and social contacts of every infected patient, or appropriate drug treatment.

And those in charge, such as Dr Alexey Priymak of the Russian Ministry of Health, said that the rising TB death toll stemmed not from a failed approach to tuberculosis control but from inadequate financing of that old model.

'Underlying it all is a struggle for the survival of these huge, hulking old hospitals and institutions,' Richard Bumgarner, deputy director of WHO's Global Tuberculosis Program, insisted. 'They charge patients now for things that were free, and discharge them when the money runs out. Therein lies the reason for the resurgence of TB. The Russian health minister doesn't see this. TB is Ebola with wings, and she is busy creating it.'

At Priymak's urging the Ministry of Health lobbied successfully in 1996 for Duma passage of a tuberculosis five-year plan. Three billion dollars (eighteen trillion roubles) were allocated for expenditure starting in 1997 on upgrading the existing TB infrastructure. Even if the government only actually came up with 30 per cent of the allocation it would more than double spending on the disease. And if Yeltsin's people didn't come up with the funds, Priymak warned, 'By 2002 the annual new caseload officially in Russia will be 200 000, and the incidence in children will increase 100 per cent.'

In fact, Priymak's system had already failed to cure at least 249 000 TB cases by 1996. It was an idle threat. But it worked, politically.

And it infuriated Western Europeans, who felt certain that Russia's drug-resistant bacteria were crossing their borders. By 1998 the Copenhagen office of WHO had documented that 25 per cent of all Russian TB cases involved multidrug-resistant forms of the bacteria.

'Tuberculosis is at our [European] doorstep, and it is uglier and more frightening than ever,' Dr Arata Kochi, WHO Tuberculosis Programme director, concluded.

In fact, it had already crossed Europe's threshold, and forms of tuberculosis found in Russian and Baltic states were cropping up all over Scandinavia. More than half of all TB cases documented in Sweden, Denmark, and Norway in 1996 to 1999 were seen among emigrés from the Baltics and Russia, Dr Nils Pederson, of the Statens Serum Institut in Copenhagen, said. By 2000 Russian-originated drug-resistant strains of TB bacteria were turning up all over northern Europe, according to WHO.

Yet Priymak and the Russian government refused to yield. Open public health warfare ensued, pitting Western and Communist policies against one another in a battle that could cost tens of thousands of lives and spread untreatable forms of tuberculosis across all of Europe.

There were dissident voices within the old Soviet tuberculosis system. The loudest and most influential was that of Priymak's former teacher, director of Russia's largest TB clinical research centre, in Moscow. Operated by the Russian Academy of Sciences, Dr Alexander Khomenko's huge TB facility was independent from the Ministry of Health—and from Priymak's influence. The former teacher and student locked horns in a battle over the future of Russia's tuberculosis epidemic, and there could be little doubt that the winner would influence not only Moscow's approach to TB but also the attitudes of counterpart health agencies in Kiev, Minsk, Alma-Ata, and capitals of other former Soviet states. Khomenko, who served as the USSR's representative to WHO in Geneva from 1965 to 1970, favoured the DOTS approach.

Khomenko had watched the incidence of TB rise throughout the former Soviet Union by 10 to 15 per cent a year every year since 1990. He had seen budgets crumble to the point where he, earning $400 a month, was one of the most highly paid TB doctors in the nation. And even more worrying, he asserted, was the phenomenal increase in drug resistance.

Under his direction, the Ivanovo Oblast, a region north-east of Moscow, was trying the DOTS approach, and it had already reduced its TB rate by 8 per cent since 1995. As part of a continuing experiment the laboratory capacities of Ivanovo's TB hospital were vastly improved, and drug sensitivity tests were performed on sputum samples from the region's patients. More than half—58.1 per cent—of all samples contained mycobacteria that was partially resistant to one or more antibiotics. One out of every eight patients in Ivanovo carried a multidrug-resistant strain of TB.

At Khomenko's Moscow facility most patients had drug-resistant TB—that was one of the reasons they made their way from as far as Vladivostok, searching for last-ditch treatments that might save their lives.

In 1996, for example, Paulina Mahachela brought her twenty-one-year-old son, Khoubanov, all the way from Dagestan, a mountainous Russian state on the Caspian Sea. A champion weightlifter with Olympic dreams, Khoubanov felt fatigued and weak in March 1996—doctors in his hometown of Makhachkala diagnosed tuberculosis. By then the young Muslim man already had enough TB bacteria in both lungs that X-rays revealed bilateral damage.

'For one and a half months he stayed at home, and he seemed all right,' Paulina, a short, middle-aged brunette, recalled. Because she is a physician—though not a TB specialist—Paulina was confident that home treatment with four antibiotics would be sufficient.

But she didn't know Khoubanov was infected with drug-resistant TB. Nobody did because none of the Dagestan hospitals had equipment to conduct drug sensitivity tests on his sputum samples. Worse yet, the young, dark-eyed man developed a toxic liver reaction to the only one of the drugs that was effective against his TB.

Hospitalized in Dagestan, Khoubanov's condition by August 1996 was dire. When doctors switched him from the four drugs he had been taking to expensive cephalosporin antibiotics Khoubanov had a severe allergic reaction to the medicine. That's when Paulina decided it was time to pool the family's financial resources and bring her son to Moscow—to the famous Dr Khomenko.

'By then he was resistant to all available drugs,' Paulina said. And X-rays revealed that both his lungs were completely infected. Khomenko's staff felt there was no option—in November the patient was rolled into the operating theatre.

When the surgeons opened up Khoubanov's lungs, they were stunned. Inside his left lung was a 'giant cavity', one of the surgeons recalled—hard as a rock, the formation was full of tuberculosis bacteria. And all but the lower lobe of his right lung was similarly infected. The surgeons removed the cavity and half of the man's right lung.

For 130 days, Khoubanov's remaining lung musculature refused to function and the man's life hung on little more than his mechanical ventilator and Paulina's prayers. His weight fell precariously from 84 to 53 kilos, and Khomenko's staff feared every day that the young man would die.

But during the worst of Moscow's 1996 winter, Khoubanov's lungs spontaneously started working again. When some of his strength was restored doctors noticed that it was his right lung—which had been surgically reduced by half—that was doing all the work. X-rays revealed that TB had once again claimed his left lung.

So on May 14, Khoubanov's entire left lung was surgically removed, leaving the man with only 25 per cent lung capacity.

In the spring of 1997 Khoubanov lay lethargically in an isolated room in the intensive care unit, breathing through a one-inch-diametre hole cut in his trachea. Painted daily with emerald disinfectant the hole gapes at horrified visitors. When he can gulp enough air through his mouth, Khoubanov covers the disturbing hole with a piece of gauze bandaging. If breathing becomes particularly difficult doctors insert a ventilator tube directly into the aperture.

Khoubanov tries to speak, but cannot muster enough air across his voice box to make clear noises. Paulina knowingly leans over, placing her ear directly over his tracheal hole, her mouth inhaling what her son exhales. She—and the staff—do this many times a day. And no one wears masks. The protective gear is in such short supply that it can only be used during invasive and surgical procedures.

'The doctors are very enthusiastic but they don't have enough money or drugs,' Paulina says.

'It's true,' one of the physicians adds. 'It's only due to the relatives that he survives.'

Since Khoubanov was diagnosed in March 1996 the Mahachela family has spent 80 million roubles on drugs (about $14 000) and 55 million on surgery (some $4000). Paulina could not recall how much she has spent on hospitalization and housing for herself in Moscow—perhaps another $4000. Even an American family would be hard pressed to come up with $20 000 in cash—for Dagestanis it's almost unimaginable. The typical Dagestani family with employed heads of households survives on about $2400 a year. Khoubanov's tuberculosis has not only destroyed one and a half of his lungs and bankrupted the Mahachela family but also left his entire clan in debt back home in Dagestan.

Such severe measures—and patient expenditures—weren't even possible for most of the region's TB patients. Most said Dugarova, in Buryatia, were 'jobless, homeless, and poor'. And it was precisely because of the poverty of both the patients and TB treatment system that Dugarova sided with Priymak, not Khomenko, and opposed DOTS.

'Okay, it's cheaper, it's cost-effective. And maybe other areas have fruit and vegetables all the time, but not here,' Dugarova said dismissively. 'If these drugs are available, okay, but they aren't. We haven't even got vitamins, so come on!'

What did Dugarova have for TB treatment? Sacks full of isoniazid powder intended for injection but given orally in capsules. Old supplies, Soviet made, that Stiblo had analysed and said 'is just like sand'. She also had two other basic antibiotics and, occasionally, a third. Supplies varied, so patients rarely got a steady, consistent course of treatment. And consistency, experts said, was the key to avoiding development of resistant strains.

'We don't interrupt therapy, but we may get down to just one drug,' Dugarova admitted.

At the Buryatia 'sanatorium'—the three log cabins, packed wall-to-wall with patients—Dugarova declares that 'at least there is running water,' though the rooms are ice-cold in the winter. Between the children's cabin and one of the adult log hospitals long clothes-lines are stretched; the children's hand-washed bed linen flaps in the crisp mountain wind.

In the adult wards patient beds are stacked so closely together that plump Dugarova cannot make her way between them. The hospitals have no pajamas or linens—these, the adult patients must provide for themselves. The dining hall consists of three hot plates and a few tables. 'I want to go home,' cries sixty-three-year-old patient Yekaterina Chernykh when she spies Dugarova.

In the intensive care ward—so designated not by virtue of any better technology, but because the patients are sicker—four men lay inert, their tableside meals untouched. Three have advanced pulmonary TB, the fourth has tuberculous meningitis.

'They are all going to die,' Dugarova whispers. 'These forms of TB—I never saw them, even in the fifties. They are, of course, sentenced to death. We cannot treat them. No way. We would like to give them four drugs and some protein but we have no money, and they have no money. They are sentenced.'

One of the attending nurses had been eavesdropping on Dugarova's conversation. On hearing the chief physician's somber pronouncement she silently bows her head, ties a wad of gauze bandaging around her mouth and nose, and tiptoes to the bedside of a twenty-one-year-old man. Dugarova looks on impassively as the nurse gently strokes the bony body outlined by a red blanket.

Thousands of miles away in Tartu, Estonia, Heinart Sillaustu, president of the Estonian Society of Respiratory Medicine, denounces such practices as 'old-fashioned, inflexible and overstaffed. The Soviet TB system was one in which the Party dominated everywhere.'

Sillaustu warmly greets visitors into his comfortable home, serving tea and offering data via a home slide show. Retired, Sillaustu devoted decades of his life to challenging the Soviet view of tuberculosis. When he began in 1953 Estonians suffered tuberculosis at a rate of 417 primary cases per 100 000 citizens. Through a combination of Soviet methods and his own uniquely Estonian brand of Stiblo's DOTS approach Sillaustu managed to push TB rates down to their nadir of 21 cases per 100 000 in 1992. But since then TB had been climbing back up, reaching 44.5 primary cases per 100 000.

'In Russia they didn't give the real data,' Sillaustu says, 'but these numbers are real,' illustrating that although public health lost some ground after the fall of communism in Estonia, no tragedy on the scale of the Russian debacle occurred.

Still, Sillaustu continues, nearly 20 per cent of all Estonian TB cases are drug resistant and the average age of tuberculosis patients has shifted down, from fifty-five to sixty years in 1981 to, in 1996, an average of thirty, 'the productive workforce,' he notes. Regrettably Sillaustu wasn't making much headway with Estonian politicians because the officials would always point to Byelorussian and Russian TB data and say, 'See, we're not so bad off.'

'But I say to them, "Let's not compare ourselves to Russia—we are rid of Russia! Let's compare to our neighbours, Finland,"' Sillaustu said, noting that Finland had one-fifth of Estonia's TB rate.

'Our politicians just don't understand,' Sillaustu says, shaking his balding head. 'We must have money to build facilities to carry out DOTS. If we don't, we will be unable to control TB.'

So much in the region hinged on Russia. If that behemoth country didn't change its TB public health policies, few politicians in other former Soviet countries were likely to support DOTS and WHO policies.

Realizing that, in 1997 Viktor Aphanasiev was preparing to do battle with Moscow. It was a high-stakes game the St Petersburg physician was playing, but he said lives were on the line. Lots of lives.

As director of tuberculosis services for Leningrad Oblast (or state), Aphanasiev had grown tired of following the Ministry of Health rules and watching the death toll from TB rise. He was going out on a limb—defying national TB director Alexey Priymak's orders and siding with the World Health Organization and Western Europeans. He was going to treat his patients with DOTS.

'Without a doubt we will have this DOTS, with the support of our governor,' the forty-something robust Aphanasiev declared. 'Whatever it takes!'

Since the fall of the Soviet Union in 1991 the TB rate in Leningrad Oblast had doubled, antibiotic resistance had developed in the microbes, the death rate had soared, and all the money for TB services had run out. It had been so long since the staff received full paychecks that much of the patient care was handled by retired health workers who lived off their meagre pensions.

In 1996 Aphanasiev ordered drug-resistance tests on sputum samples from 1160 St Petersburg patients—nearly every one contained microbes that could completely resist treatment with one or more of the quintet of drugs available in the city.

'Drug resistance is our greatest fear. If you face this problem in America, well, what about here,' Aphanasiev exclaimed. 'It's one more reason to try DOTS.'

Aphanasiev and his assistant Dr Tatiana Dolubava succeeded in gaining financial and political support from the Leningrad Oblast's newly elected governor, and hoped to get further funds from nearby, worried Sweden.

With adequate funding Aphanasiev hoped to purchase enough antibiotics to be able to put nearly all TB patients on out-patient therapy taking five drugs a day, confirmed by an observing nurse or TB official every day. The dynamic Dolubava/Aphanasiev duo wanted to get away from following the old Soviet approach of mass X-ray screening, forced sanatorium incarceration of those who have TB, and long rounds of treatment with injections of two or three drugs a day.

'I'm not happy—we administer three drugs now. And we still have active TB,' Aphanasiev said. 'Yes, we see a decrease in mortality, but we get an increased morbidity [illness] rate . . . from the point of view of epidemiology it's terrible because it increases the chances of spreading TB.'

But switching from the Soviet model that was favoured by powerful Priymak carried huge risks. It could result in even further constraints on St Petersburg's already all-but-non-existent budget.

'We are in a very difficult position,' Dolubava explained. 'We have to have courage to deviate. . . . As the philosophers say, you cannot enter the same water twice. We cannot keep working as we did in the 1930s. Conditions have changed.'

In the fall of 1996, billionaire American financier George Soros set up a $12.3 million grant with the Manhattan-based Public Health Research Institute (PHRI), aimed at offering technical assistance and advice to stem Russia's TB crisis. PHRI, in collaboration with Médecins Sans Frontières and the London-based MERLIN group, set up a pilot DOTS project in Tomsk Prison in Siberia, demonstrating that appropriate antibiotic therapy had a cure rate more than double that of traditional Soviet approaches at a cost savings of $2 million for the prison in a single year.

PHRI also conducted training workshops throughout Russia, showing their counterpart microbiologists how to do drug-resistance assays on tuberculosis samples.

But the Tomsk Prison success still wasn't enough to persuade Priymak and the Russian TB establishment, PHRI's Dr Alex Goldfarb said in 1998. 'It's a vicious circle. . . . It's not just resistance to DOTS, it's something that is combined with the severe economic crisis. All of the people are primarily concerned with saving their jobs. We said in Tomsk they could decrease costs by about 50 per cent, and use the money to pay [unpaid] salaries,' Goldfarb continued.

But the Tomsk doctors still resisted, 'because all they think when you say, "restructuring of TB services" is that it means non-payment of salaries.'

Cracks in Russia's anti-DOTS resolve began to show, however, as other tuberculosis control officials followed the examples of Khomenko and Aphanasiev, openly defying Priymak's policies. With the August 1998 economic crisis came still more fissures in the old system, prised wider by Western pressure placed directly upon President Yeltsin.

Later in 1998 the same organizations initiated a $100 million campaign to tackle Russian drug-resistant TB. And on October 28, 1998, the White House convened a meeting attended by some of the most powerful leaders of the capitalist world, focused on Russia's tuberculosis situation.

The gathering's paramount concern was that Russia adopt DOTS strategies, install drug-resistance laboratories, and remedy its prison problem. Despite such international pressure, money, and expertise, Russia's epidemic continued to expand. In early 1999 the International Red Cross issued a bulletin: 'a serious tuberculosis outbreak is killing one person every twenty-five minutes in Belarus, Moldova, Russia and Ukraine.'

As the twenty-first century dawned tuberculosis was raging out of control all across the former Soviet states, and drug-resistant superstrains had emerged regionwide. Even in Ivanovo, where WHO had executed its pilot DOTS project, drug-resistant TB rates had more than tripled since 1996, topping 10 per cent of all diagnosed tuberculosis cases. And in Kemerovo, where Europeans tried DOTS in Siberian prisons, drug resistance rates in 1999 exceeded 20 per cent.

Once considered a triumph of global public health, tuberculosis had become the world's great shame. All systems of control had failed. As Harvard University TB expert Dr Paul Farmer put it, the globalized economy had brought 'into relief the flabby relativism of the public health *realpolitik* that leaves us with a double standard of therapy': immediate multidrug treatment for the infected affluent, and inadequate treatment of the poor. The latter was leading to the emergence of drug-resistant microbes which, in turn, imperiled the whole world, rich and poor alike.

VII

Oh no,
They've gone and named my home
St Petersburg.
What's going on?
Where are all the friends I had?
It's all wrong, I'm feeling lost like
I just don't belong.
Gimme back,
Gimme back my Leningrad.
—Leningrad Cowboys

I like Edgar Allan Poe. His poems are about death. Live fast, die young.
—Aruslan Kurcenko, age twenty-seven, after injecting heroin in Odessa

Tuberculosis, diphtheria, typhoid fever, cholera, alcoholism, malnutrition—all are diseases that worsened after 1991 but whose rises predated the demise of communism. The Soviet Union's public health infrastructure had rules and regulations for each of these illnesses, but whether these structures were working to contain them was another matter. In any case, though, the ailments were familiar, as were methods of preventing and treating them.

Not so with the new public health catastrophes of the post-Soviet era.

The first of the new scourges surfaced during the Gorbachev years but did not reach catastrophic proportions until well into the Yeltsin era.

His slides were amateurish, handmade. His voice quivered. The notes he clutched made loud fluttering noises over the conference amplification system as his trembling hands struggled to hold the papers still. Dr Viktor Zhdanov wasn't an officially invited speaker to the Second International Conference on AIDS, held in Paris in 1986. But he clearly was the bombshell speaker.

The elderly Russian scientist, dressed as he was in a frumpy suit and well-worn shoes, stood out in the fashionable Paris crowd even before he spoke. After his brief speech the hall of some five thousand AIDS experts buzzed with amazement, for Zhdanov had openly defied Soviet authorities by revealing that Moscow's claims that it had virtually no incidences of HIV or AIDS cases were untrue, and small outbreaks of the virus were appearing in various parts of the vast nation.

Though the audience at the time understood that Zhdanov's action was a courageous one, few realized exactly who the scientist was. Even fewer had any idea what happened to the venerable old researcher after he returned to Moscow.

When seventy-two-year-old Viktor Mikhailovich Zhdanov returned from Paris in 1986 the Soviet secret police force, the KGB, 'hounded him relentlessly,' one source said. His stature as one of the Soviet Union's most prominent virologists didn't protect him. Despite membership in the prestigious Soviet Academy of Sciences, his position as head of the Ivanovski Virology Laboratory in Moscow, his receipt of four orders of Soviet honour, his discovery and development of the first live measles vaccine— despite all these accomplishments Zhdanov was targeted for 'destruction.'

'He was denounced as a CIA spy,' Dr Eduoard Karamov of the Ivanovski Laboratory recalled bitterly. 'He died less than a year after he returned from Paris, and I have no doubt that, despite his age, the witch hunt gave him that stroke.'

Soon after the Paris meeting the KGB and top Communists in the Soviet scientific establishment mounted a campaign that was a textbook example of how intellectual voices were silenced under the old regime. It began with a series of unsigned articles in Soviet scientific journals questioning Zhdanov's credibility as a scientist, and his loyalty as a Soviet citizen. Many of those articles, Karamov said, were written by men who Zhdanov considered his best friends.

Zhdanov's most dangerous enemy proved to be the affable leader of the Soviet Academy of Medical Sciences—and post-1991 head of the Russian equivalent agency—Dr Valentin Pokrovsky. A seemingly jolly man who enjoyed his vodka and readily hugged visitors, Pokrovsky was, several sources insisted, very close to the KGB.

Pokrovsky set up a commission within the Academy to investigate claims made against Zhdanov, most of which were filed in the form of unsigned letters. The commission summoned Zhdanov to appear on a Tuesday morning to defend himself—an order the senior scientist found so astounding that he appealed to his friend, Pokrovsky, for an explanation. Pokrovsky ordered him to go.

On the Monday night Zhdanov suffered a stroke after, Karamov insists, 'five phone calls hounding him to go' before the commission. Despite his stroke Zhdanov appeared before the commission, 'where they were tearing him to pieces,' Karamov said.

Just days later Zhdanov, age seventy-three, died.

And a few weeks following that it was announced that Valentin Pokrovsky's son, Vadim, was the head of a new HIV/AIDS laboratory and clinical centre in Moscow. In the 1990s that facility was called the Russia AIDS Centre, still headed by Vadim Pokrovsky.

After several rounds of vodka at a reception in the Russian Academy of Medical Sciences Valentin decried the social changes that seemed to be spawning Russia's AIDS epidemic as 'this wild dance of unharnessed democracy.'

His son, Vadim, told a visitor that nothing short of a resurrection of socialist rule could prevent an HIV cataclysm.

At the Leningrad Republican Infectious Disease Hospital, located in the Russian countryside near St Petersburg, a city of 4.5 million, the sorry history of the Soviet HIV explosion in Russia could be seen at once at a Salvation Army prayer meeting.

A ten-year-old girl demurely bows her head, a large pink bow in her hair, as she prays. Beside her a nine-year-old girl, her hair filled with carefully entwined artificial flowers, shifts impatiently in her seat. Across from them two tough-looking men in their midtwenties nibble on the free meal, only half-listening to an ongoing Bible reading.

In all, nearly thirty people sit around a large lunch table. Ranging in age from six to fifty, they represent a cross section of Russian society. And they're all infected with the human immunodeficiency virus.

'See little Misha over there? The twelve-year-old boy?' whispers Svetlana, a thirty-two-year-old Salvation Army volunteer who is also HIV positive. 'He says, "It's okay, I'll get married when I grow up and my HIV will go away."'

Some of the adults in the room, like Svetlana, got HIV through heterosexual intercourse. Others—probably the majority—were infected through contaminated needles they shared with fellow opiate users. And one, Nikolai, got the virus through homosexual sex.

But the children were all infected in Russian hospitals in a series of transmissions known within the health-care system as the 'Elista incident.'

The Elista tragedy signified for many a substantial rip in the fabric of basic health-care. In conversations over several months in Russia, Georgia, and Ukraine, many people spoke vehemently of avoiding minor surgery and dental visits because they feared getting AIDS via reused or contaminated instruments. They also feared repressive measures—including military quarantines—that were routinely imposed upon HIV sufferers during Soviet times. Physicians told of the dangers they faced caring for their high-risk patients.

The chain of tragic events known as the Elista incident began around 1982, when a sailor who had worked in Africa unwittingly acquired HIV. He passed it on to his wife, and she, in turn, infected her fetus.

In May 1988, the child was admitted to Elista's paediatric hospital with a variety of intractable infections, all without apparent causes. The baby died soon afterward, still undiagnosed. Meanwhile, the baby's mother, by now twenty-three, began to develop the same type of unusual infections.

The mother went to Moscow for treatment, where she ran into a woman with similar symptoms, who had also lost a child at Elista. When the two mothers compared notes, they determined that their children had been in the neonatal ward at the same time, and had suffered the same type of infections. At the mothers' insistence, doctors finally added up the coincidences and gave both HIV tests, determining that the country's first AIDS outbreak was under way. A joint Russian/UN probe later found that by the time the last mother and child in the chain were infected, in 1994, about 250 cases had occurred through hospital injections with recycled syringes and catheters, the mothers via bites from breast-feeding babies.

In the Soviet health system, healthy babies, or those suffering minor ailments, routinely received up to three hundred injections yearly of vitamins and antibiotics that were given with needles used on one patient after another all day long. And babies who were very sick typically received implants of recycled, poorly sterilized catheters.

'There was just one case to begin with,' said Dr Saladin Osmanov, of UNAIDS. 'But the terrible medical practices were enough to create an outbreak.'

And the outbreak didn't end at Elista. Some of the HIV-positive babies were shipped to other hospitals in the Russian cities of Rostov-on-Don, Volgograd, and Stavropol before their diagnoses were clear. And doctors in those facilities, repeating the same health-care practices, passed the virus around their paediatric facilities as well.

After Elista, Soviet authorities panicked, stepping up mandatory HIV testing to levels unheard of elsewhere, and allowing doctors to screen their patients without consent.

They could, indeed, use the testing to isolate individual infections. But since the rate of infection remained tiny, the Soviets felt no pressure to follow with infection control efforts that would have ensured adequate supplies of sterile syringes and protective equipment, not to mention extensive retraining of caregivers.

Instead, Soviet leaders created centres for the quarantine and study of HIV-infected citizens who—like those gathered in prayer in St Petersburg—faced futures of near imprisonment and boredom. The job of tracking down Soviet HIV cases fell, as did most public health responsibilities, to SanEp, which executed the task in classic Soviet fashion. No one had a right to refuse HIV tests, and no nation conducted as many involuntary screenings as did the USSR. From the moment the first HIV case was identified in Moscow, and with even greater vigour following the 1989 Elista incident, HIV testing was executed at a phenomenal pace. Between 1987 and 1995 some 165 470 049 Russians alone were subjected to state-mandated tests. Records on the numbers of non-Russian Soviets who were tested are not available but surely would substantially increase that toll of 165 million.[17] Testing in Russia peaked in 1992, when 24.4 million people, or one out of every 6.8 citizens, were screened by the state.

But, like so many SanEp approaches to public health, it was an extraordinarily inefficient strategy. Between 1987 and 1991 some seventy-two million HIV tests were performed in Russia, netting 522 cases of infection; more than half of them stemmed from the Elista incident. In order to conduct all of those tests—138 000 for every single Russian case identified—the Soviet Union had to maintain an enormous central laboratory in Moscow dedicated to manufacturing test kits and analysing millions of blood samples every year. Further, SanEp field workers had to round up all of those blood samples and ship them to Moscow. Most of the tests were conducted on blood donors, pregnant women, prisoners, and Soviets who travelled outside the country—tests were mandatory upon reentry.

In 1996 Russia spent about $1.75 million on testing. But 1997 opened with a smaller HIV/AIDS budget, unpaid doctors and nurses countrywide, and hospitals with empty pharmaceutical shelves. Far from being able to afford $10 000 to $40 000 a year to treat HIV patients in ways that met US standards, or to continue a nearly $2 million testing program, Russia couldn't even find the wherewithal to buy television advertising time on national television to promote AIDS education.

The same policies, including extensive, expensive involuntary testing, were the rule throughout the former USSR.

Svetlana was nineteen years old when the Chernobyl nuclear accident occurred. A Ukrainian, Svetlana lived near the power plant and was exposed to enough fallout that she suffered immediate radiation sickness. For four years Ukrainian physicians gave Svetlana blood transfusions, hoping to replenish her vital red and white blood cell populations that were killed by radiation.

In 1993 Svetlana, then living in Kiev, tested positive for HIV, sparking a panic among the apparatchiks responsible for Soviet blood supplies. Tens of thousands of donors thought to have given blood during the post-Chernobyl years were retested in a frantic search for the source of Svetlana's HIV.

But she knew that it hadn't come from the blood.

'I know who I got it from,' Svetlana, a tall, robust, blue-eyed blonde adult recalled. 'And he has passed away. He was from Italy. His sister wrote to me from Italy and told me that he died of AIDS. I realized that I was in danger and sought medical assistance.'

Nevertheless, Soviet public health officials insisted on retesting the Ukrainian blood supply. And Svetlana, who had already suffered years of hardship resulting from

Chernobyl, was shipped off to the Republican Infectious Diseases Hospital outside St Petersburg, where she lived throughout the rest of the 1990s. Her Ukrainian family was permitted to visit, but the long journey from Kiev proved an expensive one in the post-Soviet period, and Svetlana soon realized that the Elista incident survivors and a handful of adults who contracted HIV infection from other sources were to be her only comrades. She watched the tiny Elista children grow up—and, in eighty cases, die—acting as their surrogate aunt and occasional nurse.

'The children are charming,' Svetlana tells visitors. 'Their mothers are making matches between the little boys and girls, so someday the HIV-positive children can grow up and marry.'

Svetlana lowers her voice to a whisper: 'Most of the children don't know about their diagnosis.'

Since 1989 the youngsters, most of whom arrived as newborns, have known no other world save the ramshackle hospital, its personnel, and the views of distant dacha fields and a river that they can see from their windows. Life perked up a bit for the youngsters in 1993 to 1995 when diphtheria cases—thousands of them—filled the hospital. But since that epidemic's end the hallways of Republican Hospital have grown silent, and the only additions to their sad quarantine colony have been drug addicts and their babies, most of whom have come from Kaliningrad. All of them are HIV-positive.

Nikolai Nedezelski, a handsome twenty-seven-year-old, was diagnosed HIV positive in 1991 in Moscow.

'I got it from my Russian partner,' says Nikolai, who is gay. Eloquent and schooled in the ways of European AIDS activitists Nedezelski spent his days visiting quarantine centres, such as the one in St Petersburg, and lobbying for humane policies. He also was one of the only HIV patients in all of Russia in 1997 who was receiving state-of-the-art combination drug therapy—the result of frequent trips he managed to make to Los Angeles and Paris. He wanted all of his fellow HIV patients in Russia to get the life-extending drugs, but due to an arcane set of Soviet laws still on Russian books, only infected residents of Moscow could obtain even one such drug. Outside of Moscow and St Petersburg no one received the full cocktails commonly used in Western Europe.

In 1995 Nikolai was selected by his HIV-positive peers to plead their case to the international community at the Paris Summit on HIV. He pulled no punches, telling the conference that 'in Russia it's still a political disease. Everything related to treatment and prophylaxis is political. Society says, "Why spend money on prostitutes, homosexuals and drug users? ... Why should we provide combination therapy... the people will die sooner if we don't. Good."'

Nikolai's speech was aired on Russian television.

'When my mother watched my speech on TV she said, "I'm so glad you were born in these times rather than earlier. In the old days the gulag would be crying for you,"' Nikolai recalled.

In a sense, however, the gulag did still call to Russia's HIV patients, as the laws of the post-Communist state forbade most of their sexual activity, condemned infected drug users to the tuberculosis-infested prison system, and greatly limited their access to treatments.[18]

Mikhail Ivanovich Narkevich, chief of AIDS Control for the Russian Ministry of Health, says that in retrospect Elista and the tragedy of the St Petersburg colony 'taught us a lot. If not for that tragedy I don't know how many more people would have been infected in Soviet hospitals.'

After the breakup of the Soviet Union each of the new, independent countries muddled through for a while, largely ignoring HIV in favour of more immediate public health crises, such as diphtheria and tuberculosis. If not for the Elista and Romanian paediatric cases the region's HIV rates would have, in the global scheme of things, been negligible. Even including those roughly 2300 cases didn't put Russia, Georgia, Lithuania, Poland, or any of the other former Communist nations in apparent HIV jeopardy.

Until 1996.

'That was the year the situation got worse,' Narkevich insisted. Actually, it was sometime in May 1995.

'It's clear it came from Ukraine to Russia,' Vadim Pokrovsky added. 'The question is how it got from the Ukraine to Belarus, and from Belarus to Russia. It is an A clade virus—not the B clade that we saw before—so we know it was new. But where did it come from?'

The 'where' might never be clear, Narkevich countered, but the 'how' was horribly obvious. It rested with *narkomania*, or drug abuse: between May 1995 and 1996 the number of Russian intravenous drug users found infected with HIV increased nearly a hundredfold. And Russia's *narkomania* crisis was running a few laps behind the drug-use explosion in Eastern Europe, Belarus, and—most importantly—Ukraine.

It's Monday night at 7 p.m. and Artur is ready to 'walk the thread' through Odessa's prime narcotics neighbourhood, Palermo. The plan is for him and pal Oleg to score enough opium poppy straw and the necessary solvents to be able to cook up a batch of *chorny* sufficient to get two people high.

The energetic—perhaps hyper—Artur zips his coat up high against the cold wind and fog and heads first to a block of large concrete apartment buildings near the Ukrainian city's railway lines. After two years of shooting opium into his veins, the twenty-one-year-old knows exactly where to go.

He moves swiftly, cutting his way through the thick, bone-chilling fog, into one of the many look-alike Soviet communal housing buildings, and bounds up ten flights of urine-soaked stairs. Artur knows that the lift doesn't work—few do in this city of post-Communist decay. As he catches his breath on the top floor Artur unzips his jacket, removing an empty plastic water bottle and eight *hryvnya*—about $5.50. He approaches a specially constructed steel chamber that securely seals the apartment behind it off from the rest of the world. There are two cutout holes along the side of the steel fortress: through a two-inch by two-inch hole, Artur passes his money; into the other, slightly taller slot, he places the empty bottle. Artur presses a loud buzzer and waits.

A hand appears, withdrawing the money and bottle. Five minutes later a door opens in the steel, revealing an inner steel cage behind which lies still another door—the one originally built for apartment 10A. An elderly gypsy woman, dressed in a long-flowing multicoloured skirt and equally colourful but clashing silk blouse, silently returns the bottle to Artur, passing the now-filled object through the cage bars, along with a syringe filled with acetic anhydride. As the steel barriers slam shut in successive loud clanks, Artur sniffs the contents of the bottle, verifying it is the paint remover solvent he expected.

Ten minutes later Artur climbs into the backseat of an old Lada, nods to Oleg, and the pair drive the unpaved, pot-holed road into the neighbourhood dubbed Palermo. The Gypsies keep the road rough, Artur explains, so that the police cannot make any surprise raids. About halfway into the Palermo neighbourhood, where there are some ten thousand Gypsies and their 'slaves'—drug addicted Ukrainian adolescents who work for nothing more than daily hits of narcotics—the road becomes impassable.

'Now we walk,' Oleg announces, getting out of the car and disappearing into the dense, ice-cold fog. Artur follows, and the pair 'walk the thread,' as the local addicts put it, winding their way rapidly along the alleyways that zigzag between large, cinder block gypsy fortresses. Each fortified home has high, thick walls around it with small, ground-level, hand-size holes designed for passage of drugs and cash.

It's dinnertime, dark, and moonless. Few people are outdoors. A pair of colourfully dressed Gypsy girls look Artur and Oleg disdainfully in the eyes as they pass. A fashionably dressed Gypsy man polishes his 1996 BMW sedan. A middle-aged woman pops her scarfed head out of a gate and shouts a command to her German shepherd. The dog runs in the opposite direction, its tail between its legs.

Oleg and Artur pause in front of one of the fortress-houses from which blasts loud rave music, its techno-pop beat reverberating off the neighbours' walls. The men whisper to each other, and it is decided that Oleg should hold back, letting Artur approach their preferred dealer alone.

Across the muddy road from the pulsating house, Artur walks up to an eight-foot-high steel gate and shouts, 'Luba! Luba!' Middle-aged Luba, her shiny clothes of many colours billowing in the night air, comes out of the house and peers at Artur. They exchange words, but she turns him away. Artur is stumped.

From the opposite direction a new 1997 Ford Taurus arrives, the driver steps out, and he, too, calls to Luba. As the driver passes cash to the Gypsy, Artur again presses her for poppy straw. Luba tells him no—she doesn't recognize his close cropped hair and dark jeans. Artur looks like a cop.

Suddenly the aggravating music stops in the house across the dirt road. A fourteen-year-old boy wearing a Sony Walkman steps out of his house, recognizes Oleg, and calls out to Luba in Russian: 'They're okay, I know this guy.'

Luba nods, disappears into her house, and returns with two packages. She sells one to Artur, but as she passes the other to the Taurus driver the wily German shepherd appears, leaps at Luba's outstretched hand, and steals the poppy straw. In an instant the sneaky dog disappears into a neighbour's house.

Artur and Oleg, anxious now that they are in possession of the rough opium stems and dried bulbs, race back to the car.

At 8 p.m. they arrive at the apartment of Oleg's grandmother, whom he calls simply, Babushka.

'Don't worry, Babushka,' Oleg says, 'nothing bad will happen.' The grandmother, seeing she has no choice, lets the young men enter her tiny apartment but immediately telephones Oleg's mother, Svetlana.

Artur sets to work in the kitchen, removing his shirt because 'it's going to get hot in here. You'll see.' While Oleg calms his grandmother and almost instantly present aunt and mother, Artur scrubs a set of cooking pots and a meat grinder with steel wool.

'The first step,' he explains, 'is to remove all the fat from the poppy straw. We must get it out because it will induce human allergies. We have to scrub all the fat off these things.'

Artur toils in Babushka's hundred-square-foot kitchen, with its peeling white ceiling and walls, warped lime green linoleum flooring, four-burner gas stove, sink, table for one person, and minifridge. And in the living room Oleg comforts his pretty blonde mother, whose transparent blue eyes are brimming with tears. He promises Svetlana that he will not inject the drugs Artur is making in the kitchen—'if I slip down again I want to die,' he tells his mother. The widow, who lost both her father and husband last year to heart attacks, acknowledges that Oleg has tried to stop. But she is unconvinced.

'I learned two years ago that he had been addicted for three years already,' Svetlana explains, nervously tugging at her dress and fingers. 'It wasn't noticeable. He managed to keep himself together and I couldn't see it. He graduated from university and had a prestigious position.'

Oleg nods: 'It's true, I had a good job—five hundred dollars a month. More than twice the average wage in Odessa for men much older than me. I was married, optimistic.'

Oleg avoids his mother's reddened eyes. Silently, she slips into the kitchen and watches Artur, who is now dripping with sweat despite the chilly night air, grinding up the hard dried poppy pieces into a coarse powder that spills over yesterday's Ukrainian newspaper. 'If you have an intelligent son, you really grieve when he becomes an addict,' Svetlana whispers, her voice breaking on the word *narkoman*.

By eight-thirty all the poppy straw has been ground to a powder and Artur dumps it into a small tin cooking pot, along with some baking soda and about three table-spoons of Odessa's notoriously contaminated tap water.

'This will infuse into the poppy straw under heat, breaking it up,' Artur explains, displaying skills that under different circumstances might have made him a good organic chemist. It must be steadily stirred, he says, as he wipes sweat off his brow and the high gas flames heat up the kitchen, turning the poppy straw into a paste.

Ten minutes later danger begins.

Now Artur and Oleg will perform the extraction steps, which involve highly flammable solvents. Both men have seen plenty of friends be severely burned by accidents at this stage; some have even died as their kitchens were engulfed in flames. Artur decides to proceed in a slower, but safer manner, using a frying pan full of boiling water as a barrier between gas flames and the opiate concoction that now cooks with three cups of paint thinner and acetone. He must stand over the high heat stirring constantly, or the mixture could explode in flames.

Within minutes the kitchen fills with a powerful stench and the chemical fumes make everyone in the room gasp for air, their eyes watering. Oleg opens the windows, hangs a blanket over the kitchen entry to prevent the fumes from escaping into the rest of the minuscule apartment, and sends Svetlana to the living room.

The three distraught women sob in the spartan living room. Stripped of all valuables long ago—sold by Oleg for drug money—the room has the feel of a prison cell. Babushka cries out between sobs that all the neighbours will smell the acrid stench and know that drugs are being made in her apartment. Svetlana and her older sister murmur that Oleg claimed he stopped taking drugs two months ago—how can they believe him now?

At 9:05 Artur removes a stinky, hot brown liquid from the stove and pours it through a cloth into a tin bowl. The stench nearly overwhelms him, and Artur comes dangerously close to spilling the boiled opiate extract on himself. As it passes through the cloth the liquid takes on a greenish hue.

Artur puts the tin bowl into the jury-rigged double boiler and cooks it another twenty minutes until nothing remains but a thin dark green film reminiscent of pond algal scum. He grabs the syringe full of acetic anhydride and carefully injects it into the pot, producing yet another vile vinegarish odour. He stirs slowly, his tattooed wrist rotating round and round, bearing the Russian phrase, GOD BE WITH US.

By 9:46 the process is complete, and a dark brown/green puddle of about five cubic millimetres beckons from the tin bowl. From 250 grams of poppy straw, three cups of water, about a litre of solvent, and a few drops of acetic anhydride, this is it—enough opiate extract, called *chorny*, to get two addicts high. The cost: about $10 and three hours of dangerous labour.

At the urging of his family, having sworn that he was only making the concoction to demonstrate to his visitor how *chorny* is made, Oleg 'proves' he is no longer an addict and dumps the final drug into the kitchen sink. Artur watches silently, no expression on his tense face. A cold wind blows into the kitchen, dispersing the sickening fumes. Oleg's eyes fill with tears, and it is unclear whether he is regretting dumping the opiates, or merely reacting to the gaseous stench.

A few days later, the air still damp with Odessa's early April chill, a visitor crosses the train tracks and lingers for a while on a knoll overlooking a vast open meadow and, beyond, Palermo. A steady stream of adolescents pours past, their pace quickening as they eye Palermo and descend into the open field. It's easy to tell which of the youngsters have been using *chorny* the longest, as they no longer possess clothing and shoes adequate against the early spring chill and shiver uncontrollably. Those more recently inducted into the opiate world haven't yet sold their winter coats and boots for a few *hryvnya*; enough, perhaps, for another hit of *chorny*.

The opium concoction he's been shooting into his veins for two years no longer satisfies Sasha, a pale, wiry, twenty-year-old labourer. 'Even so,' he says, 'I can't quit. Something keeps drawing me back here.'

He pauses a moment to watch a cluster of other adolescent drug addicts scurry past into Palermo. 'It doesn't matter anyway,' he adds. 'I'm HIV positive. Whether it's from drugs or AIDS, soon I will die.'

Many of the friends Sasha grew up with have already died—of overdoses, alcohol, and drug-related violence, tuberculosis, AIDS, suicide. Now he is awaiting his turn.

When the Soviets fell in 1991, experts say, former KGB agents colluded with drug dealers, and new criminal war lords rose to power throughout the region—gangsters who took advantage of the turmoil inherent in the historic change to target a generation of alienated young men and women, people like Sasha. Drugs were suddenly cheap and readily available, prostitution became a huge regional industry, and the stage was set for the birth of a regional AIDS epidemic of third world proportions.

'This isn't just an explosion,' suggested Dr Alla Soloviova, a Ukrainian working for UNICEF in Kiev. 'This is an A-bomb.'

In 1996 some 7000 new HIV cases were registered in Ukraine. And one international agency projected that by 2001 they would have 20 000 AIDS cases, perhaps a quarter million accumulated HIV infections, and 4000 new AIDS cases a year erupting after that. These were startling numbers for a country that recorded only 214 cumulative HIV cases prior to 1994.

'Imagine the impact on the health-care system then,' said epidemiologist Luiz Loures of UNAIDS, which made the turn-of-the-century prediction.

It wasn't until mid-1996 that health experts in Odessa began to understand why the HIV 'A-bomb' was exploding so dramatically in that city, as well as the rest of Ukraine. At that point, volunteers such as Odessa attorney Sergei Minov opened a discreet needle exchange centre in Odessa and began questioning young people about their habits. What they found, Minov explained, 'was a nightmare.' Nearly all drug users said that they frequently shared needles and syringes, and that they typically pulled some of their own blood into the syringe after the initial injection in order to flush any remaining narcotics out.

It also became clear that the Gypsies of Palermo and organized drug gangsters elsewhere in the region were selling their poppy straw in forms already contaminated,

Minov said. This was because the drugs were mass-produced, then checked for potency by young addicts who took free narcotics in trade for these life-threatening tests. To test the samples, the slaves, as these addicts were called, repeatedly dipped their personal syringes into large pots, and often pulled the plunger in and out several times.

Finally, Minov said, local addicts reported that Gypsy children were ordered by the drug suppliers to collect used syringes: the supplier would 'fill them with narcotics and put them back in circulation.'

This practice ended, Minov said, when he and other volunteers put the word out among the addicts that he wanted to talk to the 'Gypsy Baron,' who led the poppy straw trade in Odessa. Weeks passed.

Then one winter morning in 1996, he said, two large limousines came to Minov's apartment building, bodyguards leapt out, and the lavishly dressed drug lord knocked on Minov's door. Minov told him that selling contaminated opiate and syringes was 'bad business' since it would quickly kill off his clientele.

The drug lord, whose identity Minov had sworn to keep secret, saw the wisdom of the lawyer's comments and forbade the children from collecting used syringes.

One small victory in an 'A-bomb' war.

But the shooting field in front of Palermo was covered with used syringes, and desperate teen addicts often plucked an unbroken one off the ground for a quick *chorny* injection, if need be.

Down on the shooting field young people huddle in small groups, trying to find uncollapsed veins into which to inject one another. Pain writ upon their grimacing faces the teenagers poked and prodded one another, desperate to get the drug into their bloodstreams. So viscous is the opiate compote that the users needed 10 and even 20 cc needles—volumes far in excess of the 1 cc syringes used to inject heroin in North America or Western Europe.

Minov and the staff of a small drug addiction clinic called Trusting Spot collected thousands of syringes found in the Odessa shooting field in January 1997: fully a third of them tested positive for HIV.

'It's an explosive outbreak,' Grigory Baavsky, a UNAIDS epidemiologist working in Odessa, says. 'Every month we find six hundred new HIV cases. . . . In Odessa we have three thousand registered drug addicts. The real number is ten times that—'

Minov interrupts: 'That's in a city of 1.1 million people. Think of that—thirty thousand for sure, out of 1.1 million.'

Baavsky drew a chart, plotting the mounting Odessa HIV toll since the first cases appeared in 1995. He draws dotted lines, extending to 2012: 'Within fifteen years the whole Odessa society could be up to 70 per cent infected,' he says.

UNICEF's Soloviova, a pretty, intense blonde, says that blood tests performed in the spring of 1995 revealed that nearly three-quarters of Odessa's intravenous drug-using population was HIV positive. Even she has a hard time believing the data, realizing that the virus overwhelmed the community in less than six months. Surveys of the drug users indicate that nearly all of them are under thirty years of age, have completed their schooling, and are unemployed.

Back in 1995 Soloviova attended a regional UNICEF meeting, where she pleaded with her fellow United Nations employees to commit resources to what she foresaw as an AIDS crisis.

'The policy makers said, "Oh, only three hundred cases in all of Ukraine? We have so much more cardiovascular disease, cancer... this HIV isn't a problem."'

The next year Soloviova pleaded her case again, directly to UNICEF chief Carol Bellamy. By then Soloviova had numbers that revealed a sudden surge of cases in Kiev and Odessa, 'and it was like a bomb went off. They said, "My God, is it really so?"' Soloviova recalled.

Soloviova set to work, discovering that none of the governments in the area had any public health strategy for dealing with HIV. And, she said, 'The speed of this epidemic is the fastest in all of Europe.'

Even at the Plague Laboratory, once the bastion of SanEp efforts in Ukraine, Doctors Lev Mogilevsky and Elena Yugorova believed the numbers of HIV cases in teens and young adults were huge.

'Our main task is to save the younger generation,' Mogilevsky sternly says. 'If we manage to pull them out of the reach of the Mafia structures, we will win this battle.'

Stopping the Mafia, Gypsy gangs, and other narcotraffickers in the region would be tough—perhaps impossible, psychiatrist Pavel Bem said. Handsome, long-haired, thirty-four-year-old Bem was one of Eastern Europe's leading experts on drug abuse, and chair of the Czech Government Anti-Drug Commission. Bem insisted that regardless of what factors were driving the region's young adults toward lives of drug addiction—and he felt a complex array of issues was involved—the real crisis for governments in the region was how readily, and cheaply, the killer products were available.

Almost without exception, narcotics and amphetamines could be purchased easily and openly, even in rural areas of Siberia or the frozen Arctic Circle. And intricate networks of gangsters and Gypsies, working with traditional drug traffickers from Nigeria, Afghanistan, Pakistan, and the Asian Golden Triangle, were moving across the newly porous borders behind the once-Iron Curtain.

'If you look at stable economies [such as the United States] there has been little increase in drug use in recent years,' Bem said. 'But these new economies are great opportunities for organized crime. And they are holding their prices way down at introductory levels.'

Following universal rules of marketing, drug traffickers were creating clienteles in the region by selling everything from raw opium to heroin at rock-bottom prices, more than tenfold lower than equivalent drug sales in New York City.

The cheapest high was *vint*, an extract of ephedrine allergy pills that were chemically oxidized to ephedrone, a powerful hallucinogen. In Moscow *vint* sold for three dollars.

And the *vint* sellers were elderly babushkas who supplemented their meager Russian pensions by gaining free pharmaceutical ephedrine, as was their right as senior citizens who allegedly suffered allergies or hay fever. The women did the chemical extractions in their kitchens, loaded the *vint* either on sugar cubes or inside syringes, and sold the addictive concoction to teenagers—at a 200 per cent profit above the babushka's total costs.

The primary selling spot for *vint* was Lubyanka Square, directly across the street from the headquarters of the Russian police force formerly known as the KGB.

The low cost and ready availability of these drugs explained why unemployed youngsters could afford to be high all of the time—even on top-grade heroin.

And youngsters' desire to inject the deadly drugs, Bem said in fluent English. 'It has something to do with the information overload and increasing demands on certain values and abilities. If you look at young teens today, to build a career and to be valuable to society it means you have to fulfil a lot of very difficult tasks ... to be effective. And a lot of young people say, "We cannot do it! We cannot fulfil this demand. We are not counted. It's senseless." The technoculture emerging has no sense of grounding—you are flying somewhere in space. It's not a way to understand, it's only a way to feel. As a psychiatrist I would call it a separation from authentic feelings. It's something the older generation—the parent—is not able to understand.'

The upsurge in drug use was most pronounced in the industrial areas that were erected, for the most part, during or immediately after World War II, as the USSR built itself into a superpower. Millions moved to such cities during the 1960s and 1970s, mostly voluntarily; the pay was good, and Moscow gave its top industrial centres highest priority for shipments of fresh food, new clothing, televisions, and consumer products. In times of great scarcity for the rest of the USSR, workers of Novosibirsk, Noril'sk, Kemerovo, or Narva had tropical fruit in February.

But with the collapse of the USSR came a tough transitional economy in which the antiquated, inefficient industries of the past closed down. And that new openness allowed television images and magazines that showed the startled residents just how horribly sharp the contrast was between their bleak existences and that which was available to those in Moscow who could afford to buy the dreams of the West. Once elite, the ugly, dirty cities became little more than filthy centres of disappointment, envy, unemployment, alcoholism, and drugs.

In Estonia, for example, the Russians built a heavy-industry complex in the old medieval village of Narva, located a literal stone's throw from Russia's northwestern border. Prior to 1991, Narva averaged a population of 81 000 people, most of them Russians who were given priority job status over the native Estonians. It was a prosperous city.

But by 1998 only 75 000 people remained in Narva, nearly all the cement, textile, and metal factories were closed, and officially 39 per cent of the population was unemployed. Located at the same latitude as Helsinki, Finland, the city saw no sunlight for three months out of the year, and then was entombed in snow.

'Democracy is good, but it's better when you have something for young people to do,' moans Narva's Deputy Mayor Viktor Veevo. The burly Estonian-born Russian estimates that three thousand young people in Narva are drug addicts—about one out of every five residents aged fourteen to twenty-five years.

In Narva the incidence of hepatitis B and C increased 400 per cent between 1992 and 1996, according to Dr Olev Silland, director of Narva's hospital. And he is sceptical of Veevo's estimate of the number of intravenous drug users in the city—it's far more, he says, than three thousand. Perhaps more like ten thousand, or one out of every 7.5 residents of the beleaguered city.

HIV numbers were still low in Estonia, but Dr Lea Tammai, the elderly epidemiologist of Merimetsa Hospital of Infectious Diseases in Tallinn, couldn't believe what was happening with hepatitis. In 1990, she said, the incidence of hepatitis B in Estonia was 6.9 per 100 000 people; hepatitis C was 2.6 per 100 000. By 1996 that was up to 24.5 per 100 000 incidence for hepatitis B and hepatitis C incidence had doubled.

Two floors of the hospital were full of hepatitis cases, all of them intravenous drug users.

At Narcology Hospital No. 17 in Moscow deputy director Tatiana Lysenko sees addicted boys every day. They come now in droves, their young bodies sickened by the drugs—and by hepatitis. Her 3300-bed facility in Moscow is full, and she, like her counterparts from Odessa to Vladivostock, has no idea what to do about it. Since 1982, when Narcology Hospital No. 17 opened, Lysenko has been the SanEp representative inside the massive facility, and during Soviet times her job was fairly straightforward. Narcology, or the medical discipline that dealt with *narkomania*, had extraordinary powers then to seek out drug users and incarcerate them in hospitals like No. 17—sometimes for years. Lysenko never had to resort to persuasion, methadone—which was, and remained after 1991, illegal across most of the region—behaviour modification, or any of a long list of tactics Western physicians working with narcotics and amphetamine addicts used. Until 1991 Lysenko, and hundreds of health-care workers like her, simply called in the police and locked up the users. And the patients cold-turkeyed, repented, underwent political re-education, and either learned the error of their ways or were sent to prison. It was simple.

But after 1991 and the collapse of Communist rule narcologists had no idea what to do.

'Drug use estimates from the [Russian] Ministry of Interior say there are about two million intravenous drug users, 300 000 long-term users,' UNAIDS Moscow representative Zdeněk Ježek said. 'Ten to 15 per cent of the Russian population has some experience with intravenous drug use.'

Ježek, a white-haired Czech scientist who had worked all over the world for the United Nations, was flabbergasted. He found public health officials regionally were stuck in the old Soviet ways of thinking, completely unable to grasp how to stem the tide of hepatitis and HIV in new, democratic social systems.

Ježek grabs a stack of charts and tables, telling a visitor that these very tables had been shown to one government official after another, usually with no effect. One chart shows, for example, that in 1995 only 0.3 per cent of Russia's known HIV cases were intravenous drug users. But by December 1996, Ježek said, '61.2 per cent of all HIV was in intravenous drug users. To plot the rate of growth in this population we have to use a log scale.'

In May, Dr N. F. Gerasimenko, of the Russian Academy of Medical Sciences, announced that new HIV cases there rose eightfold between 1995 and 1996 to around 1500, and the Ministry of Health said it expected 800 000 people to be infected by the turn of the century, or about 5 per cent of the country's projected population. By comparison, only 0.3 to 0.5 per cent of the US population is thought to have contracted HIV or AIDS between 1979 and 1999.

Like Ukraine, this rapid HIV expansion was occurring in a country that just a few years before was labelled an 'AIDS-free zone' by Russian health officials citing exhaustive state-mandated HIV testing, which failed for years to turn up significant signs of the pandemic.

'We are now experiencing a true explosion of HIV in this region,' UNAIDS director Dr Peter Piot insisted. 'We see the same potential as we saw in North America sixteen years ago, which makes us worry that we're really not learning from our mistakes.'

Belarus state epidemiologist Vladimir Yeremin offered this chilling example: the economically depressed industrial city of Svetlogorsk, population 72 000, had zero detectable HIV cases until January 1997. Then, suddenly, there were eight hundred, all among young drug users, and Yeremin estimated that one out of every nine residents of the squalid city were infected.[19]

Worse yet, scientists at UNAIDS in Geneva identified eight of the ten known HIV subtypes circulating in a region stretching from Belarus to Vladivostock, from the Baltic states in the north to the Eastern European nations along the Danube and Dneiper Rivers. And this, in turn, prompted concerns that it would be here, in this well-travelled region, that the disease would recombine genetically, taking on new forms.

HIV was one of the world's most rapidly mutating viruses, and it responded quickly to changes in its target human population. For example, most infected drug users and gay men in the world carried the B subtype of HIV, whereas female prostitutes in Africa and Asia predominantly had the C, D, A, and E subtypes.

But only a tiny minority of the world's AIDS population moved in social circles that allowed them exposure to widely divergent HIV subtypes, so few people in the 1990s carried two or more subtypes in their bodies at the same time. When such superinfections occurred, HIV had a golden opportunity: it could trade genetic chunks of its

RNA from one subtype to another, creating new genetic forms that could include the ability to infect a wider range of cell types, outwit certain drugs, or cause more rapid illness.

And, true to forecast, a new form of HIV did emerge in Russia's Kaliningrad during 1997. The new strain represented a blend of B and A clade viruses. The A clade was identical to a strain previously seen among intravenous drug users in Odessa; the origins of the B clade were unknown. The new virus contained the genetic capabilities of both clades.[20]

'It's unbelievable,' virologist Saladin Osmanov of the UNAIDS Programme in Geneva said. 'It now seems that the East will be the mixing pot for all of the elements of the last fifteen years of HIV worldwide: subtypes, sex, intravenous drug users, nosocomial [hospital spread]. This is it.'

All this viral diversity implied that HIV had entered the region several times, from different parts of the world. Osmanov said that there were at least five epidemics in the region—reflecting five separate times and places in which particular strains were introduced.

It was questionable whether all five would continue to develop; experts said it was clear that beyond the narcotics-driven dominant epidemic lay a burgeoning heterosexual epidemic that could be more explosive than seen anywhere—including Thailand, which went from a handful of cases in 1989 to a 70 per cent infection rate in prostitutes in 1991.

'You really need to understand the nature of sex networks in Eastern Europe' to understand the potential in the region, explained Dr Luiz Loures of the UNAIDS Programme. 'Clearly the rates of multiple partner sex are higher than in Western Europe. And though no one knows the size of the sex worker population, it's large and growing.'

'It's all very dynamic,' he added, 'and the situation is hard to forecast right now.'[21]

Despite such grim information, Ježek said government officials still declined to take appropriate steps to slow the spread of HIV among intravenous drug users.

'The government sees drug users as criminals,' Ježek explained. 'During the Soviet period drug use officially did not exist. So all of these people were underground. And if people are underground you cannot reach them, cannot educate them.'

The strongest anti-AIDS programme in the region was in Prague, the Czech Republic. There, Dr Marie Bručkova ran a national AIDS laboratory that collected and analysed blood from individuals who voluntarily gave samples in confidential or anonymous settings. Those infected got free treatment, counselling, and safe-sex education.

Meanwhile, on-the-street AIDS education was carried out through needle exchange centres with support from the nation's president, Vaclav Havel, and safe-sex education had been introduced into school curricula.

Since mid-1997 the Czech Republic had identified only 318 citizens with HIV, 95 of whom had developed AIDS, and Bručkova described the national mood in terms of AIDS as 'alert, but not in panic mode.'

The Georgian government, which was deeply cash poor as a result of post–civil war economic despair, couldn't match the Czech campaign in size but followed a similar approach, at least in intent, said Dr Tengiv Tsertsvadze, who headed up the Caucasus nation's anti-AIDS efforts, coordinated through a small laboratory in Tblisi, the capital city.

The education and voluntary testing programme was carried out in collaboration with Dr Jack Dehovitz of Downstate Medical Center in Brooklyn, Tsertsvadze proudly said, noting, 'It's a very civilized programme.'

But there were other problems in this war-torn country that doctors like Tsertsvadze had to contend with—including a highly questionable public blood supply. In Tblisi, for instance, fewer than half of all blood transfusions involved sera or plasma that had been screened for HIV or hepatitis contamination.

According to Tsertsvadze's staff only seventeen thousand of fifty thousand blood bank donors were tested in 1996, and at least half of the nation's emergency blood donations weren't tested at all—for HIV, or any other virus. Only 3 per cent of the nation's blood donations were screened for hepatitis B or C.

'In old times we had blood banks,' Tsertsvadze said. 'But not anymore.'

Blood banks in Georgia were, in fact, rather sorry affairs: Tsertsvadze said that about 5 per cent of the donations were hepatitis B positive, and an equal percentage carried hepatitis C. But he admitted that C testing was rare and 'nobody knows the real number of cases.'

Sources in Western embassies warned visitors that Georgia's blood supply was absolutely unsafe and urged them to undergo even emergency procedures that might require transfusions outside the country.

It was not hard to see why. The central blood bank system of Georgia fell apart from 1992 to 1995 during its civil war. In its place emerged a chaotic hotchpotch of hospital banks and blood donation clinics, all of which paid donors, thus attracting alcoholics and drug users in need of quick cash. One such clinic in Tblisi had only sporadic electricity to ensure safe storage of its three refrigerators full of whole blood and two small freezers of plasma. Most of its blood was 'donated' by professional donors who came as frequently as doctors allowed them, to give a few pints in exchange for 12 laris (about $9.60)—which they in turn used to purchase a pint of booze or hit of opium extract, blood bank director Bella Kvachantivadze conceded.

Two such donors, Yuri Nevandovski and Viktor Yakovlev, reeked of alcohol as they stuck their arms through a portal in a glass wall. On the other side of the barrier a nurse drained their blood. After which the men pocketed their laris and staggered off in search of strong Georgian wine.

Although some other countries in the region had better blood banking systems, only a handful had resources for universal screening of donors for hepatitis B and C, HIV, or any other dangerous viruses. Given the extraordinary explosion of these viruses occurring in the intravenous drug-using population, and the local practice of paying donors for providing blood or plasma, this seemed an extraordinary regional public health time bomb.

Nowhere was that possibility as scary as in Russia. Across the entire eleven-time-zone length of the vast nation, hepatitis, in particular, was emerging from obscurity into a full-fledged epidemic. In the short run, treatment costs were minimal, as there was not much Russian hospitals could do for viral hepatitis cases short of nutritional support and gamma globulin shots to boost patients' immune systems. Ten years down the road, however, Russia, and the other Eastern countries, will face tough economic choices as the advanced cirrhosis and liver cancer cases appear.

In the United States, advanced hepatitis-associated disease could make an individual a candidate for antiviral and cancer chemotherapy or liver transplantation—if the local board overseeing priorities in organ donations was willing to give a precious transplant to a virally infected recipient. But such procedures were extremely costly and required advanced medical technology. A six-month course of antiviral chemotherapy for hepatitis C cost $200 000 and was fully effective in less than 20 per cent of all cases.

If Russia's medical system advances far enough by 2007 to be able to handle such cases, it is still unlikely to find treatment affordable for any but the richest patients who can pay their own costs.

Officially in 1996 Russia had a combined hepatitis incidence of 26.7 cases per 100 000 adults and 5.9 cases per 100 000 children, according to the Ministry of Health. This represented a doubling in officially recorded hepatitis cases since 1992.

But in a report filed at the close of 1996 by the Russian Academy of Medical Sciences to President Boris Yeltsin, the toll of hepatitis appeared far graver and was described as 'unfavourable'. In 1995, it stated, more than 52 000 Russians were hospitalized for viral hepatitis, primarily types B and C. The incidence of type B, alone, topped 36 per 100 000 Russians. Combined viral type hepatitis was said to be far higher, but no reliable estimate of numbers could be given because so few tests were performed for types C through G.

When the Soviet Union fell apart in 1991, fewer than 6 per cent of all hepatitis cases in Russia were among intravenous drug users. By 1995, however, 21 per cent of all Moscow hepatitis hospitalizations were drug users, as were 40 per cent of those in St Petersburg.

The underreporting of hepatitis infections was a serious problem, aggravated by two factors: the lack of appropriate laboratory test kits to allow diagnosis and patient failure to seek medical assistance before their infections had reached acute phases. Often the young drug users, oblivious to their health needs, were canary yellow from jaundice and suffered fully-fledged cirrhosis by the time they sought treatment. Since most non-A hepatitis infections were asymptomatic for weeks, even years, the number of reported hospitalizations represented only a fraction of actual viral infections. In no part of Russia had scientists carried out systematic surveys of drug-using adults and teenagers to determine the genuine, asymptomatic infection rates.

In the southern Siberian city of Novosibirsk, officially registered numbers of hepatitis B and C cases did soar, approaching 180 cases per 100 000 in 1997, according to Dr
Tatyana Boyko, deputy president of the Public Health Commission. And Novosibirsk
Oblast Hospital infectious diseases expert Dr Evgeny Bocharov said that whenever he
tested hospitalized *narkomani* for the viruses, 'It's everywhere. It's a common cold
already. We've seen a fivefold increase just since 1995.'

Once these viruses found their way into a hospital—via a drug-using cirrhosis
patient, for example—they could spread to the general population with terrifying
efficiency if appropriate precautions were ignored. That was why Bocharov shouted
when asked about the hepatitis risk in his Novosibirsk hospital: 'Shortages, shortages,
and more shortages! We have no latex gloves, syringes, anything!'

At the large Oblast Hospital in Odessa, Dr Vasiliy Gogulenko was similarly distressed
about contamination, particularly because, he said, 'To be infected we [health-care
workers] need to have less than a drop of blood exposure. It takes only 10^{-9} viruses per
millilitre of blood to cause hepatitis C infections.'

Senior nurse Lila Brynchuk said that nurses on the hospital's surgical staff openly
complained because it was illegal for health-care workers to go on strike in Ukraine.
They wanted the state to pay for protective hepatitis B vaccines, which cost twenty
hryvnya, or about 15 per cent of a nurse's monthly wages—if she got paid at all.

Fear of treating drug-addicted patients had nearly paralysed the staff of Odessa's
infectious disease hospital, chief Dr Konstantin Servetskiy said, 'Because we have no
financial possibility to purchase gloves for our staff.'

The health-care providers also feared for their patients, because they could not
afford to test blood routinely for hepatitis contamination. At the Institute of Oncology
and Radiology, Dr Grigory Klinenyouk would do anything necessary to protect the
forty children who were under his treatment for cancer—including giving pints of his
own hepatitis-free blood on a regular basis to the leukaemia and lymphoma patients.
He had to bleed himself and his nurses dry, the dedicated young doctor said, 'Because
unfortunately for the recent months the institution cannot find funds for hepatitis
testing. Even HIV tests can only be done if indicated' by donor symptoms.

At a clinic in Kiev, Alexander, a television repairman by trade, sits in the converted
seventeenth-century Ukrainian monastery that serves as that country's primary AIDS
hospital. The forty-six-year-old father of three speaks of his room as his 'cage' but says
he appreciates the kindness of the staff.

One of the nurses—a woman who has treated HIV patients for more than two
years—rolls up Alexander's sleeve and takes a blood sample. Although she's not wearing protective latex gloves, she uses her forefinger to apply pressure on the site of injection after she removes the needle. Then, still bare-handed, she injects the blood into
a test tube, manually removing the needle from the syringe.

When her supervisor, Dr Alla Vouk, is questioned about the incident later, she flatly
denies that any of her staff ever performs blood-related procedures without appropriate

precautions. Her denial is unaltered by a visitor's insistence that these events were eyewitnessed, and photographed.

Throughout areas of the former Soviet Union witnessing an upsurge in HIV, health providers seemed woefully behind the times. Although concerned about their own safety, many were seen routinely without protective attire performing procedures that put them in direct contact with patient blood.

Meanwhile, some continued to demand the right to decrease their personal risks by performing HIV tests without patient approval, and refusing care to those who were infected. It was a discussion painfully familiar to American nurses, physicians, and dentists, who collectively confronted the same issues and debates more than a decade earlier.

One crisp June morning in St Petersburg Dr Aza Rakhmanova, chief infection specialist for the city, rushed between the numerous buildings of Botkin Infectious Diseases Hospital, heading for the Neurosurgery Institute. The month before, the short, plump woman recalled breathlessly, 'Surgeons did brain surgery and afterwards realized the patient was an HIV-positive drug user from Kaliningrad. And the surgeons weren't wearing gloves! They claim that the brain is a fine structure and gloves impede their work. I told them it's a crime!'

Rakhmanova disappeared into the Neurosurgery building, where she would deliver the sorry message that first-round testing had turned up some tentative HIV-positive results in six of the surgeons and nurses who were in that operating room. The tests will have to be repeated, probably several times over coming months.

Ironically Rakhmanova has just come from her AIDS ward, where she dispensed treatment that would be sophisticated even in New York City, epicentre of the North American epidemic. To twenty-eight-year-old Costa she suggested adding anabolic steroids to his protease inhibitor combination therapy to enhance the man's metabolism.

'It makes sense,' she said brusquely. The patient was left wondering how to pay for still more drugs, as Rakhmanova strolled next door to the room of a long-haired bearded man who was sitting on the edge of his bed and slowly, tentatively spooning food into his mouth.

'How is the invirase?' Rakhmanova asks. Timour Novikov looks up, his eyes fixing on a spot a few inches shy of the doctor's position. As he carefully slides his borscht soup aside, Novikov smiles and says, 'I can swallow the pills—it's not too difficult.'

Novikov, an artist, lost his eyesight recently when an opportunistic viral infection invaded his brain, causing encephalitis. Now he sells his paintings to pay for the protease inhibitors that have restored some of his weight and his ability to walk.

As Rakhmanova and her staff move from room to room making patient rounds they know when it is necessary to wear gloves—and when it is not.

But outside the rarefied world of a handful of such modern AIDS-specialized hospital settings, ignorance reigns. At the Kiev AIDS Clinic, for example, thirty-eight-year-old postal worker Viktor has had AIDS for three years. He won't take AZT—the only treatment available in Ukraine. Instead he sees a popular Kiev healer, 'who has invented an apparatus to measure biocurrents from my body. She charges the currents with a piece of tin, which we call a bullet. And the bullet counters my negative biocurrents.'

Viktor opens his shirt to reveal a bullet-shaped piece of tin taped to his chest.

And in Odessa, where abortions are the preferred form of birth control, doctors make extra cash by performing the procedures outside the hospitals. 'In that case the physician doesn't know that [the patients] are HIV positive,' prominent obstetrician Igor Boychenko said. 'And she may be treated with the same tools and instruments as the next woman.'

As the HIV toll mounted at a frightening pace in the former Soviet Union, Eastern Bloc governments found themselves in the unique position of having a small window of time to take public health actions that might forestall medical disaster. But despite nearly two decades of vivid AIDS history and experience from around the world the authorities were unable to agree upon courses of action, lacked funds to support the few steps they are willing to take, and had no experience—with any medical problem—in modern approaches to public health.

In some places, such as the Baltic nation of Estonia, freedom and candid discussion were considered the ideal approaches to stemming an HIV tide. But in many other parts of the former Communist world top AIDS doctors and politicians claimed that only a return to totalitarian control of society could stop the virus.

'From my point of view it's necessary to bring back socialism,' Vadim Pokrovsky told a visitor to his HIV research and clinical care facility in Moscow. 'This psychology of socialism is more acceptable for Russians—the so-called democratic way is not realistic at the moment. The sense of working for society is very important for young people. In the present moment they don't understand, and the result is drug addiction, prostitution, and so on.'

Extreme as that may sound Pokrovsky was reflecting a sentiment popular among members of the Russian and Ukrainian public health elite—most of whom gained entry to the top circles of science and medicine during the Soviet period when such stature could only be obtained with membership in the Communist Party. These leaders looked at their countries in the post-Communist world and saw lawlessness—an anarchy that microbes easily exploited. And they said they saw a state of disorder that needed to be arrested by classic Communist means: secret police, Young Pioneers and other rigid youth groups, large prisons, and harsh penalties.

Noting that the 'world community forced us to comply' with its notions of human rights, Russian Ministry of Health official Belaeyev said his country was compelled to abandon methods that had kept HIV in check for a decade. Now, he insisted, it was hard to believe Russia was supposed to follow AIDS control measures promoted by American human rights advocates.

'It's more than 500 000 AIDS cases in the USA. That's not a good example for us!' Belaeyev insisted.

By the end of 1998 the Russian Ministry of Health had to acknowledge two things: nearly all new HIV cases were among young intravenous drug users, and the ranks of said narcotics and amphetamine injectors had swelled dramatically. The Ministry's Onyschenko said that 90 per cent of all new HIV cases—those diagnosed since January 1996—were intravenous drug users. And, he noted, there were officially one million intravenous drug users in Russia in early 1998. Where spot checks were performed around Russia, from 20 to 70 per cent of the nation's intravenous drug users were HIV positive in 1998, which would indicate, assuming all of the above numbers were reasonably accurate, that between 200 000 to 700 000 intravenous drug users in Russia carried the virus. Given that Russia's infection rates were, until 1996, among the lowest in the world, such numbers, if accurate, pointed to one of the pandemic's most rapidly evolving epidemics. And expensive: nearly all of those cases were young adults who would, had they been healthy, have formed the backbone of Russian economic development in the early twenty-first century.

At the close of 1998 UNAIDS estimated that 270 000 people in Eastern Europe and Central Asia were HIV positive. This was certainly a conservative guess, probably a gross underestimate. Given apparent infection rates in the intravenous drug users regionally it was hard to imagine that HIV numbers were of such moderate size. As of the end of December 1997, 7 per cent of the Russian military tested positive for HIV infection. That was roughly 105 000 men, or more than a third of the UNAIDS estimate.[22] As the twenty-first century dawned, the pattern of drug behaviour and spread of HIV seen in Odessa and Kaliningrad in the mid-1990s was repeating in hot spots across the region. The results were HIV wildfires, fuelled by shared narcotics needles, in Moscow, St Petersburg, Irkutsk, Krasnoyarsk, and scattered outposts in the Baltic nations of Estonia and Lithuania, as well as Siberia. Addiction rates as high as 50 per cent were common among teens and young adults in these hot spots, and statisticians were hard pressed to calibrate the explosive spread of HIV by 2000.

In most respects the region's HIV epidemic appeared in the late 1990s to be following the tragic model set by Thailand a decade earlier. In 1988 HIV rates in all population groups in that South-east Asian nation were quite low, with fewer than 3 per cent of any group testing positive for infection. In early 1989, however, surveys of Bangkok intravenous drug users jumped ominously, with just over a third testing positive: eleven months later half of them were infected. And by the end of 1991 intravenous drug users all over the country were infected: less than 15 per cent had escaped HIV.

Lagging just a few months behind that intravenous drug epidemic was an upsurge in HIV seen in prostitutes and their male clients. Nationwide in mid-1989 less than 4 per cent tested positive. Twelve months later the infection rate in prostitutes was 10 per cent. And six months after that a remarkable 70 per cent of the prostitutes in tourist mecca Chiang Mai were infected. By the end of 1991 upward of 90 per cent of the lowest-class prostitutes—those who served more than five customers every day out of hellish brothels—were infected nationwide. And by 1992 HIV had so thoroughly spread into the general population that life expectancy for the year 2000 was expected to plummet by an average thirty years and the population was predicted to see shrinkage, with twenty-five million fewer Thais than would have existed in the absence of HIV.

All of that in a time span of just two and a half years.

For Eastern Europe's HIV epidemic to follow that tragic pattern either a high degree of promiscuity in the adolescent populations across the region or substantial prostitution need exist.

Although the end of communism may not have signalled a rise of genuine democracy in most countries in the region, it did generally usher in a freer atmosphere among young adults. With that came a rise in adolescent and post-adolescent promiscuity. In the absence of readily available condoms, or male willingness to use the protective devices, this 1960s-style free love atmosphere was woefully cavalier in the face of a 1990s HIV pandemic.

But in every country in the region the sexually transmitted diseases data tracked wrong: the genders were out of synch. Women had far higher disease rates than the men in their age groups. And that was because more and more of the girls weren't having sex with boyfriends but with older adult men who had money. And it was paid sex.

Dr Jaromir Jirašek, for example, was at the end of his rope. He had done everything he could to stop the prostitutes, pimps, and their German customers from taking over his little Czech town. But under the new post-communist Czech constitution any attempts to ban prostitution represented illegal violations of human rights.

So Jirašek and his fellow citizens of the small Bohemian village of Dubi were forced to turn a blind eye to the Ukrainian, Slovakian, Russian, Bulgarian, Romanian, and Gypsy girls who stood half naked in glass booths along the E-55 motorway, wiggling to an unheard rhythm, presenting their 'goods' to the drivers of passing BMWs, Audis, and Mercedes.

Dubi is just twelve kilometres from the German border, not far from Dresden. The tiny town is one of many strung along E-55 that during the 1990s had become little more than brothels, strip joints, roads full of streetwalkers, parklands littered with discarded underwear, and school playgrounds strewn with sex leaflets written in East German dialect.

But the forty-something Jirašek was no prude. His office was adorned with naked pinup girls and, he said with a wink, the doctor knew how to have a good time. A middle-aged man with a sharply receding hairline and wire-rimmed bifocals, Jirašek spoke sitting in front of a large calendar depicting Miss June—a naked blonde sporting bandolier criss-crossed shell casings and holding an AK-47 rifle. His objections to the new, yet already titanic, prostitution industry were those, he said, of a physician.

'We're seeing syphilis, gonorrhoea, soon HIV,' Jirašek explained. 'Since 1989 it started with pimps here with two, maybe three, girls in a car. And later they bought houses right on the motorway... and by a year ago the situation was one of girls lined all along the side of the motorway—in a huge line [several kilometres long]. And Germans drove by and chose which one. And they had sex in these houses, in the forest, in the cars—anywhere.

'Sometimes local people are involved, but the business is run by foreigners. And they don't provide health-care to their prostitutes in the vast region. They're all over the Czech Republic, all over Eastern Europe, in fact, and when one [prostitute] gets ill they just replace her. That's it.'

Since the 1989 Velvet Revolution of Czechoslovakia, the 1990 fall of the Berlin Wall, and then the 1991 collapse of the Soviet Union, prostitution in the vast region had transformed from a tightly controlled cottage industry into a multibillion-dollar, multinational enterprise controlled by organized crime rackets that transported tens of thousands of women—and in all too many cases girls and boys—from the poorest formerly Communist countries to pockets of plenty along the borders of wealthy Western Europe and the Middle East. The scale of these operations was staggering. It was globalized sex—and globalized sexually transmitted diseases.

The International Organization of Migration had struggled since 1991 to keep track for the United Nations of the woman-smuggling operations out of Eastern Europe. The trafficking of women, the IOM's Marco Gramegña said, was so massive and so rapidly expanding that the agency could provide only approximate estimates.

'These [ex-USSR] women are the new merchandise,' Gramegña explained. 'And it is a new form of slavery. I would say it is following exactly the model we see in India. These women are given a contract—a phony contract—for legitimate jobs in Western Europe. The trafficker charges her bank account or debits her future earnings for her plane tickets and lodging. When she reaches the destination the trafficker seizes her passport, plane ticket home, documents, and tells her she must work as a prostitute until she earns back her debt. And of course she never does.'

In this manner about a half million women from Eastern Europe and the former Soviet Union had been smuggled into Western Europe and forced into prostitution by 1995, Gramegña said. And thereafter the scale of the operation escalated, with up to 300 000 more women trafficked into Western Europe annually, most of them from Russia and Ukraine. By early 1998 the 'slave prostitute' trade was netting at least $20 billion a year in Western Europe and untold additional amounts in the Middle East and Asia. No one knew how many more women from the region were being smuggled into China and Japan, or south-west into the Middle East. But it was possible that the combined scales of those operations nearly matched that of the Western European smuggling enterprise.

At the international level, Gramegña noted, the crime syndicates involved in the trafficking of women and girls were also key players in narcotics and weapons smuggling. Some of the business was handled by decades-old Mafia gangs, but there were 'new Russian ones. And they are investing financially in [legitimate] Western European businesses—they are Europe's new nouveau riche.'

'A Mafia man told us that the girls are bought as slaves and every mark or dollar they earn is taken away from them,' Jirašek said. 'They are beaten. Their identity papers are taken away from them. And they can't go anywhere without a guard who keeps them from running away.' Every Bohemian official and physician in the area confirmed that more than 95 per cent of Bohemia's prostitutes were non-Czech women lured to the area under false pretenses, such as alleged disco dancing jobs, by organized crime figures. The women came from Ukraine, Russia, Belarus, Slovakia, Bulgaria, and Romania and were, in the word most commonly used to describe their plight, 'slaves.'

The prostitution syndicates appeared to be beyond regulation, out of police control. In little Dubi, for example, two of the more than twenty brothels were situated either side of a police station. Gypsy and Russian women dressed in hot pants and spiked heels called out to cars twenty-four hours a day in plain view of the police. Prostitutes also worked in front of local schools and parks, angering helpless parents.

'Since 1985 we have seen a thousandfold increase in syphilis,' Dr Alesander Moroc of the Central Hospital in Ustí Nad Labem said. Ustí, also a Bohemian town, is about a twenty-minute drive from Dubi. Moroc is the city's clinical expert on sexually transmitted diseases (STDs).

'Sixty-eight per cent of the syphilis is among fifteen- to twenty-four-year-old females. And often we see syphilis in late pregnancy women. They come in during the second half of pregnancy when nothing can be done. Before 1995 we never had any, but now we do see congenital syphilis here,' Moroc said. 'In one case the baby died right away, but normally the child is healthy looking, but serologically positive.... Often these kids are lost to follow-up' and go untreated.

The other major STD, gonorrhoea, was also on the rise, but 'we see a paradox that gonorrhoea rates appear to be decreasing as syphilis rises,' Moroc explained. 'This is because general practitioners treat the gonorrhoea and don't report the cases.'

Syphilis was harder to diagnose and treat—it required more extensive antibiotic therapy—so patients typically sought clinic or hospital assistance and ended up as registered cases. Gonorrhoea, in contrast, could be treated with a single penicillin injection. So privacy-conscious people sought discreet care for their gonorrhoea, leaving the disease woefully underreported.

Worse, widespread self-medication or physician misuse of antibiotics resulted in mutant strains of gonorrhoea that are drug resistant.

'Resistance to penicillin is actually the norm now,' Moroc said, noting that there was no drug-resistant gonorrhoea in Bohemia prior to 1991. In Dubi, Jirašek said that only three physicians were licensed, and none of them would treat the prostitutes. So, he concluded, the pimps were obtaining penicillin and other antibiotics through black market suppliers.

A 1992 Czech government survey of Ustí prostitutes showed that 30 per cent carried either syphilis or gonorrhoea. Rates were believed to have doubled since then, Moroc said, but the pimps forbade the women from participating in such studies.

A plump, middle-aged man with sparse black hair, Moroc has a face filled with warmth and sincerity. It emits genuine pain when he reveals that 68 per cent of all female syphilis cases reported in the Czech Republic in 1996 came from his hometown district of Ustí.

Moroc shakes his head.

'There were surveys done among the prostitutes and it showed that the women are forced NOT to use condoms by their pimps because they make more money,' Moroc said.

It was impossible to interview prostitutes in Bohemia: none would talk. Even taking photographs drew protests and threats. Jirašek said a German photographer who took photographs in 1996 on E-55 was shot at but escaped unharmed.

Gynaecologist Pavla Vitagfásková worked with Prague-based Pleasure Without Risk, a non-governmental outreach group that tested for HIV and STDs among Czech prostitutes. Rates of infection weren't as high in Prague as in Bohemia, she said, but they were climbing steadily. Worse yet, even her group couldn't get past the pimps and Mafia to educate and test the prostitutes.

'From time to time the girls get beaten,' Vitagfásková said. 'The pimps don't want us talking to them. And some of them are only sixteen. There's an area around the main railway station where there are many homeless women. They often come from Slovakia looking for jobs and can't find any. The girls are sick, homeless. They have sex in toilets. Sometimes merely for a bowl of soup. We found there a Slovakian woman with secondary syphilis.'

In Ustí chief epidemiologist Dr Josef Trmal, of the Regional Institute of Public Health, found evidence in 1997 that the Bohemian STD epidemic 'seems to have gone well beyond the prostitution circle to all sexually active young adults. We've seen an increase in the numbers of people seeking STD counselling and treatment and most of them are teenagers and very young adults.'

'We do see a connection between drug abusers and prostitutes,' Trmal said. 'With girls it is a strong problem—dual drug use and prostitution. Some girls said they were prostitutes only when under the influence of drugs.'

'For five hundred deutsche marks you can buy a [slave] girl from Turkish dealers,' Trmal continued. 'The pimps are buying the girls and then forcing them to be prostitutes forever. The girls are on drugs, they don't have documents.'

Nationwide the Czech syphilis rate jumped from 50 cases per 100 000 in 1986 to 320 per 100 000 in 1996, according to Dr Bohumir Kriz, head of the National Centre of Epidemiology and Microbiology—the Czech equivalent of the Centres for Disease Control and Prevention. In 1995, Kriz said, the Czech Republic saw its first congenital syphilis case ever entered into public health records: 'Terrible,' he exclaimed.

In every sizeable Russian city prostitution strips or neighbourhoods emerged in which complex networks of young prostitutes, female pimps, and male gangsters serviced both local and travelling business clienteles.

On an ice-cold night in front of Moscow's Red Square pretty Ula lures customers with her teenage charms. Dressed in a Dolce & Gabbana black jacket, tight black patent leather trousers, high-heeled boots, and a fluorescent pink mohair skin-tight sweater Ula looks like a teen queen from suburban Americana. She says she is eighteen, but blushes, betraying a poor ability to lie. She doesn't look a day over fifteen. She left her family home in frigid Syktyvkar, about five hundred miles north-east of Moscow, during the summer of 1996 to better herself, Ula says.

Now she stands in front of the Intourist Hotel, greeting men who drive up beside her. The moment they arrive Ula's stern thirty-five-year-old *mamochka*—her pimp—rushes up and negotiates a place, a price—the details of Ula's next hour's work. If the men meet the right price Ula gets 50 per cent of the take, which for one hour of sex in the hotel or back of a Moscow disco comes to $150 to $200. Her female pimp, who insists the girls call her by the affectionate Russian term for 'mommy', takes the other half of the income. A typical Moscow *mamochka* works ten to twenty girls a night, earning on exceptional nights more than $5000. On a dreary winter night like this, however, even the *mamochka* has to hustle hard to get enough customers to cover her overheads: bribes to the hotel and payoffs to local thugs who sit in a warm Mercedes ready to beat up any overtly kinky customers or men who try to cheat the girls with inadequate payments.

A few blocks away Marina pimps her six girls in front of Russia's legislative building, the Duma. The blue-eyed brunette is well bundled-up against the cold—after all, she's not selling her body. She ran into 'some financial troubles' last year, Marina says, so at age twenty-four during the winter of 1997 she took on the title of *mamochka*. A dozen other competing pimps race Marina to cars as the men pull over. Duma security guards dressed in combat fatigues watch but do nothing.

'That's the Duma across the street. If they can't do anything how can we?' asks the tall guard, who says his name is Sasha. 'It's been like this since 1980 when the Olympics happened. Now it's more open. People used to be afraid, but now we have democracy.'

His short partner—also named Sasha—laughs, adding, 'That's democracy for you!'

Prostitution in Moscow was far from subtle. The girls, their *mamochkas*, and the protective thugs could be seen day and night along main roads, in railway stations, in front of the state's sacred Red Square and Duma, inside discos and casinos, and in hotel bars. In Moscow's most exclusive nightclubs high-class hookers charged $1500 for a night's 'entertainment'. At the opposite end of the economic scale were women along Moscow's Ring Road who demanded $50 a night—or, lower still, illegal immigrant girls, homeless, who serviced their customers for a railway station $2 kiosk meal.[23]

In the daytime abandoned or runaway children dashed among cars in Moscow's heavily congested streets, hawking prostitute pamphlets and 'hot sex' tip sheets. Tiny ten-year-old Natasha, who clearly hadn't bathed in days and said she lived on the streets, darted among cars around Pushkin Square hawking a guide to Moscow prostitutes.

'Gimme fifty thousand roubles [about $8],' Natasha demanded. 'It tells you addresses, prices, and so on.'

A Fagin-type figure skulked along the pavement shouting out to Natasha and several other apparently homeless little girls. 'Hurry up! Sell more! Watch for the police!'

Natasha shot a frightened look at the man, said she was afraid of the police, and dashed off down the stairs of Chekov Metro station.

Little Natasha apparently could not read. Had she been able to she would have known that the book, written by Edvard Maksimovsky, was subtitled *An Anti-Brothel Guidebook*. In page after depressing page Maksimovsky detailed the horrors of the lives of Moscow's sex workers, underscoring the coercion and fear that both brought the women into the trade and compelled them to remain—despite the obvious risks to their health and well-being. For example, Maksimovsky wrote, 'In 1993 when the spring Moscow River ice melted there were six women's bodies found. That was a warning to all the girls: this is the fate of those who try to quit.'[24]

The police often sat among the *mamochkas*, enforcing traffic regulations and parking laws—only rarely arresting the prostitutes, and never busting their clients. Because September 1997 marked the 850th birthday of Moscow the mayor moved the most blatant Red Square–area prostitution out of the city centre. Although that temporarily decreased the visual assault of Moscow's trade in flesh, it did not affect the industry's health impact. And, of course, the prostitutes were displaced for only a few weeks.

In 1988 Russia had a total of 5704 registered syphilis cases, according to the Ministry of Health. In 1996 a staggering 386 935 cases were registered—a sixty-eight-fold increase in eight years. And this vast figure was most certainly an underreported total, according to a study conducted in 1996 by Dr Adrian Renton of Westminster Medical School in London. Joint British-Russian analysis revealed that the old Soviet system of tracking down and forcibly registering all the sex partners of identified syphilis cases had virtually collapsed, along with the rest of the health-care system. Further, in many parts of Russia the Dermatovenereology Service, as it was called, ran out of funds for drugs and now charged patients up to $300 for a twenty-eight-day course of syphilis treatment.

Wishing to avoid having their names on lists and lacking funds to pay the state doctors, more and more syphilitic individuals were either going underground for treatment or not being treated at all. Even under the best of conditions syphilis could be hard to diagnose in women because the infection hides far inside their reproductive tracts and may lurk there—contagious to her fetuses and sex partners—for years before causing obvious hard-to-treat symptoms in the female. As the old system of syphilis screening deteriorated in Russia the risk to both women's health and to general public health rose.

But even the officially registered—grossly underreported—numbers were chilling.

In 1995 the national syphilis rate in eighteen- to nineteen-year-old boys was 359 per 100 000; girls in that age group had an astonishing 922 syphilis cases per 100 000. (By way of comparison the combined male/female syphilis rate for that age group in the United States was 13.7 per 100 000.)

For 1996 the overall national syphilis rate was 221.9 cases per 100 000—thirty-seven times the US rate. And in the city of Moscow, with a population roughly the same size as New York City, twenty thousand cases of syphilis were officially reported. The entire United States of America, with a population of over 260 million, had fewer than seventeen thousand syphilis cases that year.

What most troubled demographers when they looked at the syphilis numbers was how sharply the slope of the climbing curve of cases veered upward—almost at a ninety-degree angle. In 1994 the incidence nationally was 81.7 per 100 000—by 1995 it was 172 per 100 000. In 1996 it reached 221.9, and syphilis topped 330 cases per 100 000 in 1997, making Russia's syphilis rate one of the top ten worldwide. Even far outside Moscow rates were soaring. For example, in the medium-size Siberian city of Irkutsk syphilis reports jumped 78 per cent from 1995 to 1996, reaching a rate of 422 cases per 100 000 people of all ages in the city, according to Irkutsk Oblast official data.

Watching this nervously from their offices in Geneva, Switzerland, officials with the UNAIDS Programme were convinced the official Russian figures understated the true syphilis rate by 10 to 20 per cent. By 1998 UNAIDS was regrettably reporting that one out of every four hundred Russians had syphilis, rates of the disease were five hundred times greater than those seen in Western Europe, and since 1991 congenital syphilis rates had risen thirtyfold. And they saw the same deeply disturbing STD trends in other former Soviet states, particularly Ukraine.

In Ukraine the STD epidemic was being driven by the activities of young people aged thirteen to twenty-one years. Although the Ukrainians who were over thirty had seen a steadily soaring syphilis rate since 1990, it was still below 180 cases per 100 000. Among adolescents, however, rates weren't soaring, they were rocketing sky high—especially in girls.

According to the Ukrainian Ministry of Health there were about 600 syphilis cases per 100 000 in girls fourteen years old and younger. And since 1993 fifteen- to sixteen-year-old girls had syphilis rates that fluctuated between 1550 and 2000 cases per 100 000. That meant one out of every fifty sweet-sixteen girls in Ukraine was not only sexually active, but also had seen enough male partners to have acquired syphilis. Estimated combined syphilis and gonorrhoea rates in teenaged boys and girls in 1995 was 4500 cases per 100 000. But most of those teen syphilis cases were girls.

'I always make my customers use condoms,' claimed a fourteen-year-old girl dressed in hot pants, knee-high boots, and a fur bolero jacket. She laughed and gave a knowing wink to another teenaged prostitute working in front of Odessa's Philharmonic Hall. The girls all claimed to use condoms, but the truth was they merely charged more for customers who refused to use the protective latex devices.

The girl in hot pants, who declined to give her name, was part of a well-organized contingent of fifty prostitutes who solicited customers in front of the stately Philharmonic

Hall, charging $50 for a 'quickie' or $100 for an all-night dalliance. On the complex hierarchical scale of Odessa's vibrant sex industry the Philharmonic girls were middle class, according to psychologist Valeri Kiunov, who mapped out the sex trade for the UNAIDS Programme and Odessa State University. During Odessa's cold winter months about two thousand girls worked as prostitutes. But in the summer when the beachside city was a popular Ukrainian vacation spot the prostitute population more than doubled.

Kiunov has found six distinct social strata of prostitutes. Most of the youngest girls—ages eleven to seventeen years—worked as what he called 'chaotic prostitutes', flagging down customers on the streets after school two or three times a week. They typically earned $39 to $50 a week and used condoms.

A second group, averaging twenty-six years of age, worked through female pimps and tended to have steady customers. Kiunov said two-thirds of these women had at least one STD during his three-year study (1994 to 1997).

The most promiscuous groups, called 'the Pacifiers', tended to congregate around factories and large workplaces where they serviced twenty to forty clients a week. The mean age of the group was nineteen years, and nearly all of them had an STD during any given year.

Lucky girls worked their ways up to the Philharmonic crowd or the top rung—call girls toiling for gangsters who ran high-class operations inside all of Odessa's London-skaya and other elite hotels.

But the most vulnerable group, Kiunov said, was also the largest, accounting for more than half of Odessa's sex workers. They worked particular streets, averaged eighteen years of age, and, he said, 'agree on everything. And they are the most likely to get beaten, raped, have sick stuff done to them. They can't afford condoms [which cost twenty-five cents each], and when you talk to them about "safe sex" they think it means avoiding beatings. They have no idea you're talking about STDs and AIDS.'

Half of that group injected local opiate concoctions, and in recent years the average age of these prostitutes had been dropping.

'Last summer I saw nine- and ten-year-olds working in this group,' Kiunov said. Some seven- and eight-year-olds even worked during school recesses doing what they called 'hot sex'—quickies performed with adult men behind food kiosks for about two dollars.

The regional STD explosion was staggering,[25] and no government or United Nations agency possessed a public health strategy for tackling the problem.

'The situation in Moscow is grim,' epidemiologist Nikolay Briko of the Moscow Medical Academy said in 1998. 'Syphilis rates in the Russian Federation have increased fiftyfold over the last seven years. Special anxiety is caused by a fortyfold rise in syphilis cases among children and teenagers and a thirtyfold rise in congenital syphilis.'

The highest levels of syphilis—in some cases more than two thousand times the US rates—were in 1998 seen among girls aged sixteen to twenty.

'We consider assistance from the international community essential,' Dr Leonid Barabanov of the Belarus Ministry of Health said. 'Unfortunately our government does not have adequate financial, technical, or human resources to fight the STD epidemic on its own.'

At the Geneva headquarters of UNAIDS public health experts were scrambling at the close of the 1990s to come up with strategies that could prevent the seemingly inevitable marriage of the prostitute-driven STD epidemic and burgeoning HIV/ hepatitis crisis in intravenous drug users. With syphilis levels astronomically high, predominantly in girls aged fourteen to twenty years, and HIV/hepatitis rates soaring in boys and girls of the same ages, an AIDS catastrophe seemed tragically inevitable.

German scientist Karl Dehne tried out of his tiny UNAIDS office to coordinate prevention efforts across twelve time zones. Dehne's bleary eyes and jerky body movements betrayed lack of sleep, and the urgency in his voice showed genuine anxiety.

'They don't know anything [in former Soviet countries] about outreach, behavioural change, counselling. They say, "Information! Information!" When I say, "Information isn't enough to change behaviour," they reply, "Well what else is?" Imagine—they have no methodology at all for outreach.'

And why should they? During the heyday of SanEp, 'outreach' consisted of forcibly rounding up the public and submitting everybody to whatever intervention was deemed worthwhile. The narcologists were only trained to imprison patients. The venereologists were taught how to maximize shame in order to limit spread of disease. Nowhere in the region's public health toolbox were the skills of peer education, persuasion, and non-judgemental behavioural intervention.

'They tell me to find the people there, but it's just not there,' Dehne exclaimed. 'There are several million prostitutes there and not one prostitute outreach program.'

Having done such work for years in Africa Dehne was stunned by the Eastern European dilemma: in no African country had he ever encountered such severe public health skills limitations and social obstacles to averting drug and sexual diseases crises.

'I think we have a window of opportunity here and I'm still hoping we can prevent an epidemic calamity. It's very new,' Dehne said. Then his shoulders slumped and he concluded, 'But I'm afraid I'm not really winning.' A few months later Dehne, distraught over the situation, left UNAIDS, forming a private organization dedicated to training Russians and other former Soviets in public health outreach skills.

Brazilian researcher Luiz Loures had an office down the hall from Dehne, and although he had faced tough obstacles to AIDS prevention in Latin America he, like Dehne, was finding the former Soviet nations a dismal challenge.

'First of all,' Loures said, pointing to charts and tables strewn across his data-cluttered desk, 'look at the economics. Ukraine, for example. In 1992 it ranked sixty in the Human Development Index,' a United Nations Development Program Scale in which higher numbers indicate greater progress in all facets of social and economic advancement and infrastructure. 'By 1993, a year later, it was down to nineteen. By 1994—seventeen.'

Now, Loures continued, add an overlay of a quarter million intravenous drug users and millions of teenaged prostitutes and it was obvious that Ukraine would have twenty thousand full-blown AIDS cases by 2001.

UNAIDS director Dr Peter Piot, a Belgian, had been battling HIV since the virus first surfaced in the early 1980s. He had witnessed the evolution of epidemics in one nation after another. And he knew from experience that only one thing could avert disaster in the former Soviet region: 'political leadership'.

'Fundamentally the problem everywhere is public health leadership. Without leadership and political commitment [AIDS prevention] is not going to happen,' Piot concluded. So in late 1997 Piot travelled the region, meeting with Yeltsin and other heads of former Soviet states. He went to the Davos economic summit, and the powerful G-8 meeting in 1998. He pleaded with the world's most powerful political leaders, asking that they draw a line in the sand along the former Iron Curtain, saying, 'No more HIV.'

At the G-8, Yeltsin, multi-national corporate leaders, World Bank, and all of the leaders of the Newly Independent States nodded in agreement, issued bold resolutions, and lent written support to Piot's UNAIDS efforts.

But in concrete terms, they did nothing.

VIII

It is characteristic of Russia that the majority of people were reconciled to the fact
that the guaranteed salary was wretched and the guaranteed medicine was awful.
People who are not used to living in conditions of freedom are now feeling nostalgic
for what they have lost.
—Andrei Sinyavsky[1]

Given all the infectious disease scourges that physicians suddenly faced in the 1990s hospitals could no longer view themselves as cavalierly as they had during the previous decade. Under the Soviet require medical care was farmed out to unique, specialized centres: alcoholics and drug users to narcology clinics; tuberculosis patients to the sanatoriums; infectious diseases patients to contagion clinics located in rural areas where the patients' germs couldn't cause urban epidemics. Even common colds and minor flu cases landed in isolated facilities where workers were spared having to work while ill, but removed from their families until well. In this way the Soviet public health planners believed risk was segregated, and thereby limited: the society at large need not fear syphilis, TB, or diphtheria because all of the carriers were routinely rounded up and placed in sequestered facilities.

It was a system with much in common with Soviet political control. Possessors of deviant ideas were similarly rounded up and held in gulags lest they might contaminate the masses with their subversive notions. For nearly seven decades it worked.

But by the 1980s, well before the USSR fell apart, hospitals were facing new threats about which the physicians and doctors knew very little: antibiotic-resistant bacteria; untreatable multidrug-resistant tuberculosis; hepatitis B and C. And after 1991 the trend accelerated, adding a host of once-controlled ancient infectious diseases and the new scourge of humanity—AIDS—to the mix. The microbes did not respect the hospital segregation system: infectious diseases would not oblige physicians' demands that they turn up only in designated facilities. And the patients were increasingly reluctant to abide by the sequestration system, preferring to stay at home among loved ones rather than bide months, even years, of time in isolated medical gulags—particularly as funds for the facilities diminished and hospitalization often involved stays in boring, ice-cold rooms with little to do, and even less to eat.

Thus, the 1990s signalled the region's need for a sort of shock treatment for public health in which SanEp either disappeared or transformed into a seriously beneficial epidemiology and surveillance service. And one in which the notion of sequestered patients and diseases was abandoned in favour of strict, across-the-board infection control standards in all health-care facilities, wherein it was assumed that *every* patient might be a microbe carrier, therefore precautions needed to be standardized and universal. No emergency room physician, for example, could confidently treat *any* patient in 1999 without wearing protective gloves, gown, and goggles or glasses—not when the region was in the grips of so many profound epidemics caused by organisms that could be contagious in the absence of obvious symptoms.

The new era also signalled an urgent need to decrease the amount of time patients spent in hospital, both to decrease costs and reduce risks. Patients ultimately lived longer if they spent less time in medical facilities, where they were exposed to other patients' bacteria and viruses.

In the community, public health's image needed to change overnight, from its old Soviet authoritarian and paternalistic structure into one that recognized the individual's right to refuse vaccines, found funds for repair of water supplies, adhered to appropriate antibiotic use, offered intravenous drug rehabilitation services, promoted safer sex through use of condoms, and other preventive interventions that could protect the society at large. The individual right of refusal could no longer be overcome with the power of the state: only the powers of persuasion, peer education, health marketing, and common sense would do.

But it was no easy matter to transform an entire, gigantic infrastructure. Though the Soviet Union no longer existed, its public health apparati and apparatchiks still did.

The system—most of which was executed in 1999 as originally designed in 1937— worked like this: medical students and future epidemiologists were trained from the age of eighteen onwards in different institutions, and rarely interacted. Once the epidemiologists were professionals, they joined SanEp, where they were trained to 'function as policemen who came to hospitals and brought grief,' said Russian-trained

Dr Elena Bourganskaia of American International Health Alliance in Washington, DC. 'So physicians learned to see epidemiologists as threats.'

'The surveillance of infections is not lab-based at all,' Bourganskaia said. 'And it's passive. They [SanEp] wait for physicians to report [hospital-acquired] nosocomial cases. But in the old system physicians were punished if they were related in any way to an infection. So you basically have to be out of your mind as a physician to report cases.'

Under Communist dictator Josef Stalin's rules, every system in the Soviet Union had to be monitored by a parallel, Communist Party-controlled organization. For the medical system, that organization was SanEp. And survival as a hospital administrator was absolutely contingent upon supplying SanEp with rosy reports, not word of an outbreak of antibiotic-resistant staphylococcus in your cardiac postoperative ward.

Worse yet, SanEp's entire procedural structure was based on false biology. Its concept of infection was an environmental one not that dissimilar from the ancient Greek concept of 'miasma', meaning 'bad air'. Germs flew about in the air, and illness arose as a result of filthy environments. Soviet hospitals were required to expend enormous amounts of manpower scraping off samples of whatever film or muck might be on the walls, ceilings, and floors. And hospital microbiology laboratories devoted 70 to 90 per cent of their resources to scrutinizing these samples for bacterial contamination.

If contaminants were found, SanEp marched in and someone took the blame.

If diseases spread within a hospital then a mad scramble was initiated, in search of the dirty wall or floor responsible for the spread of the microbes.

If patients failed to respond to first-line therapy then treatment typically followed an empirical course: Plan A didn't work, switch to Plan B. Rarely were patient samples sent down to the laboratory with instructions to find out why Plan A had failed.

'Virtually no one in [the former Soviet Union] is a clinical expert in diagnosis, management, and prevention of nosocomial [hospital-acquired] infections,' said Dr Ed O'Rourke, an infectious diseases expert at Boston's Children's Hospital, who, during the 1990s, shuttled around Russia and other former Soviet countries trying to spread the gospel of Western-style infection control.

'We talk about the abuse of antibiotics here, but here it's usually using overpotent drugs for simple infections,' said O'Rourke, who was also on the faculty of the Harvard Medical School. 'There they simply add one on top of another without any particular rationale.... And when the patient worsens they just add another drug to the regimen.'

O'Rourke's main message was that more patients would survive simple bacterial illnesses, fewer such illnesses would be acquired inside hospitals, and everyone would save both lives and money if they stopped using antibiotics and conducting hospital hygiene in the manner they were taught under the Soviet regime.

There was no way to quantify the extent of nosocomial infections and antibiotic resistance in Russia or any other ex-Soviet country. The first—hospital-spread disease—couldn't be quantified because the old Stalin-era infrastructure of infection control was so punitive that doctors rarely reported cases. The second—drug resistance—couldn't be quantified because few clinical laboratories had adequate supplies or skills to perform drug sensitivity tests.

Nevertheless, it was obvious that the spread of drug-resistant microbes was proceeding at an alarming pace, and the sorry saga of Irakli Sherodzle—the streptococcus-infected Georgian teenager—was becoming more commonplace every day.

At the Russian Ministry of Health's Central Microbiology Laboratory in Moscow, doctors Nina Semina and Viktor Maleyev screened bacterial samples drawn from patients all over Russia. Their approach allowed them to determine what sorts of mutant microbes were out there, but not how frequently they were causing human disease. Despite the drawback, they had already found unnerving evidence of rapidly expanding antibiotic resistance.

Since 1993 the Moscow scientists found new drug-resistant strains of staphylococcus, klebsiella, pneumococcus, salmonella typhi (the cause of typhoid fever), shigella (dysentery), and cholera. By 1994, more than 10 per cent of all staphylococcus samples sent to their laboratory were methicillin-resistant and 3 per cent of all pneumococci were penicillin-resistant.

'It's becoming a real crisis now,' Maleyev said.

In Ukraine the picture was similar, Dr Anatoly Shapiro, of the L. V. Gromashevski Epidemiology and Infectious Diseases Research Institute in Kiev, said. 'Our physicians, maybe this is a drawback in their education, but their first thought isn't to go to the laboratory. They'll just prescribe and see what happens.... And now Ukraine is flooded with new Western antibiotics; the physicians don't understand them—cephalosporins and such.'

Streptococcus and pseudomonas bacteria developed widespread multidrug resistance throughout Ukraine, Shapiro said. And ampicillin was no longer effective against enterococci. With each additional layer of antibiotic resistance the bugs got harder—and far more expensive—to treat. As physicians escalated their weaponry from simple penicillins to powerful broad-spectrum antibiotics, it was a little like starting out with an expert sniper and ending up using an all-out aerial strategic bombing campaign. The collateral damage, in the form of ravaged stomach, intestines, liver, kidneys, and other organs increased and had to be managed by physicians, often with other drugs. In a country like Ukraine, physicians were unfamiliar with such antibiotic collateral damage and didn't know how to treat it. And although all sorts of alternative antibiotics were readily available after 1991, patients had to buy them, with cash—cash few possessed. As a result, many bacterial infections were economically incurable.

Microbiologist Vera Ilyina of the Novosibirsk Oblast Hospital had tracked antibiotic resistance in Siberia since 1994. At that time so many untreatable infections suddenly turned up in the region's children that, she said, 'It was a real problem. We were begging for humanitarian aid.'

The American Merck, Sharp and Dohme pharmaceutical company donated laboratory supplies for bacterial sensitivity assays, and Ilyina discovered that staphylococcus all over the hospital—indeed, all over Siberia—was acquiring resistance to methicillin, a crucial antibiotic. She also found evidence that streptococci were resistant not only to the third-generation cephalosporin drugs—the kinds Rovena searched for in Georgia for poor Irakli—but also to the even more expensive new fourth-generation cephalosporins, drugs that weren't even available in Siberia until 1993.

At that point, she began hunting around the massive Novosibirsk Oblast Hospital, trying to find sources for these new, lethal microbes. She looked for connections among the infected patients and noticed that those with drug-resistant strains tended to have spent a long time on a mechanical ventilator in the burn ward, or were babies in the neonatal intensive care unit.

But in the spring of 1997, her inquiry ground to a halt when she ran out of money to buy the culture medium to complete her study.

That was a perfect example, Dr Mikhail Yan said, of the degree to which the medical community of the former USSR suffered in the 1990s for having been isolated from the rest of the scientific world for seven previous decades. After all, it was very well known everywhere else that burn units, neonatal ICUs, and mechanical ventilators were key sources of nosocomial infection. But it was not because something was 'growing' there; it was because the patients and equipment in all three sites were subject to a lot of contact with the ungloved hands of doctors, nurses, orderlies, and family.

'We have been very cut off from international experience,' Yan, a Buryatia Republic state epidemiologist in Ulan Ude, explained. 'WHO bulletins, medical journals, scientific books—we haven't seen them, ever. And we don't know what has been working elsewhere. Information is simply not available.'

How bad was the information gap? Think of hand washing.

From the poorest to wealthiest of hospitals in most of the rest of the world, doctors and nurses understood that they must scrub their hands and forearms thoroughly with disinfectant soap before touching any patient or device that will come in contact with a patient. In lieu of hundreds of scrubbings a day health providers ideally wore latex disposable gloves, donning a different pair for each patient or procedure.

The reason for all this gloving and scrubbing was that human hands were the primary vector of person-to-person bacterial transmission. Lack of attention to hand cleanliness guaranteed that, for example, the staphylococcus on Mrs Jones's arm would get to Miss Smith's mouth by hitchhiking on the unwashed hands of Dr Brown when he examined the Jones wound and then put a thermometer under Smith's tongue.

It seemed obvious. Yet it was revolutionary thinking to doctors and nurses trained under the old Communist regime.

'I can't tell you how surprised I was by their lack of infection control,' Howard Cohen, former executive director of Coney Island Hospital in Brooklyn, said, referring to hospitals in Odessa, Moscow, and Kiev. 'In the operating room they had commonly used soap bars, commonly used towels. Surgeons were going from one patient to another without washing. . . . They thought airborne infection by bacterial spores was the key. They really didn't appreciate that the key was dirty hands.'

In some operating rooms in Russia and Ukraine devices that looked like upside-down umbrellas hung from the ceiling. Inside were ultraviolet lights. The contraptions were designed to zap 'flying' bacterial spores, doctors explained, which then 'fell dead' into the umbrella, sparing the patient any risk of infection.

'Three years ago when I first went there my initial impression was—my god!—they sacrificed their entire population for the sake of satellites in space and their military. For seventy years they sacrificed public health,' said Regina Napolitano, Coney Island Hospital's infection control chief.

For example, the cash-strapped Children's Hospital No. 17 in St Petersburg had stopped purchasing both paper towels and rubber gloves. The staff, oblivious to the crucial need for clean hands, either stopped scrubbing or did wash (especially after using toilet facilities), but shared cloth towels with dozens of co-workers a day.

In the Siberian Oblast of Irkutsk, infection control was hampered in all the hospitals by 'shortages, shortages and more shortages,' cried Dr Tatyana Boyko, deputy president of the Committee on Public Health. The lack of latex gloves, paper towels, disinfectant soap, and disposable devices such as catheters has, she said, sparked a 30 per cent increase in sepsis among newborns since 1995—with most cases being fatal.

In Ossetia, an autonomous region inside Georgia, a hernial resection surgical procedure was underway. Some of the staff in the operating room wore no masks or gloves—including the scrub nurse. And midway during the operation she collected bloodied instruments, carried them to a wash tub filled with water that had been in place, uncovered, for hours. She dunked the instruments in the water, gave them a quick shake, and returned the surgical equipment to the surgeon's table. Within seconds one of the haemostats the nurse had rinsed was inside the patient's intestines, holding tissue aside while the surgeon probed the hernia.

Napolitano said that in every hospital she visited in the region, 'There were no [infection] barriers that we would consider acceptable for preventing blood-borne infection. They were reusing needles, gloves were scarce.'

Dr Gennady Onyschenko, who was in charge of all infectious diseases issues for the Russia Ministry of Health, was dismissive of the problem. He was well aware, Onyschenko said, that some Russian hospitals were diverting scarce resources from purchase of such things as latex gloves to doctors' salaries and fancy high-tech equipment purchases. But the Russian nation 'has everything: reagents, test kits, gloves, enough for our patients. We are not importing anything. In principle, we are self-sufficient.'

Furthermore, Onyschenko insisted, antibiotic resistance was a trivial issue in Russia, noting, 'There are much more important ones to think of here.'

On the contrary, however, the nosocomial and drug-resistance problem in the region was massive, but went largely unseen because of the very nature of the Soviet system of SanEp.

In addition to resistant bacteria, the enormous, antiquated medical facilities were spreading—rather than halting—hepatitis B and C, HIV, and other blood-borne diseases. Though comparisons with conditions in Africa always drew rage from health providers in the former Soviet region, it was hard to avoid reflecting on Kikwit's Ebola virus outbreak or other epidemics that were propelled on that continent by the medicinal reuse of syringes and poor hospital infection control. There was a difference, however: most trained African physicians knew what decent infection control entailed but lamented the poverty of their facilities and paucity of appropriate supplies. In Russia, Turkmenistan, Moldova, and the rest of that region, however, even where supplies were plentiful they were not properly used, and standards of infection control were not maintained.

Whereas most hospitals and physicians remained entrenched in old SanEp thinking after 1991, a few were beginning to step away from it.

Coney Island Hospital's Napolitano spent a lot of time in Odessa Oblast Hospital in Ukraine during the 1990s teaching New York standards of hospital infection control to her counterparts in Odessa. And staff from the Ukrainian facility rotated through Coney Island, where they felt at home because 45 per cent of the patients spoke Russian. After four years of such an exchange, sponsored by American International Health Alliance (AIHA), chief Odessa physician Vasily Gogulenko was proud to say he had reduced the average length of patient hospitalization from fifteen to eleven days and decreased the death rate by an amazing 29 per cent.

AIHA hoped that the Odessa hospital experience would serve as a lightning rod, sparking reform across the region.

But O'Rourke said change 'doesn't just spring up like wildflowers [because] the whole concept of infection control has been so punitive.... The system here is still find the scapegoat and punish them. The focus is always to get the bad guy and throw him in the slammer.... So infection control is a bunch of rules, it's not a thought process.'

Bourganskaia said it all boiled down to thinking about biology. Doctors prescribed combinations of antibiotics in Russia, for example, that made no sense because they all targetted the same aspect of the bacteria rather than hitting a microbe at two or three different vulnerable points. But they didn't actually understand how antibiotics worked, she insisted, so the precious drugs were almost universally misused.

'We calculated that they could save millions of dollars if they just changed that practice,' Bourganskaia said. 'Similarly, if hospital administrations realize that infection control improves quality of care and saves money, then maybe they can change. If they can just change the way they think about what they do, and how they do it.'

The former Soviet states need not view Bourganskaia's critique as a sellout to the West. They need only look slightly westward, to the Czechs, for a clear illustration of this principle.

The Czech Republic not only performed the job of infection control well—it did it better than the United States and nearly all Western European countries.

The Czech Republic had the lowest antibiotic-resistance rates in disease-causing pathogens in the former Communist world and was rivalled by few nations in the world for the number one slot, overall. Many antibiotics that had been rendered useless in the United States and former Soviet Union because of widespread drug resistance still worked as well in Prague and the rest of the Czech Republic in 1998 as they had twenty years earlier. And some of the most worrying forms of antibiotic resistance, such as enterococcal resistance to vancomycin, never emerged in Czech hospitals.

'We are an island, you could say, in terms of resistance,' said Dr Anna Jedličková. 'Slovakia and Hungary—all our neighbours—are much worse off. So we are in very good shape.'

Though the Czechs were governed by many of the same SanEp-type health policies that were the law in the Soviet Union, the country's microbiologists and physicians strived to be more scientific and, as best they could, follow Western European trends.

The nation's microbiologists, caught up in the spirit of resistance that permeated Czech life in '68, broke with Soviet policies and set up their own system. They didn't know what the West was doing to control new bacterial infections, but they realized that the Soviet model was a disaster.

Cut off from the West, the Czechs invented their own unique system. By law all uses of antibiotics had to be cleared by a control microbiology laboratory such as the enormous one that Jedličková ran in Prague. Physicians could not just prescribe the drugs, prompting emergence of resistance bacteria. Instead, they had to submit sputum, blood, or infected tissue samples to the laboratory for analysis, where the precise nature of the infection would be determined.

If, for example, the laboratory diagnosed streptococcus, the physician was told, 'Okay, it's streptococcus. Here is a list of three antibiotics we recommend you use.'

The 'recommendation' was actually a command, and the central laboratory in Prague periodically modified drug-use guidelines according to observed trends in bacterial mutations and resistance. Policies often varied regionally in the country, reflecting differences in the local bacterial ecologies.

Hospitals were also told which disinfectants they could use, and what equipment needed sterilization. This, too, reflected constant vigilance on the part of the microbiology laboratories, searching for trends in microbial resistance to chlorine bleach and other antiseptics.

'And we introduced a specialized laboratory of sterile controls,' Jedličková said. 'It is unique. It will detect the sterility of the environment and of autoclaves and disinfecting machines.'

Ironically, the entire system nearly toppled following the successful 1989 Velvet Revolution that overthrew the Czech Communist dictatorship.

'Some doctors thought that antibiotic use policies were undemocratic,' Jedličková said. 'These people wanted to abolish the [microbiology] centres. But fortunately common sense won. Even the opponents to antibiotic centres started to understand that bacteria don't recognize democracy.'

Soon a new challenge faced Jedličková and her fellow microbiologists—free market medicine. The Czech government was easing its way out of nationalized medicine into a mixed economy of health-care similar to that in the United States. This meant private practices, managed care, health maintenance organizations, and personal health insurance were all swiftly replacing five decades of Soviet-modelled socialized medicine. For the microbiologists this signalled a loss of control.

Jedličková was still able to dictate antibiotic and infection control practices for the prestigious three-thousand-bed University Teaching Hospital in Prague, but her wide influence over the private prescribing practices of individual physicians was quickly evaporating.

The impact was felt most sharply in treatment of syphilis, gonorrhoea, and other sexually transmitted diseases, according to Czech Deputy Minister of Health Dr Miroslav Čerbák. Fuelled by both the desire to protect patients' sexual privacy and the enormous amount of money that could be made in off-the-books treatment of prostitutes and their customers, Czech doctors were risking their licences and prescribing drugs without seeking microbiology laboratory testing and approval.

In Russia the lessons of modern science had yet to permeate most medical and public health facilities—except, of course, at the Kremlin. That was why you'd never be able to convince Texan J. T. Peoples that Russia had a medical system in chaos.

'Hell no!' Peoples declared in his Beaumont, Texas, twang. The sixty-year-old American Embassy electrical engineer said his major symptom on May 9, 1997, was 'Death!'

'I figured I only had a few hours,' he recalled. Diverticulitis and a perforated abdomen had Peoples doubled over in agony. But he was lucky. As an American Embassy employee Peoples qualified for admission to the most advanced facility in all Russia, the Kremlin Hospital, otherwise known as Moscow Central Clinical Hospital.

It's no wonder Peoples felt right at home in the Kremlin Hospital—he practically was. The fully renovated luxury floor on which Peoples recuperated from surgery had wall-to-wall American pile carpeting, walls papered in American synthetic fabrics, lovely American sofas on which patients rested while watching American television, American nurse Marianne Hess on staff to provide that down home touch, American magazines to read. And in case all of this is too subtle there was an American Stars and Stripes standing right next to the Russian tricolor in the front lobby.

A plaque on the wall read: 'Training for the unit has been provided by the following health-care members of Premier Health Alliance, Chicago, Illinois, with the support of the United States Agency for International Development and American International Health Alliance.'

This was where Russian President Boris Yeltsin received his heart treatments and check-ups. Seventy per cent of the patients were deputies in the Duma, senators, or members of Yeltsin's cabinet and top staff. The remaining 30 per cent of the patients were either Western embassy personnel like J. T. Peoples, or wealthy executives from the newly privatized major corporations and banks of Russia, according to cardiology unit director Dr Marina Ugryumova.

'We have some rich people that can be treated here,' Ugryumova said. 'But we do not want robbers and killers treated here because we have serious security concerns.'

In other words, if you had enough money you could be treated where the American flag flew—unless your money was blatantly ill-begotten.

The Kremlin Hospital had always offered a better class of care. But it wasn't easy to get into the facility—and never had been. The elite central Moscow compound, with its well-manicured grounds and expansive buildings, was surrounded by a perimeter of walled security. Entry was closely monitored by armed guards, video cameras, and gated driveways.

As would be expected, considering the clientele. It was here that President Leonid Brezhnev was treated for his strokes during the 1970s and final cardiac death in 1982. And his successor Yuri Andropov died in the Kremlin Hospital two years later of kidney failure; his successor, Konstantin Chernenko, was treated here for heart failure, hepatitis, and multiple other health problems the following year, dying in 1985.

But by the 1980s the hospital had become little more than a high-security, fancy geriatric care centre, catering for the Soviet Central Committee and Politburo dinosaurs. It stopped advancing, Ugryumova said, because treatment of the septuagenarian elder statesmen of Russia was too predictable, and easy.

Then in 1996 the world learned that president Boris Yeltsin was suffering life-threatening heart disease. No facility in Moscow was up to Western standards for the quadruple bypass cardiac surgery Yeltsin desperately needed. But it was unthinkable that the president of the Russian Federation would disgrace his nation's bruised, but proud, health-care system by seeking treatment overseas. So the US government hastily renovated not only the Kremlin Hospital's physical appearance and equipment but the structure and skills of its staff as well.

The result was a facility so many cuts above what was generally available in Russia as to seem from another planet.

The region's hospitals and medical clinics outside the hallowed Kremlin walls ranged from appalling to astonishingly horrible. Most were staffed by personnel who rarely—if ever—were paid. Supplies of all kinds were scarce. Physical maintenance had long since been abandoned, and many health structures were poorly built in the first place. So everywhere hospital administrators had for more than a decade patched and painted peeling walls, cracked floors, caving ceilings, and shattered windows.

And, remarkably, little thought was given to patient mobility. Central planners in Moscow dictated that the region's hospitals have lifts of one size but trolleys of another—incompatible—length. In many hospitals patients had to be carried up and down stairs by relatives in order to reach X-ray machines or other diagnostic and treatment equipment. Virtually no hospital was wheelchair accessible. Beds were rarely more than basic, non-adjustable affairs. For some procedures—notably, abortions and childbirth—anaesthesia and painkillers were used minimally, if at all. And in general pain management was not a priority.

The situation only worsened after 1991, as lifts broke down, compelling ailing individuals to climb stairs in order to get from test sites to their hospital beds. Food fell into short supply, with most hospitals stating frankly that families needed to provide rations for their ailing relatives, much as they would in India or Zaire.

The old Soviet medical system was titanic in size but utterly lacking in efficiency or cost-effective management. Like the polluting, inefficient industries that shut down after 1991 all across the region, the Soviet model of health-care simply could not function in the New Reality. In Russia, for example, there were 10 280 hospitals, 1601 clinics, 6107 out-patient centres, and 450 university teaching hospitals. For a population of 147 million people in 1995 Russia had nearly two million hospital beds, for a patient-to-bed ratio of 1:118. The average hospital stay in Russia in 1995 was *seventeen days*.

A fee-for-services form of medicine had emerged in which patients' ability to pay (or barter) determined the extent and quality of their care. To a certain degree this had always existed. During the Soviet period—particularly during the Brezhnev years—patients were expected to provide their surgeons and physicians with under-the-table cash or services, such as free auto repairs or caviar and vodka. But the situation spun into marketplace chaos after 1991, with doctors and nurses demanding arbitrarily set payments for everything from cardiac surgery to changes of bedpans.

Dr Yuri Komarov of MEDSOCECONOMINFORM noted that by the late 1990s nearly 100 per cent of all health-care in the Caucasus nations (Georgia, Armenia, Azerbaijan) was paid for directly by the patients: cash up-front for every single service.

'We are still living in lawless countries,' Komarov said. 'We are still at the mason's stage, building we don't-know-what,' as a health-care system. More than 80 per cent of the annual 1997 Russian state health-care spending, for example, went to hospitals, which used it largely to maintain their inefficient, overly large staffs.

'We need to change that around,' Komarov insisted.

In Turkmenistan the 1990s witnessed radical changes in health-care as reformers like Annageldy Gaipov, of the Ministry of Health, pushed successfully for complete elimination of Soviet-era priorities. Average in-patient hospitalization was reduced by 4 per cent from 1994 to 1997, Gaipov said. The number of physicians on the national payroll was slowly reduced, first by making medical school admission far more difficult and licensing fewer new physicians, and then by eliminating duplicate medical departments. The number of in-patient beds was cut by a third. And all priorities for state-funded medical care shifted from lengthy, tertiary care in hospitals to public health.

The result? From 1990 to 1997 Turkmenistan decreased its maternal mortality rate by 10 per cent, Gaipov said, its measles rate by a third, its anthrax rate by 60 per cent, and eliminated all cases of polio by 1996.

'We're pretty confident that we're on the right path,' Gaipov said, grinning.

But it was a comparatively easy path for little Turkmenistan, population 4.5 million, to follow. The challenge of health-care reform was greater in nations with more difficult geographic or population obstacles. In Kazakhstan, for example, the population was so spread out that human density averaged just 1.5 people per square kilometre, Dr Bakhyt Tumenova, social affairs director for the city of Semipalatinsk, said. Amid rising economic chaos many of the rural clinics had turned into lawless entities in which health providers extorted patients for huge sums of money, or refused care. To counter this trend, Tumenova said, the state created a competitive bidding system, privatizing the small clinics and forcing them to compete.

In Georgia health reform ran smack in the face of resistance from the medical community, as providers realized that many of them would be unemployed by the time reform was completed. Georgia had about thirty-seven thousand physicians and fifty-five thousand nurses on the state's payroll in 1990—enough, experts say, to meet the public health and medical needs of a nation of sixty-five million people. But Georgia had only five million citizens. Like all Soviet states, Georgians overdiagnosed illnesses and hospitalized far too many people.

For decades Georgia's health-care system was based on enormous facilities such as the Republican State Hospital, located in downtown Tblisi. The twelve-story, two-thousand-bed concrete facility was so full during the 1980s, doctors said, that patients often lay upon trolleys lining the hallways.

By 1997, however, a visitor found all of the hospital's lifts broken, and scaled ten stories of concrete stairs, littered with bloody bandages and medical detritus, before finding any patients. Around them was evidence of little more than decay: swathes of linoleum flooring curled up and bubbled in waves of self-destruction, holes gaped in the plaster walls, and stretches of assorted types of tapes covered cracks and holes in most of the windows, proving inadequate in the face of gusts of icy winds. The thirty-year-old hospital was disintegrating.

As the Soviet state issued dictums from Moscow, local government workers had no choice but to follow—or, at least, appear to obey. In the case of health planning Moscow's orders always focused on two things: goals for percentage reductions in various infectious disease rates and construction of hospitals.

'In old times they would write with these five-year plans, "1957: must build one thousand new beds." And two thousand the next. This was the nature of planning. All of this was *not* improving health in the country,' Minister of Health Avtandil Jorbenadze, a forty-something, dashing, dark-haired man, said. With policies that were driven by pursuit of gigantism—always assuming that bigger meant better—the Soviets set their health system on an upward spiral they could not afford. Building more hospital beds meant staffing the ever-larger hospitals and polyclinics with more trained personnel to tend to those beds. By the 1960s it was obvious to everyone in the medical system that supply far exceeded demand, so the Soviets simply expanded the list of medical conditions that required hospitalization and lengthened the recommended durations of hospital stays.

'In the old days we lived in a country with a strange system of health-care,' Jorbenadze said, chuckling. 'And not all of it was bad. But we had an excess of technical and capital investment. After 1991 we had to imagine the main role of the state, health-care, and people in our new society. And we had to evaluate our resources and needs. And, most of all, we had to change this vertical system into a horizontal one, with partnerships among the state, managers, and employees.'

Critical to any reform, according to Jorbenadze, was the elimination of SanEp. In its place he hoped to create a system of public health and disease control that was clearly rooted in sound science. He dreamed of the US Centers for Disease Control and Prevention, which—at least in Jorbenadze's fantasies—used epidemiology as a scientific tool for providing a data-driven basis for health policy. It was Jorbenadze's ambitious goal for Georgia.

And it would be a tough one to meet.

IX

In order to renovate our state apparatus we must at all costs set out first, to learn, secondly, to learn, and thirdly, to learn, and then to see to it that learning shall not remain a dead letter, or a fashionable catch-phrase (and we should admit in all frankness that this happens very often with us), that learning shall really become part of our very being, that it shall actually and fully become a constituent element of our social life.
—V. I. Lenin, 'Better fewer, but better,' March 2, 1923

When hard-line Communists staged their failed coup against Soviet President Mikhail Gorbachev in 1991 the job with the highest prestige in the land was Scientist. The twenty-storey, white marble Russian Academy of Sciences was built just four years before the coup out of anodized gold aluminum and titanium and featuring cut-crystal light fixtures: it was designed as a paean to scientific discovery. The giant white edifice cast an impressive shadow over the Moskva River. On top of the building was an odd five-storey-tall golden aluminum and titanium construction that glistened in the noon sun.

But the strange, massive pseudosculpture on the Academy headquarters was a poor disguise for an unbelievable mistake. Convinced Soviet science would one day rule the world the Communist Party architects planned a building of more than fifty stories in height, and spent a fortune on Georgian marble and fantastically expensive titanium to proclaim its glory. But less than halfway up the engineers noticed that the building was sinking. Laden with marble, the construction was heavier than the Moskva River landfill site could bear. To cover their abominable oversight in failing to conduct a geological assessment before designing the gigantic mess the architects simply halted construction and created the strange aluminum/titanium 'sculpture' to cover the partially built twenty-first to twenty-fifth floors.

Years after the collapse of the USSR the Academy headquarters had a sad look to it, reminiscent of an abandoned American shopping mall circa 1975. Footsteps echoed across the emptiness of the meeting halls and reception areas, unreplaced light bulbs left dark cavernous shadows, and behind the leather-gilded doors lay hundreds of empty offices.

The scale of the Soviet scientific enterprise was staggering before 1991. What it may have lacked in quality was certainly offset by quantity. In Russia alone there were 250 civilian scientific institutes employing sixty thousand scientists. In some institutes—particularly outside Novosibirsk—scientists often functioned with a sort of privileged sense of freedom, able to indulge intellectually in ideas that would land any other Soviets in gulags.

That was then.

After 1991 everything changed.

The average Russian scientist in the late 1990s earned 500 000 roubles a month, or about $88—if he or she was paid at all. Once the best paid members of the Soviet society, Russian scientists had fallen dramatically in prestige and earned only 80 per cent of the median national income, according to Boris Saltykov of the Russian House for International Scientific and Technological Co-operation. In Russia the number of employed research scientists and technicians dropped to just 1 300 000—down from 3 400 000 in 1985. During the 1980s scientists were bedecked with Orders of Lenin and praised as socialist heroes. But as the twenty-first century approached, according to the Centre of Science Research and Statistics in Moscow, scientists ranked among the lowest professions in public esteem, just 1 per cent above the military.

At least fifteen thousand Ph.D. scientists left Russia between 1991 and 1996, forming the largest peacetime brain drain in world history.

The Russian scientific collapse was mirrored in most of the other nations of the former Soviet Union and Eastern Bloc—with the striking exception of the tiny Baltic States. Even before the USSR collapsed East German scientists got sobering glimpses of the price they were going to pay for decades of isolation from their more advanced West German peers. In 1989, months before the fall of the Berlin Wall, the Iron Curtain weakened enough to allow some 400 000 Germans from the East to visit the West, and 1 per cent of her scientists moved to the West. Those scientists who went west told colleagues back home that they found their skills woefully backward. In particular, the almost complete lack of computer skills and knowledge of computer-driven research tools put the Easterners twenty years behind. And after the fall of the Berlin Wall the West German scientists were shocked to see how completely the Communist Party controlled Eastern science, allowing dogma to carry greater weight than such seemingly irrefutable foundations as the law of physics.

Czechoslovakia awoke from its 1989 Velvet Revolution to the realization that most of its fifteen thousand scientists had been cowed or jailed after the Soviet invasion of 1968. Only the Communist ideologues in the ranks of Czech and Slovak scientists had, for twenty-two years, received lavish research funding and prestigious academic positions.[26]

Georgia's ten-thousand-strong Academy of Science was in a state of utter chaos after the country's civil war, from 1991 to 1994. Virtually all of its research institutes went without electricity, resulting in destruction of all frozen laboratory samples and what little computer-stored information had existed. So desperate had economic conditions become that by 1996 laboratories were stripped by thieves of equipment, copper wiring, electric transformers, even light bulbs.

Hungary's scientific establishment shrank swiftly, as federal funding all but disappeared and the National Academy of Sciences was forced to reorganize. Between 1985 and 1996 Hungary lost 27 per cent of her biologists and chemists: some moved west, some simply had no choice but to find new ways to earn a living. Poland, Bulgaria, Romania, Latvia, and Lithuania followed similar courses.

Ukraine suffered particularly, as more than 70 per cent of the country's scientists prior to 1991, were employed by the Soviet military.

Sadly, the sinking of the titanic Soviet science came at the time when the health and survival of the region's populace hinged on innovation, research, and course corrections in the directions of medical thinking. Though money was absent, solutions rested less with cash infusions than with fundamental changes in the ways policy makers, hospital administrators, physicians, nurses, epidemiologists, and biomedical researchers thought about what they did.

'Basic research science has fallen apart. And even before [the collapse of the USSR] the quality of research was very low,' Elena Bourganskaia said in 1997. 'You can't trust the results. There are no case-controlled studies. There is very little appropriate statistical methodology. And the research need is huge! They have to change what they're doing, but they can't just base practices on American or French data. Their practices must be appropriate to the setting.'

Bourganskaia, at the age of twenty-seven, embodied the tragedy of Russia's loss. Trained as a doctor in Moscow, the pretty, energetic Bourganskaia spoke fluent English, was earning two PhD's at large American universities, and was curious about her world, energetic in her work, sophisticated in her views of the role of modern science in public health, ambitious, and personable. She worked, however, not in Russia but in the United States and will only return for a visit, she said. She was Russia's loss, and America's gain.

'The concept that you need data to determine the efficiencies and efficacies of your practices—it's not a concept that's in use. Medical school training does not include the scientific method: hypothesis, study, data-driven solution. You never see denominators in reports. . . . Everything was a 'science' in the Soviet view—history was a science, politics was a science, philosophy was a science. Any academic can be called a scientist. And the stuff that gets published is horrifying!'

Bourganskaia's wish list for Russian scientific research included the establishment of key laboratories that could determine the extent of antibiotic resistance in disease-causing bacteria and develop appropriate treatment strategies. And she wanted to see tests carried out to determine if many medical techniques in general use across the region actually worked—or worse, caused harm.

At Children's Hospital No. 5 in Moscow microbiologist Valery Stroganov would have loved to tackle some of Bourganskaia's questions. But the thirty-four-year-old scientist had a more basic problem: he couldn't get a decent culture medium to grow bacteria in, and he couldn't get appropriate biological supplies even to conduct simple screenings for antibiotic resistance.

'That's why Russian microbiologists don't have the possibility of clearly interpreting the results of their work,' Stroganov said. 'We don't have any tools.'

In Ukraine, Russia, Belarus, and Estonia physicians concerned about HIV and hepatitis were desperate for information about drug abuse: were the bizarre concoctions used in the region—which could include such hellish chemicals as acetone—more addictive than the counterpart narcotics popular in the West? And how do you prevent and cure such addictions?

'The drug users come to us and ask for help. They are injecting heroin and opium dissolved in acetone and paint thinner,' Dr Svetlana Danks of the AIDS Information and Support Centre in Tartu, Estonia, said. 'The answer is we just don't know. Like with everything else, we just don't know.'

Danks wanted to see more carefully controlled scientific testing done on several methods suggested within the region, but this hadn't been a priority with regional governments. And money was not available.

In the old days, the Soviet Union's Gamaleya Institute was the nation's top medical science facility. After 1991, however, Gamaleya rented out most of its land and office space to small-time entrepreneurs, a beer brewery, and a parking garage in order to pay its taxes, heat, and electrical bills, said its director Sergei Pozorovskii.

'In the old days we were guaranteed funding. Okay,' said Gamaleya scientist Henry Dolgov. 'But some of the work may not have been the best. Today we must compete for funds. Well, we have to learn the grants process. We have to learn to compete. That's the way it is.'

In Moscow physicist Michael Alfimov was doing his best to create a competitive grants process for Russia modelled on the way the National Science Foundation in the United States dispensed funds that it received from Congress. Since 1994, Alfimov—who spoke fluent English—had led the Russian Science Federation, basing it closely on the NSF in Washington, DC.

The main problem for Alfimov was that the Russian legislature kept reneging on its promised funds for science. In 1996, for example, the Russian Science Foundation received fifteen thousand grant proposals, of which three thousand were judged by panels of experts to be worthy of funding. The Duma promised nearly one trillion roubles ($200 million), but by December 1996 the RSF had only received 170 million roubles ($340 000).

By 1998 Russian spending on science had fallen from a 1991 level of $11.6 billion to $1.5 billion, prompting Science Minister Michael Kirpichnikov to say that 'today's situation is the worst it's ever been for Russian science. And the most difficult times are in the future.' And, true to prediction, funding for scientific research fell further still, in 1999 sinking to just a half billion dollars. The average research grant was a mere $5000.[27]

Many outside organizations, including George Soros's Open Society, the Howard Hughes Medical Institute, US National Institutes of Health, and the European Union, sank substantial funds into the region's scientific enterprises, picking out the most promising researchers and awarding reasonably sized grants. But the scientists still had to toil within the political economic realities of their countries, which often proved impossible.

Russia's 1996 minister of science, Boris Saltykov, said that at the core of all the flaws in the region's scientific enterprise lay one key point: until 1991 more than 75 per cent of all Soviet scientific research—in all subject areas—was controlled by the Soviet military. The military closed science off from the rest of the world, rewarded those ventures that had potential strategic applications, and created a vast scientific bureaucracy in which, Saltykov said, 'Obedience and tolerance for bosses' views were valued higher than freedom of creative works.'

The dominance of the military also explained why Soviet leaders rarely funded research done in universities, a key component of scientific progress seen in Western society.

This may not have been altogether bad, given the quality of some of that science. For example, the man in charge of all psychiatry and psychology research in post-Soviet Ukraine, Dr A. P. Chuprikov, published numerous studies claiming that colour-tinted glasses, laser surgery of the brain, and insulin-induced comas all could cure schizophrenia. An independent panel of Dutch and Canadian psychiatrists judged the work 'reminiscent of the KGB/psychiatric circuit' and 'a direct violation of Human Rights,' not to mention shoddy science.[28]

Such shoddy psychiatry had immediate implications for public health. As drug abuse, alcoholism, and suicides sky-rocketed regionally the legacy of absurdist approaches to psychology rendered the profession ill-equipped for the challenge.

In Georgia, for example, psychiatrist George Nanieshvili, head of the nation's largest psychiatric service, sadly watched the suicide toll mount among Georgian men, particularly forty- to sixty-year-olds.

'Why? Of course, the social situation,' Nanieshvili exclaimed during a discussion in his dark, ice-cold, unheated, and unelectrified office. 'Because traditionally the father takes care of the family. With the [post-Soviet] change the man has to bring food to his family but he cannot. And the man's reaction is . . . to commit suicide.'

In Nanieshvili's institute a middle-aged woman who declined to give her name was recovering from a complete nervous breakdown. It wasn't having her home seized by rebels in Georgia's breakaway district of Ossetia that made her crack. Nor did four years of living in a squalid refugee encampment inside a former hotel in Tblisi. Even the kidney stones diagnosed in one of her three children and the heart and lung problems in another didn't put the woman over the edge. Or the complete bankruptcy of her family of six, all of whom lived in one 400-square-foot room.

What did it was the fire, she said. It started when refugees in the apartment below made a mistake while cooking dinner on a hot plate and the flames soon devoured her apartment. She jumped from a second-storey window, breaking her leg. And as she watched the fire eat up all that remained of her former life in Ossetia—her family photographs, embroidered clothes, bits of hand-me-down jewellery—the woman suffered a complete nervous breakdown.

The stress caused by the former Soviet Union's transition from communism to capitalism was producing such pronounced psychiatric difficulties, Nanieshvili said, that it could be likened to Leningrad Syndrome—the sociopsychiatric state experienced by the population of St Petersburg during World War II when German troops surrounded the city for more than a year in a siege that left millions starving or dead.

And this psychological burden had to be borne by societies that, in many cases, almost completely lacked any tradition of psychotherapy or modern psychopharmacopoeia. Indeed, during the height of Soviet totalitarian control over the vast region psychiatrists worked hand-in-hand with the KGB and police, certifying that individuals who held dissident views were insane and should spend the rest of their days in Siberian gulags and asylums.

Dr Semyon Gluzman of Kiev, Ukraine, spent ten years in a Siberian gulag. His crime? He found that noted Ukrainian General Petro Grigorenko, who opposed the use of nuclear weapons, was 'sane and the doctors committed an act of injustice,' Gluzman recalled. Grigorenko spent the 1970s in an asylum for challenging the concept of a 'winnable' thermonuclear war.

'The KGB used psychiatry for political purposes,' Gluzman said in his Kiev office. 'And that was doable because psychiatrists were inadequately trained. Most psychiatrists just aren't ready for modern practice. It was very important in Ukraine [during Soviet days] to explain everything very simply, without ambiguity and forever. That's why it was impossible for a psychiatrist to say, for example, "we don't know what schizophrenia is." We had to say, "It is X disease and it was discovered by the Soviets and it will exist forever." In the mid-twentieth century Western doctors realized it's better not to treat an unknown disease, but to help the patient lead a normal life. In the Soviet system it was forbidden to use the term *psychologist*. And psychologists were forbidden to participate in treatment.'

During the seventy years of Soviet rule of the Ukraine, no Western psychology or psychiatry books, articles, or journals were allowed in the country. The pioneering works of Freud and his followers were ignored, as was the striking 1970–1980s revolution in the understanding of the chemistry of the brain and the development of drugs that could adjust specific chemical imbalances. Most psychiatric disorders were simply classified in one of five boxes: psychoses, senile dementia, schizophrenia, neuroses, and mental retardation. Notably absent was the world's most common psychiatric disorder, depression. It was assumed that the only individuals who could be depressed under communism must be anti-Communists, not depressed.

Throughout the former USSR and Eastern Europe psychiatry and psychology had suffered similar fates and were proving woefully inadequate to meet the tasks of the post-Soviet era.[29]

Dr Toma Tomov of the Medical University in Sofia, Bulgaria, said that the real question was, 'How does the Self gain esteem if the social organism is sick? That requires facilitation—it means coming to terms with reality.' A reality that included the knowledge that everything you were taught to believe about the world, and your place in it, was wrong. It was, many psychiatrists argued, a situation that induced regional mass paranoid psychosis.

Even in the Baltic States, which were only occupied by the Soviets for forty-six years and retained strong Western traditions, the psychiatric profession was controlled by Soviet ideology and was struggling to cope with what Dr Lembit Mehilane called 'a nation suffering a broken heart.'

Mehilane, who was on the faculty of Estonia's prestigious University of Tartu, catalogued the tragedy: a doubling in suicide rates between 1988 and 1994 with six thousand suicide attempts in the tiny nation during 1994, alone. In 1996, he said, there were more than sixty thousand cases of clinical depression diagnosed in Estonia, or one case in every twenty-five people. Only 53 psychiatrists had private practices in the country, 170 were inside hospitals, and nationwide there were only 40 clinical psychologists.

Classic psychiatric disorders such as psychoses and schizophrenia did not increase in frequency after 1991—and would not be expected to, experts insisted, as they were usually genetic in origin. The increase was primarily in depression. After all, millions of workers in all imaginable professions were toiling in expectation that someday they would be paid. No one had a count of these people. The Russian government conceded only that 'trillions of roubles are owed' in back pay; the Ukrainians and Byelorussians gave even fewer clues. Laid-off workers, who comprised anywhere from 28 to 50 per cent of the region's potential workforce depending on where you looked, wouldn't be collecting welfare or getting unemployment checks.

The smart ones were getting by, working in the massive unofficial economy of trading and hustling, smuggling and small-time entrepreneurship. The World Bank estimated, for example, that the Ukrainian unofficial economy in 1996 topped $10 billion, which, given that its official net private capital flows were only $247 million, may have far exceeded the size of the official economy.

Increasingly, then, survival depended on skills that most people raised under communism didn't have: individual initiative, monetary flair, and competitive instincts. Those who couldn't cope were suffering nervous breakdowns, depression, alcoholism, drug addiction, and suicide.

'I think that's the main reason for this psychological crisis,' Gluzman said. 'For us, having grown up with a Soviet mentality, we don't realize we have to pay a price for freedom. Secondly, the average Soviet person sees it as freedom for *oneself*, not freedom for the whole society, *for everybody*. And third, not everyone realizes that a better life can come as a result only of very hard work.'

Totalitarianism was obviously a terrible, repressive force. But it also offered predictability and stability. No surprises. Steady checks, repeated habits. 'In old socialist times we weren't comfortable but we were in a cage—and this cage protected us,' Georgia's Nanieshvili said. 'Don't think I am a Communist, but a totalitarian system offered stability.'

There might not have been much on the shelves of the USSR but everyone had money—just in case some mouldy beets turned up at the market. Now the reverse was true: in even the most remote Siberian outposts Pepsi and Coke vied for consumer loyalty and Norwegian salmon competed on the shelves with local sturgeon.

But most of the population could only look. They hadn't enough cash to buy.

Genuine psychiatry disappeared as a profession prior to World War II.[30] During the 1960s and 1970s Soviet psychiatrists were obsessed with psychic research: extrasensory perception, evidence of UFOs, telepathy, telekinesis, astrological birth control, psychotronic generating devices, pyramid power, and unusual uses of acupuncture. Joseph Stalin was an admirer of psychics, as was Nikita Khrushchev. The Soviet Navy spent enormous sums of money training sailors to psychically communicate with submarine captains, thus allowing Moscow to issue orders to its fleet without using radio signals that might be intercepted by NATO or US eavesdroppers. The line between vaudeville-style magicians and Soviet Academy of Sciences members was fine in this area, perhaps undetectable.[31]

By the 1980s the parapsychology of the previous decade, coupled with the extraordinary KGB-granted power psychiatrists had over the lives of Soviet citizens, pushed many members of the profession to extraordinary heights of grandiosity. Some psychiatrists, particularly in Ukraine, Siberia, and Belarus, came to see themselves as religious figures. Around them grew cults, featuring everything from medieval black magic and doomsayers to faith healers and a colourful variety of pseudo-Christians.[32]

Even at the once-prestigious Russian Academy of Sciences' Institute of Clinical Immunology in Novosibirsk scientists were absolutely convinced that stress, combined with pollution, had wiped out the Siberian people's immune systems. But they were curiously unable to offer a shred of laboratory evidence for this assertion—no T-cell measurements, lymphocyte counts, allergy test results, or other standard tools used in the West. Pseudoscience was hardly unique to Soviet psychiatry: all biomedical fields suffered from a fair amount of hocus-pocus.

The Immunology Institute, which had suffered devastating budget cuts during the post-Soviet years, survived in large part off treating the public's perceived immune deficiencies, on a fee-for-service basis. Thirty-year-old Sivieta, for example, suffered chronic bronchitis and headaches for three years. The institute treated her with injections of pig spleen extracts that were intended to boost her antibody production.

Former gulag judge Leonid, at sixty-eight, was having trouble breathing. So he was living in the institute and undergoing immune system treatments that included consumption of *Topim ambur* Siberian herbal bread—patented by the institute—and foam made from an oxygenated form of a green liquid, the contents of which clinical director Dr Valery Shirinsky declined to name.

'But it will lift you,' Shirinsky declared. 'It will raise you—lift your immune system. You must feel high! Your spirit must be light.'

And every patient spent time in a device ubiquitous in Soviet-era medical facilities: hyperbaric chambers. The patients were sealed, prone, into contraptions that created a sensation of pressure akin to that achieved in deep-sea diving. There were chambers designed for people of all ages and sizes—even newborns. And though no controlled, valid scientific studies were ever presented to an inquiring visitor, physicians all across the region affirmed that these chambers boosted immune responses, through unknown biological means.

Dr Yvan Hutin was part of the enormous Russian scientific diaspora. Working with the CDC in Atlanta, Hutin documented a pattern in Eastern Europe of overuse of medicinal injections, and resultant spread of hepatitis B and C. In Romania and Moldova Hutin found that people had four to six therapeutic injections annually, typically given as treatment for such vague diagnoses as simple fever, the blues, mild diarrhoea, and stomach aches. Vitamin supplements and antibiotics were, typically, the injected substances given with little or no basis in science.

And given with nonsterile needles.

Many of these injections were part of the theory of 'weak children' so popular among paediatricians from Budapest to Sakhalin. Overall, the theory held that living creatures—plants and humans alike—'reacted' to their environments, eventually, if all went well, 'adapting'. But adaptation was hampered, according to the view, if the living being was weak, and *all* of the region's children were, by the 1990s, as per popular belief, severely weakened; therefore, they were unable to 'adapt' after 'reacting' to such things as pollution, vaccines, common colds, and allergies.

This adaptation concept originated with the work of an obscure Ukrainian agronomist, Trofim Denisovich Lysenko. Born to an impoverished peasant family in 1889, Lysenko rose after the Bolshevik Revolution because of a series of experiments he conducted in 1925 in Azerbaijan. The effort boiled down to one tantalizing assertion:

under appropriate conditions plants could be forced to adapt to frigid surroundings, providing ample yields of vegetables. In subsequent years Lysenko claimed to have experimentally 'adapted' strains of peas, barley, wheat, rice, and oats—all of which could thrive in Siberia.

The peasant agronomist was catapulted to the most vaunted levels of Soviet scientific power overnight because he fulfilled two of the Communist Party's needs: he promised he could increase food production and he represented a heroic peasant figure at a time when Stalin needed to coax Soviets to turn their backs on traditional intellectuals in favour of the new proletariat leaders of thought and science.[33] The Marxist thesis of human malleability through social change was threatened by Mendelism, bolstered through Lysenkoism.[34] In 1927 his ascendancy to dominance over all Soviet biology and medicine began with a well-placed article singing Lysenko's praise in *Pravda*.

By 1929 Lysenko had enough power to be able to hold sway at all large genetics gatherings in the USSR, where he adamantly pushed his concept of 'vernalization', in which crops could be coaxed to grow in climates and during seasons in which they did not usually thrive.

Lysenko unabashedly extended his vernalization theories to human beings. Chromosomes, and the DNA they held, had no relevance to the nature of offspring. Indeed, Lysenko argued, they were mere artefacts:

> When a nuclear dye such as gentian violet is used, the whole preparation is heavily stained. Chromosomes become visible at a certain point in the removal of the dye. But when this process is continued, the chromosomes simply disappear. Hence the chromosomes are just temporary pictures observed during the removal of the stain.

When Lysenko was reshaping Russian genetics, based on 'vernalization' and 'adaptation', every college student in Europe and North America was imbued with the writings of Darwin and Mendel. The West's geneticists were thoroughly convinced; the Soviets were not.

By 1945 Lysenko was Stalin's darling, so powerful that he had received eight Order of Lenin medals, the highest honour in the Soviet Union, was a deputy in the Supreme Soviet, became director of the Genetics Institute of the Soviet Academy of Sciences, and in 1945 received the ultimate honour 'Hero of Socialist Labour'.

And as Lysenko's power grew, terror rose among the Soviet Union's legitimate scientists. The purges began in 1932. One by one the nation's leading geneticists were packed off to gulags or summarily executed, as Lysenko purged from the halls of Soviet science all 'Morganist-Mendelists'. His power extended to Poland and much of Eastern Europe, where scientists who believed in chromosomes—literally, simply believed in the existence of chromosomes—were obliterated.[34] In their places Lysenko promoted quacks and sycophants who decried every single aspect of what were then the frontiers of biological sciences in the West.

It is impossible to overstate the impact Lysenkoism had on Soviet medicine, science, and public health. Not only did this ideology set Soviet biology on a course backward into the eighteenth century, but the belief system also created a legacy of death that would continue to affect public health policies regionally well into the 1990s and early twenty-first century.

Consider this: if one asserted that chromosomes, and modern genetics, were irrelevant it would be impossible to comprehend such things as viruses, antibiotic resistance, immunology, and inherited disease. Thus, Lysenko's coterie insisted that viruses formed spontaneously out of organic matter. And clusters of viruses spontaneously became bacteria. And, conversely, by placing the antibiotic crystals of penicillin in a slurry one could spontaneously grow *Penicillium* fungi.

By the time Lysenko finally fell from grace in the USSR in the 1960s scientists outside the Soviet Union had delineated most of the elegant biochemistry and molecular biology of DNA, inheritance, cell function, mutations, antibiotic resistance, viral structure, cellular infection by viruses, the existence of promiscuous DNA plasmids, protein chemistry, hormone interactions with cells, and—fundamentally—the 'central dogma', elucidated by Francis Crick in 1956. Its simplicity belied the dogma's essence: life boils down to DNA, which is transcribed into RNA, then translated into a chain of amino acids, forming a protein.

In 1965 every college biology student in the non-Soviet world knew these simple truths.

Yet not one word of *any* of it appeared in a medical school or graduate biology text in the USSR or most of Eastern Europe until the late 1970s, and Lysenkoists still held prominent positions in regional science in the 1980s.[35]

With Lysenkoism as a framework it is easier to understand the public health policies of SanEp, Soviet hospital administrators, and physicians. If, for example, bacteria could spontaneously arise from dirt on a wall it made sense to create a SanEp police force tasked with penalizing doctors who failed to keep their hospital walls well scrubbed. If viruses spontaneously arose from organic matter there need not be concern about reused syringes. Why worry about inappropriate antibiotic use or radiation exposure if chromosomes are irrelevant artefacts?

The Lysenko legacy was crippling.[36] As American scientists geared up for the dawning 'biotechnology century' in 2000 their former Soviet counterparts were struggling to catch up, begging for research funding, and devouring scientific literature for so long denied them.

'Our biomedical science really is in not-bad shape, largely thanks to Lysenko,' said leading Estonian scientist Endel Lippmaa sarcastically, 'since it was forbidden to investigate the molecular basis of life, then, obviously, it was fashionable [in Estonia] *because* it was forbidden.'

To see how science could be practiced properly in the 1990s the former Soviet nations needed to look no further than to tiny Estonia. Although molecular biology and genetics remained in the Dark Ages in most of the Soviet Union, the rebellious Estonians dove into genetic engineering and cellular studies with relish.

'We were able to establish quite serious research which percolated even to medicine,' Lippmaa said proudly. 'But why should you compare us to *them* [Russia]? After all, our country was an occupied country. It is their hard luck if they have rotten science, not ours.'

This turn-your-back-fast-on-Russia attitude was pervasive in Estonia, and explained why the tiny nation salvaged its scientific enterprise so quickly. In 1991 it looked 'like all the most senior thirty-five- to forty-year-olds were going to leave Estonia. And science here would collapse like in Moscow,' Dr Richard Villems, director of the Estonian Biocentre in Tartu, said.

As soon as Estonia's *kroon* stabilized against the deutsche mark in late 1993 Villems and his colleagues took decisive action to save science.[37] They used available funds to, as Villems put it, 'buy back' scientists who had left, luring them with new laboratory equipment and guaranteed good salaries. And they asked the Royal Swedish Academy of Sciences to conduct an impartial review of all of Estonia's science, grading the work and helping the tiny nation spot its weakest areas. Instead of bolstering the weak, Estonia sunk resources into enhancing its strongest areas, making them competitive with European and American science.

The key to Estonia's success was its willingness to not only build up strong departments but also eliminate those that produced the poorest science. In 1970 Estonia had seventy-two research institutes; in 1990 that was pared down to forty-seven. In 1970 anyone who gained membership in the Estonian Academy of Sciences was guaranteed funding, regardless of the quality of his or her research. But in July 1991 the government created a grant and peer-review system that dispensed funds based on research quality, much as was done in nearby Sweden.

The big winner was medical science, which included molecular biology. In 1990 medical science received 7.7 per cent of all grant funds—by 1995 it had gained 16.5 per cent and was expected to grow further, largely at the expense of engineering and agricultural sciences.

With only 0.3 per cent of the population of the former Soviet Union, in 1996 Estonia won 14 per cent of all grants dispensed to the ex-USSR by the European Union, Villems said with no small amount of pride.

Toivo Maimets, the vice rector of the University of Tartu, said the challenge then was to translate that new scientific vigour into changes in the way medicine and public health were practiced in Estonia.

'The fights are sometime quite active,' Maimets laughed, 'because physicians were quite conservative, wedded to old Soviet ways. The problems are deep. The medical community is quite closed. It doesn't let new ideas—troublemakers—in.'

'I personally have problems when I take my children to doctors,' Maimets continued. 'They prescribe an antibiotic and I ask, "How do you know this is the right one?" And they say, "Well, that's what I usually prescribe." They have no idea if it's the appropriate drug, biologically."

Maimets, who spoke fluent English and had studied tumour biology in Britain, was doing research on the p53 oncogene, looking at a relationship between expression of that gene and infection with human papilloma virus.

It was research that would have been unimaginable for a Soviet scientist.

By the end of 1999 it seemed that Estonia wasn't the only country in which there was a scientific renaissance. Billionaire George Soros sank hundreds of millions of dollars into supporting such science, in hopes of halting the brain drain from the region. Hungary, the Czech Republic, and Poland all saw science blossom out of painful pruning processes similar to that experienced by Estonia's research community. But the blossomings were few and isolated, still surrounded by the old, tired Soviet-era debates, inefficiencies, dogmas, and ideologies.[38]

X

What is to be done?
—V. I. Lenin, 1902

In the end public health—its failures and hopes for its future—was tightly bound with the social, political, and economic status of a nation. And in the once-Soviet and Eastern Bloc nations on the eve of the twenty-first century the precarious futures of each were tied, to varying degrees, to the most problematic among them: the Russian Federation.

Prognostications worked overtime at the turn of the century trying to predict Russia's future.[39] Most Western observers, in the end, concurred with Washington analysts Yergin's and Gustafson's perspective:

> Russia's path to capitalism in the twenty-first century does not...start from nowhere. Rather it marks Russia's return to a journey that it abandoned, under duress, in 1917. By 2010, the post-Soviet transition will be far from complete. Russia could well run off the road in the meantime, once or more than once. But a democratic Russia is possible; a non-imperial Russia is possible. A capitalist Russia seems almost certain.

Perhaps. But it also appeared likely that the Russian Federation would de-federate, splintering into wayward provinces that followed the course of Chechnya: Dagestan, Samara, Novgorod, Krasnoyarsk, Vladivostock, Saratov. Russia's federal government was imploding under the weight of its own corruption, incompetence, and lawlessness. It had long since lost control of the far-flung provinces. Vladivostock, for example, stopped passing tax roubles to Moscow in 1996, and its governor ran Russia's easternmost Pacific oblast as if it were his own private domain. Boris Yeltsin's longtime rival, Alexander Lebed, was similarly inclined as governor of Krasnoyarsk, which bisected the nation north-south through the centre of Siberia.

At the local level laws were passed that flouted contradictory federal legislation. Public health law, what little there was at the federal level, was flagrantly ignored at the local tier. Lacking federal roubles to pay such basics as salaries and electricity few health policy and administration leaders felt much cause for allegiance to Moscow. And the forecast called for more pain.

Sadly, public health desperately needed centralization, as none of Russia's constituent parts had, by themselves, the essential tools of the trade: vaccines, pharmaceuticals, databases, sterile medical equipment, qualified scientists.

The rest of the region had its own problems, which were generally less severe as one progressed westward. But a collapse of the rouble, Russian hyperinflation, a civil war inside Russia—any of these events could have profound ripple effects across the length and breadth of the former Soviet world.

Any simplistic answer to the demographic puzzle was useless. The regional trend towards declining life expectancy and rising premature mortality was, in the end, due to a complex constellation of factors, both Soviet in origin and unique to the post-1991 transformation.

The Soviets under the despotic rule of Stalin created public health, from its outset, as an ideological tool. The practice of public health was executed in a manner that stressed, in every facet, the primacy of the collective over the individual. At times—even, perhaps, frequently—public health was a cruel mistress of the state. Certainly its leadership was devoutly Communist, its scientific underpinnings rested more on ideology than on any set of experimental facts.

The collapse of the Soviet Union foisted its former socialist states into the world community, which had three impacts. First, long-sealed exit doors were opened, allowing for a record-breaking brain drain that stripped the region of most of its brightest scientific and medical minds. Second, doors also opened inward, allowing both the aspirations and sins of the external world entry into the long-sequestered societies: the populations for the first time realized their comparative material poverty, experienced resentment and avarice, and discovered drugs and other ways to dull the pain of that awakening. Third, the legacy of Soviet-era science, psychology, public health, and human rights left the professionals, their infrastructures, and individual citizens without the tools to cope with the New Reality: narcology, TB sanatoriums, SanEp, venereology, KGB-affiliated psychiatry, and Lysenko-devastated biology could not protect the health of a free public.

The Soviet public health infrastructure, in short, required authoritarianism. In the absence of centralized despotism and the intrusive powers it extended to public health authorities, the fundamental flaws in the system were frighteningly exposed.

The anguishing transformation, even anarchy, of the post-1991 years in the ex-Soviet region did not, of course, occur in a global vacuum. A New Reality greeted every nation on earth at the same time, spawned by the end of the fifty-one-year Cold War and rise of globalized capitalism, a key feature of which was shared excruciation. It was not an equitable participation in pain: Americans felt little, Europeans got off light, but Asia, Africa, Latin America, Canada, and all of the former Soviet sphere of influence suffered economically and socially.

Globalization did involve shared risk, however, as escalating drug markets had ways of spilling over into other nations; prostitute slave markets became sources of exported sexually transmitted diseases; new mutant strains of bacteria that could defy modern medical options swiftly spread beyond country or regional borders; tuberculosis was an airborne transmitter; disease-ravaged regions often spurned mass human migrations to other regions of the planet; and instability in any strategic part of the planet could reverberate with geopolitical impact across the globe.

'In sum, those specializing in geopolitics, economics, and the military who ignore these issues or put them into a "who cares?" pocket do so at the hazard of not understanding what is going on and its consequences,' Murray Feshbach said. 'Perhaps the Russian population will be dead or so ill that there will be no solution to the economic, military, and political problems of the country. Neither the past system managers nor the current leaders should take any solace in blaming the others; both are or will be responsible.'

The region's old guard fought tooth and nail against change, as the agents of the West pushed their agendas into the vacuum. It was not always a pretty picture. Private North American and European insurance, health management, and pharmaceutical companies swarmed over the region during the 1990s, hoping to clinch lucrative deals that would commit the new societies to mixed economic structures of health. Government agencies marched in from the West to preach the gospels of health management organizations, managed care, global pharmaceutical patent protection, and social marketing. The World Bank and an assortment of United Nations agencies tried carrot-and-stick approaches, hoping to lure the region's governments toward Western models of reconstruction in exchange for substantial interest-free or low-interest financial aid. They met with varying degrees of success, particularly in their overall push toward health insurance-based systems.

'In general, given the chaotic nature of the economic reform and democratization processes, Russia may simply not be ready for a market-based insurance scheme at this time,' wrote a top team of American public health experts. 'Certainly, it must have seemed persuasive to Russia's health-care decision makers, in light of the failure of socialized medicine to fulfil its mandate, to embrace "insurance" as a kind of antimodel. Many Russians, however, are now realizing that at least some elements of the old system, with its "assurance" of universal health-care at state expense, may be worth preserving until "insurance" can fulfil its promises.'

'We don't know, actually, where we're going, or what is happening, especially in science,' Dr Alexi Savinykh of Moscow's MEDSOCECONOMINFORM think tank explained. 'We now have a blanket made of pieces—a quilt. Each local government is free to do whatever they want. . . . And as to public health and health-care, it's not an easy question. We have *no* standards for the current time.'

In Georgia Minister of Health Avtandil Jorbenadze eagerly embraced American models of public health and health-care. But he admitted that public health was getting short shrift, as most funds still went to the nation's overly large hospital system. Less than forty cents was spent per capita on public health during the 1990s, Jorbenadze acknowledged.

He leaned heartily on American advisors, Jorbenadze said, laughing. 'It was part of building a new state with market economic relations and democracy.'

Which echoed clearly the US government's position on public health in the newly independent nation. 'We're here to do democracy building,' a top US official working in the region said. 'We are *not* focusing on health sector reform.'

Smugly the official added that 'the public health leadership of this country is not looking [to Russia] for ideas—it's looking West. That's what matters.'

Perhaps.

But the moves were tenuous, at best. WHO advisor to Georgia, Dr Archil Khomassuridze, acknowledged that his country, for example, had embarked on a distinctly American-style reform of public health and health-care.

'The country is on a path of progress, but they are *only* at the beginning,' Khomassuridze said. 'It could still slip back. If war breaks out again. If there is a cataclysm in Russia. Remember: if Russia sneezes Georgia catches pneumonia.'

Estonia's minister of social affairs, Jaan Ruutmann, drank his morning coffee from a US government coffee cup emblazoned with Old Glory. In his spacious office, decorated in wood and pastels, the raffish, robust Ruutmann spoke sternly about changes in his Baltic country. Since 1991 he had imposed strict accounting and financial controls on the nation's hospitals—the first time most administrators had ever been required to tell the government how they spent their money.

Key to public health was assuring that those hospitals spent adequately on basic preventative services, such as immunization, STD screening, surveillance of diseases, and health education. Though Ruutmann felt that 'it's obvious' that spending on prevention ended up saving money by avoiding severe diseases in the future, he was uneasy. He could see profiteering emerging in the Estonian health system. As the insurance industry moved in, more and more doctors seemed to be after short-term, high-yield medicine, rather than the less profitable preventive health measures.

In the Czech Republic the pendulum had swung too far in the direction of managed health and private insurance, complained Dr Victor Kayak, who had the largest private pulmonary medicine practice in the nation. The hallways of his Prague clinic reverberated with the sounds of tubercular coughing. Between 1995 and 1996 he saw a 35 per cent increase in tuberculosis cases at a time when government public health authorities recorded only marginal increases in TB levels.

'How would they know?' Kayak, visibly exhausted, asked. 'In the Czech Republic it's a question of financing of health-care. Our government and Ministry of Health didn't even consider TB.... The state should finance bringing TB under control. But it doesn't. We are now financed through insurance reimbursement and that's not enough for TB.... It's a horrible situation!'

Terribly upset, the tall, lean doctor, dressed in his spotless laboratory coat, had eagerly embraced the new democracy, even the new health economy. But now, he nearly shouted, public health was pushed aside, 'and the government is giving up all of its responsibilities.'

The last thing we need, he mumbled, is your American system.

CHAPTER 4

Preferring anarchy and class disparity

The American public health infrastructure in an age of antigovernmentalism.

Public health is purchasable. Within natural limitations a community can deter-mine its own death-rate. . . . No duty of society, acting through its governmental agencies, is paramount to this obligation to attack the removable causes of disease.
—Dr Hermann Biggs, New York State Commissioner of Health, 1913

Government is not the solution to our problem; government is the problem.
—Ronald Reagan, presidential inaugural speech, January 20, 1981

As the scientific case for public health becomes stronger, politics and popular support has not kept pace. Public health programmes in the United States—and the situation is similar in many other countries—are either not being improved or, in many cases, are being allowed to wither. . . . Overt resistance to public health is rare. On the contrary, public health has been subject to the death of a thousand cuts, some of them noticed, others not.
—Daniel Callahan, The Hastings Centre, 1998[1]

The twenty-first century dawned with America's public health system in disarray. Some might argue that there was actually no system *per se*, but a hotchpotch of programmes, bureaucracies, and failings.

As incredible as it might seem, given America's breathtaking prosperity at the close of the 1990s, most of the problems and crises noted in the health apparati of central Africa, the Indian subcontinent, and former Soviet Union could also to a certain degree be found in the United States. American public health leaders of the 1990s were struggling to ensure that the nation's food and water were safe, that diseases like HIV and hepatitis C didn't overwhelm the populace, that the country's children were appropriately vaccinated: item by item the travails of the rest of the world were also America's. And America had its own additional problems, reflecting unique political and economic dimensions of the society.

If the former Soviet states suffered from an overemphasis on the public health needs of the collective, at the expense of the individual, America at the end of the twentieth century was reeling under the weight of its newfound libertarianism: the collective be damned, all public health burdens and responsibilities fell to the individual. It was an odd paradigm and an about-face from the attitudes and sense of duty that had formed the foundation of American public health at the dawn of the twentieth century. Whereas the 1991 end of the Cold War brought public health chaos and despair to the losing side, for the American victors it unleashed a national me-first sentiment that flourished during the country's most phenomenal and lengthiest period of economic prosperity.

Less than a decade after the fall of the Berlin Wall, the middle class of the United States had become blasé about the word *millionaire*, the New York Stock Exchange scaled heights that would have been unimaginable in the 1980s, and few citizens of the United States seriously doubted that the New World Order hailed in 1991 by then-president George Bush meant anything less than American dominance over the global marketplace.

It seemed, in short, a good time to be smug—if you were a fortunate American.

The nineteenth-century and early-twentieth-century creators of America's public health systems would have found this emphasis on individualism amid such grand prosperity shocking. For them, the health of a community was the key measure of its success, and if pestilence and death stalked even one small segment of the population it was a stark indication of the community's political and social failure. They were zealous in their beliefs, imbued with a sense of mission and, in most parts of the country, empowered by law to execute their plans—even if such efforts entailed battles with governors, mayors, or legislative politicians: 'The public press will approve, the people are prepared to support, and the courts sustain, any intelligent procedures which are evidently directed at the preservation of the public health,' New York City health official Dr Hermann Biggs declared in 1900. 'The most autocratic powers, capable of the broadest construction, are given to them under the law. Everything which is detrimental to health or dangerous to life, under the freest interpretation, is regarded as coming within the province of the Health Department. So broad is the construction of the law that everything which improperly or unnecessarily interferes with the comfort or enjoyment of life, as well as those things which are, strictly speaking, detrimental to health or dangerous to life, may become the subject of action on the part of the Board of Health.'[2] If disease raged, the objective, in short, was to stamp it out by any means necessary.

These crusaders would find it amazing to witness the erosion of America's public health infrastructures during the later twentieth century, the low status ascribed to public health physicians and scientists, the legal limitations placed on their authority, and the disdain with which Americans viewed their civil servants. In the early 1890s America led the world in designing and executing the primary missions of public health; in the 1990s, the same nation turned its back on most of the key elements of the enterprise known as Public Health.

For example, American hospitals had once been death traps from which few patients emerged in better health than they had been in when they entered. Public health zealots of the late nineteenth century cleaned up the hospitals, ordered doctors and nurses to scrub up, and dramatically reduced death rates.

But a hundred years later, although Zaire might have been the only nation with the dubious distinction of having twice spawned Ebola epidemics out of its hospitals, it was hardly alone in an apparent state of helplessness before wave after wave of hospital-acquired (nosocomial) infections. Throughout the former Soviet Union infection control—or the lack thereof—was in a calamitous state. In the poor regions of the world resource scarcities could always be blamed when dangerous microbes passed from one patient to another via the hands of a physician, who, ironically, had sworn to the first maxim of medicine: do no harm.

But scarcity could hardly explain why nosocomial disease was, like a dark horseman of death, sweeping over American hospitals. Nor could lack of resources justify the apparent helplessness and impotence with which public health officials greeted the tidal wave of mutant, drug-resistant superbugs.

Even in wealthy America, hospitals were places where many patients became more ill than they had been when they checked in, catching diseases on the wards. By 1997, 10 per cent of *all* patients who spent more than one night in the average US hospital acquired a non-viral infection nosocomially, carried to their fragile, ailing bodies on contaminated instruments or the hands of medical personnel.[3] The more severely ill the patients, the greater their likelihood of being nosocomially infected. This was simply because individuals in an intensive care unit recuperating from, for example, open-heart surgery were subjected to far more potentially contaminated needles, shunts, devices, and manipulations than were, say, women recovering from childbirth. In intensive care units the odds that any given patient would be infected in this way approached fifty-fifty. And all too often those infections were fatal.[4]

A few hospitals in the United States cooperated with the CDC to form the National Nosocomial Infection Surveillance System. Their research work showed steady increases in the percentage of drug-resistant organisms that could defy conventional treatments in every population of common hospital microbes during the 1990s.[5] A University of Iowa-run Sentry Antimicrobial Surveillance System in Europe, Canada, and Latin America spotted the same trend, as did a WHO global surveillance network that monitored the emergence of mobile rings of DNA that carried drug-resistance genes. These rings, called plasmids, were readily shared among bacteria, even across species.[6]

For reasons nobody could quite pin down, New York City had the highest rates of drug-resistant bacterial diseases and deaths in its hospitals.

'We seem to be leading the nation on this, which is a dubious number-one position, to say the least,' the city's health commissioner, Dr Margaret Hamburg, said with a sigh. Hamburg's assistant commissioner, Dr Marcelle Layton, said in 1997 that the city faced an unparalleled scale of public health challenges that might be contributing to the steady rise in drug resistance her staff had observed over ten years.

'There are fifty-three thousand people per square mile in New York City,' Layton said, and 'about two hundred thousand of them are HIV-positive. A quarter of the population lives below the poverty line. One point three million have no health insurance.'

Layton stopped and shrugged her shoulders, her body language saying, 'What can we do?' And, indeed, public health officials all over America were stymied, as they anxiously watched death tolls rise, the bugs mutate, vital drugs become useless, but lacked any powers to stop what seemed an inevitability: the arrival of the post-antibiotic era. And nowhere was that terrible prospect looming more precariously than in the nation's hospitals.

Unfortunately, hospitals had become physicians' sacred grounds, not to be tampered by public health authorities. A century earlier Layton's counterparts could have marched in and shut down any hospital that, like Kikwit's Ebola-spreading General Hospital, created epidemics. Not so in the 1990s. Instead Layton and her counterparts nationwide counted death tolls and issued warnings.

The numbers were appalling. One of the key sources of nosocomial infection was contaminated intravascular catheters. Such devices were placed in nearly all post-surgical patients. If contaminated with pathogenic bacteria or fungi the result was blood poisoning, or septicaemia. Twenty-five per cent of the time such septicaemia episodes during the 1990s proved fatal. For the 75 per cent of patients who survived, nosocomial infection added an average of $33 000 in medical costs. In 1996 there were an estimated four hundred thousand nosocomial septicaemia survivors in the United States whose total additional treatment cost was $13.2 billion.[7]

By the end of the 1990s somewhere between one hundred thousand and one hundred fifty thousand Americans were dying each year, from infections caught inside US hospitals. The deadliest of nosocomial microbes were the newly emerging, mutant bacteria that could resist antibiotic treatment.

The crisis brewing in New York City during the nineties involved four ubiquitous pathogens: *Enterococcus faecium*, *Enterococcus faecalis*, *Streptococcus pneumoniae*, and *Staphylococcus aureus*. The enterococci were troublesome, but not usually lethal, intestinal bacteria that produced digestive problems, diarrhoea, and bowel and colon pain and spasms. If an individual was highly stressed or immune deficient—as were the cases with most hospitalized individuals—these bacteria (particularly *faecium*) could be lethal.

Streptococcus and staphylococcus caused far more concern. Streptococcal pneumonia bacteria were leading causes of ear infections, disease-associated deafness, pneumonia deaths, and what was commonly called streptococcus throat. Severe streptococcal infections could result in bacterial colonization of the meningial tissues, leading to meningitis and life-threatening infections of the central nervous system. In the pre-antibiotic era, 30 to 35 per cent of all *S. pneumoniae* infections were fatal.

In 1996 *S. pneumoniae* was the leading cause of pneumonia in the United States, producing four million adult cases annually. Out-patient treatment costs alone exceeded $1 billion a year. And for patients over sixty years old such infections were, despite vigorous antibiotic treatment, fatal about 7 per cent of the time.

Staphylococcus aureus was the cause of wound infections, sepsis (blood poisoning), toxic shock syndrome, bedsores, osteomyelitis bone disease, endocarditis heart infections, boils, abscesses, and bacterially-induced arthritis. Because some strains of the organism exuded powerful toxins, staphylococcal infections could be terrifying, escalating in a matter of hours from little more than a small, pus-producing contamination of a wound to life-threatening blood poisoning and cardiac arrest. It was mainly because of staphylococcal infections that tens of thousands of soldiers' limbs were amputated during the Civil War and World War I.

Staphylococcal bacteria tend to cluster in tight groups, like grapes on a vine. Under stress, the organisms can expel the water from their cytoplasm and go into a dormant state as hard, dry 'beads'. In that state they are virtually invulnerable and can survive in air, water, food, soap, soil—almost anywhere. Streptococcus are also spherical, but instead of forming clusters, they tend to gather single file, forming long chains, like pearl necklaces. They, too, are capable of resisting environmental stress by expelling water and going into a dormant state.

New York's troubles with these organisms were severe in the late nineteenth and early twentieth centuries, but had virtually disappeared with the arrival of the penicillin era. However, these were among the first microbes to acquire penicillin resistance, and all over the city by the early 1990s Dr Hamburg's department was finding streptococcus that was resistant, or completely impervious, to penicillin.

A citywide survey of seventy-three hospitals found that penicillinase-resistant infections in all age groups of patients had soared from 8 per cent in 1993 to more than 20 per cent in 1995, said Layton in a speech to the 1996 American Public Health Association meeting in Manhattan. The incidence of resistant streptococcus was highest in children under one year of age, with eleven cases per 100 000 New York City infants occurring in 1995.

That year, Hamburg noted, only one antibiotic vancomycin was still universally effective against New York City streptococcus *pneumoniae*: . It was also the only treatment for drug-resistant staphylococcus—MRSA (methicillin-resistant *Staphylococcus aureus*)—which by 1993 represented a third of all staphylococcal cases in the United States.[8]

And there was the rub: three different species of common bacteria had acquired powerful drug-resistance capacities simultaneously. And all three left medicine with the same last-resort drug: vancomycin.

The critical concern was that the vancomycin-resistant enterococci (VRE) would share their resistance genes with streptococcus or staphylococcus. Test tube studies in the early 1990s showed that VRE resistance genes were carried on mobile transposons, or plasmids, and that the changes they mediated in the enterococci could also be carried out in streptococcal or staphylococcus bacteria.[9]

Remarkably, some enterococci actually became 'addicted to vancomycin,' Rockefeller University microbiologist Alexander Tomasz said. The bugs could not only *resist* vancomycin, they actually evolved to *depend upon it*.

Looming over New York City in the mid-1990s, then, was the prospect that, within a hospitalized patient who was infected with enterococci, some VRE would share its dreaded genetic machinery with staphylococcus or streptococcus, resulting in a terrifying, highly contagious superbug.

It was a nightmarish public health prospect.

'We're just waiting for the other shoe to drop,' Dr Hamburg said nervously. Hamburg's staff, together with Tomasz and scientists from the local Public Health Research Institute and area hospitals, formed the BARG—Bacterial Antibiotic Resistance Group—in 1993 to watchdog microbial trends in the area. And Hamburg warned the area's hospitals in the strongest possible terms that their infection-control standards needed to improve or they would soon see death rates soar due to drug-resistant microbes. The New York State Department of Health toughened infection control guidelines, too, and ordered that every single hospital employee in the state—from intake receptionist to brain surgeon—had to undergo state-certified infection-control training every year, beginning in 1994.

As part of that first year's training, infection-control nurse specialist Kathleen Jakob warned an audience of health providers at Columbia College of Surgeons and Physicians in Manhattan that lapses in infection control usually were the unintended results of becoming overly habituated to the hospital environment. 'People outside the medical profession have a very hard time discussing rectal abscesses over dinner,' Jakob said, drawing guffaws from the medical students. 'We don't. We don't see our environment the way visitors do. We get so used to it that we don't see risks, the chaos, the filth.'

But when it came to controlling the spread of tough bacteria inside hospitals, the time-honoured Semmelweis technique for scrubbing hands before touching patients—an insight that had revolutionized medicine more than a century earlier—had more than met its match. Now microbes such as *Staphylococcus* were capable when dormant of living on tabletops, curtains, clothing, even in vats of disinfectant. Despite strict scrubbing, careful health workers could pick up such organisms when their uniforms brushed against a patient's wound or sheets, and then carry the bug to the next patient's bedside.

Of the more than fourteen thousand germicides registered in 1994 with the US Environmental Protection Agency (EPA), few could kill such bacteria in their dormant states, and some required hours of soaking to guarantee disinfection. Indeed, some bacteria had acquired additional supercapabilities to resist disinfectants and soaps. They could, for example, shunt all chlorine-containing compounds out of their membranes, rendering all bleaches utterly useless.

The only cleansers guaranteed to kill dormant bacteria were quaternary ammonias and formaldehydes, Jakob told her Columbia audience. And those compounds were associated with cancer and birth defects, so the EPA discouraged their use on neonatal and paediatric wards.[10]

An alternative to cleansing was cooking the germs in autoclaves, flash sterilizers, gas chambers, and steamers. But there, too, hospitals were encountering problems because of the tenacity of the bacteria, the sloppiness of personnel, and new medical equipment that was extremely difficult to clean. Additionally, some bacteria mutated to tolerate high temperatures, forcing either longer or hotter sterilizations.

The only way hospitals could track lapses in infection control was to monitor the organisms found in their sicker patients and run laboratory analyses to determine which—if any—antibiotic could still kill those microbes. If highly resistant bacteria were identified, tests were carried out on patients in nearby beds. If they were infected with the same bacteria, a stern-faced Jakob told her anxious audience, 'It's a sure sign that a break in infection control took place somewhere on the ward.'

At that point, every piece of equipment on the ward, every millimetre of surface area, each television set, chair, bed—*everything*—had to be scrubbed thoroughly with effective disinfectants. Patients had to be placed under quarantines (ranging from total, air-lock isolations to remaining in their rooms, away from other patients), all ward personnel had to be tested to determine whether any of them carried the mutant bacteria in their bloodstreams, and all staff operational procedures needed to be scrutinized to determine where lapses might have occurred.

Sometimes the microbes—particularly MRSA—proved so tenacious and resistant to disinfection that hospitals had no choice but to shut down the ward, strip it of all organic matter (rubber, cotton, wool, silicone, plastics), repaint all walls, retile all bathrooms, and apply new linoleum to all floors.

Only after that mammoth task was completed, and all equipment had been replaced, could the once-contaminated wards be re-opened.

Such procedures were very expensive and almost always led to patient lawsuits against hospitals. And all too often the carrier of resistant microbes turned out to be a nurse or doctor who unknowingly harboured the germs in his or her blood; harmless to the health-care worker, but lethal to the susceptible patient. So it was in the hospitals' and health providers' interests, whether they recognized it or not, to take tedious steps to avoid such extreme contamination.

It sounded straightforward, but even at an elite institution such as Columbia-Presbyterian—one of America's best hospitals—preventing spread of VRE and other drug-resistant organisms was all but impossible.

For example, at Columbia-Presbyterian Hospital, nurse Janise Schwadron was handling post-surgical intensive care patients. When word came that the patient in 'contact isolation' had to be taken downstairs for a CT scan, Schwadron sighed, 'What a pain.'

In addition to recuperating from lung transplant surgery, the patient was infected with a mutant strain of enterococcal bacteria resistant to *every* antibiotic used for its treatment. To protect the rest of the hospital's patients, moving the patient to radiology was quite a job. Everything that touched the patient had to be disinfected before and after making the move. Schwadron ordered up three helpers. Then—dressed in head-to-toe protective gowns, latex gloves, and gauze masks—they began scouring every inch of each piece of equipment before changing the patient's bedding. Hours later, after the CT scan room had also been disinfected and the transplant patient was back, Schwadron relaxed. A simple diagnostic test that usually involved just two employees and an hour's time had taken up more than six hours' time for five employees, as well as a heap of expensive protective gear.

Hospital staff were only part of the problem. Schwadron was also responsible for watching others who entered the transplant patient's room, from family members to attending physicians—reminding them to follow proper precautions and, if they failed to do so, ordering them off the ward.

Some of the patients seemed to do everything they could to make matters worse. For example, Columbia-Presbyterian had a patient the nurses called 'the Wanderer'. Normally, patients who insisted on walking the halls and popping their heads into other patient's rooms were nothing more than a nuisance. But the Wanderer was infected with VRE. If, in her travels, the Wanderer were to meet with another patient infected with a mutant version of either staphylococcus or pneumococcus, they could easily infect each other, their bugs could share genes, and both patients could end up carrying completely drug-resistant staphylococcus or pneumococcus infections.

In the late-nineteenth-century day of public health pioneer Hermann Biggs, recalcitrant, belligerent patients like the Wanderer would have been restrained, placed in quarantine, or locked up for the good of the community. But in 1994 such actions weren't legal. The only power nurses had over the Wanderer was the power of persuasion—and this patient wasn't heeding their pleas. Indeed, she had slapped a nurse who tried to push her away from nibbling food off another patient's tray.

Public health had lost so much power and authority by the 1990s that Commissioner Hamburg's options did *not* include the three steps that offered the greatest likelihood of slowing the spread of deadly drug-resistant bacteria. All evidence indicated that physicians' overprescribing of antibiotics was driving up drug resistance, but years of successful American Medical Association lobbying had stripped public health authorities of all powers to affect doctors' prescription practices. Ideally, Hamburg would like to have put vancomycin in some special legal category, requiring doctors to seek the Department of Health's permission before using the precious drug. That might preserve its usefulness a few years longer, but she and her colleagues nationwide were powerless to implement such a stopgap measure.

The second and third options were to order forced confinement of patients who carried highly drug-resistant strains of bacteria and mandatory testing of medical personnel on a routine basis to ensure that they weren't unknowingly infected with such bugs. But there, too, Hamburg's legal powers were minimal. Inside hospitals all over America there were modern 'Typhoid Mary' doctors who flatly refused to undergo tests to see if they were carriers of drug-resistant bacteria.

One New York City burn ward—the largest burn treatment centre east of the Rockies—had an outbreak of MRSA, which was *extremely* dangerous for burn patients because so much of their bodies were exposed, unprotected by skin. Every single person who worked on the ward, except for its chief physician, was tested. All came up negative as MRSA carriers. The physician refused to be tested. When that physician transferred to another hospital, that hospital, too, experienced a MRSA outbreak. But Hamburg's department could do nothing legally to compel the physician to undergo testing or treatment to cleanse the lethal bugs from his body.

When the legal authorities of public health were stripped during the mid-twentieth century, nobody anticipated that hospitals would become centres not only for disease treatment but also for disease creation. VRE first appeared in the United States in 1988 when it was reported in three New York City hospitals. But a survey of twenty-four hospitals in New York City, neighbouring Long Island, and Westchester County found it had surfaced in every single one by the beginning of 1994.

Nationally, cases of VRE increased twenty-fold between 1989 and 1993, and about 7.9 per cent of all 1994 enterococcal infections involved the mutant bacteria, according to the CDC. That was up from less than 1 per cent just four years earlier.

Hospital by hospital, it was extremely difficult to obtain information on VRE rates—nobody wanted their institution labelled a centre of drug-resistant bacteria, and public health authorities were powerless to order hospitals to be candid about their nosocomial infection rates. So Hamburg had to cut deals with the hospitals, promising to keep secret the details of their VRE rates in exchange for gaining access to their laboratory records. Publicly, she said, the department could never reveal that 'Hospital X has this much VRE'. We will say, 'Overall, there's this much in hospitals in the city'. That's the only way we could do it.

All but three hospitals in the New York metropolitan area declined to provide an inquiring reporter with their VRE details. Those three hospitals all reported steadily climbing VRE rates.

One institution that was very open about its VRE situation was Cabrini Hospital, a private facility in Manhattan that in 1993 published a detailed rundown of VRE cases detected on its wards between 1990 and 1992. Over a thirty-six-month period, Cabrini treated 2812 enterococcus cases, 213 of which were vancomycin-resistant. More important was the trend over time. In 1990, 85 per cent of all enterococcal infections were fully vulnerable to vancomycin. By the end of 1992 only 25.8 per cent of all enterococcal infections treated in the hospital remained fully susceptible to the drug.

'We have been living in an era when if you got sick, there was always a pill to take,' said Rockefeller University's Tomasz in later 1995. 'We are approaching an era when that will no longer be true.'

'Every bacterial species you can name has increased its level of drug resistance over the last twenty years. . . . It is probably the number-one public health issue in the United States,' the CDC's expert, Dr William Jarvis, declared in 1995. And, he insisted, if VRE ever shared its resistance genes with staphylococcus or streptococcus, 'it would be a catastrophe.'

By 1997 the trend regarding MRSA and VRE was clear in New York City and nationwide according to Dr Louis Rice of Emory University. 'If we want to control resistance in the community, we have to control it in the hospital first, because that's where it starts.'

And the larger the hospital, the more MRSA and VRE lurked on its wards, Rice continued. In 1997 hospitals with fewer than two hundred beds had MRSA in 16 per cent of their staphylococcal-infected patients, but hospitals with more than two hundred beds had a 27 per cent incidence of MRSA. The implication was that infections spread more readily in the chaotic atmosphere of large, generally public hospitals.

Once these organisms surfaced in a hospital, 'infection control is not going to be the answer,' Rice insisted. 'I'm not all that optimistic that we're going to be able to control this.'

When resistant organisms emerged on a ward, drastic clean-up and escalated infection control could slow their spread, Rice said, but hospitals also needed to take radical steps to change their prescription practices; for example, completely stopping vancomycin use when VRE emerged. Still, he acknowledged, even that didn't always work. One hospital reacted to its first MRSA outbreak by ordering an immediate stop to the use of methicillin, telling doctors to instead use mupirocin on their staphylococcal patients. In a year, staphylococcus infections in that hospital went from involving 2 per cent to 64 per cent mupirocin-resistant organisms.

New York-Cornell Medical Centre had a similar experience with drug resistant *Klebsiella* infections: switching all antibiotics simply led to emergence of multidrug-resistant *Klebsiella*.

On the other hand, changing drug-use practices had, indeed, lowered bacterial disease rates in some other settings, Rice said, indicating that when it came to controlling mutant bugs in hospital ecologies, 'one size definitely doesn't fit all'.

At Queens Hospital in New York City, Dr James Rahal had discovered that the nature of the mechanism a resistant organism used to get around antibiotics was a key determinant of how tenacious that organism could be: were plasmid transposons the key to its resistance or was it actual mutations of the bacteria's DNA? The latter, Rahal argued, were the toughest to eradicate once they emerged. After all, plasmids could pop *out* of microbes as readily as they popped *in*, making resistance a transient event. But if a germ mutated, if its *chromosomes* were altered, resistance was permanent not only in that individual microbe but also in all its progeny for generations to come.

For example, Rahal said, the percentage of *Klebsiella* infections in his hospital that were resistant to ceftazidime went from 6 per cent in 1988 to 37 per cent in 1995. Those were transposon forms of resistance and were moderately controllable through drug switching and standard infection-control measures. But in 1995 a new strain of chromosomally resistant *Klebsiella* emerged in the hospital—a form that had mutations in its primary DNA—and by Christmas of that year *every single Klebsiella* bacterium they found in the hospital was fully resistant not just to ceftazidime, but to the entire cephalosporin class of antibiotics.

At that point, the hospital ordered a cessation of the use of cephalosporins to treat *Klebsiella* infections. And then a strange thing started happening: resistance emerged in an entirely different microbe population. The hospital decreased its total cephalosporin use, for all purposes, by more than 80 per cent during 1996, and increased use of the expensive alternative drug imipenem by 59 per cent. That cut *Klebsiella* drug resistance down by nearly half. But it prompted emergence of imipenem-resistant *Pseudomonas aueriginosa*, a pneumonia-causing organism.

'So the problem just shifted from one microbe population to another,' Rahal sadly concluded.

With the clean-up being so difficult, and new superbugs emerging in the best hospitals in America, 'I suppose that we're back in the preantibiotic era now,' said Dr Matthew Scharff of Albert Einstein Medical School in the Bronx. Speaking before a 1993 gathering of the Irvington Trust, an investment banking group that funded medical research, Scharff said patients who underwent cancer chemotherapy, transplant surgery, radiation, or who had AIDS commonly died of what, for other people, were fairly benign fungal or bacterial infections, even though they received high intravenous doses of antibiotics. *Staphylococcus, Meningococcus, Pneumococcus, Cryptosporidium*—all those germs could devastate such people.

'In the absence of our own immunity, even antibiotics cannot kill these agents,' Scharff said, adding that even otherwise healthy individuals were at increasing risk from some diseases because the bugs had acquired drug resistance.

The evidence was clear on the cancer and AIDS wards of large hospitals in the greater New York area, Scharff insisted. Some 10 per cent of all people with AIDS died from cryptococcus—a ubiquitous fungus found in bird droppings. Once it got into their brains, the microbe caused meningitis. Similarly, a variety of bacterial infections were essentially incurable in cancer lymphoma patients—former First Lady Jacqueline Kennedy Onassis died in New York as a result of such an infection.

Scharff thought that doctors in public health pioneer Hermann Biggs's day, before the invention of antibiotics, had had at least a partial solution to the problem: antisera. In the early twentieth century, physicians injected samples of the bacteria that were infecting their patients—say, pneumococci, which caused pneumonia—into a horse.

The horse made antibodies against the pneumococci. The doctors withdrew blood from the horse, separated out and purified the antibodies, and injected the resulting antiserum into their dying patients.

'About thirty per cent of the time it worked,' Scharff said. But it was also often toxic because humans developed acute allergic reactions to horse proteins that were residual in the antisera.

At the close of the twentieth century, however, technology existed that would allow scientists to make pure human antisera in mice or in test tubes. So-called monoclonal antibodies were in use for other medical purposes, and Scharff's group had already made anticryptococcal monoclonal antibodies and proved that they worked in immuno-deficient mice.

'I think we should look back at this,' Scharff argued. 'We have to. We have nothing else.'

Few New York physicians were willing to accept Scharff's dire view of the situation. Bad as antibiotic resistance problems were, *something* usually, eventually, worked— most of the time. Or so they argued in the late 1990s.

Not so, said the New York State Senate's Committee on Investigations in early 1999.[11] That committee issued a report concluding that hospital-spread infections in New York City alone in 1995 had caused 1020 deaths and $230 million worth of extra patient hospitalization and treatments. Chaired by Senator Roy Goodman, a Manhattan Republican, the committee drew its conclusions from evidence presented by Nobel laureate Dr Joshua Lederberg and Tomasz, both of Rockefeller University; Dr Willa Appel of the New York City Partnership; and rheumatologist Sheldon Blau of the State University of New York Medical Centre in Stony Brook.

Based on testimony and studies presented to the Senate committee, its report charged that between 1975 and 1995 the number of days patients were hospitalized nationwide rose 36 per cent due to hospital-acquired infections. In 1995, the report continued, 1.7 million people in the United States acquired infections in the hospital that proved fatal to eighty-eight thousand of them and added $4.5 billion to the nation's health costs.

Further, the report charged, cost-containment measures under managed care were severely exacerbating the problem because nursing staffs were overworked and so tired that they made mistakes; and more hospitals were cutting costs by replacing skilled nurses with poorly trained nurses' aides. Within the New York City Health and Hospitals Corporation, for example, nursing staff was cut by 21 per cent from 1994 to 1999.

Even worse, 70 per cent of all such hospital-acquired infections involved drug-resistant organisms. In metropolitan New York City alone, 7800 patients acquired drug-resistant staphylococcus infections during hospital stays in 1995: 1400 of them died as a result.

About half of all hospital-acquired infections could be eliminated by simply imposing stricter hygiene regulation inside hospitals and reducing the rate at which doctors prescribed antibiotics.

'Some five years ago I entered a good, prestigious hospital,' Blau said, 'for a routine angioplasty. . . . I developed a hospital-acquired, drug-resistant staphylococcus infection, and I was so close to dying that last rites were said.' Blau charged that his infection resulted from spread of staphylococcus within the hospital by doctors and nurses who failed to wash their hands and instruments between patients. And, he said ominously, 'the next time you're in the hospital visiting a relative, you see how often the doctor washes his hands'.

'This is a shocking thing,' Goodman said. 'It's almost unbelievable that something as basic as the washing of hands is being ignored by doctors.' Incredible as it might seem American doctors were, apparently, almost as likely to shun essential infection-control procedures as were their counterparts in Siberia.

The Senate report scolded New York hospitals: 'Health-care workers seek to heal us and, first and foremost, must do no harm. Yet their failure to consistently follow even the simplest hygienic practices is a major reason for the contraction of bacterial infections in hospitals. Good long-term financial incentives exist for hospitals to insist on strict infection-control procedures; yet short-term financial considerations have militated against the consistent use of such procedures.'[12]

Four decades earlier Lederberg had won a Nobel Prize for demonstrating how bacteria evolve, eluding antibiotics. In the 1950s he warned the scientific and medical communities that, unless carefully used, antibiotics would become less useful with time simply because the microbes were master mutators. By the close of the 1990s evidence supporting his prognostications was abundant, but public health actions aimed at preventing the otherwise inevitable end of the antibiotic era were nearly non-existent. A dignified man, Lederberg rarely expressed public anger. But he was, nevertheless, enraged. He felt that the solutions were many and attainable, but lack of social, political, and economic will was blocking every rational path toward restoration of hospital safety and drug efficacy against resistant bacterial populations.

'We're running out of bullets for dealing with a number of these infections,' Lederberg pronounced soberly, slowly shaking his white-bearded head. 'Are we better off today than we were a century ago? In most respects, we're worse off,' he pronounced.

Citing declining government support for public health, increasing globalization of humanity and its microbial hitchhikers, and the rise of managed care in America, Lederberg held out little hope for the future. 'The world really is just one village. And our tolerance of disease in any place in the world is at our own peril,' he insisted. 'Patients are dying because we no longer have antibiotics that work. And there's no way we're going to eradicate all of these organisms. We have to learn to live with them, as moving targets.'

It *was* possible to develop new antibacterial drugs, Lederberg insisted, if the pharmaceutical industry were so motivated. And it *was* possible to control the spread of resistant bacteria, if public health authorities were sufficiently funded and empowered to do so.

'But to say public health is going to be left out in the cold by Washington is an understatement,' the visibly angry Lederberg continued. 'It's already out in the cold. Public health—that system is very close to being in a shambles at this time.'

It took centuries to build a public health system, and less than two decades to bring it down. Once the envy of the world, America's public health infrastructure at the end of the twentieth century was, indeed, in a shambles.

I

Hot, dry winds forever blowing,
Dead men to the grave-yards going:
Constant hearses,
Funeral verses;
Oh! what plagues—there is no knowing!
—Philip Freneau, written during the great yellow fever epidemic, Philadelphia, 1793

Public health—the discipline, the profession, the infrastructure that bears that name—was born at a time when hospitals were little more than warehouses for the dying, and the biggest enemy of humanity's healthy well-being was human behaviour. In New York, political corruption, slavery and racism, urban squalor, and gross wealth disparities all gave microbes fantastic opportunities to spread, killing nearly half of all children before they reached their twelfth birthdays. In the Midwest, profound ignorance and medical corruption were key culprits. Out in the far West of America, where the climate limited microbial possibilities, religious and racial biases, coupled with boomtown growth that outstripped the pace of infrastructure development, left public health leaders bereft of popular support for their activities well into the twentieth century.

Yet the foundations of public health were built out of such trials, and the very tools of the trade that nurses on Columbia-Presbyterian's wards needed to apply in hopes of controlling the Wanderer and VRE had been developed more than a century previously. Indeed, as early as 1629 American colonists in Virginia realized that they couldn't protect their people's health unless they had numbers—hard facts, entered dutifully by quill into log books: births, deaths, illnesses, and marriages were, by law, recorded, chronicling the vital statistics of the colony.

Colonial leaders also recognized, despite their lack of any theory of contagion, that great epidemics followed the arrival of ships with ailing crews and passengers. While the Great Plague ravaged London in 1665, the port cities of the Americas held British ships offshore in strict quarantine. This set a striking precedent: thereafter each colony instituted increasingly strict quarantine regulations, detaining ships and even incarcerating their crews on islands offshore for periods of time deemed safe, for the sake of the public's health.

Despite such early public health efforts, the colonial cities were visited periodically by epidemics of such magnitude as to seem terrifying in retrospect. For example, smallpox—which had arrived in 1689 aboard a slave ship—hit New York in wave after wave of deadly assaults beginning in 1679.

In addition to smallpox, New Yorkers and other colonials suffered and died in enormous numbers from measles, scarlet fever, yellow fever, typhoid fever, malaria, and a host of other diseases, nearly all of them infectious. The waves of disease and death could not be explained rationally, though colonial leaders blamed satanic, anti-Christian forces of various kinds. That religious rationale yielded to the miasma theory, which saw malodorous and malevolent forces in the environs that, on occasion, enveloped humanity.

Despite the ravages of smallpox, the disease that sparked the greatest fear, claimed enormous numbers of lives, and ignited public health policies for decades to come was yellow fever. Depending on the strain of virus and the level of immunity in the local population as a consequence of prior yellow fever epidemics, death would claim anywhere from 5 to 50 per cent of everyone infected.

Unbeknown to the Americans of the seventeenth and eighteenth centuries, the yellow fever virus was passed from one person to another by *Aedes aegypti* mosquitoes. It wasn't actually a new disease, but it seemed so to the American Indians and white colonials, particularly because it appeared unique in claiming whole families, not just the children. Both the virus and its *Aedes aegypti* carrier were native to West Africa, and, like smallpox, they made their way to the Americas via slave ships. Fear of yellow fever prompted passage of new, tougher quarantine laws and creation of offshore detention centres for ailing crew, passengers, and slaves.

During the 1743 yellow fever epidemic that claimed an estimated 5 per cent of New York City's population, an immigrant physician from Scotland began to see the light. Dr Cadwallader Colden recognized a crucial connection between homes located around filthy standing water and higher incidences of disease, surmising that poor water supplies, inadequate diet among the city's poor children, and general filth caused yellow fever. In a series of striking essays,[13] Colden drew the old miasma theory of disease toward a new concept—what would eventually be dubbed sanitarianism. With some subsequent refinements, sanitarianism would become the key framework for all American public health activities for more than 150 years.

In practical terms, Colden's yellow fever theory translated into a call for clean water and improved sanitation in New York. Both were tough goals for a city that, remarkably, lacked any source of fresh water except that drawn from wells, and had long failed to enforce its rubbish and waste regulations. Physicians generally ignored Colden's 'notions' as they were dubbed, as well as those of other medical thinkers of the day.

Desperate to control the economically devastating scourges of smallpox and, in particular, yellow fever, the New York State Legislature in 1796 passed the nation's first comprehensive public health law. It created the office of a State Commissioner of Health, a New York City Health Office, pest houses for isolation of infected citizens, vigorous maritime quarantine regulations, and a system of fines for failure to comply with quarantine and sanitation ordinances.[14]

Yellow fever fear inspired a wave of similar organized public health activity elsewhere in the United States. In 1798 Congress ordered the creation of the United States Marine Health Service, conceived of as an agency that would monitor sailors and protect American ports from incoming disease. Two years later the nation's capitol was built upon a large swamp located between the strategic states of Maryland and Virginia. Immediately overrun by yellow fever, smallpox, viral encephalitis, and a host of other diseases, Washington, DC, constituted a public health disaster from the moment of its conception. In 1802 the District of Columbia enacted a series of public health ordinances modelled on those in New York.

In 1805, facing yet another summer yellow fever onslaught, New York City created the nation's first Board of Health. Armed with a budget of the then-considerable sum of $8500 and authority to do whatever it deemed necessary to stop yellow fever, the board set out to sanitize the city. The board worked in tandem with John Pintard, the country's first city inspector.

Both Pintard and the Board of Health were strongly supported by New York's powerful commerce class in 1805. But as the city's efforts paid off, and yellow fever diminished, the popularity of public health measures ebbed. By 1819 the Board of Health's budget had fallen to a mere $500, and the business community was lobbying for its elimination.

The clash between New York's wealthiest men of commerce and its civic authorities over public health was a classic conflict between pursuit of short-term profit and prevention of often longer-term threats to the populace. Men of commerce, most of whom depended directly or indirectly on foreign trade and shipping, recognized the need for strict health measures during epidemics, even where such steps as quarantines impeded their business operations. But in the absence of crisis the economic impacts of such activities far outweighed any perceived health benefits, and opposition arose from the commercial sector.

This theme—of tension between business and health sectors—repeated itself so frequently in following decades in America as to constitute a primary motif of the nation's struggle for population health.

By 1819 commercial sector pressure brought New York's Board of Health to its knees, curtailing not only its activities but even its meetings. And, predictably, the city suffered another yellow fever epidemic in 1822. By 1835 the power of the Democratic Party organization called Tammany Hall—a corrupt political machine that would manipulate New York and national politics for more than a century—was virtually synonymous with entrepreneurial interests in the city. Tammany seized control of the board, stacked it with cronies, and corruption set in.

In 1850 New York City death rates (driven predominantly by infectious diseases) were 10 per cent higher than those estimated for 1750. Clearly, the public's health was failing. This was not progress.

Ironically, New York City's health laws and its Board of Health became models for the nation. If Tammany corruption rendered those laws unenforced in New York, and staffed Gotham's Board of Health with fools and cronies, the structures were still sound ideas. So much so that, propelled by the fear of yellow fever and cholera, cities all over America adopted New York's Board of Health laws: Washington, DC, Boston, Chicago, New Orleans, and dozens of other cities all created boards of health between 1810 and 1840 that were nearly identical in structure and intent to that originally designed in New York City in 1805.

On the East Coast, the combination of waves of impoverished immigrants (primarily from Ireland)[15] and overall urban disorder was driving the public's health downward. Epidemics regularly swept over the cities, claiming huge tolls among the poor.[16] None of America's densely packed cities had appropriate infrastructures: safe water, decent housing, paved streets, sewer systems, ample safe (not rotten) food, and public health control of contagion. In 1850 the average US male life expectancy was thirty-six years, female was thirty-eight years. Huge epidemics were part of the problem: in 1853, for example, 11 000 residents of New Orleans died in just two months of cholera. But the real factors holding down life expectancy were the huge maternal and child mortality rates.

In 1857, twenty-four out of every fifty-four pregnancies in the United States resulted in postpartum puerperal fever, an infection that physicians and midwives did not understand. As a result of puerperal fever, nineteen of every fifty-four pregnancies proved lethal to the mother. Given that most women at that time gave birth to more than six children, the risk of premature death over the course of their reproductive lives was enormous.

Child mortality was also astronomical. In 1850 children growing up in large American cities had about fifty-fifty odds of reaching the age of five without succumbing to disease or malnutrition. Odds were even worse—three to one against them—for children of the poorest urbanites: immigrants and African-Americans.

What was missing from American urban society—but would soon appear—was a middle class. Prior to the Civil War, most of the country's cities were largely populated by the working poor, entrepreneurial poor, and desperately poor. A small, elite group of urbanites possessed enormous wealth and employed large numbers of servants. They and the poor lived parallel but rarely intersecting lives.

In the absence of a strong, civically invested middle class, the cities became centres of political corruption. And the public's health worsened.

This theme of public health—the need for support from a sizeable middle class— would resonate throughout the future history of America. In the absence of a middle class, the rich simply lived separate and unequal lives, maintaining spacious homes along clean, tree-lined boulevards and raising their families through private systems of health, education, and cultural training. That a city might starve, politically and economically, in the absence of the elite's interest and finances seemed of little but occasional Christian concern to them. And the poor lacked the education, money, and skills to choose and run an effective government.

American public health would improve in tandem with the rise of the urban middle class, which paid taxes, supported cleanliness and public education, recognized and abhorred corruption, and, as home owners, had an investment in their cities. This was the interest group that would put into practice public measures based on the notion that 'cleanliness is next to Godliness'. In 1820 such a social class was virtually non-existent; by 1850, pockets of middle-class professionals and small businessmen were surfacing in most American eastern cities. And following the Civil War, the middle class steadily expanded in America, becoming the dominant force in municipal and regional political life by the mid-twentieth century.

In 1842 two crucial documents were published that compelled urban leaders and physicians to consider health in the light of the social, particularly class, context of industrialization. In London, Dr Edwin Chadwick published *Report on the Sanitary Condition of the Labouring Population of Great Britain*, a remarkable survey of the country's living standards right down to the numbers of people using any one privy and the odour of particular London neighbourhoods.[17] Under twentieth-century labelling, Chadwick would be considered an epidemiologist and perhaps a demographer, and a very good one at that. But his contribution went well beyond dry, statistical accounts of English filth, poverty, and pestilence. Chadwick correlated the three.

Chadwick called for organized public health, and he defined its mission as one of sanitary clean-up. An old-fashioned miasma thinker, Chadwick believed that if one lived amid filth, disease would be one's constant companion. Thus, the way to rid England of pestilence and premature deaths was to give her a good scrubbing. In the 1840s this was an astonishingly revolutionary insight.

Chadwick's counterpart in the United States was New Yorker John Griscom, who published *The Sanitary Conditions of the Laboring Populace of New York* in 1842 and his battle cry, *Sanitary Reform*, in 1844.[18] Griscom's goal was slightly less ambitious than Chadwick's: he didn't hope to scrub clean an entire nation, just New York City.

By the 1840s New York and most other large American cities were horribly crowded, disgustingly dirty affairs. Horse manure formed a thick, redolent layer over all of the streets, dead animals were usually left for days wherever they fell, tenement refuse was piled high in every vacant space, and everyone, save the rich, had to walk through this filth daily.

By 1845 Griscom had followers in the form of a loosely organized civic group known as the sanitarians that advocated New York cleanliness. Their call soon spread across the United States, with the ranks of sanitarians swelling swiftly to include Christian leaders, civic activists, politicians, some doctors, and the growing middle classes. Their target was filth, which generally was seen to be associated with immigrants. Like England's Chadwick, the American sanitarians weren't particularly interested in raising the standard of living of urban workers. In fact, many nativist sanitarians blamed the poor for their own poverty; they labelled slum and tenement residents lazy, idle, and immoral.[19]

The early sanitarians in America were also reluctant to rely on government to fulfil their dreams of hygiene. Most Americans in the 1840s were staunchly anti-government, as well as anti-intellectual.

Doctors themselves were hardly a sophisticated group anywhere in America during the first four decades of the nineteenth century. The oldest American medical school, established by Benjamin Franklin in Philadelphia in 1765, graduated only a handful of doctors every year, and most American 'physicians' hadn't undergone any training at all. In 1780, for example, there were about four thousand doctors practising medicine in New York City, only four hundred of whom had ever obtained a medical degree. Though medical schools had been established in New York and Boston before the American Revolution—institutions that would eventually be known as Columbia University College of Physicians and Surgeons and Harvard Medical School—few practitioners ever availed themselves of such academic training. And, as the typical sojourn in medical school lasted a mere nine months, with the bulk of that time spent studying Latin and philosophy, even those who did have training were ill-prepared for handling epidemics. In 1869, the president of Harvard University would denounce his school's medical training as 'not much better than a diploma mill'.

It was widely believed in the early nineteenth century that the best physicians were French. US medical men tended to ignore European advances in their profession for years: the Semmelweis technique of sterilizing the hands by thorough washing before touching patients was developed in 1840, but was not practiced in the US until well into the 1890s. Neither did they jump on two other crucial European developments for decades. In 1848 they paid little heed when the British parliament passed the Public Health Act. This legislation compelled every city and town in the United Kingdom to construct water systems, sewers and proper drainage, and surface primary roads: a feat accomplished in just over twenty years.

American health leaders also failed to take note of Dr John Snow's 1853 insight that by removing the pump handle (and thus the source of contaminated water) from the well in a London neighbourhood with an especially high cholera rate, that neighbourhood's cholera epidemic promptly slowed. Though Snow had no concept of the bacterial cause of cholera, he realized that filthy water carried the disease.

Despite the early sanitarians' best efforts, and perhaps in part because of antigovernment sentiment throughout America in the 1850s, truly awful epidemics continued and were just beginning to ignite action. In Providence, Rhode Island, Dr Edwin

Snow harangued the city government for months until, in 1850, he won passage of the nation's first compulsory vaccination law, mandating smallpox inoculation of school children. Many years and court challenges would pass before such laws would take hold elsewhere in the United States. And resistance to vaccination, despite its clear efficacy as a disease prevention strategy, remained as one of the themes of public health 150 years later.

Just as yellow fever had pushed the first public health measures in America, the terror of cholera was enormous, and it became the impetus for both change and inappropriate panic in the mid-nineteenth century. When rumours spread of cholera's arrival to a region, cities sought, and usually obtained, authority to forcibly detain the disease's victims in hospitals or pesthouses—facilities that functioned as little more than holding cells for ailing individuals, generally those from the poorest classes. Though such measures surely violated all concepts of personal liberty and usually proved lethal to the sufferers, quarantine enjoyed a fair amount of popular support, primarily because cholera was such a horrifying disease.

The sanitarians missed the message of John Snow's Broad Street pump. Rather than accept the possibility that a contagious agent might lurk in unclean water, the sanitarians continued to insist that filth, in and of itself, was the cause of disease. Spurred by fear of cholera, however, their zeal for cleansing was boundless.

While civic leaders targetted pigs, dirt, and horse manure, more advanced notions of disease were percolating overseas: talk of Charles Darwin's *On the Origin of Species* was on everyone's lips. Rudolf Virchow in 1858 published *Die Cellularpathologie*, which drew from his extensive laboratory studies to demonstrate that human illness functioned at the cellular level. The following year in Paris, Dr Claude Bernard published the first modern book of human physiology. And in 1862 Louis Pasteur had published in France his theory of the existence of 'germs' which, he argued, were key to fermentation. But America was focused on the Civil War. Most of the 535 000 deceased soldiers were victims of disease or the hideous health-care practices that resulted in the amputation of most injured limbs and proved fatal to 62 per cent of those with chest wounds and 87 per cent with abdominal wounds.[20]

While public health improved in most other north-eastern cities, except among soldiers, New York's stagnated. In New York City the Civil War had heightened tensions between immigrants, African-Americans, nativists, and politicians. Under Tammany Hall's control both the city inspector's office and the Board of Health were inept, corrupt, and stacked with Tammany sycophants. In 1865, at war's end, Francis Boole was Tammany Hall's man in charge of the New York City Inspector's Office. In a matter of months Boole hired 928 public health 'inspectors,' all of them cronies who either did nothing for their wages or used their inspectorial authority to blackmail the owners of restaurants, bakeries, slaughterhouses, produce markets, and private hospitals. The Board of Health was similarly inept, corrupt, and controlled by Tammany.

In far off Minnesota, Dr Charles Hewitt was fighting his own war on corruption. His targets were not, however, the likes of 'Boss' Tweed and his Tammany thugs but the state's physicians. A native New Yorker, Hewitt knew what constituted quality medical care in the 1860s, and what most certainly did not. In 1858, shortly before it became a state, Hewitt set to work mapping the demography of the territory's population, health, and disease. In his travels he was astonished by what passed for medical care.

'There is so little fact and so much theory, that I am sometimes tempted to think a medical practice founded upon the honest experience of *one* practitioner of sterling common sense would be safer and more successful than a practice based on what is vauntingly called "the united experience of centuries,"' Hewitt wrote in 1856.[21]

Convinced that many Minnesota physicians were unintentionally killing their patients with toxic tinctures, salves, and potions, and that the doctors were worsening public health catastrophes such as smallpox epidemics through inept handling of patients, Hewitt went on a professional rampage. In doing so he aroused the ire of most of the state's medical practitioners. Despite attempts by rival doctors to discredit him, Hewitt's words resonated with average Minnesotans who were sick to death of paying doctors for hocus-pocus, snake oil, and Christian homilies. Hewitt used his popularity to force the state's political leaders to create a Board of Health and a rudimentary vital statistics system to track Minnesotans' births, deaths, and diseases.

Hewitt became Minnesota's first secretary of the State Board of Health and began behaving like a government official, ordering hand cleansing among health-care workers, smallpox vaccination across the state, and quarantines of the sick. He told the state's politicians that if they gave his office legal support the legislators could, in return, trust in him: he would stop epidemics and slow disease. It was a trust Hewitt never betrayed, though the politicians often failed to keep their side of the bargain.

In 1877 Hewitt began a disease detective tradition that one hundred years later became one of the state's claims to fame. Smallpox had broken out and, not satisfied with issuing pamphlets calling for immunization, Hewitt set out to find the source of the outbreak—the index case. In so doing, Hewitt demonstrated that well before the issue was settled in the East, he favoured a contagion—rather than the sanitarian— theory of disease origin. Although Hewitt certainly supported clean cities, such filth could hardly explain the spread of smallpox in his sparsely populated, largely rural state. No, Hewitt reasoned, smallpox was caused by *something* that was spread from person to person.

Though he didn't know what, exactly, that 'something' was, he felt certain that only the existence of a communicable, deadly entity of some sort could explain why quarantine could effectively slow epidemics. Hewitt soon spotted a connection between the first 1877 case of smallpox in Minnesota and a recently constructed railway line that connected St Paul to neighbouring Wisconsin. He discovered that the first case in the state, was in a woman who had caught the disease in Wisconsin, boarded the St Paul and Sioux Railroad, and travelled to Mankato, Minnesota. She unwittingly spread the illness to fellow passengers on the train who, in turn, took smallpox to towns all over the state. At all railway stations on the state's borders, Hewitt established checkpoints where physicians examined passengers and crew for signs of smallpox. He stopped the epidemic in a matter of days, leaving only seven dead Minnesotans in its wake. It was, by 1877 standards, a spectacular feat.

Once again Hewitt used the smallpox victory to castigate the physicians, telling them that it was high time they accepted his contagion theory of disease and commenced some local detective work whenever measles, scarlet fever, or other microbial scourges surfaced among their patients. In the post–Civil War nineteenth century, however, physicians—like Tammany Hall—typically held public health in open disdain, seeing it as little more than a combination of meddlesome government and sanitarian scrubbers. Hewitt had already alienated scores of doctors by exposing their medicinal frauds. Now he dared to demand that they accept his belief system, seeing diseases as ailments caused by as-yet-undiscovered, mysterious, contagious elements, the spread of which was preventable. In Minnesota, and all across America, doctors balked at the notion. They felt their autonomous powers over patients were being threatened. And they resisted the population-based activities of Hewitt and his compatriots. The healers, it seemed, opposed the would-be preventers of disease.

Friction between healers and preventers, between would-be curers and sanitarian scrubbers, and, eventually, between independent doctors and government regulators formed another lasting theme of American public health. A century and a half later this tension limited Dr Margaret Hamburg's ability to control antibiotic-resistant diseases in New York, as she was powerless to change physicians' prescription practices. In the 1860s Hewitt ran Minnesota public health services but was at odds with organized medicine. All over America men like Hewitt had to challenge the American Medical Association and individual physicians.

The severity of such tension varied across the nation because American public health grew up in an entirely different manner from its counterpart in Europe. In Europe public health policies were promulgated from the top down, developed from an essentially federal (or royal) function: American public health, in a manner characteristic of its fervor for democracy, arose from the local level, and no two cities or states had precisely the same policies. In some regions, medical systems grew alongside those of public health; in most, they followed separate, often oppositional, courses. Not only was there no genuine federal leadership in public health in nineteenth-century America, few states had laws and policies that extended to all of their counties and cities. In New York and Massachusetts, for example, New York City and Boston were the tails that wagged their state health dogs.

On the East Coast the large cities grew larger and more crowded, so their public health needs revolved around essential urban services, such as sewers and surfaced roads. Out on the prairie, men like Hewitt were focused on quarantines and epidemic control; in the far West health wasn't even on the political agenda. The climate was benign, Anglos were, generally, far healthier than they would be in the cities of the East, and nearly the *only* thing on the western agenda was land and the mad scramble to bump Indians and Spanish descendants off it, in favour of Anglo, or Yankee, control. By 1865, at the end of the distant Civil War, the destitute *Californios* were huddled into the state's first ghettos, located in neighbourhoods of Los Angeles such as Chavez Ravine.

Bad as these barrios were, they paled in public health significance when compared to the new ghettos of the East's cities. Waves of impoverished immigrants were flooding into New York, in particular, only to be warehoused in such states of squalor as would be unimaginable a century later. Indeed, the quality of drinking water, sewer conditions, the safety of local produce, and housing all worsened considerably for New York workers by 1866, compared to those in 1776. Any disease adapted for spread via human waste and contaminated water would find the ecology of 1866 Gotham highly favourable. That year, fed-up citizens bypassed Tammany and created a new Metropolitan Board of Health. Spurring its creation was word of virulent cholera epidemic in Paris.

Having spotted cholera from Europe aboard a ship in New York City's harbour, the new board—ardent sanitarians all—ordered immediate cleaning of every street and sewer in Manhattan and Brooklyn, among other measures. Crucially, board member Dr Elisha Harris made the bold contagionist assertion that cholera infected people as a result of contact with water that was contaminated with faecal matter from other cholera victims. He knew, of course, of John Snow's Broad Street pump experiment in London, but Harris went a critical step further, mixing the Snow observation with Semmelweis's hand-washing insights.

Harris told New Yorkers to wash their darned hands with soap and clean water.

By summer's end, though cholera had ravaged Paris and London and would wreak havoc throughout the United States, there were few deaths in New York.

Despite such successes, Tammany-controlled judges and attorneys plagued the Board of Health for decades with lawsuits and injunctions, blocking as many quarantines and other actions as possible. The goal was to eliminate board enforcement of violations committed by Tammany-allied businesses or by Irish owners of tenement buildings. To gain public support for their obviously self-interested efforts, the Tammany machine rallied Irish tenement residents, telling them—falsely, of course—that the rules and regulations were being used prejudicially against their neighbourhoods and that quarantines bypassed 'niggers'—the Irish immigrants' key enemies—in favour of targeting those who had recently arrived from Ireland.

A similar tension between immigrants and blossoming public health departments surfaced in other American cities as the flow of poor Europeans moved west. It was to highlight another perennial theme of public health, one that would haunt America well into the twenty-first century: tension between the health concerns of native-born Americans and the fears and suspicions of recent immigrants.

In the mid-nineteenth century the US-born population often saw immigrants as little more than sources of disease and filth, readily blaming them for all epidemics and, indeed, supporting sanitarian interventions that prejudicially targeted the newly arrived poor. Even when prejudice was not behind health department actions, political leaders could readily tap immigrant apprehensions, guiding the newly arrived Americans to see discrimination where it did not exist. Throughout the nineteenth century public health leaders tended, on balance, to side with the needs and biases of the native-born population. The imbalance persisted, during the twentieth century for example, prompting federal officials to designate Haitian immigrants a 'risk group for AIDS'. And the same public health agencies would underplay issues that preferentially afflicted immigrants, such as the impact of pesticides on the health of Mexican farm workers, the remarkably high infant mortality rates seen in Latinos living in Los Angeles, and a plague outbreak among Chinese immigrants in San Francisco. Throughout the twentieth century, public health leaders had to tread a fine line between the exigencies and suspicions of the immigrant communities and those of the native born.

II

It is in health that cities grow: in sunshine that their monuments are builded. It is in disease that they are wrecked; in pestilence that effort ceases and hope dies.
—Annual Report of the Commissioner of Health, Milwaukee, 1911

In retrospect, the turn of the century now seems to have been a golden age for public health, when its achievements followed one another in dizzying succession and its future possibilities seemed limitless.
—Paul Starr, *The Social Transformation of American Medicine* 1982

The revolution was about to begin. Genuine public health was gestating and would soon be birthed by the likes of Minnesota's Hewitt and New York City's Hermann Biggs. The profundity of Biggs's insights, in particular, proved so deep and powerful that a century later they guided New York City leaders through the horror of an epidemic of drug-resistant tuberculosis.

The ideas were sparked in far-off Europe, but it was in America's atmosphere of middle-class democracy that genuine systems of population protection were spawned.

In Europe during the late nineteenth century a great intellectual revolution was underway that enabled disease to be defined and, with that, relegated to the status of problems humanity might solve.

The great debates of the past—spontaneous generation, miasma theory, sanitarianism versus contagion—were resolved, or took on new themes, as science stepped into the picture. And if public health suffered from any intellectual sins amidst the confusion of disease delineation information they were arrogance and hubris.

On the eve of this great revolution, however, a host of essentially non-scientific measures had, by the 1880s, already vastly improved the public's health. Sewer and privy construction, improved drinking water quality, quarantine policies, street cleaning, enforcement of safer food, meat and milk production standards, proper roads—each of these measures had had its impact. In addition, the railway and lorry-driver transport networks that developed in post-Civil War America radically improved people's diets as fresh crops made their way into city centres in bulk and at prices most working families could afford. While many children still lacked protein-rich and adequately varied diets, there was no doubt that fewer of them were nutrient deficient and malnourished in 1875 than had been so two decades earlier. In addition, many cities—notably New York and Boston—set up distribution stations that handed out fresh milk to poor children. That alone had a profound impact on the strength and stature of urban youngsters.

Though housing in city areas remained atrocious for many of America's poor, sanitarians were doing their utmost to improve the squalor surrounding tenements and slums.

Death rates from yellow fever, smallpox, and cholera, three chiefly adult diseases, fell as swamps were drained, window glass installed, sewers built, vaccination improved, and, perhaps, because nutrition was enhanced. The impact of such measures was limited, however, before the advent of vaccines, and plagues, such as the 1878 yellow fever epidemic that killed at least twenty thousand people in the Mississippi Valley, were yet to come.

Also still to come were ebbs and flows in the great scourges of childhood: measles, whooping cough, diphtheria, typhoid fever, and scarlet fever, each of which, just forty years later, claimed comparatively minor numbers of American lives.

With the devastating yellow fever epidemics at centre stage in the 1870s, and the then slow pace at which information travelled, it was hard for US sanitarians and health leaders to take note of the staggering scientific advances that were occurring across the Atlantic. Further, the sanitarians, among whom Christian moralists predominated, were slow to note advances in science. But advances there were indeed.

Antiseptics were discovered in England in 1870 by Dr Joseph Lister, who found that by pouring carbolic acid on a wound or a suture site, infection would never take hold there. Beginning in 1876 doctors Robert Koch in Berlin and Louis Pasteur in Paris were racing to identify the individual germs that caused disease.

In 1880 Pasteur published his landmark *Germ Theory of Disease*, in which he argued that all contagious diseases were caused by microscopic organisms that damaged the human victim at the cellular level—as Rudolf Virchow had argued—and spread from person to person.

In Berlin, Paul Erlich went a step further, discovering that animals that survived an infection had substances in their blood that could successfully fight off the disease in other affected animals. He called the agents of ailment toxins and his newly discovered substances antitoxins. So enthusiastic was Erlich about the miraculous powers of antitoxins that he dubbed them 'magic bullets'.

Between 1880 and 1889 the rival Berlin and Paris laboratories discovered the bacteria responsible for tuberculosis,[22] cholera, and diphtheria; they developed a vaccine against rabies; and they named the mosquito responsible for spreading yellow fever.

Among the most progressive public health leaders in America it was understood that if the identity of each great microbial killer was established, diagnostic tests, vaccines, and cures wouldn't be far behind. Suddenly there was a rationale for vaccination, which they had long encouraged but had never been able to explain to sceptics.

Even more profound was the shift in perspective from outward, mysterious miasmic origins of disease to microscopic. In Minnesota Hewitt lobbied the state legislature in 1888, to raise funds to purchase the region's first microscope. Similarly, New York City's health leaders realized that the age of laboratory-informed decision making had arrived and constructed the nation's first public health laboratory.

However to grasp the revolution then under way, men like Hewitt and his New York counterparts sailed off to Europe to sit at the feet of the great Koch and Pasteur.

All over America there were individuals inside local health departments who wholeheartedly embraced Pasteur's germ theory of disease, revelled in the new-found possibilities of their laboratories, and, practically overnight, changed the methods, strategies, and tactics of government public health. Past measures of disease prevention and epidemic control may have been effective—at least in some cases—but they lacked scientific explanation. Without a clear rationale for draining swamps or vaccinating children, health advocates had little choice but to await an epidemic and, capitalizing on the public's hysteria, twist the arms of politicians and men of commerce in order to obtain the desired laws and funds.

The germ theory changed that. While funding continued to ebb and flow with the tide of politics and the level of public concern about contagion, support for prevention efforts became more sustainable. Advocates could now use their new laboratories to provide scientific evidence of a specific contamination or infection. In addition, they could prove to sceptics that a particular intervention was, indeed, responsible for lowering germ levels in the social milieu where it had been applied.

In short, public health suddenly had an empirical basis that rested upon demonstrable facts.

Nowhere was the impact of germ theory more powerfully felt than in New York City, which, in a few short years, metamorphosed from one of America's sorriest, most cesspoollike excuses for a metropolis into the world's paragon of government action on behalf of the public's health. Chief among the architects of this change were Drs T. Mitchell Prudden and Hermann Biggs, both of them firm adherents to the germ theory of disease.

Biggs and Prudden had been appointed to the city's new bacteriology laboratory in 1885 by President Grover Cleveland. The nation's leaders feared that escalating waves of 'filthy, dirty foreigners' arriving daily in New York harbour would import further epidemics. As most immigrants passed through New York harbour, President Cleveland reasoned that he ought to place a pair of top scientists inside the city's laboratory.

Theophil Mitchell Prudden was, at the time of his federal appointment in 1885, a thirty-six-year-old graduate of Yale Medical School. The son of an immensely wealthy New York family, Prudden was one of the rare members of his social class who dedicated his life to science. Educated at the best of America's schools, Prudden was well-versed in Europe's bumper crop of scientific discovery and imbued with a youthful zeal over Pasteur's germ theory. During the early 1880s he studied in the best laboratories of Germany and Austria and even worked beside Robert Koch.

Hermann Michael Biggs was ten years Prudden's junior but already an impressive presence on New York's medical landscape. A native of the city, Biggs had trained in medicine at Bellevue Hospital. Though his scholastic experience paled in comparison to that of Prudden, his uncanny political skills more than compensated. More than any other individual in America in his day, Biggs understood the intimate relationship between politics and public health and could successfully manoeuvre around corruption, complacency, and cronyism. In less than twenty years, backed by the power of the germ theory, Biggs moved public health from near the bottom of New York's ladder of political clout and public esteem to the top.

Although the nation's first bacteriology laboratories were actually established elsewhere (in Laurence, Massachusetts; Ann Arbor, Michigan; and Providence, Rhode Island), it was the New York City bacteriologists who reshaped both their usefulness and their authority. Prudden proved to be the intellectual giant, Biggs the street-savvy political force.

In 1888 the city's Board of Health named Biggs and Prudden 'consulting pathologists,' appointing them as city employees. The pair immediately set to work to formulate, and back up, public health measures based on laboratory science.

The duo swiftly dispensed with tubercular cow's milk, built up both the size and influence of their laboratory, and began confronting the child killer diphtheria. They invented a screening test for cholera—the first that could identify human carriers of the deadly bacteria. And when the disease arose in Hamburg in 1892[23] and spread across Europe with terrifying ferocity, claiming upwards of three thousand lives a day, Biggs and Prudden used their test and powers of quarantine to identify the first carriers that arrived in New York that summer on ships from Europe. The handful that escaped their grasp were tracked down by an army of health department staff and volunteers who hunted through every housing unit in search of diarrhoea victims and filled privies and toilets with disinfectants.

Thanks to these actions, in 1892 only nine people died of cholera in New York City, compared to tens of thousands who perished from Vladivostock to Lisbon to London.

It was a phenomenally successful demonstration of the strength and dynamism of germ theory-based public action. The forces of sanitarianism worked in tandem with the laboratory-based scientific efforts of Biggs and Prudden. The impeccably dressed Dr Biggs, in particular, became an overnight sensation and, at barely thirty years of age, the hero of New York.

The Gay Nineties, as the 1890s were called, were times of social change that bene-fited public health. Some such changes arose from a growing civic pride—parks, good roads, public transport. Some were the result of mass activism on behalf of labour and the poor. The anti-tenement movement focused scrutiny on the lives of slum dwellers, lives made unbearably grim by the appalling conditions of their crowded, pestilent, unmaintained dwellings, workplaces, and schools. In addition, union agitators, anarch-ists, socialists, and Communists were all gaining strong followings. Social movements were growing across the industrialized Northeast and Midwest. Even in the Pacific states of the far West, socialists and anarchists were finding favour among poorly paid labourers.

Chief among the demands shared by all these geographically and ideologically dispar-ate movements were the calls for greater occupational safety and improved housing.

The most influential social activist of the day was Danish-born photographer and writer Jacob August Riis. In 1890 Riis published his masterpiece of text and photo-graphs, *How the Other Half Lives*. It gave his appalled readers both a visual image of tenement hell-holes and a vivid description of their odours, sounds, and claustropho-bia. In the worst of them, located on what was called 'Lung Block', could be found the city's densest concentrations of infant mortality, tuberculosis, and pneumonia.[24] Lung Block had four thousand inhabitants, ten times more than lived on any average New York block. Crammed five or six to the room, its inhabitants witnessed 265 cases of tuberculosis during the 1880s for a case rate of 6.6 per 1000 people—possibly the highest in the world at that time. Riis estimated that there were 1.5 million people living in such New York City tenements in 1890, or about 60 per cent of the population of metropolitan New York.

On an entirely different front, a variety of organizations were demanding improve-ment in the lots of women and children—the right to vote, to birth control, to abor-tion. Margaret Sanger, for example, published and distributed pamphlets on birth control, decrying the extraordinary death toll among women who, despite the continu-ing risks of puerperal fever and other pregnancy-associated ailments, were expected to give birth to six or more children.[25]

Social unrest and discontent continued to grow, further polarizing urban America during the next ten decades. For the expanding middle classes and the old, native-born elite of eastern cities, these movements were cause for considerable consternation and evoked two key responses: anti-immigrant sentiments and capitulation to nominal reform sparked by fear of all-out social unrest and disease contagion. These responses continued to cast a shadow on the public's health into the twenty-first century.

For the middle class had embraced to an extreme the idea of a germ theory of disease, becoming germ-phobic. Whereas the wealthiest city dwellers may have abhorred germs, they could avoid the riffraff or escape to distant estates. The middle class, however, felt trapped. For them, everything from public library books to dust could harbour lethal germs. Germicide sales boomed, as did the installation of indoor plumbing, flush toilets, and modern kitchens that included iceboxes to keep food fresh.[26]

This germ phobia and resolute commitment to stamping out the bugs ultimately fuelled support for grand public health schemes. Because the middle and upper classes were convinced that the poor—particularly immigrants—were the source of all truly terrible microbial scourges, they were willing to pay the price in higher taxes for *biological*, as opposed to *class*, warfare. The sanitarians supported provision of some health hygienic services to the working people in America's cities. By 1890 in New York City, for example, nearly a quarter of all health care was provided free by tax-supported municipal dispensaries, and in 1887 the Board of Aldermen had agreed to install toilets in all of the city's state schools. But the sanitarians also imposed a moral judgmentalism that openly expressed disdain for the religious, family, and cultural lives of the poor.

Harper's Weekly put the matter of class tensions starkly in 1881 with a cartoon depicting a conversation between the goddess Hygeia and a top-hatted man of wealth. Pointing to streets of filth and poverty, Hygeia berated the man, saying, 'You doubtless think that as all this filth is lying out in the back streets, it is of no concern of yours. But you are mistaken. You will see it stealing into your house very soon, if you don't take care.' By 1890 the message was hitting home. The public health revolution began.

Projects of enormous scale, particularly water and sewer works, to improve communities' health, were undertaken at the behest of the wealthy and middle classes.[27]

With so many social forces swirling about his public health world in Gotham, Biggs and his colleagues set the immodest goals of completely eliminating diphtheria and tuberculosis. Though Biggs declared a 'War on Consumption' in 1893, he first set his sights upon diphtheria and, like Minnesota's Hewitt, made the journey to Europe to learn from the masters of microbiology. The New Yorker settled into the laboratory of Louis Pasteur, working beside Émile Roux.

Upon his return to New York in 1894, Biggs immediately set to work with his staff building a diphtheria antitoxin production facility and lobbying for funds. The Hospital for Sick Children in Paris had just begun using diphtheria antitoxin with remarkable results—an immediate 50 per cent reduction in paediatric death rates. Seizing upon that evidence, Biggs did something almost unheard of in 1894: he held a press conference. And for weeks he systematically and deftly manoeuvred several of New York's many newspapers into supporting his diphtheria antitoxin laboratory. By early 1895 Biggs's charitably funded laboratory was the world's largest diphtheria antitoxin producer and was also mass-manufacturing smallpox and anthrax vaccines and a host of other 'magic bullets'.

Soon, distraught immigrant mothers from the tenements were turning up in dispensaries demanding 'magic bullets' for their ailing children. And diphtheria death rates in New York City plummeted, going from an 1875 high of 296 per 100 000 people to 105 per 100 000 in 1895 to 66 per 100 000 five years later. By 1912 New York's diphtheria death rate fallen to just 2.2 per 100 000 residents per year.[28] Soon every city in America was buying antitoxin from the Biggs laboratory.

With such diphtheria success at his back, Biggs set full sail into the seas of tuberculosis, which was then overwhelming New York's tenements. In an 1897 speech before the British Medical Association Biggs outlined his War on Consumption strategies, tactics, and biases and received worldwide press attention for delivering the first clearly delineated strategy for attacking the disease. Many of his comments, delivered to a hall full of openly sceptical physicians, became the often-quoted battle cries of TB fighters worldwide and remained so a century later. At just thirty-six years old, Hermann Biggs was already the undisputed leader of the new public health movement:

> The government of the United States is democratic, but the sanitary measures adopted are sometimes autocratic, and the functions performed by sanitary authorities paternal in character. We are prepared, when necessary, to introduce and enforce, and the people are ready to accept, measures which might seem radical and arbitrary, if they were not plainly designed for the public good, and evidently beneficent in their effects. Even among the most ignorant of our foreign-born population, few or no indications of resentment are exhibited to the exercise of arbitrary powers in sanitary matters. The public press will approve, the people will support, and the courts sustain, any intelligent procedures which are evidently directed to preservation of the public health.
>
> The most autocratic powers, capable of the broadest construction, are given to them under the law. Everything which is detrimental to health or dangerous to life, under the freest interpretation, is regarded as coming within the province of the Health Department. So broad is the construction of the law that everything which improperly or unnecessarily interferes with the comfort or enjoyment of life, as well as those things which are, strictly speaking, detrimental to health or dangerous to life, may become the subject of action on the part of the Board of Health.

It was a declaration of war, not just against tuberculosis but against any group or individual who stood in the way of Public Health or the sanitarians' Hygeia.

But while easterner Biggs was exercising his 'autocratic powers' on behalf of public health, residents of the far western states were sneering at, or ignoring, Hygeia. In Los Angeles County, poor J. L. Pomeroy, first to hold the title of health officer, tried hard to impress upon the leaders of his county's many towns that 'it must be clearly recognized that diseases recognize no boundary lines, and that the health and social problems of the rural areas ... are closely associated with those of urban areas'.[29] Pomeroy (a practical, though uninspiring physician) conducted health surveys in 1915 that indicated that his county's equivalent of New York's tenement population was its non-white population. Among the Mexicans and Mexican-Americans, for example, infant death rates routinely exceeded 200 per 1000 births (compared to 80 for whites), and in 1916 it was 285 per 1000—that is, nearly one-third of their babies perished in infancy.

From its quite late inception in 1915,[30] organized public health in Los Angeles was more a county than a city function, and, also from the beginning, took on the role not of Biggs's anti-disease crusades but of a service provider. Rather than ruffle feathers with great Biggs-style campaigns, Pomeroy's county team concentrated on racing to give the ever-burgeoning towns and cities of Los Angeles the basics: food and water inspection, vaccines, and medical care. It made sense at the time, as the basics were desperately needed and the epidemics that ravaged the East were less severe in the mild climate of the West. Besides, Pomeroy won little support from apathetic Angelenos for much else.

The still-sparse population and favourable climate were Pomeroy's only allies, holding Los Angeles death rates well below those of most of the United States: 7.9 per 1000 residents per year. In contrast to New York City[31] and similarly dense eastern cities, most of Los Angeles's deaths were among people over fifty years of age. Children under ten years of age accounted for just 14.5 per cent of the total. Most of them succumbed to diphtheria, measles, or whooping cough—and to smallpox.

Pomeroy found that delivering vaccines often ran into a wall of resistance. The nation's strongest anti-vaccination movement arose in his county and consistently blocked all attempts to impose both compulsory immunization of schoolchildren and some uses of diphtheria antitoxin. Though more than two million people lived in Los Angeles County by the end of the Roaring Twenties, fewer than a hundred thousand took advantage of free vaccination programmes; most of the population actively opposed immunization.

Anti-vaccine organizations sprouted up all over California during the early twentieth century, driven by Christian Scientists, opponents of the germ theory of disease, and groups generally opposed to government interference in personal affairs. As a result, smallpox rates rose steadily at a time when most of the country saw the disease disappear.

Elsewhere in America, vaccine opposition hit its peak in the 1890s, but in the far West it was still an effective obstacle to public health in the 1930s. Despite a 1905 Supreme Court ruling that the rights of individuals to opt for or against a medical procedure were far outweighed by the powerful need to protect the community as a whole, as each new vaccine was developed and health authorities pushed to add it to the list of compulsory child immunizations, a nationwide pattern of opposition was repeated. It surfaced, for example, when New York City passed a compulsory diphtheria vaccination law in 1920, when typhoid fever immunizations were introduced during the same period, following initial rounds of polio immunization in the early 1950s, and later with measles, rubella, whooping cough, chicken pox, and hepatitis vaccines.

As early as 1905, another critical and lasting theme of public health began to emerge, largely from the far West: the needs of the community versus the rights of individuals. In the twentieth century, public health leaders and courts tended to interpret—and reinterpret—appropriate balances between those often opposing needs, usually falling into positions that reflected the cultural and political moods of the nation at that time. Because during the early part of the century, bacteriology-based public health was perceived as extraordinarily powerful and the background of disease was obviously grim and urgent, both public health leaders and the courts tended to tip the balance far in the direction of community needs. By the end of the twentieth century, the scales had swung to the opposite extreme, favouring individual rights.

Between 1901 and 1930 New York City officials routinely deployed police officers and zealous nurses or physicians to the homes of those suspected of carrying disease, and force, or the threat thereof, was commonly used to overcome vaccine refusers. In some cases, police officers pinned the arm of those who refused while a city nurse jabbed it with a vaccination needle.

Biggs often spoke of the 'absolute preventability' of disease, proudly noting that nowhere else in the world had 'sanitary authorities granted to them such extraordinary and even arbitrary powers as rest in the hands of the Board of Health of New York City'. He used that power to search out TB sufferers and (forcibly if necessary) place them in sanitariums. He also used it to find and destroy contaminated food and drugs. No hearing, no appeals. The payoff was in steadily declining death rates.

The most notorious example of Biggs's willingness to push the legal and ethical envelope in order to protect the collective health of New Yorkers was the case of Irish immigrant cook Mary Mallon. In 1902 Germany's Koch proved that healthy people could, for years on end, be contagious carriers of *Salmonella typhi*, the bacterial cause of typhoid fever.[32] Biggs and an army of disease detectives sleuthed their ways through a series of typhoid illnesses and deaths, finding Mallon to be the common link, and a laboratory-proven carrier.[33] They incarcerated her on an island in New York's East River until she pledged to stop working as a professional cook, as it was fostering her spreading the disease. But after her release Mallon illegally returned to that profession under a pseudonym. When Biggs's staff tracked the belligerent and thoroughly uncooperative woman down, they exiled her to that island again, this time for the rest of her days. She would forever be remembered as Typhoid Mary.[34]

Moving westward, however, there was a gradient of discontent with such forceful public health measures, with Los Angelenos in extreme opposition. Remarkably, such adversity for public health came during a time of spectacular scientific and social success for the profession.

In 1900 the American Public Health Association began to professionalize the calling by giving advanced degrees. By the time the Panama Canal was finished in 1913, the US military effort to drain that country's swamps had virtually eradicated malaria and yellow fever from the Canal Zone, and similar drainage campaigns were under way all over North and South America.

Their imaginations fired by the bacteriology revolution that was in full swing, US philanthropists endowed other bold campaigns. John D. Rockefeller created a scientific foundation bearing his name that in 1906 declared war on hookworm.[35] Ten years later Rockefeller's foundation put up millions of dollars to create the Johns Hopkins School of Public Health in Baltimore. It opened seven years after other philanthropists had funded the creation of the Harvard School of Public Health.[36]

A foundation set up by the steel tycoon Andrew Carnegie aimed to improve the quality of education in the 160 medical schools of the time. Abraham Flexner, who was put in charge of the effort, in 1910 wrote arguably the single most influential indictment of medical education ever published in the English language.[37] The Flexner Report, as it was called, not only revealed in truly gruesome detail the abominations of medical training at the time, but recommended detailed steps for repair, with the ultimate goal of transforming American medical schools into rigorous centres of science.

The primary benefit of this for public health care came from the far higher level of belief in germ theory and vaccinology among graduates of the improved medical schools. And hospitals were transformed from nineteenth-century warehouses that merely isolated the diseased from the community into genuine treatment centres.

But as physician skills and hospital quality improved, medical costs rose. And with that came the debate over what, if any, role government should play in the provision not only of essential public health services, but of medical treatment. New York City already had public hospitals, funded by tax dollars. Out west, Los Angeles County was well on its way toward being the *sole* provider of medical care in its region. But no state, and certainly not the US Congress, had yet addressed the question of where responsibility for paying for medicine lay. Debates over government provision of universal health coverage began in 1912 and have continued—unresolved—into the twenty-first century.

Over time, the nexus of basic research science was shifting continents. In the 1820s France had led the Western world's race of medical discovery. By the 1840s, it was Germany that dominated medical sciences and, with the exception of the Pasteur laboratory, produced most of the key discoveries of the latter half of the nineteenth century. By 1910, however, the American output was, by far, dominant, with most of the discoveries emerging from laboratories in New York City.[38] By the First World War's end, US science, which had escaped war on its own territory, was in a position of dominance and, in many fields of research, remained there throughout the twentieth century.

Everything, it seemed, was working in favour of public health. The germ theory crusaders were at the zenith of both their power and respect in America. It seemed no disease could go unvanquished by the scythe of their science.

Until 1916. And polio.

The microbe responsible for polio was not successfully isolated and grown in laboratories for more than forty years. Until then, it shared with smallpox, rabies, and yellow fever—like polio, all viral diseases—the dubious honour of being an infectious disease whose microbial agents could be indirectly demonstrated to exist but not seen or understood. Science, and with it public health, had hit a major obstacle.

Only decades later did experts understand that it was the triumph of turn-of-the-century public health that had caused polio: the microbe was ancient, but the disease was not. Before sanitarians set to work cleaning up the water, infants were exposed to minute, immunizing doses of the virus from the moment they were weaned. Disease-free water meant that such childhood exposure to the polio virus was much rarer. The generation born after 1900 in cities like New York, Boston, Chicago, Paris, and London had little, if any, immunizing exposure to the microbe.

All it took to spark an epidemic, then, were a few days during which water supplies were inadequately filtered—a common occurrence during the hot summer months when bacterial growth and lower water levels increased the concentration of microbes.[39]

On June 6, 1916, New York City paediatricians reported the year's first cases of poliomyelitis—found among residents of the densely populated waterfront area. By the month's end, cities all over the United States were witnessing their worst polio outbreaks. Recognizing that they were facing an enormous epidemic, the New York City Department of Health and the US Surgeon General turned to a new solution—publicity. They reached out to the nation's newspapers, civic organizations, and schools urging hygiene as the best defence against polio. On the eve of the Fourth of July holiday the Surgeon General declared that 'a state of imminent peril to the Nation' existed.

The public health leaders of America did everything they could imagine to try to control the child killer. In Gotham, teams of nurses, police at their sides, scoured the tenements. And all households containing a poliomyelitic child were placed under quarantine.

All over the city signs were nailed over entry doors:

INFANTILE PARALYSIS (POLIOMYELITIS)

Infantile paralysis is very prevalent in this part of the city.
On some streets many children are ill. This is one of those streets.
KEEP OFF THIS STREET

It was decades before scientists understood that quarantine was of no use in epidemic polio control. A child's own parents, siblings, or friends might be dangerous sources of contagion. Only a vaccine could prevent polio and that innovation took four decades to come.

Though polio seemed in retreat in 1917,[40] it resurfaced with a vengeance. And polio was just the first of several new challenges between 1916 and 1919 that severely undermined the nation's admiration and belief in public health. Public health's germ theory-based zenith had been reached in less than twenty years, thanks to bold political manoeuvres, strong science, and equally impressive strategic planning.

Now it began its downward spiral.

While men were fighting World War I in the trenches of Europe, in America temperance leagues, largely led by Christian women's groups, successfully pushed Congress to pass the Eighteenth Amendment to the US Constitution. The new law prohibiting nationwide 'the manufacture, sale, or transportation of intoxicating liquors' reflected widely publicized middle-class moral indignation over what was portrayed as an epidemic of drunken fathers and husbands—generally pictured as working-class.

Though the impetus for Prohibition was not public health, it was obvious that alcoholism was unhealthy, not only for the drinker but, potentially, for the entire family.

Popular evangelist Billy Sunday predicted a rosy future as a result of Prohibition: 'The reign of tears is over. The slums will soon be a memory. We will turn our prisons into factories and our jails into storehouses and corncribs. Men will walk upright now, women will smile, and children will laugh. Hell will be forever rent.'[41]

On the contrary, Prohibition spawned a public health catastrophe fuelled by a massive crime network. Customer demand for alcohol never waned and in cities like New York, Prohibition actually increased both alcohol consumption and the use of narcotics. And although federal authorities chased trucks loaded with bathtub gin, physicians openly prescribed as alternative sources of recreational levity medicines rich in morphine, opium, laudanum, belladonna, absinthe, marijuana, and cocaine— all of which were sold and swapped in ellicit liquorshops (speakeasies).[42]

Nationwide, crime rates jumped 24 per cent during the first year of Prohibition. Jails filled to 170 per cent of capacity. Bribery and extortion of government officials swiftly became so commonplace as to barely raise eyebrows among news readers.[43]

In 1919 the New York City Department of Health sadly reported that there were at least a hundred thousand drug addicts in Gotham, primarily users of opium or cocaine. As the era swung into the Roaring Twenties, the numbers of alcoholics and drug addicts rose. Newly appointed Commissioner of Health Dr Royal S. Copeland fought to place all matters related to drug addiction within his department and turned Riverside Hospital into an addiction treatment centre. But the police, many of whom were addicted to Prohibition-related graft, fought Copeland. By 1920 his drug treatment funds had dried up and Riverside, having managed to rehabilitate fewer than 5 per cent of its patients, was closed.[44]

Another continuing theme of public health had emerged: the battle pitting those who would medicalize drug and alcohol addiction against those who would criminalize it. Though in coming decades public health witnessed an occasional victory, Americans generally opted for law enforcement approaches to illicit drugs. After the repeal of Prohibition in 1933, concern about alcoholism rarely enjoyed such a powerful spotlight again, but anxiety about illicit drugs swelled steadily throughout the century.[45]

Bad as America's new love for addictive substances was, the real disillusionment with public health was incited not by opiates and alcohol but by another virus: influenza. The swine flu pandemic began during the summer of 1918 in Kansas and circled the planet three times in eighteen months.[46] By early 1920 the virus had claimed an estimated twenty to twenty-five million people worldwide.[47]

In November of 1918, every one of the 5323 hospitals in the United States was overwhelmed; nearly all of their 612 251 beds were filled. On the eve of the pandemic in 1917, the national death rate due to influenza was 164.5 per 100 000 annually. It soared to a staggering 588.5 per 100 000 in 1918 and stayed high until 1921.

So overwhelmed were public health authorities that virtually all of their other activities had to yield to influenza control. With quarantine out of the question—there were simply too many flu cases—health departments had little to offer. Otherwise helpless, they counted the numbers and raced about collecting bodies. Other forces stepped in to fill the vacuum: in the absence of a clear understanding of the influenza virus, every manner of crackpot and quack sold elixirs, masks, vapours, alcoholic tinctures, and hundreds of other items.

For health officials from New York to Los Angeles, the 1918–19 epidemic was another awful slap in the face of their otherwise triumphant achievements. Polio, drug and alcohol addiction, and influenza each highlighted crucial shortcomings of the sanitarians. There were, after all, limits to their power over the microbes and the social forces of disease.

In its 1920 annual report the New York City Department of Health struck an almost plaintive note that was in sharp contrast to Biggs's braggadocio of the previous decade:

> While a very few years ago, the slogans, 'Safety First,' and 'Health First,' had been popularized to a very considerable degree, one might term the present state of affairs in practically every civilized country as showing an attitude which may be characterized as indicating consent to permit a 'Health Last' policy to govern. These observations are not irrelevant as a matter of stock-taking. This low ebb of interest in social welfare activities ...is reflected in the progress of public health activities. The trend of times makes evident the need for sane, aggressive leadership, in such things that promote human welfare....

The trust that citizens had placed in their public health leaders seemed somehow unwarranted. Recent triumphs over diphtheria, yellow fever, and cholera were overshadowed in the collective memory by the apparent failures.

And it was becoming increasingly obvious that even the public health triumphs of the early twentieth century had not been universal in either their implementation or impact. Pomeroy's Los Angeles County officials quietly logged the three-fold differential in mortality rates between Mexican-American and white infants, but conducted no studies that might reveal why the disparity existed. Even in the heyday of Biggs's authority in New York City, the roughly ten-year difference in life expectancies between white immigrants and native-born African-Americans constituted little more than a set of statistics dutifully logged year after year.

For a century, health-oriented intellectuals in England and the United States had speculated upon the relationship between poverty and disease, variously concluding that it was either the squalid environs of the poor, the nature of their home life, or 'familial tendencies' (a.k.a. genetics) that determined their medical misery.[48] In the United States the added factor of immigration clouded the picture, and native-born white health leaders found bigoted explanations for the poor health of recently arrived, impoverished workers. Anti-Semitism, stereotypes of Irish and Italian traits, anti-Catholicism, and other prejudiced perspectives offered easy explanations— albeit, as history has shown, incorrect ones.

The spectacular monetary gap between America's richest and poorest citizens was impossible to ignore at the turn of the century.[49] The top 1 per cent of America's income earners made more money in 1920 than did the bottom 50 per cent. Inescapably obvious to public advocates of the day were both the painful poverty of the people on society's lower rungs and its contribution to the paucity of healthy options available to them.

But at the turn of the twentieth century it was also common in both England and the United States to subsume concern about poverty beneath the thick layer of moral indignation that ascribed alcohol and drug use, sexually acquired illnesses, and psychiatric difficulties to the moral weaknesses or inferiority of poor people.

The germ theory crusaders of the early twentieth century, however noble their cause, were also incapable of confronting the roots of racial and economic disparities in health. With the rise of social Darwinism during the 1920s, explanations for racial variations in life expectancy and health shifted from the search for moral weakness to evolution and, in primitive form, genetics.[50]

The concept of 'racial immunity' to disease was a popular one among physicians and many public health advocates, but not among statisticians and demographers, who saw a very different picture in the disparate mortality rates. 'I do not believe that there is such a thing as *absolute* racial immunity to any disease,' wrote Metropolitan Life Insurance actuary Louis Dublin.[51] 'The Negro death rates for practically all diseases in the prevention or cure of which care and sanitation are of paramount importance are much higher than among the whites: but this does not prove that the Negroes are, *inherently*, more susceptible to such diseases—or, for that matter, that they are less resistant to them. It is probable that their higher death rate is due more than anything else to ignorance, poverty, and lack of proper medical care.'

In the West the gulfs between the races—Mexican-Americans, Chinese-Americans, and whites—were equally gargantuan. Mexican-Americans had, by the turn of the twentieth century, become the region's main unskilled labour force and by 1920, up to a third of all Mexican-American households in Los Angeles County had absentee fathers, and the mothers, who on average had more than four children, typically toiled in a distant Caucasian household.[52] Many factors probably contributed to their far-higher mortality rates, compared to whites,[53] but no one in the Los Angeles County Department of Health during the 1920s had the time or inclination to study the matter.[54]

Throughout the twentieth century, American public health leaders struggled with questions of race, genetics, ethnicity, and economic class, unable to define their relative impacts on individual and population health. And that debate, coupled with social exclusions from the health system, formed a critical, lasting, and shameful theme of US public health.

III

By the thirties, the expansionary era had come to an end, and the functions of public health were becoming more fixed and routine. The bacteriological revolution had played itself out in the organization of public services, and soon the introduction of antibiotics and other drugs would enable private physicians to reclaim some of their functions, like the treatment of venereal disease and tuberculosis. Yet it had been clear, long before, that public health in America was to be relegated to a secondary status: less prestigious than clinical medicine, less amply financed, and blocked from assuming the higher-level functions of coordination and direction that might have developed had it not been banished from medical care.

—Paul Starr, 1982 [55]

On October 29th the New York Stock Exchange crashed after several days of sharp declines, hurling the world into the Great Depression of the 1930s. Paul de Kruif, a bacteriologist who had become the best known science writer of his day,[56] travelled the country in the months following that black October day. His eyes were opened to a reality of poverty and disease that he—indeed, nearly all scientists of his day—had never before seen. Nearly boiling with rage, he wrote:

I don't know why it took me so long to see that the strength—and life-giving results of the toil of those searchers were *for sale*; that life was something you could have if you bought and paid for it; which meant you could have your share of it if you'd been shrewd, or crafty, or just lucky.

It still puzzles me why for so long I found excuses for our ghastly cartoon of a civilization—that's great...that's ruled by the Calvinistic humbug that God has predestined suffering and that suffering is good; that awards its searchers prizes, smirks congratulations at them, and allots the real benefits of their science to the well-heeled few; that turns its face from millions in pain, or hidden-hungry, or dying with an absolutely possible abundance of life-giving science all round them.

De Kruif turned completely from a public health booster who believed science would conquer humanity's worst diseases to the profession's sharpest critic. Amid national poverty on a scale America had never previously witnessed, de Kruif saw that years of ignoring the public health needs of the poor or, worse yet, blaming the poor for their own illnesses, were now undermining the very successes he had once loudly trumpeted.

In his travels across America, de Kruif saw a patchwork quilt of health; some communities were seemingly unaffected by the Depression whereas others experienced resurgent tuberculosis at levels he called 'murder', and crippling rheumatic fever epidemics among children (New York City's rate rose twenty-fold between 1929 and 1934). Government cutbacks had curtailed vaccination programmes in many states, prompting surges in diphtheria that de Kruif decried as 'damnable'. There was also soaring child malnutrition.

In 1935 a *New York World Telegram* editorial declared: 'One hundred and thirty-five thousand pupils in New York City's elementary schools are so weak from malnutrition that they cannot profit by attendance.... This is almost one in every five of the children enrolled—18.1 per cent in all.'

Sarcastically, de Kruif asked, 'Should children eat? Why keep them alive?'

Then he turned his formidable anger to birth issues, chronicling the 'fight for life' in grossly substandard Depression-era hospitals. All across North America, he argued, basic standards of hygiene had disappeared from hospitals. Mothers were again dying of puerperal fever at rates last seen before Semmelweis's great discovery about hand washing. Babies were succumbing to 'childbed fevers' as they were tended by nurses who changed one nappy after another without washing their hands. Syphilis and tuberculosis rates were soaring and, according to the National Tuberculosis Association, by 1937 TB was costing the nation $647 million a year in medical care and lost productivity. Yet hospitals had no funds to combat these scourges and departments of public health were on the edge of collapse all over the country. 'Let's face it,' de Kruif said, 'with the poverty of our hospitals and universities deepening and becoming more desperate, with our rulers, comptrollers, budget-balancers bellowing economy, there is small chance that this wherewithal will be forthcoming to train the new type of death fighter.'

Public health leaders, so recently America's heroes, were shunned, impotent, even forced to act as apologists for government and industry. The Charles Hewitts and Hermann Biggses of the world were long gone. Into their place stepped bureaucrats.

The Great Depression killed more than lives and economies: it rang the death knell for the public health revolution. The functions of public health were only saved through federalism, creating ever-larger national programmes staffed at all tiers of government by often lacklustre physicians and bureaucrats.

But when the stock market crashed in 1929, the federal public health effort was a jumbled mess involving forty different agencies that answered to five different cabinet secretaries. A total of five thousand US government civil servants worked in public health programmes of some kind. It was hardly a force equal to the challenge.

In the United States in the years following the crash every critical indicator of population health worsened, just as they did sixty years later in Eastern Europe following the collapse of the Soviet Union. Suicide rates among men soared, especially among unemployed men aged fifty to sixty-four years. And suicide rates, overall, went from 12 per 100 000 men and women in 1925 to 17.4 per 100 000 in 1932—the highest rate ever recorded in US history. Between 1929 and 1936 overall life expectancy for men and women combined rose slightly, but that masked a sharp decline of more than five years in life expectancy that occurred between 1933 and 1936.

During the Great Depression, the incidence of death from certain communicable diseases increased significantly nationwide, among them were scarlet fever, diphtheria, whooping cough, measles, influenza, and pneumonia. In some regions, tuberculosis and typhoid fever death rates also peaked during the 1930s. Worse, hospitals all across America closed. The problem, of course, was that the patients were broke and, regardless of whether they were government institutions or private facilities, the hospitals simply couldn't cover their operating costs. And with no money in their pockets, patients shunned the prestigious and private hospitals in favour of free care in government-owned facilities.

It is difficult to overstate the impact the Great Depression had on the lives, and health, of the American people. Unemployment ran between 10 and 40 per cent in most cities, with industrial centres hardest hit. Sales of consumer products and capital goods collapsed because overnight the consumer market disappeared. Farmers were forced to lower their prices so much that they couldn't cover the costs to harvest and transport their products. Over a quarter of a million farms were closed by 1932. Construction came to a complete halt.[57]

Entire industries closed their doors. Their former employees turned to relief offices where, increasingly, the city officials in charge turned them away. City coffers were empty. Hardest hit were the African-American, Mexican-American, and American Indian populations amongst whom unemployment ran as high as 60 to 75 per cent.

Also devastated were the beneficiaries of earlier public health triumphs: America's unprecedentedly large population of retired people over the age of sixty-five, which represented 5 per cent of the nation's population in 1929. Few of them had pensions or sources of income during the Depression. More than ten thousand banks collapsed nationwide between 1923 and 1932.

Local governments sought all sorts of solutions to the crisis, few of which were judicious or, in the end, effective.

The alternative to suicide for many families was relocation. Between 1929 and 1940 the nation's demography shifted radically as millions of people moved from one place to another in search of jobs. Many of them had been uprooted by the devastating dust storms of 1935, a result of decades of over-farming the soils of Arkansas, Texas, Oklahoma, and the Great Plains.

Many of these refugees went to California, where they were supremely unwelcome. Conservative Californians placed great faith in their native son, Herbert Hoover—the first westerner ever elected to the presidency. Even as the Great Depression worsened, most civic leaders accepted as wise policy Hoover's 1932 assumption that 'it is not the function of government to relieve individuals of their responsibilities to their neighbours, or to relieve private institutions of their responsibilities to the public.' It was a sentiment to be heard from California-spawned presidents well into the future.

Class war was brewing in the West. 'Hoovervilles', clapboard housing slums loaded with dust bowl refugees and itinerant workers, sprang up outside every large western city. Labour organizers, from anarchists with the Industrial Workers of the World (IWW) to Eugene V. Debs socialists, found fertile soil amid the outrage. Trade unionists throughout California staged demonstrations and all manner of protests against the 'capitalist bosses'.

Los Angeles's leaders responded to the mounting tension by targetting Mexicans and Mexican-Americans for mass deportation, beginning in 1931.[58]

In this topsy-turvy atmosphere, all aspects of governance were strained, and public health was no exception. On the eve of the stock market crash, the County Department of Health had 400 employees; ten years later it had 419. During that time the population it served swelled from about 677 000 people to 900 000, though the numbers involved some guess work, as on any given day nobody really knew how many Mexicans, 'Okies', or Mexican-Americans were living in the county. Department reports from the time have a breathless quality to them, as if even the moments spent hammering at a typewriter were precious. An American Public Health Association assessment of the department's performance in 1930 found it 'severely wanting,' as its beleaguered staff raced about the vast county barely able to meet the populace's most basic health needs.

Even in times of prosperity during the 1920s, when Dr Pomeroy had planned for a network of health clinics spanning the vast county, his dream had been quashed by the weighty opposition of the local American Medical Association, which would brook no competition from government. By 1935 most of Pomeroy's planned health-care system lay in shreds, the victim not only of AMA assault but, probably more significantly, of attack from a new and growing group: red baiters. Provision of health services for the poor, even in times when most Los Angelenos were suffering, was considered 'socialistic' by the county's elite, and they followed the Los Angeles Times's lead in denouncing alleged abuse of tax-supported services by the so-called undeserving poor.

In the midst of such chaos, whooping cough, diphtheria, typhoid fever, puerperal fever, maternal and infant mortality, and tuberculosis rates all rose during the Great Depression. And in 1934 when polio struck hard in Los Angeles, the health department couldn't cope.

This polio strain was unusual in that many cases involved adults, few victims suffered paralysis, death rates were low, and most had what appeared to be encephalitis.

County health officials were at a loss to explain how the disease was spreading, why it was causing such bizarre symptoms, how it could be stopped, or what treatments might work.[59]

By the epidemic's height, public health authority had completely broken down. Fearing infection (which had passed to many health workers) public hospital staff abandoned their posts, leaving remaining personnel so overwhelmed that stretchers and trolleys, laden with waiting patients, stretched around the block and for hours on end ailing children wailed and victims called in vain for assistance.

For years afterwards, the LA County Department of Health spoke with a meek voice and was rarely able to gain recognition or cooperation from the region's political leaders, physicians, or general populace.

And it was not alone. Counties, cities, and states all over the United States fell apart between 1929 and 1933 as tax revenues disappeared. In some areas, physicians volunteered their services for epidemic control duty. But before the presidential election of Franklin Delano Roosevelt, most public health departments in the United States had either already shattered, as was the case in Los Angeles County, or were teetering on the brink of collapse.

One significant exception was Minnesota, which had swung so far to the left during the Great Depression that Roosevelt's Democratic Party became its targeted right wing. Just weeks after the stock market crashed, Minnesotans elected Minneapolis leftist Floyd Olson to the governor's seat, putting his Farm Labour Party in power. That party considered social programmes, such as those for public health, of paramount importance and dismissed opposition to public welfare as part and parcel of some dark capitalist plot. 'As long as I sit in the governor's chair,' Olson said, 'there is not going to be any misery in the state if I can humanely prevent it. I hope the present system of government goes right down to Hell.' To that end, public health programmes gained prominence during the Olson years and were pushed toward provision of medical and disease control services for rural farmers and the urban poor.

Long after the reign of Farm Labour ended in the 1940s its impact on Minnesota politics and public health could still be felt. And for six decades Minnesota was famous for both its high rates of graduated income taxation and strong tax-supported social programmes, including public health and provision of medical care for indigent and poor working Minnesotans.

By the end of Roosevelt's nearly four-term presidency, public health in the United States had been federalized. Each municipality and state offered its own unique brand of health services and programmes, but what was once totally based on local revenues became dependent on dollars from Washington. And with that beneficence came Washington-dictated policies and increased power and influence for the US Public Health Service (USPHS).

The USPHS was initially a tiny federal force with authority strictly limited to the main ports of entry into the United States—particularly New York's Ellis Island and San Francisco's Angel Island—and to national contagion catastrophes. That changed after a showdown in California in 1901, just after *Yersinia pestis*, the plague, struck San Francisco's Chinatown.[60] It was no doubt brought by sea from Shanghai or Hong Kong. Angel Island USPHS microbiologist Joseph Kinyoun analysed the blood of Chinatown patients and rats and confirmed the presence of *Yersinia pestis*. He immediately alerted California and federal authorities.

Governor of California Henry T. Gage dismissed Kinyoun's findings as hogwash. Republican Gage would brook absolutely no such obstacles to California's development and population expansion. So he simply said there was no plague in California.

After an eighteen-month Kinyoun/Gage standoff, an independent review commission confirmed the presence of *Yersinia pestis*. And for the first time in US history, federal health authorities took charge of an epidemic control effort, without a request from or support of state leaders (but at the urgent behest of San Francisco local health officials).[61]

In 1912 Congress granted the USPHS authority to intervene at the local level on behalf of the health of *all* Americans, not just seamen and immigrants, and gave the agency authority over basic medical research.[62] The first sweeping federal health law, the 1921 Sheppard-Towner Act gave the USPHS annual pots of money from which to hand out to state grants for well-baby programmes. This set the precedent for a new model of funding that would become the dominant paradigm of the remainder of the century: money would filter from federal sources down to the states and cities and would arrive already earmarked for implementation of policies that had been decided by federal health authorities and congressional politicians.

Given that, unlike in Europe, public health in the United States had originated at the local level and matured as a patchwork quilt of very diverse infrastructures, each with different rules and authorities, the imposition of such top-down policy making was odd. It proved impossible to come up with suitable general health policies and, over the coming decades, local public health authorities had conflicting opinions about the federal generosity: they wanted the money but might dispute the policy to which it was attached.

The Sheppard-Towner Act was an indisputable boon, however, to the forty-one states that made use of the funds during the 1920s.

In 1926 the National Health Council, a consortium of private medical and public health organizations, submitted a report to Congress describing public health in the United States as a feeble and disjointed array of largely leaderless efforts that fell under five different cabinets of the executive branch. Some five thousand civil servants, working in forty different agencies, played a role in setting public health policy and executing actions of one kind or another. The USPHS was hardly alone, or even in charge.

At the Democratic Party nominating convention in 1932, Franklin Delano Roosevelt had called for a 'New Deal for America' in which banks and finance were regulated and the state extended its charitable hand to rescue the masses from their dire straits. Upon taking office in 1933, Roosevelt surrounded himself with a coterie of advisors, swiftly dubbed 'The Brain Trust' by the press, and set to work creating his New Deal. Congress passed nearly every piece of legislation the White House sent it, and by the end of 1933 America was taking the first tentative steps out of the Great Depression.

The New Deal's impact on the nation's public health infrastructure was profound and proved lasting. A dozen agencies were created between 1933 and 1938, each of which affected the health of Americans. And most of these agencies in some form, became permanent components of the US government.

No state turned its back on what the New Deal offered (not even Minnesota), but no one made better use of it than New York City's dynamic mayor, Fiorello La Guardia.

Even before he ascended to New York's throne, La Guardia told Roosevelt that he would happily allow the president to use Gotham as a testing—and proving—ground for every New Deal programme. He made this promise even though his 1933 victory was not assured.

During the Roaring Twenties Tammany's grip on the health department was absolute, even defying Hermann Biggs' attempts at reform after his 1923 elevation to New York State Commissioner of Health Dr Frank J. Monaghan's thoroughly corrupt leadership of the health department in every way undermined the very programmes that had made New York City a national public health model.

But Tammany's greed finally went too far, becoming too blatant even for remarkably corruption tolerant New York City. Private citizens' organizations dug up enough dirt to force Monaghan out in 1925 and his successor, Dr Louis Harris, discovered still more evidence of astounding fraud, patronage, and extortion. One ring of restaurant inspectors alone had been extorting $3 million a year from eating establishment owners who were compelled to pay five dollars 'protection' a week. A $1 million fund for contagion control had simply disappeared.

Harris—by all accounts an honest man—ordered a long list of firings and indictments followed. But the department's credibility with the public had eroded severely. In 1928 the private Welfare Council of New York published its *Health Inventory of*

New York City, which was highly critical of the health department. It said that nearly every programme was in a shambles. The damage done by Harris's predecessor was simply overwhelming.

Into this Great Depression quagmire stepped the man known as the Little Flower, Fiorello, and after 146 years in existence, during seventy-seven of which it criminally manipulated New York City and the National Democratic Party, the Tammany machine was finally vanquished.

The conversations with Roosevelt's Brain Trust paid off less than a year after La Guardia took office and a hallmark of his tenure was his uncanny ability to match New York's needs with Roosevelt's New Deal agenda. New Deal money paid for mosquito abatement and marshland drainage, a study of New York's rising air pollution problems, and a 'full-scale assault on VD'.

Between 1935 and 1937 the New York City Department of Health underwent a construction boom, providing new laboratories, clinics, and offices—all thanks to federal dollars from the Public Works Administration (WPA). La Guardia boasted, 'We have cleaned politics out of the Health Department in just the same way that we're chasing microbes, germs, and bugs out of our city.'

One New Deal–funded study revealed in 1937 that in New York City as in Los Angeles (though through different mechanisms) the Great Depression had taken a far greater toll on non-white versus white residents. Mortality rates among New York African-Americans and other men of colour were 473 per cent higher than among white men. And infant mortality among non-whites was double that of white babies.

In his final term in office, after the end of the Depression, La Guardia awoke to a startling realization: despite fifteen years of economic hardship for the people of New York, hospitals and doctors there had become very prosperous—so prosperous that city employees could no longer afford health care. So in 1944 La Guardia set up the first municipal health insurance programme in the United States. The city covered half of all health expenses for employees earning more than $5000 a year and fully covered costs for lesser-paid city workers.

But long before La Guardia took the nation down the path of health insurance, the AMA kicking and screaming in protest each step of the way, he and Health Commissioner Dr John Rice used New Deal money to transform public health activities in Gotham. In the department's 1938 annual report, Rice acknowledged that the very mission of public health had changed. Though scourges of contagion, notably syphilis, tuberculosis, bacterial pneumonia, meningitis, and polio, continued to plague the population, 'diseases which influence mortality rates' could no longer absorb most of the department's energies. Rather, said the prescient Rice, in the future public health would need to 'include consideration of physical and mental disorders which affect the general health and well-being of the community'.

By that time one out of every five dollars spent by the New York City Department of Health was of federal origin. Given that just four years previously the city's public health effort hadn't received a nickel from Washington, that was a marked change of affairs. And in 1940, for the first time, the department faced a funding crisis that proved an ominous indicator of things to come: changes in White House policies had trickled down the funding ladder through an array of New Deal bureaucracies in Washington and suddenly New York faced a 21 per cent cut in Public Works Administration revenues. Doctors and nurses in many divisions saw their incomes halved overnight as they were reduced to part-time status. This also proved a harbinger of future weaknesses in America's public health safety net.

Dependency can be a terrible thing, especially if the terms of a dole are dictated entirely by the donor. In coming decades public health programmes grew increasingly reliant upon Washington's largesse and, therefore, more vulnerable to the whims and priorities of faraway politicians over whom they had little or no influence. Without the political savvy of a Hermann Biggs or the supportive political hustle of a Fiorello La Guardia, few localities proved immune from the tug of war with Washington.

However, the New Deal's impact on public health was remarkably positive and the benefits often came from surprising sources. The health of American Indians improved as a result of changes in their land rights under the Indian Reorganization Act of 1934. Mortality decreased among farmers and 'Okie' farm workers as a result of New Deal agricultural programmes. Rural areas saw their food poisoning rates go down as the Tennessee Valley Authority brought electricity to tens of thousands of households, allowing installation of refrigerators. Eight million workers suddenly had money with which to feed their children, thanks to employment with the WPA. Hookworm infection rates declined as southern families earned enough to provide their children with shoes.

The 1934 congressional elections swept so many Roosevelt supporters into the House and Senate that Republicans formed an impotent minority. Despite its tremendous popularity, Roosevelt's Brain Trust met its match when the administration moved to create health insurance and Social Security programmes. Roosevelt's plan was to create a 'cradle-to-grave' social insurance programme that would cover every American's health, medical, and pension needs and would be financed through a payroll contribution system. Roosevelt imagined a system that would serve as a safety net for unemployed workers, offer prenatal care to their pregnant wives, and provide a living wage for retired people. As he conceived it, every American, regardless of race or class, would come under the US Social Security umbrella.

That was going too far.

Southern political leaders said they would never vote for a law that might carve cents out of the paychecks of white workers to pay unemployment benefits to 'Negroes to sit around in idleness on front galleries.' The Republican Party said the Roosevelt plan was overtly socialist and, by said definition, had to be blocked.

And, of course, the American Medical Association chipped in again, with its leaders opposing all of the health insurance provisions of Roosevelt's Social Security proposal.

In the face of dogged opposition, the finally adopted Social Security Act of 1935 compromised or defeated all of Roosevelt's original intentions for it and was a deeply flawed piece of legislation. As the AMA had hoped, it had no provisions for health insurance.

Thus, for the second time in US history, the possibility of universal health care based on compulsory insurance was raised—and defeated. And the primary force responsible for vanquishing it was, in both cases, the AMA.

Paul de Kruif, who was highly critical of the compromises struck in the Social Security Act, eventually concluded that the only hope of salvaging public health in the United States rested with further federalization and creation of a large corps of USPHS officers. He advocated creation of something not unlike the future US Centers for Communicable Diseases.

In *The Fight for Life* de Kruif wrote:

> Why cannot our US Public Health Service be entrusted with co-ordinating in the instances of these now-preventable plagues, the people's fight for life? You hear the wail that this will breed a new bureaucracy. Let this then be remembered: we have an army and a navy supported by the government, by all the people—to defend our nation against threat of human invasion that becomes real not once in a generation. They are bureaucracies, granted.
>
> But is it anywhere advocated that the army and the navy be turned over to private hands and the defense of our country be left to us individuals armed with scythes and shotguns, because the army and navy are bureaucratic? . . . Who then objects to the organization of a death-fighting army against the far more dangerous subvisible assassins in ambush for all the people—always? . . .
>
> If you allow our death-fighters—we can assure you they are competent— the money to wipe out such and such and such deaths that cost us billions to maintain, within a generation there will no longer be this drain upon the wealth of our nation.

IV

There is no reason to doubt, of course, the ability of the scientific method to solve each of the specific problems of disease by discovering causes and remedial procedures. Whether concerned with particular dangers to be overcome or with specific requirements to be satisfied, all the separate problems of human health can and will eventually find their solution. But solving problems of disease is not the same thing as creating health and happiness.

—René Dubos, 1959[63]

At 7:55 a.m. on December 7, 1941, the Japanese air force attacked the US naval fleet based in Hawaii, thus compelling American involvement in World War II.

Although the military economy created jobs and brought the Great Depression to an end, it also skewed government spending toward the war front. For many parts of the country, the sudden shift of federal funds away from domestic spending proved painful—local governments had grown accustomed to New Deal dollars.

The Minnesota Department of Health, for example, had planned on a 1942 budget of $764 134, of which 60 per cent ($453 496) was to come from federal funds. Most of that federal contribution, however, was diverted by Washington to the war effort. In addition, tens of thousands of public health professionals—doctors and nurses— were recruited to the war effort, thus depleting domestic services of vital personnel.

On the other hand, the war propelled vital public health research, resulting in bold new programmes for control of insect-borne diseases (notably typhus, yellow fever, and malaria), bacterial infections, and venereal diseases. And by the end of the 1940s, Americans had shifted their concern from microbes to two chronic killers: cardiovascular diseases and cancer. Commensurate with that shift came a slow change in how people in the United States viewed their physical milieu: once considered a constantly threatening miasma of germs, it began to seem controllable, even subservient, to human exigencies.

By 1941 Roosevelt's New Deal had vastly improved the nation's health. Per-capita health spending, having plummeted in the middle of the Great Depression by 120 per cent, surpassed pre-crash levels in 1941, reaching nearly $4000. Life expectancies for whites rose from the despairingly low 61.1 years of 1934 to 64.8 years for babies born in 1941—a net gain of 3.7 years of life. Non-white Americans gained two years of life during those years, rising from a 1934 level of 51.8 years to, in 1941, 53.8 years. One clear reason was food: Americans in 1941 were at last able to afford to eat as much as they had in 1929, before the stock market crash. Tuberculosis, scarlet fever, typhoid, and malaria death rates all improved markedly—the latter two were halved.

After Pearl Harbor, the challenge for local authorities was to maintain 1941's rosy health picture amid wartime staff reductions and scarcities and in the face of new, war-related health crises—all at a time of enormous social movement and upset.

Roles were shifting in America as women filled employment positions vacated by drafted men and blacks, migrating en masse from the South to military production centres of the far West and Midwest, entered the industrial workforce on an enormous scale. Economic wealth followed the war industry and the number one beneficiary of World War II government spending and financial growth was Los Angeles County. Most of California's $19 billion in military contracts went to Los Angeles, which by the war's end was the nation's second-largest industrial centre and had the largest and most modern industrial infrastructure in the entire world.

Between 1940 and 1945 the population of California grew 135 per cent from 6 982 000 to 9 491 000, and most of that increase occurred in Los Angeles County.

On July 26, 1943, the burgeoning, industrious, and unsettled metropolis of Los Angeles experienced Black Monday. It was the fourth day of horrible air pollution in the region and the worst Los Angeles had ever endured. As the *Los Angeles Times* described it: 'With the entire downtown area engulfed by a low-hanging cloud of acrid smoke, yesterday morning city health and police authorities began investigations to determine the source of the "gas attack" that left thousands of Angelenos with irritated eyes, noses, and throats. . . . Visibility was cut to less than three blocks in some sections of the business district.'

A word was invented to describe that haze: *smog*. Though by the 1950s smog enveloped cities from Rio to New York, Los Angeles was the first to suffer its ongoing assault. On 'good days' the nauseating mass was blown eastward by winds from the Pacific, but on Black Monday the cleansing winds didn't blow for days on end and the smog formed brown layers of carbon monoxide, ozone, and industrial effluent.

Three years later, when smog had become a nearly permanent feature of Los Angeles, Ed Ainsworth wrote in the *Los Angeles Times*: 'The recent rain washed the once-celebrated air of Los Angeles and gave Southern California an unaccustomed view of an object known as the sun . . . through the pall of "smog" which settled over Los Angeles in 1943 and has persisted with exasperating firmness ever since, it hardly ever was visible to the naked eye.'

Near the oil fields of Long Beach the peculiar haze was regularly redolent with sulphur and methane, prompting local residents to talk of 'rotten egg days.' Eastward toward Fontana around the steel mills, smog tasted vaguely metallic in the back of residents' throats. In the posh San Gabriel Valley towns of Pasadena and San Marino, the eyes first sensed smog's arrival, producing tears uncontrollably. Children who ran and played outside were soon overcome by aching lungs and powerful headaches.

In the mad haste to grow, grow, grow that had been Los Angeles's hallmark since Anglo estate agents first began advertising it to potential buyers from the Midwest during the 1890s, the county had given little thought to the fact that it lay in a basin and was subject to periodic, prolonged air inversions.

By 1941 Los Angeles no longer had its Big Red railway system, and it was criss-crossed by roads, boulevards, and motorways used daily by hundreds of thousands of motorists. Long before the car took hold in the rest of America, Los Angeles had developed a car commuter culture.

Black Monday and the subsequent wartime smog were the result of combined industrial and auto emissions. And, for the always understaffed and beleaguered County Department of Health, smog was a nightmare that stretched the department to its limits.

By the time the war ended, Los Angeles County had more than 4 million residents and over four thousand square miles. Forty of its forty-five incorporated cities contracted with the County Department of Health not only for public health but also for medical services.

Dr Roy O. Gilbert, who took over as Los Angeles County health officer in 1945, made it clear that the primary task of public health remained communicable diseases control. Unable to obtain special funding with which to address the smog problem and lacking solid scientific evidence that the irritating gases constituted a public health crisis, Gilbert simply added 'air pollution' to the long list of duties for the department's Sanitation Section.

In 1947, four years after Black Monday, California enacted its first of many pieces of legislation aimed at reducing the presumed health risk of air pollution. The law gave health authorities the right to declare smog alert days. On heavily polluted days, the Los Angeles County Department of Health would issue warnings requesting that residents avoid driving, stay indoors, and keep children from running and playing. In some Los Angeles school districts, smog alerts prompted principals to ban all forms of student exercise; during breaks youngsters were told to lie down indoors. Powerless to control the sources of smog and lacking funding for research on air pollution measurement, the health department could do little more.

Over the next decade researchers worldwide analysed smog and concluded that it contained a host of chemicals considered dangerous to human health: cyclic hydrocarbons, carbon monoxide, nitrous oxides, sulphur dioxide, benzpyrene, ozone, and lead. Public anxiety about smog increased when some of its contents were found to cause cancer in laboratory animals. But it was decades before the sources of smog were effectively reduced. In the meantime, public health leaders stood by helplessly, convinced, as Columbia University's George Rosen wrote in 1958, that 'the atmosphere of the modern industrial community is a carcinogenic sea, polluted and made murky by many sorts of individual waste. In such an environment it is hardly possible to avoid daily contact with cancer-producing agents.... However, inherent difficulties have so far prevented a full epidemiological and technical solution of the problem.'

In California air pollution standards would not be set until 1956, and the car was not formally identified as the primary source of smog until so designated by the Air Pollution Control Board of Southern California in 1959. For the remainder of the decade pollution control officials, petrol distributors, and car manufacturers sparred over standards for car engine design, fuel, and emissions. Particularly striking was the comparatively minor role public health leaders eventually played in the struggle against smog, a battle largely waged through political and regulatory action at the federal level.

It was well over a decade before such things as chemical pollution and smog were linked to a growing public—and public health—concern about cancer, and there was also a time lag after the war before the growing incidence of heart disease became alarming.

During the war years Minnesota remained a comparatively clean, if freezing cold, state where the incidences of nearly all communicable diseases continued to fall. The most dramatic mortality shift for wartime Minnesotans was due to heart disease.

When the Japanese struck Pearl Harbor, Minnesotans were dying of heart disease at a rate of about 270 per 100 000. By the time the war ended and the troops had returned home, in 1947, the cardiovascular death rate had increased dramatically, reaching 309.7 per 100 000. It was the largest increase in heart disease Minnesotans had ever seen.

The state's Department of Health had long accepted that heart disease was its populace's number one killer, yet did little to try to control it. In part the inaction was because, like its counterparts all over the United States, the Minnesota State Department of Health was constructed around a communicable diseases model and had little idea how to tackle chronic ailments. In addition, at the time, most physicians thought of heart attacks and strokes as inevitable components of old age. They were wrong, as the sharp increase in deaths among younger men, aged forty-five to fifty-four years, indicated.

Public health leaders in the state had little knowledge at the time of the relative roles smoking, poor diet, and lack of exercise played in the cause of heart disease. Minnesota was at the front end of a radical change in American lifestyles in which a host of factors were interacting to increase the risks of cardiovascular diseases. Machinery had made Minnesota's farmers more sedentary; the car had made everyone more sedentary; and diets were changing. Supermarkets appeared and offered processed foods high in the fat, sugar, and salt that improved sales. Treats, laborious to prepare at home, suddenly became abundant.

Tens of thousands of men had acquired a taste for chain-smoking while on the World War II battlefields. Cigarette sales soared in the 1940s and 1950s and smoking suddenly became socially acceptable in virtually every setting from offices to churches, schools to cinemas, hospital waiting rooms to doctors' offices. Every medium, even the *Journal of the American Medical Association* and many other leading medical publications, ran cigarette adverts. In fact, public health leaders in the 1940s saw no reason to attack America's love affair with the cigarette.

During the war years, the biggest source of public health consternation in all cities that served as staging and leave sites for military personnel was the escalating venereal diseases rate. In New York's case, the battle against gonorrhoea and syphilis consumed the city's communicable diseases control resources, leaving few dollars or health personnel to fight the old scourges of tuberculosis and childhood diseases.

Nationally, syphilis and gonorrhoea rates had been rising steadily since the turn of the century and no public health agency had developed an effective strategy for venereal diseases control.[64] At the end of World War I national syphilis rates averaged 113 per 100 000. By the end of World War II average syphilis rates had reached 450 per 100 000, with the highest incidence among military men.

Gonorrhoea had shown an overall rising trend since 1900, though national rates had fluctuated. During the middle of the Depression, gonorrhoea had averaged 121 cases per 100 000 Americans. In 1941 the rate rose to 146.7 per 100 000, and in 1944 it reached 236.5 per 100 000.

From the earliest days of organized public health, Americans had exhibited a peculiar inability to cope with the conjunction of three fearsome factors: sex, disease, and death. In colonial America and later in the United States, even non-sexual diseases were traditionally framed in moralistic terms.[65] Reflecting the general American predilection for Christian moralism, social condemnation of individuals who suffered from venereal diseases was far more extreme in the United States than in Europe. And, as a direct result, individuals with syphilis and gonorrhoea were more likely to hide their ailments until the diseases reached physically obvious, and completely incurable, tertiary stages. Secrecy, of course, required that there be no change in one's behaviour lest a spouse question why a partner no longer desired sexual intercourse. So shame supported the spread of gonorrhoea and syphilis.[66]

In the 1930s hospitals all across America had a policy of refusing to treat venereal diseases on the grounds that the patients were immoral. It was as if the alleged lack of morality was, itself, contagious. Even the AMA—usually a staunch opponent of government-provided health services—offered no resistance to the creation of public health VD clinics, isolated from the hospitals and staffed by government doctors and nurses.

Congress passed the Venereal Disease Act in 1935, giving the USPHS authority to conduct research on syphilis and gonorrhoea. A year earlier, New York State's health commissioner, Dr Thomas Parran, was taken off CBS Radio for uttering the word *syphilis* on the air. Shortly thereafter, Roosevelt appointed Parran his Surgeon General, and the New Yorker made VD one of his primary causes.

For many years the highest rates of syphilis and gonorrhoea had been seen among African-American men, a fact that reinforced the white racist view of profligate, rampant sexual activity among blacks. Because of the racial stereotyping and moralism surrounding sexual diseases, African-Americans resented all discussion of syphilis and gonorrhoea in their communities.

One of the highest syphilis rates in the entire world was in Macon County, Alabama, where in 1932 Dr Taliaferro Clark of the USPHS discovered that 35 per cent of the black population had syphilis and 90 per cent of the cases had gone untreated.

The USPHS funded Tuskegee University, working under Clark, to conduct a study of syphilis in Macon County, Alabama.[67] Under the original study design, Tuskegee was to recruit four hundred black men who already had syphilis and two hundred who did not for tests and observation. No treatment was to be provided, as it would interfere with the study's two goals: to determine the long-term course of the disease in the absence of treatment and to note the peculiarities of the disease in black men. (There was widespread, mistaken belief among physicians that blacks responded differently to the disease than did whites.) Though white physicians initiated the study, over its four decades it was executed by African-American nurses and doctors as well.

In order to lure men into the study, none of the patients was told he had syphilis— rather, they learned from the Tuskegee staff that they suffered from 'bad blood'. And for years their continued participation was guaranteed by the provision of free transportation, hot meals, medical care for non-syphilitic minor ailments, and burial insurance. Initially imagined as a six-month study, the Tuskegee experiment lasted until 1972. During that time, the Macon County men and their families were never told that they had syphilis. Nor were they provided with penicillin in 1943 when USPHS researchers discovered that it could cure syphilis. For decades the USPHS continued the study and outside reviewers approved it, until an Associated Press journalist stumbled upon its existence in 1972. A storm of publicity followed, as a result of which study participant Charlie Pollard learned he had been duped and was dying of syphilis. He retained the famous civil rights attorney Fred D. Gray, who in 1974 brought a class action suit on behalf of all the Macon men against the USPHS. In an out-of-court settlement, each of the surviving men got a paltry $37 000 in compensation.

By then, all but seventy-two of the participants were dead, most having suffered the extremes of tertiary syphilis: infection and destruction of the brain and heart and lesions all over the skin, mouth, and genitals. Thirty had died directly from syphilis and at least seventy more of complications associated with their venereally acquired infection. Never realizing that they carried an infectious disease, by 1974 the men had passed syphilis on to twenty-two of their wives, who transmitted the diseases to seventeen children and they to two grandchildren.

The travesty of Tuskegee festered in both the public health and African-American communities, widening a credibility gap that was already vast. Eventually, the divide became so great that in the 1990s all US government public health pronouncements and programmes were viewed with hostility, even outright contempt, by African-Americans of all social classes.

The legacy of the Tuskegee experiment proved to be an extreme example of a larger failure for American public health. Throughout the twentieth century there were glaring differences in the life expectancies, health statuses, infant mortalities, and access to medical care for white versus non-white US citizens. Public health leaders proved ineffectual, apologist, blatantly racist, or determinedly ignorant in these matters. By the 1960s the divide between public health (both government and academic) and the nation's minority communities had become explosive.

Because the Tuskegee subjects were functionally illiterate, they never realized that they were suffering the very symptoms that, beginning in 1936, were emblazoned on flyers and notices distributed nationwide by the US Surgeon General's office. That is also why they never learned, as did most Americans, about two landmark discoveries that could have cured their 'bad blood'.

In 1937 USPHS physician John Mahoney, working in the government's Staten Island laboratory, discovered that sulpha drugs could kill gonorrhoeal bacteria. Five years earlier, Scottish scientist Alexander Fleming discovered a sulpha compound he called penicillin. And it proved powerfully effective in laboratory tests against a broad range of bacteria.

In 1943 Mahoney showed that penicillin and other sulpha antibiotics could also kill tough spirochaetes like syphilis; a discovery that opened a new door for public health. Immediately both civilian and military physicians realized that if the promise of a cure could flush all the ashamed gonorrhoea and syphilis carriers out of hiding and encourage them to name their sexual partners, it would be possible to treat all of the cases and thus halt the spread of venereal diseases.

And by all accounts, penicillin seemed the long-awaited magic bullet promised sixty years previously by Erlich. In tiny doses the drug miraculously healed even the advanced cases of syphilis and gonorrhoea. And when supplies ran short, army doctors discovered that even the unmeasurable quantities of the drug that had passed into the urine of a treated patient could be used to cure another.

Within months of Mahoney's discovery of using penicillin for syphilis treatment, the New York City health department opened a special VD ward at Bellevue Hospital and distributed free penicillin to doctors and hospitals citywide. The city also instituted contact tracing policies under which all syphilitic and gonorrhoeal patients were forced to name their recent sexual contacts, who were subsequently tracked down, interrogated, and treated. When necessary, either because the contact's full name wasn't known or the individual refused treatment, officers of the New York Police Department were deployed. Biggs's old typhoid tactics of five decades earlier were resurrected for venereal disease.

Similar procedures were followed all over the United States after 1943, and US average rates of syphilis fell from an all-time high of 447 per 100 000 in 1943 to 154 per 100 000 in 1950, and to 43 per 100 000 by 1970.

Gonorrhoea rates, however, proved more mercurial. Unlike syphilis, gonorrhoea could respond to a single dose of penicillin and patients wanting privacy who could afford to see a private physician could remain outside the net of public health scrutiny. Amid widespread overuse of the new antibiotic by private physicians, penicillin-resistant strains of gonorrhoea soon emerged, further limiting successful control. During the 1950s rates fell as low as 129 per 100 000, but by 1970 they had surpassed the 1947 all-time high of 284.

Antibiotics allowed a similar transformation in public health approaches to tuberculosis. In 1944 the Mayo Clinic in Minnesota successfully used streptomycin to cure TB in a group of hospitalized patients and public health leaders immediately recognized that the contact tracing model could be applied to the control of tuberculosis. By 1970 the national tuberculosis rate had been cut by 91 per cent, compared to its 1944 level.[68]

The primary impact of the antibiotic revolution on other bacterial diseases, such as streptococcal pneumonia and typhoid fever, was an immediate reduction in death rates. In some cases the rates approached zero. Between 1936 and 1945 pneumonia death rates nationwide fell to less than 1 per cent of all cases, a 40 per cent drop. Though health departments continued to keep track of the bacterial diseases and distribute available vaccines, they were medically controlled by antibiotics. Physicians, antibiotics in hand, wrested authority over the bacterial domain from public health and never again relinquished their power except during epidemics. This proved a serious problem, as antibiotic-resistant strains of the old killers began to emerge.

In 1943, even before Mahoney proved penicillin could cure syphilis, there were already more than three thousand six hundred antibiotic products in some stage of development. That figure increased ten-fold over the next decade. So great was public excitement over the magic bullets that most of these products were ushered into clinical use after only a modicum of testing. As a result, side-effects were often severe and dosages uncertain. The use of antibiotics therefore actually increased national hospitalization rates, as doctors generally urged their patients to take the miracle drugs only under close supervision. Civilian hospital admissions rose during the war, from about 10.5 million in 1941 to 14 million in 1946, and most were voluntary. Thus, the antibiotic revolution increased the power of hospitals, transplanting entire fields of public health from the home or community level into the entirely physician-controlled environment of institutional medicine.

Germany surrendered in May 1945 and the Pacific effort escalated that spring. On July 16th, four months after Roosevelt had died in office, a team of physicists successfully tested the world's first atomic bomb in Alamogordo, New Mexico. For three weeks the administration of President Harry S. Truman internally debated use of the new weapon, then on August 6th the *Enola Gay* dropped its payload on the Japanese city of Hiroshima. Three days later a second atom bomb fell on Nagasaki.

Japan surrendered on August 15, 1945, bringing World War II to an end.

And within nine months of Victory in Japan Day, the first children of the largest baby boom in US history were born. By the time the baby boom had ended in 1964 the nation's women had given birth to 76.4 million babies, bringing the US population to more than 105 million.

The economy boomed, too. The US gross national product increased from $100 billion in 1939 to 1945's $212 billion. Though Americans might quibble about President Truman's performance, they were passionately patriotic at the war's end and proud of the government of the United States. Federalism had served them well, ushering the country out of the Great Depression, guiding the nation to victory in battlefields all over the world, and rewarding the citizens with phenomenal postwar prosperity.

It seemed an auspicious time to reconsider the comprehensive health plan President Truman had submitted to Congress two years earlier, only to have it languish in committee.

In 1946, however, the Republican Party gained control of Congress in national elections and Senator Robert Taft took over the relevant health committee. Taft made it clear that public health ought to be meted out to the poor as each state saw fit and the poor should accept whatever they got, on whatever terms were dictated.

Some Republicans went further, charging that 'socialized medicine' was all part of a Moscow-dictated Communist plan. The Cold War was getting under way both internationally and domestically and public health was caught in the crossfire.

The health of Americans was undergoing a great transition in the 1950s. Only a handful of infections diseases still claimed or maimed significant numbers of children every year, noteably measles, pertussis, tetanus, and polio. Though the actual numbers of polio sufferers in America and Western Europe were far higher in the early part of the century, the disease produced greatest anxiety during the 1950s, when about 32,000 people, mostly children under six years of age, suffered annually from the disease. As the numbers of paralysed and dead children mounted genuine panic set in across the country. Polio was conquered as a result of a unique nongovernmental initiative. The National Foundation for Infant Paralysis, waged a March of Dimes campaign in the 1950s to raise funds for polio research. Nearly two-thirds of Americans made donations. The foundation had a public health, not a curative medical, goal. Rather that fund the search for a treatment, it was to eliminate, via development of a vaccine, the threat polio posed.

But the virus was extremely difficult to study until in 1949 Drs John Enders and Thomas Weller, and Frederick C. Robbins created a simple way to mass produce polio viruses. By 1953 Dr Jonas Salk had a killed virus vaccine. But the key proved to be adding an adjuvant (a potentizer) developed by Dr Jules Freund at New York's Public Health Research Institute.

Gotham's Health Commissioner announced the discovery of the adjuvant to 1953, declaring the city's intention to be the first test site of large-scale human use of the Salk vaccine, and more than 80 000 six-to-eight-year-old New York City schoolchildren rolled up their sleeves for shots of either Salk's vaccine or a placebo. In 1954 and '55 tens of thousands of children nationwide enlisted as Polio Pioneers to serve as willing guinea pigs for the vaccine. The fear of polio was far greater than any parental concerns about the experimental nature of the vaccine. And on April 12, 1955—a date selected because it marked the tenth anniversary of the death of polio victim Franklin Delano Roosevelt—Jonas Salk announced that the polio vaccine was safe and effective. The reaction nationwide was jubilant. Church bells rang from coast to coast. Schools all over the country held celebration assemblies. And every news organization worldwide spread the word in elated tones.

Few doubted that Salk's vaccine was one of the great triumphs of public health. The moment the Salk vaccine went into widespread use in the spring of 1955 polio began to disappear from North America. But Salk's rival, Albert Sabin, warned, "Everybody in the public health field knows that when you reach the point where you begin to inoculate an agent into millions of children, your probelms have only just begun."

Indeed, they had. One of the Salk vaccine manufacturers, Cutter Laboratories, failed to adequately kill the viruses from which they made vaccine, thereby causing polio in 220 children and creating a national scandal that nearly wiped out political support for the national public health effort. Polio rates went down to zero in the United States when Sabin's oral vaccine was put into use in 1961. Sabin had always argued that an injected vaccine might protect the individual but would not lower the background level of polio in the community. Therefore, the risk of polio would remain, and it would reemerge as a public health threat the moment collective immunity waned.

Sabin had solid scientific reasons for insisting upon an oral vaccine. In the course of natural infection, polio viruses are ingested in water and pass from the intestine to the bloodstream and eventually to the central nervous system. Salk's injected vaccine caused the viruses to be destroyed in the bloodstream, but as long they remained in the GI tract, they were free to multiply and be passed back out into the environment in stools. As a result, the amount of polio present in a given community might not be diminished by that population's use of the Salk vaccine.

Sabin invented ways to keep polio viruses alive in crippled, nonlethal form. These attenuated viruses, mixed with Freund's adjuvant and a harmless liquid, could be swallowed. And, as they were alive, the attenuated polio viruses could make their way into the intestines and stimulate profound local immunity. The new vaccine droplets began to be dripped into the mouths of school-children in 1961. Despite the small risk of acquiring poliomyelitis from Sabin's vaccine, the oral formulation had two advantages over Salk's injectable one: it eliminated polio viruses from the environment and it erased all hazards of needle-borne disease.

With polio nearly vanquished in America and Western Europe, public health leaders realized that the burden of mortality due to infectious diseases was quickly receding to be replaced by cancer, heart disease, and accidents. Baumgartner's department recognized that in 1957, 'public health and the work of the Health Department is ever-changing, for the nature of health problems change. As one is solved, another emerges.'

Among the least popular of the 'new' problems Baumgartner and her counterparts in cities all over the United States faced was heroin. Invented in 1898 by the German company Bayer Pharmaceuticals, Inc., heroin had been in use—legally and illegally—for decades in the United States, but didn't become a serious problem until 1948, when traffickers flooded the streets of New York with it. Between 1948 and 1960 the city, and most of the country's other town centres, suffered wave after wave of what public health officials, the police, and the media termed 'drug epidemics'. With the rise in heroin use—almost exclusively by people aged fifteen to twenty-nine years, most of them men—came hepatitis, which spread among the users through shared needles and syringes.

New York City had little idea what to do with people who had become addicted to heroin. Though criminalization of the problem had been the longstanding approach, the health department tried its best to offer heroin users an alternative way to get off drugs short of going cold turkey in jail. But as Baumgartner said in her report to the city for 1960, 'There is a growing awareness that the narcotic addict should be looked upon primarily as a sick person, not solely as a criminal. But inasmuch as the physiological basis and curative treatment of the narcotic addict are still both unknown, programmes for the addict are obviously palliative and relatively ineffective.'

Surveys from the mid-1950s to the end of the century put the number of heroin addicts in the United States at, variously, between 300 000 and 1.5 million. Some law enforcement and political leaders painted a picture of heroin use that, terrifyingly, focused not upon the very real nightmare of the lives of the addicts themselves but on their alleged antisocial, even demonic, behaviour. The spectre of deranged heroin addicts roaming city streets further nudged the middle class towards the suburbs. And though in absolute numbers whites always dominated the ranks of American heroin users, the middle class imagined the dangerous narcotics user with a black face.

Indeed, heroin use did concentrate and appear more obvious in the nation's increasingly rundown African-American ghettos.

Following World War II the pace of black migration northward and westward quickened, but when southern African-Americans reached Boston, New York, Chicago, Los Angeles, Detroit, and other destinations, they found the cost of housing beyond their limited means and property segregation became an obvious urban reality. Though the administrations of Eisenhower, Kennedy, and Johnson marked a time of remarkable prosperity and economic growth for the nation as a whole, more than half of the nation's black population lived in poverty throughout the 1950s and well into the 1960s. A key reason was job discrimination. And rigid segregation in schools forced most blacks to settle for second-rate education.

During the 1950s African-Americans instigated legal actions and staged a series of both spontaneous and well-planned protests that came to be known as the civil rights movement. By 1956 Reverend Martin Luther King Jr. of Montgomery, Alabama, had emerged as its clear leader. The old gospel song that urged people to 'Hold on just a little while longer/Everything will be all right' captured the spirit of determined strength that marked the civil rights movement in the 1950s. But by the 1960s, the nation's African-American populations, particularly the young city dwellers, had become much more defiant and rebellious. One hundred years after southern whites seceded from the United States to form a confederacy dedicated to perpetuation of slavery, some African-American leaders in the North were calling for a black revolution.

'To be a Negro in this country and to be relatively conscious is to be in a rage all the time,' writer James Baldwin said in 1961.

The deep racial divide reverberated in the medical and public health systems. Dozens of blacks—perhaps hundreds, though nobody was counting—died because emergency rooms at white hospitals refused them treatment. (Among the most famous of such tragedies was the death of blues singer Bessie Smith.) In order to obtain the right for qualified black nurses and physicians to practice medicine in Newark City Hospital, National Association for the Advancement of Coloured People attorney Thurgood Marshall had to sue the state of New Jersey. Until 1940 the American Medical Association listed all African-American members with the abbreviation 'Col.' next to their names, indicating that they were 'coloured' doctors.

By the late 1950s the Eisenhower administration had made it clear to most of the states that no federally funded hospitals could deny medical care on the basis of the colour of the patient's skin. Nevertheless, a new form of segregation emerged— black patients were turned away from prestigious facilities and directed to city- and county-run public hospitals, which all but the poorest whites typically shunned.

Public health departments in the fifties were typically all white, or had black employees working only at bottom-level jobs. The most well-meaning of white leaders, such as New York's Baumgartner, were bewildered by the hostility that greeted their efforts in black ghettos like Harlem, East New York, and the South Bronx, even though for a decade the American Public Health Association had backed the all-black National Medical Association's call for an end to discrimination in health and medical practices.

By 1961 President Kennedy's Department of Health, Education, and Welfare (HEW) was deluged with claims of racial discrimination practices by federally funded hospitals, but legislation that would have empowered HEW to cut off funding to discriminatory medical facilities was languishing in a Senate subcommittee. So HEW did little more than catalogue the complaints and send query letters to the offending hospitals. The Civil Rights Leadership Conference called HEW's inaction 'a silent but nonetheless full partner in the perpetuation of discriminatory practices'.

In June 1963 President Kennedy finally introduced his version of a civil rights act, Title VI, which stipulated that acceptance of federal funds would carry a compensation for non-discriminatory practices. Growing support for Dr King and national outrage over the disgraceful actions of southern whites—particularly their political leaders— had swung the political pendulum to support for Kennedy's civil rights legislation. At last the time seemed ripe for change.

But on November 22, 1963, President Kennedy was assassinated on a campaign tour through Dallas. Five days after the tragic assassination, President Johnson told a joint session of Congress that 'no memorial oration or eulogy could more eloquently honour President Kennedy's memory than the earliest possible passage of the civil rights bill for which he fought so long. We have talked enough in this country about equal rights. We have talked for one hundred years or more. It is time now to write the next chapter and to write it in the books of law.'

Johnson's HEW secretary, Anthony Celebrezze, was immediately saddled with the hot issue of segregated hospitals. And he stalled—took no action—hoping that the Supreme Court would resolve the matter by hearing *Simkins v. Cone*, a case brought by a black man accusing Cone Memorial Hospital of North Carolina of racial discrimination. But on March 2, 1964, the Court let stand a lower court decision in favour of the hospital.

Urged by Johnson to whip up support for the civil rights bill among his fellow liberals, Vice President Hubert H. Humphrey specifically claimed the *Simkins v. Cone* decision as cause for immediate passage: 'Racial discrimination in medical facilities is at least partly responsible for the fact that in North Carolina the rate of infant mortality (for Negroes) is twice the rate for whites and maternal deaths are five times greater.'

On June 10, 1964, with bipartisan support, Johnson's Civil Rights Act of 1964 was passed by both houses. Title VI of the act eliminated all legal forms of racial discrimination in the practices of medicine and public health.

Arizona senator Barry Goldwater expressed disgust with the act, signalling a new spin on civil rights, adopted in a political atmosphere that had made overt supporters of racial segregation political pariahs. The new tack for the extreme conservative wing of the Republican Party, then led by Goldwater, was to attack federal authority for imposing socially liberalizing laws.

In 1964 President Johnson pushed passage of two other massive initiatives that would profoundly affect public health: his War on Poverty programme and Medicare. Johnsons' overall goal was to create what he called the Great Society through a federal effort akin to Roosevelt's New Deal. A key difference, however, was that whereas Roosevelt promoted large-scale federal spending during a time of tremendous economic deprivation in America, Johnson wanted a similar level of spending for social programmes at a time when most Americans were enjoying tremendous prosperity. That was a hard sell.

When Johnson declared his War on Poverty, twenty-one million people in the United States were living below the administration's poverty line. At the bottom of the heap were three social groups targetted by Great Society programmes: people over sixty-five years of age who, having been cleaned out by the Depression, had little in savings upon which to live out their final years; blacks; and women who were single parents. Among the remedial programmes Johnson pushed as part of his Great Society effort were Medicare, Medicaid, and Aid to Families with Dependent Children (AFDC).

The net effect of Great Society initiatives was the creation of a federal system aimed at offering the nation's poor, elderly, children, and immigrants an opportunity to join the American mainstream. Johnson's intention was for the programmes to act as a sort of stepladder that would put individuals within reach of prosperity. But it would be up to the individual, on his or her own, to make the final ascent. It was never Johnson's intent to create a no-load handout system or turn the federal government into a welfare state. And his programmes would no doubt have unfolded more successfully had Johnson not been irreparably involved in the Vietnam War.

Spending on the war created enormous budget deficits, draining resources Johnson had hoped to use on domestic programmes. Military spending rose from an already all-time high of $49.6 billion in 1965 to $80.5 billion in 1968. It was money the US Treasury couldn't spare and it started America on a downward spiral into debt.

'I knew from the start,' Johnson later told author Doris Kearnes Goodwin,[69] 'that I was bound to be crucified either way I moved. If I left the woman I really loved—the Great Society—in order to get involved with that bitch of a war on the other side of the world, then I would lose everything at home. All my programmes. All my hopes to feed the hungry and feed the homeless. All my dreams.'

Except for the Civil Rights Act of 1964, Johnson did, indeed, lose most of his dreams to the war bitch. Every one of the Great Society programmes he had proposed was eventually enacted by Congress in a form unrecognizable to its designer. The programmes as enacted were seriously flawed and the mistakes had profound public health implications. Medicare and Medicaid, in particular, completely reshaped American health care and public health. And the end result was not be as Johnson had planned.

As Congress and the administration debated details of these social programmes, the nation was ripping itself apart. Riots, demonstrations, generational polarization, racial conflict, and labour struggles were exploding in every corner of society.

Johnson was the chief victim of the so-called credibility gap between Washington and the people of the United States, but every member of Congress felt the sting of public mistrust and attack from many sides: the war in Vietnam necessitated a draft, which fuelled an already active student movement and turned millions of college students into angry protestors. Despite passage of the Civil Rights Act, life in African-American urban ghettos only worsened, prompting explosive riots. And many white, working-class Americans fought militant battles to protect the jobs and lifestyles they felt were threatened by hippies and blacks. Torn asunder, the nation was not in a thoughtful mood, and the sixties proved to be a reactive, rather than a contemplative, era.

As a result, Congress passed legislation aimed at massive US crises, such as lack of health care and entrenched poverty, but did so in a piecemeal fashion that reflected the conflicts of powerful lobbying constituencies and interest groups. The goals were to eliminate poverty and increase access to health care. But few political leaders stood back and asked: How? Why? An overarching vision was lacking.

Between 1900 and 1940 average US life expectancies at birth for females had risen from 48.3 years to 65.2 years, 16.9 additional years of life. Male life expectancy also increased from 46.3 years to 60.8 years, a total gain of 14.5 years. These fantastic gains were made after the germ theory revolution but before development of modern vaccines or antibiotics. They preceded most forms of treatment for cardiac disease and for cancer, short of surgical tumour removal. And the gains occurred in the absence of a vast nationwide network of hospitals.

Perhaps more striking, they were achieved in a nation that had three times declined creation of a universal health-care system and, thus, had routinely denied medical care to three generations of America's twentieth-century poor and people of colour. As early as 1911, when Britain created its national compulsory medical insurance system, American voters had signalled their desire to have some sort of government-ensured equity for access to health care. In 1919 Californians even gave the concept their voted approval. But the AMA, using the then-new pejorative 'socialized medicine', quashed that and all subsequent efforts to create universal American health care.

The great gains were therefore made not by medicine, but as a result of large-scale public health efforts that had sought to prevent infectious diseases through community intervention. As early as 1900 Hermann Biggs had proved that such interventions saved money and were therefore not simply matters of humane policy but also made sound fiscal sense. The basic philosophy had focused on the collective: the health of individuals would be protected by raising the level of health of the community as a whole. Some of the gains were the result of economic improvements and rising standards of living. Others reflected improved nutritional levels.

In contrast, between 1940 and 1965 (when Congress was debating Medicare) female life expectancy rose from 65.2 to 73.7 years, a gain of just 8.5 years. Male life expectancy increased from 60.8 to 66.8 years, a net gain of 6 years. Perhaps more significant was the trend in average remaining life expectancies after Americans reached the age of sixty years. In 1900 the average woman in the United States who had managed to reach that ripe age could expect to live an additional 24.4 years and reach the age of eighty-four. The average sixty-year-old male faced 23.1 more years of life and would live to be eighty-three years of age.

By 1940 average additional life expectancy for sixty-year-old Americans was 33.3 years for women and 30 years for men. Serious gains had been made, adding 8.9 years of elderly life for women and 6.9 years for men. By 1965, elderly women had gained another 4.2 years; elderly men just 1.7 years.[70]

A shift was obviously occurring and as infectious disease crises receded in significance, what population-based strategies might appropriately address this new era? What was to be the goal of Medicare? Was it to increase these average American life expectancies? To improve the quality of those years of added life? To equalize availability modern medicine for all elderly Americans? To increase the size of the paying medical consumer populations? To enhance the role and size of hospitals in America? To compensate physicians for services, as few might have offered free treatment for elderly patients?

The questions were never really asked or answered. Instead, political leaders simply reflected cultural trends of the day and assumed that what everyone wanted—and needed—was more medical care.

In 1965 average Americans knew that they were healthier than their parents or grandparents had been. They were taller, stronger, gave infectious diseases little thought, could have sex without fear of dying of syphilis, could swim in a public pool without pausing to consider polio, and had vast and varied quantities of food at their disposal. Newly discovered drugs or vaccines were announced almost daily. On television, doctors were portrayed as omnipresent geniuses who could save and heal the world. Overall, people living in the United States in 1965 had a remarkably optimistic, even adoring, belief in new technology.

Social problems—poverty, racism, Communist threats, the war in Vietnam, student unrest—seemed complex and controversial to Americans and there was little societal consensus on any of them. Science and technology, however, offered solutions, strategies, and miracles, especially in medicine. Americans had an almost unquestioning faith that money spent on Big Medicine was money well spent. The human body was, metaphorically, a machine that occasionally broke or, with age, deteriorated. Enough medicine could fix it.

During the late 1960s and early seventies health and environmental concerns combined in US public opinion, spawning new realms of government regulation, academic pursuit, commerce, and political activism. By the end of the Nixon administration on August 8, 1974, the environmental movement in the United States was enormous. Its impact on government could be felt by at least six federal agencies. It influenced numerous fields of public health and, to a lesser degree, medicine, including toxicology, epidemiology, health statistics, oncology, and occupational health. Environmentalist thinking had both polarizing and radical effects on public health, eventually pushing many leaders in the field into confrontation with corporate interests. Whereas public health had always been a voice for society's poor, it now joined a large US chorus protesting—largely on behalf of a middle-class constituency—corporate polluters.

With every passing 1970s day, another chemical was implicated, another pollutant named. Public panic rose and eventually left public health vulnerable to a large, and often effective, assault on its credibility.

Well before the public began paying attention to cancer, the nation's death rates had been steadily climbing. In 1900 deaths due to cancer claimed 64 of every 100 000 Americans. By 1940 that rate had nearly doubled to 120.3 per 100 000. In 1950 it hit 140 per 100 000. And in 1969 the US annual cancer death rate was 160 per 100 000. Although far more people died of heart diseases (500 per 100 000 people annually in 1969), cancer created a unique level of concern. Only about one out of every twenty-five Americans in 1900 died of cancer. By 1969 the figure was about one out of every seven, and both cancer and heart disease morbidity and mortality rates had climbed steadily since World War II.

The main cause of those rising death rates was not, however, some mysterious environmental pollution. It had been recognized and named long before the 1970s: tobacco smoking. In 1956 Deputy Director of the National Institutes of Health Dr Luther Terry, impressed by then-mountainous evidence that smoking increased lung cancer, called upon the nation to 'Stamp Out Smoking.'

Terry became Surgeon General in 1961 and launched an aggressive effort to confront the role of cigarettes in disease. He appointed a blue ribbon tobacco study panel and in January 1964 he told a televised, standing-room-only press conference of its conclusions: 'Cigarette smoking is causally related to lung cancer in men. The magnitude of the effect of cigarette smoking far outweighs all other factors. The data for women, though less extensive, points in the same direction.'

The report caused an immediate sensation both within the medical profession and on Capitol Hill. At Terry's urging, the Johnson administration ordered health warnings placed on all packs of cigarettes.

The tobacco industry waged a vigorous 'public health campaign' of its own, supporting members of Congress whose constituencies included tobacco growers whose healthy well-being, the industry said, was imperilled by anti-tobacco laws.

Clandestinely the industry funded the Tobacco Institute, a quasi-independent centre that for decades published studies finding few or no ill effects associated with cigarette smoking. Remaining unpublished were the institute's revelations not only of the ill effects from cigarettes, but of a powerful addictive response to the tobacco stimulant, nicotine. It was nearly thirty years before the institute's documents saw the light of day.[71]

In the 1970s many public health advocates and their lawyers tended to downplay tobacco's contribution to cancer and heart disease.[72] They did so not because they disbelieved evidence of tobacco carcinogenesis, but in reaction to the chemical industry, which consistently explained away cancer cases found among people exposed to their products by referring to the victim's cigarette smoking. Both sides were being less than candid.

Though tobacco use and its public health consequences became increasingly politically partisan issues, there never was a good reason why. Surgeons general ranging from left-liberal to ultraconservative consistently followed Luther Terry's precedent in striking out against the tobacco industry. Indeed, the loudest voice was the Surgeon General appointed by Ronald Reagan, Dr C. Everett Koop, a notorious social conservative who was considered the darling of the 1980s American far right. But he had a powerful public health conscience and was the cigarette industry's arch-nemesis. 'How,' he asked, 'could the tobacco industry dare to dismiss as unfounded and unproven the absolutely clear connection between smoking ... and a dozen or more serious, debilitating, exhausting, expensive, and humiliating diseases? How could it do that? The answer was—it just did. The tobacco industry is accountable to no one. ... The tobacco lobby is overwhelmingly powerful.'[73]

Most of tobacco's protectors on Capitol Hill were Republicans and Southern Democrats, who justified their opposition to smoking-related public health measures on two grounds: job protection for tobacco farmers and industry employees and philosophical opposition to any regulations that fettered free enterprise—including health laws aimed at saving tens of thousands of lives every year. The politicians were less open about reason number three for their staunch support of tobacco: money. The industry spent between $500 million and $1 billion every year from 1969 to 1999 on advertising and made generous campaign contributions. In contrast, public health had paltry advertising resources during the 1960s and 1970s, and few of its leaders appreciated—as New York's Baumgartner did—the power of Madison Avenue. Even in the mid-1980s, federal anti-smoking advertising spending amounted to a mere $70 million a year compared to the more than $900 million annual pro-tobacco advertising dollars.[74]

In 1964 Surgeon General Terry could cite more than seven thousand studies demonstrating a link between tobacco and human morbidity and mortality. By 1988 Surgeon General Koop could point to ceiling-high stacks of documents, more than sixty thousand studies, proving links between tobacco and dozens of diseases in both smokers and so-called passive smokers—people who shared aeroplanes, offices, and homes with smokers and breathed their exhaled tar, nicotine, carbon monoxide, and other insidious chemicals. These studies demonstrated clearly why and how tobacco exerted its lethal effects.

Bad as the biochemical effects of burning tobacco were, they would surely have had only minimal public health impact had it not been for nicotine. Without nicotine's addictive qualities, far fewer smokers would have become hooked. The immediate pleasurable stimulation the smoker feels is the result of nicotine's attachment to receptors located on the synapses of the brain's nerve cells. Normally, these synaptic receptors are used by the most critical neurotransmitter, acetylcholine, to send the messages that are the essence of how the mind thinks. Nicotine competes with acetylcholine to saturate these receptors. The sensation for the smoker is pleasure. Nicotine also binds hormone receptors that control release of adrenaline, one of the most powerful chemicals in the body. When adrenaline surges into the bloodstream, the stimulation can be extremely dangerous to smokers' already taxed hearts, but the smoker, paradoxically, feels more pleasure.

Neurostimulation is a greedy mistress. The brain wants more and more of it: the longer a smoker uses cigarettes, the more the brain actually changes physically, adapting to nicotine stimulation so thoroughly that it can not readily function without it.[75]

'That is what we are really talking about: not smoking, not tobacco, but nicotine addiction. Most smokers are drug addicts,' Koop concluded. And tobacco companies he added, were pushers.

During the later quarter of the century, tobacco smoking was estimated to have caused four hundred thousand deaths each year in the United States, resulting in the loss of five million years of potential life.[76] After the Surgeon General's 1964 report was released, researchers established that a long list of cancers and other ailments was associated either with cigarette smoking or with sharing a home for years with a smoker. The USPHS estimated that smoking was responsible for almost a third of all cancer deaths in the United States (nearly nine out of ten lung cancer deaths), and for one out of every five deaths due to cardiovascular diseases.

Despite their comparatively minuscule budget for raising public awareness, public health leaders tried to combat Madison Avenue's pitch for cigarettes through education campaigns, primarily in schools. But early campaigns seriously underestimated the power of nicotine addiction. The most health-conscious smokers heeded the educational warnings and quit, but several legal measures ultimately played critical roles in thinning the ranks of US smokers. The Federal Communications Commission banned broadcast advertising of tobacco products and most local and state governments eventually prohibited smoking in public. Heavy taxes were levied on cigarettes and in the final years of the century, lawsuits filed by the families of lifelong smokers who died of cancer won multimillion-dollar cases against tobacco giants, and, through legal discovery, opened doors on long-covert data gathered by the Tobacco Institute.

Between 1964 and 1989 the numbers of American smokers fell from more than 40 per cent to 29 per cent of the population. Most of the quitters were white, middle-class adults. Still smoking in numbers exceeding a third of their populations were African-Americans and American Indians.

Tobacco offered unique challenges to both public health and medicine during the 1970s. Public health had yet to find effective ways to alter human behaviour when the dire outcomes of their actions were in the future and less than certain. It was one thing to mobilize five million people to take a specific action in the face of an immediate threat such as getting vaccinated against smallpox. It was quite another to get the same five million people to alter a behaviour that most of them found quite pleasurable, particularly when the odds were relatively low that a given individual would face bad consequences. The new public health era called for just such interventions, however. Heroin injection, addictive use of prescription drugs, behaviour that spread sexually transmitted diseases, routine consumption of distilled alcohol, and smoking were all features of American lifestyles in the 1970s that, for health reasons, needed to change. And few public health leaders had any idea why these behaviours were so prevalent in society or how they could be altered.

Shortly after taking office, in January 1981, President Reagan had ordered a combination of covert and overt operations in support of pro-US forces throughout Central America: the anti-Sandinista Contras in Nicaragua and the governments of Guatemala, Honduras, and El Salvador.

As the brutal wars and repression spread, hundreds of thousands of Central Americans fled to the United States, most settling illegally in Florida, Texas, Arizona, and California. Between 1981 and 1988 Los Angeles County absorbed the largest number of these illegal immigrants, estimated to have totalled 350 000 to half a million. (When, by 1991, the wars had largely ended, few of these refugees returned to Central America.)

Most of the Salvadoreans who reached Los Angeles during those years were traumatized and terrified of deportation back to what they felt would be certain death or torture. Unlike the Mexicans and Chicanos in Los Angeles, the Salvadoreans kept their heads down, tried to be invisible, stayed away from anyone connected to government, and avoided even the health-care system except in emergencies. Since they did not qualify for Medi-Cal, the county had no choice but to provide them with free medical care, holding out no hope of state or federal reimbursement.

This greatly exacerbated the L.A. County Department of Health's already serious list of problems. By 1984 the Board of Supervisors began mortgaging government buildings to raise funds for its payroll. Cutbacks in Medicare and Medi-Cal revenues came as the patient burden increased.

Just five months after Reagan's inauguration, doctors in New York, Los Angeles, and Washington, DC, publicized word of odd deaths occurring in gay men and intravenous drug users. Parasitic pneumonias, once-rare skin tumours, types of lymphoma usually seen only in elderly men—suddenly, previously healthy young men were turning up at hospitals with these diseases and dying there.

It was, of course, the beginning of what would become the twentieth century's second worst pandemic (after the 1918 influenza), caused by the human immunodeficiency virus, or HIV. By the end of the century, just nineteen years after the first cases of the disease were reported, more than thirty-four million people worldwide had become infected with HIV. At least half of them had developed the end-stage syndrome called AIDS and at least twelve million had died of the disease. It had spread to every corner of the planet, defying both public health efforts and the scientific pursuit of genuine cures or vaccines.

There could be no greater evidence of the need for a new, global approach to public health. But when the first intravenous drug users suffering from AIDS staggered into New York City public hospitals and initial handfuls of ailing gay men begged for help from doctors in San Francisco and Los Angeles, the public health response was abysmal, even non-existent.

Though a tiny group of epidemiologists, scientists, and physicians struggled at the CDC and in San Francisco, New York City, Los Angeles, and elsewhere in the United States, as well as in Europe, to understand the new threat, their efforts were ignored or rebuffed by government.

At the top, the Reagan administration seemed utterly incapable of getting past the fact that most of the first cases of AIDS involved homosexual men. It was the first administration in the White House that had campaigned on a Christian fundamentalist platform and Reagan's constituents were avidly anti-gay. According to his personal physician, Reagan thought AIDS was something like measles: a virus that was passing through but would soon disappear without any special effort on humanity's part. That this was an inaccurate understanding of measles—a virus controlled through vigorous public health efforts—was one thing. Worse, it was a dangerously wrong perception regarding HIV.

It seems clear from the record that Reagan never fully understood that a true pandemic of an incurable disease was unfolding during his presidency. And though many of his aides did appreciate the scale of the epidemic, they agreed with the assessment of the Moral Majority's Reverend Jerry Falwell that the disease was God's retribution for immoral, sinful, homosexual behaviour. Some members of Congress shared that view and openly opposed virtually every piece of public health AIDS legislation that reached the House or Senate.

Within the Department of Health and Human Services, the technological view of public health predominated during the Reagan years. So in response to AIDS classic public health measures were shunned in favour of a completely unsupportable belief that laboratory science would swiftly solve the problem—by the turn of the century, that still had not come to pass.

Within this department, Surgeon General C. Everett Koop was the most outspoken—often the sole—voice in favour of public health approaches to the HIV crisis. He recognized that in the absence of scientific 'magic bullet' solutions, there was a crying need for public education. Armed with accurate information about how the virus was spread and how individuals could best protect themselves, the American people would, Koop reasoned, make proper choices. But the information had to be fairly explicit to be useful. And sexually active adults had to be advised to use condoms.

The mere idea of promoting condoms was anathema in the White House and within the Republican Party. Throughout US history, whenever moral issues were involved the public's health suffered. This had been especially true in the case of sexually transmitted diseases and drug abuse issues. By the time HIV surfaced in the United States, the incidence of gonorrhoea, chlamydia, syphilis, hepatitis B, and other sexually transmitted diseases had been escalating for decades. Americans opposed sex education in schools, discussion of condom use, and education about birth control, particularly for adolescents.

On October 22, 1986, in the largest public health mailing in US history, Koop issued his Surgeon General's Report on AIDS to 107 million US households. Though the report fell short of containing the explicit discussions of homosexuality advocated by many

AIDS activists, it nevertheless came under harsh attack from the Moral Majority, the Right to Life movement, and the right wing of the Republican Party—all of which interpreted it as an endorsement of the sins of premarital and extramarital sex and homosexuality.

In retrospect, what was more remarkable about the Koop mailing was not its contents but that it occurred five years *after* the epidemic was recognized and more than two years after HIV was discovered, proving that the disease was contagious. There was foot-dragging in Washington on every public health measure related to HIV: funding for basic research, public education, anti-discrimination legislation to protect infected individuals, and health-care coverage.

Because nearly all of the epidemic's casualties were young adults or their children, HIV hit the very demographic groups that were most likely to fall outside the health-care safety net after the Reagan administration's changes in Medicare, Medicaid, and special public health programmes went into effect.

AIDS activists, who were for the most part white gay men in their twenties and thirties, made the search for a cure and anti-discrimination legislation their top priorities. As the toll of HIV cases and deaths rose, and many died never having received quality care, Dr James Curran of the CDC called out for 'human resources to care for the people who are already infected.' But doctors and dentists all over the United States declined to treat HIV patients on the grounds that those individuals posed a threat. The same health providers willingly worked with patients who carried far more contagious microbes, such as hepatitis B and drug-resistant forms of staphylococcus and streptococcus, but the spectre of AIDS prompted them to break the most basic of physician's ethics.

From a public health point of view, the key AIDS priorities in the 1980s should have been: number one, identify the cause of the disease; number two, determine exactly how the organism was spread from person to person; number three, stop that spread; number four, initiate vigorous research in pursuit of both a cure and a vaccine.[77]

The record shows that number one (identification of the cause) and number two (modes of transmission) were achieved very quickly, in large part through the efforts of US federal agencies. The CDC, working closely with epidemiologists in San Francisco, Los Angeles, and New York, swiftly identified the means by which AIDS was spread and proved that the disease was caused by some form of infectious microorganism. Within months of the May 1981 recognition that a new, fatal disease had emerged among gay men, Curran's team at the CDC had determined that it was spread via anal and vaginal intercourse, contaminated intravenous needles, and contaminated blood. A little later in the epidemiology, they noted mother-to-child transmission. The main cause, the CDC said in 1982, was exposure to contaminated blood.

Even in the absence of discovery of HIV, appropriate public health measures (number three) based on those observations would have involved widespread education about how every American could avoid blood-to-blood exposure and concrete steps to decrease such risks: screening of the US blood supply, basic protective gear for hospital and clinic employees, promotion of condom use by sexually active adults, ensuring that all injections—medical or for illegal drug use—involved use of sterile needles and syringes, and closure of or strong admonishments against social settings that encouraged behaviours that put people at risk of blood-to-blood exposure.

Rational as that list appeared, implementation of every one of those measures ran up against a wall of political, social, economic, and civil libertarian obstacles. Indeed, by the end of the century incidents of blood-to-blood exposure were still commonplace in US society, and several measures that might have mitigated against HIV exposure would remain blocked. In some instances, the right laws may indeed have been passed and appropriate public health steps taken, but that happened only after much delay and argument.

The nation's most prestigious medical science body, the Institute of Medicine, issued everything from memos to tomes begging—in plaintive, nearly supplicant tones—for a viable public health response to the epidemic. In 1988 the institute urged 'the federal government to take the lead in developing a comprehensive and coherent national plan for delivering and financing care for HIV-infected and AIDS patients.' It insisted that 'present funding is insufficient for public health approaches to stem the epidemic.' And it decried the 'gross inadequacy of federal efforts to reduce HIV transmission among intravenous drug abusers....'

By the time those statements were released, some eighty thousand Americans had developed AIDS and forty-five thousand had died of the disease. It was far too late to close the proverbial barn door: simple public health measures were no longer sufficient.

What had gone wrong?

Bigotry against homosexuals and injecting drug users had blinded the general public, politicians, the medical community, and, sadly, many public health leaders to the urgency of responding to AIDS when effective action might have had a profound impact: between May 1981 and the end of 1984. Those health leaders at the CDC, and in New York City, San Francisco, and other hard-hit cities who did voice concerns and tried to implement appropriate measures were thwarted by community resistance that was both complex and overwhelming. From the Right they faced outright hostility. From most tiers of government they received shrugs or snubs. From the industries most involved in blood products and related equipment they heard cries of government interference and economic woe.

Nor did public health leaders get much support from mainstream America, which continued to be woefully ignorant about AIDS and frighteningly prejudiced. A *New York Times*/CBS poll in 1988 found that more than three-quarters of respondents had 'no sympathy for homosexuals suffering from AIDS.' A shocking 19 per cent said they had no sympathy for AIDS patients *regardless of how they acquired their HIV infection*, even if the individuals were infants or transfusion recipients.

How did public health leaders counter such public hostility? In general, by identifying with the populations of Americans who had AIDS or were at greatest risk for HIV infection, even to the extent of adopting issues that served only to distract the nation from the primary health issues involved. All disease surveillance and identification of infected individuals was made confidential or anonymous, thus protecting individuals from societal discrimination. And HIV infections were never reported; only full-blown AIDS cases were tracked, amid clearly justifiable concerns about protecting the civil liberties of outwardly well, HIV-positive individuals.

Thus, nobody truly knew at any given moment how large the public health catastrophe was, where and in which communities it was spreading, whether any public health interventions were actually slowing that spread, or if such programmes might be failing and the millions of dollars spent on them wasted. The summaries public health leaders received of the epidemic were, by definition, out of date. Epidemiologists in the 1980s and 1990s were forced by political and technological limitations to use slow-motion tools to decipher the epidemic's nuances. It was very crude.

And it opened the door to policy decisions based as much on political and emotional issues as on science. For example, as late as 1986 in New York City it was Department of Health policy *not* to tell individuals who donated blood that their sample had tested HIV positive.

'We should not share test results with people whose blood is tested,' the city's Dr Joyce Gaynor told blood bank officials in 1985. 'We should refrain until we know the significance of such a finding.'

Elsewhere in the United States, some public health officials blatantly lied to donors, telling those who had positive results that their blood was rejected because it contained hepatitis. Even as late as 1986 some refused to test blood at all.

There was not a nationally uniform FDA blood products policy until 1989, and the parameters of general testing (both of individuals and donated blood and plasma) were never made nationally uniform. Each state decided its own policies regarding those who could be tested voluntarily, or under legal mandate; whether individuals who tested positive would be informed; in what context that information would be dispensed; how—or even if—the identities of HIV-positive individuals would be followed or codified; and what systems would be in place to track the names of those who developed AIDS or died. It evolved into a hotchpotch system full of epidemiological flaws and fraught with policy confusion.

In states in which gay activists were vocal and well organized, the toughest civil libertarian restrictions were put in place. And in states with little vocal gay activism, civil libertarian protections were typically far weaker. Jesse Helms's home state of North Carolina, for example, kept records by name of all HIV-infected individuals and their sex partners. This meant that it was easiest to track the unfolding epidemic in states with the smallest HIV-positive populations.

It also meant that public health authorities working in the hotbeds of HIV at the time—New York City, Los Angeles, San Francisco, Newark, Washington, DC, Miami, and Chicago—were operating largely in the dark. For example, in 1984 all of these cities hotly debated whether to close gay sex clubs and bathhouses in order to minimize spread of HIV. At the time, Curran's CDC staff only knew of 6122 cases nationwide and 2800 deaths. Overall, Curran concluded in 1984, 'it is estimated that two hundred to three hundred thousand people in the US have been exposed to the virus.' Though the virus that would later be dubbed HIV had already been discovered, widespread use of HIV blood tests was not yet in place and epidemiologists had to do off the cuff reckoning, often in the face of open hostility from the gay community that they sought to protect.

While the bathhouse issue was under debate, epidemiologist Andrew Moss of the University of California San Francisco told that city's health commissioner, and later the superior court: 'What we expect to see is that this growth will continue until the disease has saturated the population—that is, until most of the people who are susceptible to the disease get infected—and at that point we will see the number of new cases trailing off.'

The remarkably prescient Moss said that public health policy on AIDS should emphasize at least two other factors: 'One is to make it clear to people what the truly terrifying nature of the disease is, how grave and serious a disease it is. The second is to attempt to support what you might call serially monogamous lifestyles—that is, cutting down by changing from a lifestyle with a very large number of sexual partners to a lifestyle that is closer to serial monogamy.'

Public Health Commissioner Dr Mervyn Silverman decided to close the city's bathhouses and Superior Court Judge Roy Wonder upheld his decision. In New York City, Health Commissioner Dr Stephen Joseph confronted similar difficult decisions and reached analogous conclusions.

Both men faced attempts to oust them from office as a result.

Silverman came under attack from gay activists who thought his actions discriminatory and homophobic and from Mayor Dianne Feinstein who felt he had moved too slowly and not taken drastic enough measures. Silverman was asked to resign. Joseph survived activists' attacks, but Mayor Koch did little to defend his health commissioner.

In New York the debate over how to limit spread of HIV in the gay community was ultimately decided at the state level.[78] On October 24, 1985, after months of hearings and debates, State Health Commissioner Dr David Axelrod sent a memo to Governor Mario Cuomo: 'I have concluded that establishments which allow, promote, and/or encourage sexual contacts that produce blood to blood or semen to blood contact are a serious menace to the public health and must be prohibited. . . . It applies to any establishment that caters to dangerous heterosexual or homosexual sex.'[79]

Governor Cuomo, a liberal Democrat, followed Axelrod's recommendation to close sex parlours and bathhouses and stated, 'Until the scientists find a cure for AIDS, education is our only vaccine.'[80]

Finally, America moved to public health step number four: vigorous research. There was a tremendous blind faith that Science would, indeed, find a cure for AIDS; it just needed some nudging. Many top NIH scientists, particularly at the National Cancer Institute, professed great optimism. More practical scientists, such as National Institute of Allergy and Infectious Diseases director Dr Anthony Fauci and his circle, assiduously avoided use of the word *cure*. They believed it highly disingenuous to offer hope that science could, indeed, cure a disease caused by a virus that hid inside human DNA. How could such a microbe be excised without destroying the individuals' genes in the process?

The thrust of AIDS activism, however, was focused on the search for a cure. As more of the estimated 700 000 to 1 million men and women in the United States who were infected with HIV came to realize that their time was running out, the activists' ranks swelled and militance increased. Certain a cure could be found, given an all-out effort, they attacked the drug companies, the FDA, the NIH, the White House, the Department of Health and Human Services—any institution thought to be dragging its feet regarding AIDS.

It was a first among infectious diseases: the patients were living long enough and being well enough organized to set the relevant public health agenda. Given that their lives were on the line, the primary goal was a medical one. Classic public health aims took a distant second place.

With one possible exception: needle exchange programmes. The drive to push government to supply, or at least legalize, sterile syringes for injecting drug users was the main focus of both activism and of pressure from the public health community from the second Reagan term through Bush and on throughout the Clinton administration. By 1988 some 38 per cent of all injecting drug users in New York City, for example, were HIV positive, and it seemed clear that the prevalence there among drug injectors would soon surpass that seen in gay men. Further, because many injecting drug-using women worked as prostitutes, there was considerable concern that through them HIV would reach the larger heterosexual society. Many health advocates believed that provision of clean needles was the key to slowing that part of the epidemic. These needles could be provided either through simple distribution of syringes or through street exchange programmes (in which users traded used syringes for an equal number of sterile ones), legalization of over-the-counter sale of syringes, legalization of the possession of drug-use paraphernalia, or a combination of all of the above.

Of these approaches, needle exchange received by far the most attention and also faced significant public health obstacles. First, it was opposed by Congress not only during the Reagan administration but by the Bush and Clinton administrations as well. Many state legislatures and governors were similarly disinclined to weaken in any way their restrictions on the activities of illegal drug users.

The second obstacle was then already very high HIV rate in the injecting drug-using population. Needle exchanges would probably have had a powerful impact between 1981 and 1984 when the incidence of HIV in that community was still manageable. But by Reagan's second term, many cities were reporting HIV rates of 35 to 60 per cent among injecting drug users.

Yet another impediment was the methadone and treatment crisis.

In June 1982 Reagan delivered his War on Drugs speech, declaring, 'We're taking down the surrender flag that has flown over so many drug efforts. We're running up a battle flag.'

By the end of the nineties New York City and other HIV hot spots in the United States had some good news: the death rate among people infected with the virus had plummeted. And fewer people infected with HIV were progressing to full-blown AIDS. That meant that the pool of immunologically compromised New Yorkers had shrunk, making management of tuberculosis and other institutionally spread, drug-resistant microbes easier—at least in theory.

From 1997 to 1998 the US HIV death rate dropped by 20 per cent (from 21 222 deaths to 17 047). And that was after a 42 per cent AIDS death rate decline from 1996 to 1997. The national AIDS death rate fell to 4.6 per 100 000 in 1998—a 70 per cent decline since 1995. In 1995 HIV was the number eight cause of death in the United States: by 1998 it didn't even rank in the top fifteen.

And national syphilis rates had dropped so dramatically during the 1990s that the CDC forecast US eradication of the disease in 2005. By 1998 the nation's syphilis rate was a minuscule 2.6 cases per 100 000 US residents, with more than half the cases occurring in just twenty-eight counties. (New York was not one of those counties, but Los Angeles was.) Syphilis rates were highest among African-Americans living in Baltimore, Chicago, Memphis, Nashville, Phoenix, and Detroit.

Combined, these findings pointed to a dramatic set of public health achievements in control of sexually transmitted diseases.

'Any reduction in the numbers of Americans dying from AIDS is good news,' said CDC director Dr Jeffrey Koplan. 'We should pause and fully recognize the tremendous public health accomplishment that has been achieved by reducing AIDS-related mortality from fifty thousand deaths a year in 1995 to an annual rate of just under twenty thousand.'

But was it truly a victory for public health, as opposed to one for medical care? Fewer Americans were dying of AIDS, yes, but the pace of new HIV infections hadn't flagged. The triumphant decline in mortality was achieved through widespread use, beginning in 1996, of an innovative set of treatment cocktails that held the virus at bay, but at tremendous cost. The drugs, coupled with necessary medical supervision and tests, cost successfully treated patients (or insurers, or the government) more than $20 000 a year.

Might the HIV situation at the close of the twentieth century, sceptics asked, constitute a grave public health challenge, rather than a triumph?

Internationally, HIV continued to rage out of control, having infected 47.3 million people by December 1998, 33.4 million of whom were alive in 1999. Fewer than 5 per cent of the living could possibly afford to take the life-extending drug cocktails that had proven to so impressively affect mortality rates in America. Cumulatively, HIV had killed 13.9 million people in eighteen years, outstripping the Black Death's toll in Europe from 1346 to 1350 of between 9 and 11 million people. By 1999 AIDS was the number one killer in Africa, having surpassed the continent's ancient nemeses of tuberculosis, measles, malaria, and other tropical diseases. In ten African countries more than 10 per cent of the population (of all ages, combined) was HIV positive. Globally, HIV was the number four killer and the main infectious disease in 1998.[81]

Given mounting evidence that HIV had originated in Africa decades prior to its discovery among gay Americans,[82] it seemed prudent to assume that as long as no affordable, effective treatment or vaccine was available for the people of that beleaguered continent, the virus would be reintroduced repeatedly in the United States, Canada, and

Europe in the future. Thus, it made no sense in the Age of Globalization to imagine that a slowdown in AIDS deaths in one place on earth heralded a public health victory.

But even limiting a rosy view of the HIV situation just to the United States merited warnings of hubris. A 1997 CDC survey of gay men in several US cities[83] found that the rate of new infections was still dangerously high: 6 per cent of gay men became newly infected each year, despite copious amounts of safe-sex education. Even more alarming were seroconversion rates among fifteen- to twenty-two-year-old gay males in America: in 1998 7 per cent of that group was found to be already infected and 3 per cent were thought to become newly infected each year. Nearly half the young gay males surveyed by the CDC in several cities admitted to having had sex without using a protective condom at least once during the first six months of 1998.

Nationally, at least 40 000 people were becoming infected with HIV every year during the late 1990s. That was a fraction of the 150 000 annually in the early 1980s, but in those days nobody had realized that HIV existed. Nineteen years later, after hundreds of millions of dollars' worth of HIV education efforts, hundreds of thousands of Americans were still taking dangerous sexual risks.

The problem was pop mythology. The myth: AIDS was over.

The reality: the number of HIV-positive Americans was growing daily. And it was almost impossible to predict which of the infected would stay healthy and strong and which would die. Twin brothers Eric and James proved that.

In 1987, at the age of twenty-six, Eric died of AIDS. Most HIV patients did perish at that time, as treatment was, at best, luck of the draw. His death drove his twin brother, James, to join AIDS activists in the group ACT UP. Thanks in part to the often militant voices of James and his fellow activists, the pace of HIV science quickened in the 1990s, FDA approval of new medicines was put on a fast track, and a raft of new, seemingly miraculous, treatments reached local pharmacies in 1996. Taken in combinations of three or more different medicines, the new anti-HIV cocktails, dubbed HAART, or Highly Active Anti-Retroviral Therapy, brought the first genuine hope in the epidemic's grim history.

James, a thirty-five-year-old New York Ivy-Leaguer, jumped onto the HAART bandwagon in early 1996. A few months later Steve, the love of James's life, also started HAART. And it was immediately obvious that one of them was going to be among the successes on science's scoreboard and the other was not. While Steve thrived, James got sicker and was hospitalized twice in 1998 with AIDS-related ailments.

In September of that year James complained of grogginess. Two days later he was hospitalized with sepsis. Three days later he was dead. Steve still felt healthy.

James died when more than 250 different combinations of drugs for HAART were available and many Americans and Europeans had declared the epidemic over. Though thousands like James still suffered and died of AIDS, in the wealthier world of Western Europe and North America the sense of plague emergency disappeared post-HAART, AIDS acute care facilities closed, HIV-positive individuals began worrying about their retirement funds, and gloom no longer pervaded gatherings of gay men and their physicians.

The key class of then-new drugs, called protease inhibitors, blocked the ability of HIV to package its progeny into viable infectious form. Taken alone, the protease inhibitors had proved worse than useless: they were toxic agents towards which HIV quickly mutated and became resistant. But when taken in combination with other anti-HIV drugs of classes that targetted different aspects of the virus's life cycle, protease inhibitors seemed to elicit miraculous results in the small numbers of patients observed in prelicensing drug studies.[84]

On November 10, 1996—just six months after James started taking his HAART cocktail—HIV-positive author Andrew Sullivan wrote a controversial *New York Times Magazine* piece entitled 'When Plagues End: Notes on the Twilight of an Epidemic,' and *Newsweek* ran a cover story headlined 'The End of AIDS?' *Science* magazine closed 1996 by declaring HAART the 'breakthrough of the year', and *Time* magazine named Dr David Ho, a key player in HAART development, its Man of the Year. By usual American media standards, a revolution was officially declared.

But if so, Steve said, it had cruelly passed by James and thousands of other Americans on HAART. By late 1998, more than a third of all individuals who started HAART during the exciting days of mid-1996 had failed on the therapy.[85]

A few weeks after James's death, Steve talked, with emotional difficulty, about the loss of his lover and the new reality of HIV. 'I'm a scientist by training,' Steve explained, 'so I'm always looking for evidence. Things are different, yes, but people are still dying. Another close friend died a week ago. I'm not convinced that this [HAART] will keep me going until I'm seventy. But I'm forty-one now and I think I could live to fifty. But God knows what these medications are doing to us. Are we all going to need liver transplants?'

Steve appreciated that anybody who had taken the HAART cocktails for more than eighteen months was living in a sort of Twilight Zone of uncertainty. The doctors and patients did creative battle with the virus on a daily basis, having no long-term experience or signposts to guide their extraordinary complex strategies. While some declared victory, most HIV experts and seasoned AIDS activists recognized the truth: HAART was buying time, but it offered neither a cure nor even a tolerable long-term holding pattern.

Before this realization set in, however, there had been a period of euphoria. At the summer 1996 International Conference on AIDS in Vancouver, word spread of Lazarus-like recoveries by AIDS patients taking early forms of what would become known as HAART. Top HIV researchers from all over the world gathered cautiously to discuss one new possibility: eradication. If eradication were achieved, HAART would represent *both* medical and public health victories.[86]

Propelled by the jubilant news, tens of thousands of Europeans and North Americans started taking HAART soon after the Vancouver conference. And when the international AIDS community reconvened two years later in Geneva, results, overall, still looked great as the dramatic drop in AIDS deaths attested.[87]

By the late 1990s some scientists were beginning to see beyond the starry-eyed optimism. 'Even if you take someone who has a successful response to HAART,' said Dr Neal Nathanson, 'my sense is that it won't be possible to keep someone on HAART for a lifetime. . . . I don't think the drugs alone are going to be like insulin and diabetes.' In 1998 Nathanson took the reins of the National Institutes of Health's Office of AIDS Research (OAR), overseeing a scientific budget of $1.7 million annually. He stepped to the helm just as doubt about HAART began to surface.

'My view is that every death that didn't occur in 1997 is not a cure, it's just a post-poned death,' Nathanson said, well aware of the gravity of his comments. 'I don't hear much optimism. . . . I'm afraid that the death rate may start to climb back. . . . The decline in mortality, where the graph looks like it's going to zero, that could be used to argue that we should cut back in our research. And that would be a disastrous message.'

Disastrous, Nathanson said, because he foresaw that there would soon be need for fundamentally new treatment strategies for HIV disease, yet most of the drugs in development at some twenty-five companies targetting the $5 billion US AIDS market were simply variations on the basic HAART themes. No pill-form drug that targetted HIV in an entirely new way, and no vaccine, was likely to find their way to the market-place before 2005 to 2020.

'For the next few years,' Nathanson opined, 'the only thing one can anticipate is refinements on the same drug themes.'

'I think we're probably as far away from treatment cures as we are from vaccines,' said Peter Young, vice president of HIV therapeutic developments for the Glaxo Well-come pharmaceutical corporation. The image that came to his mind was of 'a lot of people filling up sandbags' to bolster the weakening HAART dam.

An unabated stream of new HIV cases was continually flowing into a large pool of infected people—a pool that hadn't existed prior to the HAART revolution of 1996. The drugs created a dam, however, holding the HIV stream inside an ever-expanding pool, rather than allowing them to flow on to AIDS and eventual death.

'If you were trying to graph the prognosis for the [HIV] population, clearly we're not at a point where we can say we've levelled this graph off,' Young concluded with regret. 'Maybe we changed the rate of flow up to that dam. But it's a work in progress'.

Many researchers—including those originators of the eradication hypothesis of 1996—said four years later that the reservoir of hidden HIVs in apparently successful HAART patients was large and long-lived. David Ho thought patients would have to take the difficult drugs for twenty-five to thirty years to eliminate those hidden viruses. Some scientists put the figure even further out at forty to fifty years.

Regardless of the number, it was too long. The HAART drugs involved a complex and difficult regimen, were expensive and difficult to take, and increasingly were seen to cause a range of nasty, even life-threatening, side-effects. With at least 250 different combinations on the market in early 1999 and a host of new HAART drugs scheduled for future FDA approval, physicians needed to keep track of a long list of dos and don'ts. For the patients, taking HAART could become a full-time job. Some drugs had to be taken six times a day, some once, some twice. Some had to be ingested on a full stomach, others before eating. And all well-managed HIV patients also took a host of prophylactic drugs that prevented common opportunistic infections.

And HIV developed resistance to anti-viral drugs roughly the same way bacteria became resistant to antibiotics: by exploiting inappropriate human use of the drugs. But HIV did it in orders of magnitude faster than that seen with bacteria. Any use, followed by an interruption and later reuse of the same drugs, gave HIV the opportunity to mutate and clone an enormous colony of resistant viruses. And in the case of HAART, very brief interruptions, of the order of days, were enough to shift the advantage to the deadly viruses. Companies responded by developing quick resistance tests that physicians could routinely perform on patients' virus samples. If a patient was found, for example, to have HIVs that had mutated to resist indinavir, the physician might then switch the client to a cocktail that had a different protease inhibitor. Until the virus was resistant to *all* protease inhibitors.[88]

Time alone might eventually work against the HAART dam. Each time patients changed their cocktails, resistant strains seemed to emerge more quickly and they might pass those resistant strains on to their sexual or needle-sharing partners. Eventually, like James in New York, patients would run out of effective options.

Some physicians reacted to HAART failure by giving patients extraordinarily complex cocktails of up to eight antivirals, at a cost of over $60 000 a year. 'And,' said Manhattan HIV specialist Dr Howard Grossman, 'it's really well tolerated. It's amazing.'

By 2000 this 'mega-HAART', as Grossman called it, was remarkably common therapy among patients who had failed standard treatment due to the emergence of drug-resistant HIVs.

As physicians like Grossman ventured into ever wilder frontiers of HIV treatment, the grand HAART experiment was rushing forward without any guiding data. No one was keeping track. Indeed, convinced the rhetoric stressing that 'the plague is over' was valid, most AIDS service organizations saw donations drop in the late 1990s. So they had cut back on their policy and research staffs. And all over America acute AIDS care facilities shut down, breaking up teams of scientists, physicians, and nurses that used to monitor patient outcomes on a scale that offered statistically relevant information.

One of the few such facilities remaining intact in 1998 was at the University of Alabama in Birmingham, where Dr Michael Saag supervised research and care on more than fifteen hundred patients.

By the end of 1998 Saag's massive data pool was yielding heartbreaking numbers. He could see that May 1997 had been the nadir for AIDS and deaths in his population, but since that time death rates were 'clearly on the rise. They aren't dying of a traditionally defined AIDS illness. I don't know what they're dying of, but they are dying. They're just wasting and dying.'

The data had caught up with 'cure' and 'eradication'—by early 1999 both concepts were dead. The new buzz word was *remission*, a term taken from another dismal field of medicine, cancer care. By 2000 even that word had disappeared from the HIV lexicon.

At Northwestern University in Chicago, Dr Steven Wolinsky analysed viral genes found in his most successfully treated patients. His findings were abysmal: virus was always present and it seemed to mutate over time.

'The virus is not gone—it's still there years out. So the question is, is this an evolutionary question? Is there ongoing replication? Why do we always see [viral] RNA? The virus is telling me something, but I'm not smart enough to see it,' Wolinsky shrugged. 'Is the sky falling?'

'Is it?' he was asked back.

'I wish I knew,' he concluded. In other words, was the human immuno-deficiency virus following the same tragic public health route as had the bacteria that became known as MRSA, VRE, and VISA?

Emilio Emini, head of the Merck Research Laboratories in West Point, Pennsylvania, once a leading HAART optimist, agreed in 1999 that HIV had replicated and mutated in apparently effectively treated patients. It was a shared overall consensus reached in 1999 among HIV scientists: the virus *will* reproduce and mutate.

'We've said from the beginning this is a nasty little virus,' Emini insisted. 'My fundamental hope is that in the end we'll be able to make a sincere shot at a vaccine here.'

Meanwhile, said gay author and well-known New York activist Michelangelo Signorille, outside a few scientific circles, a sort of mass denial had set in. 'People were furious,... enraged that I would be saying that AIDS did not go away. People accused me of causing panic, being hysterical. People are embarrassed to talk about the fact that the drugs aren't working for them and even to say that their lover recently died of AIDS. Because of that sense of failure.'

By late 1999 there was mounting evidence that the sort of denial Signorille declaimed was leading to a resurgence of unsafe sexual activity in the gay community, posing a potential public health threat.

Researchers at the CDC developed a test that, for the first time, offered public health authorities the chance to handle HIV the same way that they had long handled syphilis. The test allowed researchers to tell who had been infected recently with the virus versus those who had been carrying HIV for years. Before the test, called a detuned ELISA, was developed, public health workers had no way of tracing the spread of HIV in their communities. It had been too hard for anyone to recall the names and addresses of all of their sexual partners, spanning years of their lives. But the detuned ELISA could pick out newly infected individuals[89]—those who had acquired HIV within the last 120 days. And nearly everyone could remember whom they had had sex with over the last four months.

Armed with such an itemization, public health authorities could, theoretically, track down individuals who appeared to be spreading HIV and interrupt the chain of transmission. The idea, then, was to do for HIV what for years had been done with gonorrhoea and syphilis.

'It's brilliantly simple,' said Dr Willi McFarland of the San Francisco Department of Public Health. 'When we heard about this we were just ecstatic because this opens up the possibility of answering questions we never could address before.'

In 1999 San Francisco was the only city in the world that routinely used detuned ELISA tests. And after about nine months of detuning thousands of Northern Californians, McFarland and his colleagues were thoroughly convinced of its use as a research tool.

About nine thousand San Franciscans had an HIV test in a city clinic every year and McFarland's colleagues in neighbouring Alameda, Marin, and San Mateo counties also administered limited numbers of detuned ELISAs in co-operative studies in 1999. What they found, McFarland said, 'blew our minds.' Despite several thousand HIV tests, not a *single* woman turned up positive for recent acquisition of HIV. Not one. *None* of Northern California's injecting drug users who were tested turned up positive for recent infection except those who were gay. *All* of the newly infected San Franciscans were gay men, most of them white and in their thirties.

McFarland wanted to learn more about those men, especially who their partners might be. But unlike New York and a dozen other states, California had no contact tracing law for HIV. And according to McFarland, any attempts to elicit partner information from the state's mostly gay, male HIV population were greeted with cries of 'sex police!'

'It raises a lot of issues—political things—and the memory of Typhoid Mary,' McFarland said. 'We were baffled by the tremendous resistance to naming names. Undermining our whole effort is community resistance.'

The AIDS service organization Gay Men's Health Crisis conducted a survey in 1998 in Manhattan of seven thousand gay men, finding that 80 per cent had undergone an HIV test within the previous three years: 13 per cent were HIV positive. That infection rate was a far cry from the 50 per cent HIV-positive rate that was presumed to be in the New York City gay community in 1980. That was the good news. The bad news was that 39 per cent of the respondents admitted to having had unprotected (without a condom) anal intercourse within the previous year.

The reason? 'Now people mistakenly feel that AIDS is over,' GMHC director Joshua Lipsman said. Because of HAART's apparent success, 'the misimpression in the public is that you pop a pill and you're fine.'

Five years before, the ravages of AIDS had been visually obvious even to casual observers strolling through gay urban centres. Along the streets, in the cafes, one could see young men who painfully leaned their frail bodies on friends, on their canes, against doorframes. And for uninfected gay men, every day brought obvious reminders of the dangers inherent in having sex without latex protection.

However, since 1996, and widespread use of HAART, gay neighbourhoods had completely transformed. They were full of healthy-looking, muscular men—whether they were HIV positive or not—who worked out in local gyms, took growth hormone and testosterone, and looked a lot more like Arnold Schwartzenegger than stick figures leaning on Death's door.

'I do think that the lessening of fear about death and AIDS has resulted in a decrease in fear about contracting HIV,' said Dr Mitchell Katz, the director of the San Francisco Department of Public Health and himself a gay man.

Meanwhile, gonorrhoea incidence in gay men rose 74 per cent between 1993 and 1996 in a national survey of twenty-six cities. In Seattle the number of syphilis cases in gay men had increased by 60 per cent and gonorrhoea by 76 per cent since 1996. Chicago saw syphilis, which had disappeared from its gay population, suddenly resurface in 1998 in a North Side homosexual neighbourhood. And gonorrhoea incidence among gay Chicagoans doubled.

According to the New York City Department of Health, Gotham's gonorrhoea rates had not risen. But syphilis rates had. Overall (in all population groups, gay and straight) there were about eighty active syphilis cases in New York City in 1998. By mid-1999, the case numbers were well ahead of 1998 and the department forecast more than one hundred for the year.

San Francisco's troubling trends were more obvious, according to its health department. In 1994 fewer than 1 per cent of the gay men who were diagnosed with gonorrhoea also had HIV. In 1998 the number of gay HIV-positive men with gonorrhoea had risen to 16 per cent, meaning, McFarland said, that more HIV-positive and HIV-negative men in the city were having sex without protective condoms.

Dr Kimberly Page-Shafer of the University of California San Francisco and Dan Wohlfeiler of the local Stop AIDS Project surveyed 21 857 gay men between 1994 and 1997. They found a steady rise in the number of gay men who admitted to having sex without a condom, until, in 1997, it reached a third of the respondents.

Another UCSF study, conducted by scientist Ron Stall, saw that by the end of 1997 half of more than five hundred men who had been questioned repeatedly since 1993 were having unprotected intercourse. 'What's remarkable about this study is that for the very first time in the history of the epidemic we are seeing very large increases in unsafe sex,' Stall explained. 'This is new. And it's on the order of a 50 per cent increase over the last two years. About half of the risk-taking is unprotected anal intercourse where the men either knew their partner had a different [HIV] serostatus or didn't know their partner's serostatus.'

'What's new is people were supposed to feel remorse about having unsafe sex,' Katz said. 'And now there's this small minority saying, "Yes, I did, and I'm not sorry."'

It was called barebacking, UCSF medical sociology graduate student Michael Scarce said. Scarce had interviewed 826 gay men nationwide who considered themselves barebackers. Most were white and the average age was thirty-six. They knew everything that the CDC and groups like GMHC and the Stop AIDS Project had to say about HIV yet they rejected the prevention campaigns, calling public health officials and prominent gay leaders 'safer sex police' and 'condom police'. They were, Scarce insisted, 'public health outlaws' and their popularity was rapidly increasing.

'And it never would have happened without the Internet,' Scarce maintained. 'Barebacking was born on AOL. It was through the anonymity of the Internet that gay men were able to be honest about what they wanted and connect with one another to get it.' Scarce had identified more than 150 list servers on the Internet dedicated to barebacking.

In 1999, Ron Stall said, the '$100 000 question' is whether gay culture had entered a radically new paradigm that called for dramatically different approaches to disease prevention. So how would the CDC's detuned ELISA contact tracing plan figure into such a picture? Scarce predicted that 'a war is coming between gay men and public health if they do contact tracing.'

As the twentieth century neared its close, it looked as if HIV would, indeed, follow the sorry courses of MRSA, VRE, multidrug-resistant tuberculosis, and chlorine-resistant microbes in drinking water.

Three different research teams published proof in 1999 that drug-resistant strains of HIV were spreading among sexually active people in the United States and Europe. The findings raised deeply troubling reservations about both HAART and the future of public health control of the epidemic. Since all three research groups discovered highly multidrug-resistant forms of the virus that had surfaced within the previous eighteen months, the fear was that observers were witnessing the beginning of a trend that could render anti-HIV treatments useless to people infected in the future.

At a 1999 National HIV Prevention Conference in Atlanta, CDC director Koplan hailed HAART as a 'tremendous public health accomplishment,' and added, 'I think you're hard-pressed not to say it's a public health triumph when people can live longer.'

But there was a big difference between antibiotic treatments for, say, tuberculosis and HAART for HIV. The antibiotics were curative, when properly used, and thus decreased the size of the contagious TB population. HAART, in contrast, was *not* curative and had greatly increased the size of the population of Americans and Europeans living with HIV—living behind the leaky HAART dam.

There, they could transmit HIV to their sexual partners, in some cases passing on mutant, highly drug-resistant forms of the virus.

'Clearly HAART was a great boon for medicine,' Thomas Jefferson University's HIV expert Roger Pomerantz said. 'For public health, though, it's a challenge, maybe an obstacle.'

By 2001, this debate would be front and centre of the global stage, with AIDS advocates and political leaders calling for widespread distribution of HAART drugs in SubSaharan Africa and other hard-hit regions of the world. In June 2001 the United Nations General Assembly, in an historic first-ever session on AIDS, passed a resolution calling for creation of a multibillion global AIDS fund, to be used for both treatment and prevention of HIV disease.

And so the twentieth century ended on a confusing, ominous note for public health in the United States. Humanity's old nemesis, the microbial world, was creating so many new challenges that scientists and doctors were hard-pressed to keep track. Globalization opened America to fantastic new economic and cultural horizons, but left her vulnerable to a higher order of microbial threat. The ageing population was increasingly likely to fill oncology and cardiology wards, just as the nation's health-care financing system was finding new, creative ways to deny access to such care. Ever more Americans were outside the system, denied health insurance and access. Politic-ally, many Americans decried anything that reeked of 'government', thus undermining support for public health.

Horribly, hospitals had been transformed in a remarkably short period of time from esteemed bastions of medical bravado to financially managed hubs for transmission of drug-resistant, lethal microbes. Tough CDC infection-control standards, coupled with decreased use of catheters and other invasive devices, brought nosocomial infection rates down in the US during 1999 in top hospitals, but spread of bacteria in medical facilities still cost America about forty-four thousand to ninety-eight thou-sand lives and up to $29 billion that year.

The sheer complexity of treatment for previously simple bacterial infections had become mind-boggling. Hospitals, physicians, and public health leaders made valiant attempts at limiting emergence and spread of antibiotic-resistant, ubiquitous bac-teria, discovering by 2000 that despite fifty years of the drugs' use they had barely an inkling of how to perpetuate their efficacy in such complicated American ecologies as intensive care units, child care centres, and prisons. Not surprisingly, new staphylo-coccus and streptococcus strains capable of resisting the last-resort drug, vancomycin, continued to crop up across America.

Though many of America's main health threats by 2000 came from outside the country, the nation's public health infrastructure was not at all prepared to deal with such external menaces. Agencies that traditionally had ignored public health, such as the CIA and the Centre for Strategic and International Studies, were by 2000 address-ing concerns about globalized infectious diseases far more vigorously and anxiously than were most public health agencies.

US public health at the end of the twentieth century had also been stymied in its meagre attempts to address racial gaps in life expectancy and other basic indicators of well-being. An average white baby boy born in America in 1980 had a life expectancy that was seven years longer than that of an African-American infant born the same year. By 1990 that life expectancy gap was slightly wider: 7.3 years. And in 1996 that gap was eight years. Public health's abysmal track record in minority communities had not, despite greater prominence of Hispanic and African-American leaders in relevant government leadership positions, much improved during the 1990s.

In New York City, for example, the African-American neighbourhood of central Har-lem had Gotham's highest overall death rate in 1998 and led the metropolis not only for most infectious diseases mortality rates but also for cancer and heart disease. The death gap between Harlem and whiter, wealthier parts of the city was of the order of 30 per cent.

Prevention of chronic killers—cancers, heart diseases—continued to stump Ameri-can public health leaders in 2000, partly because of contradictory scientific findings regarding diet and behavioural issues. But even where the science of both prevention and treatment seemed clear there were terrible failures. Topping the list were hyper-tension and obesity, both of which rose dramatically among Americans during the

1990s. In a 1999 survey in Minnesota, for example, more than half of all tested adults were hypertensive (39 per cent of whom didn't know it, and only 16.6 per cent of whom were receiving treatment of any kind).

Though health care was not synonymous with public health, by 2000 it was glaringly obvious in the United States that lack of access to medical treatment, and insurance company limitations on such care, were affecting life expectancies. The National Coaliton on Health Care announced that lethal false diagnosis rates soared during the 1990s, approaching 35 per cent of all 1997 deaths. And an estimated 180 000 Americans died annually during the late 1990s because of nontreatment or improper medical care. A University of Wisconsin study found that some managed care-dictated early hospital discharge policies during the 1990s *tripled* infant death rates.

At the close of 1999 a team of Harvard and University of North Carolina researchers surveyed the status of the United States public health system. The analysts gave detailed questionnaires to every local public health leader in the country, asking them to rate the performance of their own departments and services. On average, those polled gave themselves a 35 per cent rating out of a possible 100 per cent.

In other words, by the end of the century, public health leaders themselves said that they were only achieving one-third of the functions essential to protecting the health of the population of the United States.

It recalled the ancient dichotomy between Hygeia and Panakeia: In Greek mythology, the god Asklepios had two daughters. Panakeia was the healer and she invented cures for all manner of ailments. Asklepios's other daughter, Hygeia, taught Greeks sensible ways to live so that they would stay healthy and have no need of Panakeia's healing. Both daughter's names have lived down through the ages. Hygeia in English is Hygiene, and Panakeia has been transformed over time into a cure-all, a universal treatment, a panacea.

What would ancient Greece's Asklepios have thought of America's great bastions of health in 2000, her prestigious teaching hospitals? Strolling along hallways resonating with the sounds of beeping heart monitors and emergency audio pages, Asklepios might turn to daughters Panakeia and Hygeia.

'Where is the solution to this mess?' Asklepios might ask.

Panakeia would cast her eyes upon the plethora of high-technology devices to which patients were attached and the long lists of drugs they were receiving. She would note the spread of diseases inside the hallowed chambers of panacea. And she would be at a loss.

'Sister,' Panakeia would say in desperation, 'have you an answer?'

And Hygeia would shake her head sadly, whispering, 'Most of these suffering souls should never have been here in the first place.'

CHAPTER 5

Biowar

Threatening biological terrorism and public health.

Could it not be contrived to Send the Small Pox among those Disaffected Tribes of Indians?

—Sir Jeffrey Amherst, British commander-in-chief, American colonies, July 1763, writing in reference to an uprising among the Pontiac. Two weeks previously, smallpox-infested blankets had been distributed to the Shawnee and Delaware peoples.[1]

Above 700 Negroes are come down the River in the Smallpox. I shall distribute them about the Rebel Plantations.

—British General Alexander Leslie, July 13, 1781, writing of his plans to use smallpox against supporters of General George Washington, during the American Revolution.

The bright sunlight and glare off freshly falling, sparkling snow belied the danger of the day. The wind chill factor on this January morning in Minneapolis was −50 °F—cold enough to kill any ill-prepared fool who ventured far from shelter.

Through the glass panel of his tiny, drab government office Mike Osterholm eyed his heavily clad employees as they walked toward their respective cubicles, peeling off layers of down, Gore-Tex, and wool as they went. Peering through heat-steamed glasses one waved a good-morning greeting to Osterholm who, as befits a classic Minnesotan, cheerfully waved back and shouted, 'Cold enough for you?'

'Yup. Gonna be good ice fishing this weekend,' the young state health worker joked. They both knew he'd be about as likely to spend a day off in a tent on one of Minnesota's hundreds of frozen lakes as he would dance with the Rockettes at Radio City Music Hall.

Two eighteen-inch-wide slits of glass afforded Osterholm a few rays of winter sunlight and a glimpse of snow drifting down onto leafless trees. On the white Sheetrock walls were ominous old State Health Department signs, one reading: SMALLPOX EXISTS ON THESE PREMISES. Osterholm was in unusually good spirits, as he'd just received a remarkable telephone call.

Mike Osterholm, an epidemiologist in America's Siberia, was preparing to play a historic role in the politics of a Middle Eastern nation about which he knew next to nothing. He had just been summoned by the king of Jordan to brief the monarch about a subject that had caused Osterholm many sleepless nights: biological terrorism.

On that icy January 5, 1999 day as his staff of exceptionally astute disease-detectives were busy tracking the trail of a new outbreak of listeria food poisonings Osterholm spoke from his office with Washington, getting details of the planned meeting from the State Department and National Security Council.

King Hussein, leader of the Hashemite Kingdom of Jordan, held a position of strategic global import that far outweighed the size and economic clout of his tiny desert nation. He was the longest-ruling head of state in the latter twentieth century, having acceded to the throne at the age of seventeen. But his continued survival was in jeopardy. Just five days earlier Hussein had hastily left his six-month-long cancer care at the nearby Mayo Clinic, having not yet completed a final round of bone marrow transplant procedures. His sudden, unexpected departure, accompanied by American-born Queen Noor and eighteen-year-old Prince Hamzah, had caused consternation at the Mayo and sparked rumours of political intrigue. Now, with cancer cells coursing throughout his body, the sixty-three-year-old monarch had an apparently sudden interest in biological terrorism. It seemed to have been sparked shortly before Christmas when Osterholm, on a visit to the Mayo Clinic, met teenaged Prince Hamzah and struck up a conversation not about deadly tumour cells but about lethal microbes. The young prince, who was enrolled at Britain's prestigious Sandhurst military school, was impressed by the energetic Swedish-American.

Shortly after that chance meeting, the king and his family had made their hasty departure, stopping first in London, where the royal family owned a tastefully appointed home not far from Buckingham Palace. Even Osterholm was unaware that the king was in London, and in preparation for meeting with the monarch he was finding out about Amman, a desert city he could barely imagine from the vantage point of his American Siberia. Yet if the place seemed unfathomable the subject did not, as bioterrorism had obsessed Osterholm for nearly six years.

As he prepared to meet Hussein, he explained to a visitor that the interest began on May 11, 1993, in the CDC's Auditorium A, at precisely 1:00 p.m. He remembered such details because for the state epidemiologist the moment was an epiphany the likes of which he had never previously experienced. The topic on the agenda was possible destruction of remaining laboratory stocks of otherwise eradicated smallpox virus. During the debate information was revealed regarding former Soviet scientists who had defected to the United States and United Kingdom, giving Westerners information on a previously secret Soviet biowarfare programme. The classified word was that Soviet scientists had developed a weapon of mass destruction, made of smallpox viruses.

'And I thought to myself, "Jeez! In this century alone, 500 million people died of smallpox, and all of the wars combined were only 320 million,"' Osterholm recalled.

Like most American biologists and physicians Osterholm had always considered talk of bioweapons the stuff of silly science fiction, paranoid conspiracy fantasies, or old-fashioned red-baiting. He had never previously imagined that someone might actually use germs as weapons. And the meeting was shattering if for no other reason than it made real a concept he had for his entire life comfortably dismissed as nonsense.

After that fateful CDC meeting Osterholm had drinks with General Philip Russell, the military's highest-ranking biologist, who revealed still more alarming details: it wasn't just smallpox; it wasn't just the Russians; it wasn't even just belligerent countries that had bioweapons. Russell told Osterholm that such horrors had found their ways into the hands of groups of political zealots, armed terrorists, religious cults, and American ultraright-wing militiamen.

'And it started me on a journey,' Osterholm said. For the next three years Osterholm sat as a civilian advisor on military and foreign affairs secret committees that were focused in Washington on biological warfare and terrorism issues. He accumulated a lot of frequent-flyer miles jetting to and from the nation's capital, growing more anxious with every new secret revelation. He could tell his colleagues in the Minneapolis office nothing—even the names of his Washington committees were classified.

It was driving him crazy, Osterholm said, because the further he got into the issue, 'the more I realized we really didn't know what was going on.'[2]

Osterholm recognized by 1996 that the only effective response against a bioterrorism event would come from public health, 'and meanwhile I'm watching the infrastructure for public health in this country deteriorate.'

Never one to mince words, he soon spoke his mind in these meetings. And in Washington an emboldened Osterholm came under attack. The more he cried at secret meetings that no one was prepared, the more he was accused of grandstanding, trying to wave his ego around the capital. One New York City official privately charged that Osterholm was out for personal glory, rather than public protection.

Osterholm had retaliated, saying that he saw 'two enemies. The perpetrator. And the ones who are supposed to respond to it, who instead have blindfolded themselves. . . . Right now we are missing enough rods in public health we could not stop that [metaphoric] nuclear reaction of bioterrorism.'

By the close of 1996, having patiently sat on FBI committees, briefed Vice President Al Gore, and been through innumerable classified gatherings, Osterholm was convinced it was time to go public. He turned to Dr D. A. Henderson, one of public health's most venerable spokespersons. He urged the smallpox expert to speak out. Henderson, he knew, had the greatest credibility. The senior scientist ran a unique programme at Johns Hopkins University's School of Public Health, called the Centre for Civilian Biodefence Studies. And Henderson had been in even more classified meetings than Osterholm.

Thinking back over these events that January morning prompted Osterholm to call Henderson, who served as a sort of mentor on the bioterrorism issue. Osterholm turned to him for advice on what to tell the king of Jordan.

A week later the Minnesotan found himself seated across from the royal family of Jordan in their opulent home. Queen Noor, her son Hamzah, and the king's security chief listened and energetically partook in the hours-long discussion. Osterholm was impressed with King Hussein's vigour and keen intellect. He decided that rumours of King Hussein's imminent death were greatly exaggerated. And there was no doubt whatsoever in Osterholm's mind as he left the royal family that King Hussein, for reasons unstated, had cause for acute concern about the possible use of biological weapons inside his kingdom, or regionally in the volatile Middle East.

The king told Osterholm that he wanted to host an international meeting of world leaders to discuss bioterrorism. And Osterholm was, in turn, in awe of the Jordanian leader.

Jordan was defended against hostile neighbours on every side by an armed force of 82 250 men and 35 000 reserves. It was a tiny military force compared to those amassed around it. To the north Syria spent more than $3 billion a year building an armed force of more than 306 000 men, 392 000 reservists, and strategic missile, tank, and aircraft capability, all of it well tested in battles against Israel and in Lebanon's long civil war. To the south was the Hashemite's ancient tribal nemesis, the House of Saud, protected by a Saudi Arabian highly trained military force of some 50 000 men, including twenty air bases stocked with the most expensive high-technology aircraft, missile, and reconnaissance equipment available in the global marketplace. To Jordan's west was Israel, the only country in the region with which the Hashemite Kingdom had in recent decades waged war. With military spending that topped $8 billion annually, an army of 140 000 men and women, including seasoned combatants and highly sophisticated air and land strategic capacity, Israel was the Middle East's most significant tactical force.

Most troubling for King Hussein, however, were two things: the forces massed on his eastern flank and domestic insurgents. On the east was Saddam Hussein's Iraq, with an army of some 450 000 men, combat-seasoned fighter pilots, an ambitious SCUD missile programme, and military spending well in excess of $5 billion annually.

Domestically, King Hussein had always been plagued by would-be assassins, terrorists, attempted coups, and religious fanatics, who readily gained political and financial support from Jordan's belligerent regional enemies. Even within his own army was a 1200-man Palestinian subdivision that swore allegiance not to the king, but to PLO leader Yasir Arafat. Most of Jordan's population was Palestinians, most of whom considered themselves refugees from Israeli-occupied Palestine. On innumerable occasions during his reign the PLO and other Palestinian organizations had used Jordan as a staging ground for unauthorized attacks on Israel, carried out violent demonstrations within the kingdom, and even attempted to overthrow the king. It was rumoured King Hussein had survived more than fifty assassination attempts: publicly thirty were acknowledged by the Hashemite government.

The king did not discuss these matters with Osterholm in their London meeting, but they must have formed a backdrop to his avid interest in bioterrorism. At the close of their meeting the king, queen, and prince cordially thanked Osterholm and withdrew to their private chambers. The following day King Hussein piloted his own jet home to Amman.

Seven days later, on January 26, the king stunned the entire world by announcing that his brother, Prince Hassam, would not inherit the throne, which for thirty-four years had been his promise. Rather, the comparatively obscure Prince Abdullah, a thirty-seven-year-old Jordanian military leader and son of the king, would take control of the nation. Amid rumours of court intrigue that were described in scales of Shakespearean drama a lengthy letter from the king to Prince Hassam explained the radical change. Among the issues discussed at length in the fourteen-page missive was germ warfare. The king warned Hassam—and the Jordanian people—of the grave dangers of deliberately fomented epidemics. Echoing lessons learned in his hours with Osterholm, Hussein described bioweapons as a terrible new resource for the stateless terrorist or rogue nation. Realizing his letter would be published in Jordanian newspapers and resonate across the Arab world King Hussein pointedly warned that there could be no winners in a world of man-made epidemics.

A few hours after completing the letter the dying king boarded his jet and under US Air Force escort flew back to the Mayo Clinic. Prince Abdullah was sworn in the following day.

And then the king died.

Osterholm would never know what role—if any—his discussion with the royal family had on the king's shocking twelfth-hour decisions. He recognized some of his remarks in the king's letter and knew from the questions the royal family had posed in London that a few of his themes had got through: that new scientific technology made genetic manipulation and creation of superbugs fairly simple feats. And systems of civilian defence against bioweapons were virtually non-existent. The Minnesotan's brief moment in the world of international intrigue served, however, to confirm Osterholm's belief that he had been right a year earlier when he insisted that the bioterrorism issue be placed on the agenda for public concern.

For months he had bugged Henderson about it, pressing the older scientist to reveal to the press what they had both heard in all those secret Washington meetings. Henderson first gingerly tested the waters at the September 1997 meeting of the Infectious Diseases Society of America. He carefully restricted his comments to published information, but made reference to larger concerns he had picked up in the secret Washington meetings. Henderson stuck to historical ground, outlining the destruction and terror produced by outbreaks of smallpox and anthrax during the latter half of the twentieth century. He kept the academic litany remarkably dry, given the horror he was describing. And he concluded his remarks with an observation that stood in stark contrast to the almost nonchalant tone of his previous comments: 'The spectre of biological weapons is every bit as grim as that of nuclear winter,' a reference to the theory that use of nuclear weapons would sink the world into an ice age that would obliterate nearly every life-form on earth.

Osterholm wasn't satisfied. He pushed his mentor for more. And he got it six months later at an enormous public meeting in Atlanta.

Henderson decided that the time had come to speak his mind in the manner Osterholm had urged. It was hard to imagine the tall, barrel-chested baritone ever doing otherwise. His presence dominated any conversation, filled any room.

Seas of colleagues parted when Henderson entered a room, in deference to his leadership role in probably the most dramatic public health victory of the twentieth century, the elimination of smallpox. By his own admission Henderson, then an officer of the World Health Organization, had broken every rule in the UN bureaucratic book by the time the various strains of human smallpox viruses were vanquished in 1977. It was necessary, he insisted. After all, they were fighting to defeat a virus responsible for killing more human beings in the twentieth century than all wars combined.

Henderson had, for example, rationalized open cooperation between military and public health personnel and collaboration across 1970s Cold War boundaries. The global campaign to eliminate smallpox had been originally a Soviet idea, announced in Moscow in 1958. And the Soviets had a profound—perhaps unnerving—knowledge of the two species of viruses capable of causing smallpox. So at a time when virtually all other communication between Moscow and the capitals of the capitalist West were tightly shut, Henderson encouraged public health alliances with hands outstretched across the Berlin Wall.

When all traces of wild human smallpox had been eradicated, Henderson had to go along with WHO's diplomatic plan for dealing with the fate of remaining laboratory samples of the virus. One set went into the deep freezers of the maximum security laboratory at the Centres for Disease Control and Prevention in Atlanta, Georgia. The other was placed in frozen isolation in a Moscow laboratory that, Henderson knew, was physically less secure. He didn't much like the Moscow setting but compromised: after all, with all other known laboratory samples of smallpox scheduled for immediate destruction the WHO scheme limited global concern and security to just two sites. In 1977 that had seemed reasonable.

Henderson didn't then know that Soviet Premier Leonid Brezhnev had other plans for those viruses—indeed, for hundreds of different lethal pathogens. Twenty years later military and intelligence experts in the West confessed that they hadn't a clue about the programme Brezhnev dubbed Biopreparat until at least ten years after the smallpox bilateral accord was reached. They'd known nothing of Brezhnev's great scheme for offsetting American nuclear deterrence, nor of his absolute resolve to violate the Biological Weapons Convention signed with US President Richard Nixon in 1973.

They had no idea that by 1977 the Soviet Union was well advanced in construction of what would eventually be forty-seven biological weapons laboratories and testing sites, employing upward of fifty thousand scientists, technicians, and support staff in facilities spanning at least ten time zones. Most crucially, they knew nothing about the secret laboratories in Siberia.

By 1998, seven years after the collapse of the Soviet Union, though, Henderson was aware of at least some of the facts about Biopreparat. He confessed that it was 'damned hard' to sift fact from fiction, to know which former Biopreparat scientists could be trusted. They could all be exaggerating the situation. Or they could be hiding information that was vital—Henderson felt with no sense of overstatement—to the survival of the human race.

The horrible possibility that a politically—even pathologically—crazed group or individual could get their hands on the Moscow viruses hit home when Henderson watched televised reports of the 1993 standoff between Boris Yeltsin's government and a loose coalition of armed dissidents, ranging politically from relatively moderate members of the Duma to angry Afghan war veterans shooting guns on behalf of a return to power of the Communist Party. Like most non-Russians Henderson had no sense of what was to come when American TV networks mentioned on September 21 that Boris Yeltsin had issued a decree on reform that was found objectionable to most of the Duma. But as days passed, the standoff escalated, and Henderson's fear for the safety of Moscow's stash of smallpox grew.[3]

'I learned that they dispatched soldiers to guard the Virology Institute and at that point it seemed logical to get [the smallpox] out of there,' Henderson later recalled. But when the protectors of Russia's smallpox stash were questioned closely it appeared 'that they moved it before that,' secretly, to the former Biopreparat facility located about an hour's drive from Novosibirsk, in central Siberia. Henderson was stunned, as the Russians had never told WHO that the tubes of lethal microbes had been re-located, and no international representative had seen the new repository or could vouch for the safety of the smallpox storage.

When US intelligence officials discovered that the Russian smallpox supplies had been moved, Henderson recalled, 'They asked, "Why didn't they get permission to move it?" and I said, "We never gave them a mandate to request permission from WHO." So they moved it.'

Now, four years after Yeltsin's White House confrontation Henderson remained unsure about where all of Russia's lethal smallpox supplies were located. Had they all gone into the Biopreparat freezers in Novosibirsk? Or had they secretly been dispersed, a test tube at a time, over the years to other Biopreparat laboratories? Was it even right to think in terms of Russian test tubes of the terrible virus, or might the old Soviets have cloned and mass-produced gallons of the viruses? Such uncertainty, coupled with classified intelligence reports he'd heard, made Henderson very, very nervous.

'Until recently the subject of biological terrorism has been little discussed or written about in the medical literature or, for that matter, in the public press,' Henderson began, addressing a tense March 1998 gathering of some six thousand professionals in Atlanta for the first International Conference on Emerging and Infectious Diseases. The moment Henderson, dressed in a black-and-white check jacket, starched white button shirt, tie, braces, and black trousers, stepped to the podium a hush came over the audience—unusual in its make-up as military personnel, academics, researchers, US government scientists, investigators from all over the world, and the media mingled. Henderson casually ran his fingers through his white hair, adjusted his steel-rimmed bifocals, and continued.

'Until recently, I personally had doubts about publicizing the subject because of concern that it might entice some to undertake dangerous, perhaps catastrophic experiments,' Henderson said. 'However, events of the past twelve to eighteen months have made it clear that likely perpetrators already envisage every agenda one could possibly imagine.'

Among recent events that had escalated US, European, and United Nations concerns about biological weapons were UN inspectors' findings in Iraq, recent innovations in biotechnology that streamlined genetic manipulation of microbes, elucidation of the scope of Russia's Biopreparat programme, and evidence that some of its former scientists may have moved their expertise and products onto the international arms market. Though most of these elements for concern had been known to experts before, it was only in 1997 that the full picture—the sense of threat—coalesced in Western military, intelligence, and some scientific circles.

Until the late 1990s few experts in any field considered biological weapons a viable threat. Lederberg, who, like Henderson, was part of that scientific fraternity of advisors on the subject, said that there were several mistaken assumptions that had previously steered world leaders away from concern about virusal and bacterial weapons, and biological toxins. Paramount, Lederberg felt, was the thankful fact that no one had yet committed the biological equivalent of Hiroshima.

In the absence of a bio-Hiroshima, Lederberg argued, it was all too easy to dismiss concerns about biological weapons on other grounds: 'biobombs' were more likely to kill a protagonist's own colleagues or troops than its opponents; it was impossible to create biological weapons, making them deliverable to enemies via missiles or a localized dispersion device; it was assumed that there were sufficient vaccines and medicines invented and available to counter the effects of such weapons, should they be deployed; any nation or organization that used such weapons would be greeted with disgust and moral repugnance by the rest of the world, therefore bioweapons represented a poor choice, even for outlaws.[4]

'Each of these arguments is without validity,' Henderson insisted. 'We now know that there are nations and dissident groups who have both the motivation and access to skills selectively to cultivate some of the most dangerous pathogens and to deploy them as agents in acts of terrorism or war.'

Henderson dangled the prospect of germ terrorism before the assembled public health experts, beckoning them to get on board for a journey previously taken only in secret, largely by military and law enforcement personnel. The invitation carried risks, he knew. Military and police cultures rarely mixed well with that of public health.

But the CDC's Dr Scott Lillibridge had no such reservations, and made it clear that biological weapons were a public health issue. The event that set off the first apprehension in public health, military, and intelligence circles occurred in Tokyo on March 20, 1995.

It was rush hour. Tens of thousands of Japanese office workers were boarding Tokyo's vast underground system. Three of the main, extremely crowded underground lines came from the residential districts to the west and north of Tokyo, particularly Asakusa and Aoyama, converging in the Kasumigaseki government centre of the city. At 8:00 a.m. these trains were extremely crowded as hordes of civil servants headed to start work at 8:30 a.m.[5]

At 8:09 a.m. a small bomb detonated in Kasumigaseki station as the Eidan, Marunouchi, Chiyoda, and Hibiya underground lines converged, releasing a deadly nerve gas called sarin.[6]

Four minutes later another bomb detonated inside busy Kasumigaseki station. At least three individuals carried additional plastic bags of nerve gas on the underground, which they poked open at the same time. The simple bombs released an invisible chemical, 1-Methylethyl methylphosphonate, bringing hundreds of passengers to their knees, overcome with nausea, bleeding from their noses and mouths, and suffering headaches, a profound sense of chemically induced anxiety, coughs, and, in three cases, pulmonary oedema. The Tokyo Fire Department rushed to the scene, responding to word of bomb blasts. Many were, themselves, overcome by the gas.

Hundreds of commuters staggered out of Kasumigaseki station and made their ways to local hospitals.

In the end, 5510 people were harmed in the sarin attack, about 100 of whom required hospitalization. Twelve died.

Japanese police soon discovered the culprits were members of a bizarre religious cult called Aum Shinrikyo, or Buddhist 'Om' and Supreme Truth.[7] Led by a forty-year-old Rolls-Royce-driving, long-haired, bearded guru named Shoko Asahara, Aum Shinrikyo was on a mission to bring about the end of the world, placing themselves in dominion over the survivors. Whereas religious cults in many cultures have long forecast Armageddon, Aum Shinrikyo was determined to hasten its arrival.

Subsequent years of police investigation and court proceedings revealed that Aum Shinrikyo was an enormous organization with minimally forty thousand devotees in Japan, Russia, Europe, and the United States. Japanese police swiftly discovered that the Kasumigaseki station attack was just a trial run: the organization had stockpiled enough sarin to kill 4.2 million people in a future attack. Further, the March 1995 sarin attack followed at least two prior gassings, several botulism toxin assaults, endeavours to kill Japan's leaders with anthrax, and attempts to acquire and develop Q fever bacteria and Africa's dread Ebola virus.[8]

With a donated and earned $2 billion treasury at its disposal thanks to a computer software company it ran, the cult bought the best expertise, including former KGB agents and Russian military advisors. In 1991 cult members even solicited advice from Russia's Minister of Defence, Grachov, and Oleg Lobov, a member of President Yeltsin's advisory council. The cult was negotiating purchase of nuclear weapons materials, using Ukrainian and Russian mobsters as go-betweens with ex-Soviet military personnel. Even the isolationist and vehemently anti-Japanese North Korean government provided the cult with arms and advice.

Aum Shinrikyo's activities proved to a once-sceptical national security community that weapons of mass destruction, and in particular bioweapons, could and were being developed by groups well outside of traditional government control.[9]

A few days after the Tokyo attack a classified national security forum convened at the White House, attended by President Bill Clinton, Vice President Al Gore, several cabinet members, and a select group of scientists, defence, and emergency officials. Kenneth Adelman, vice president of the Institute for Contemporary Studies in Washington, asked Joshua Lederberg at the meeting whether there weren't technological 'fixes' that could prevent biological and chemical attacks in the United States. As an example of what he was getting at, Adelman cited the positive role metal detectors were playing in virtually eliminating terrorist attacks at airports and on commercial also planes.

Lederberg responded carefully by comparing prevention approaches for nuclear, chemical, and biological attacks:

'Well, for the most part, it is not detection and prevention but deterrence which is the keystone of our security in the nuclear area.... That breaks down when you have a kamikaze—when you have people willing to commit suicide as part of the game. Deterrence is not a feature there.'

Lederberg discussed options for detecting nuclear devices that had fallen into terrorist or rogue nation hands, noting that 'in the nuclear field there is some room for detection.'

But, he added ominously, 'It is much more difficult in the chemical and biological area—it is next to impossible.'

Were an Aum Shinrikyo type of attack to occur in America one of the key responding agencies would be the federal Office of Emergency Preparedness and National Disaster Medical System. Its director, Dr Frank Young, listened as Lederberg speculated that an effective bioattack on the New York City subway system posed the possibility of '6000 dead, 100 000 in perilous condition. Your local authorities cannot begin to cope with events of that kind.'

'That is absolutely correct,' Young responded soberly.

It was the sort of nightmarish vision the congressional Office of Technology Assessment had pictured in 1993 in a now-classic scenario: a crop duster plane, loaded with one hundred kilograms of anthrax spores, flies over the White House, Capitol Hill, the Pentagon, and much of Washington, DC, in a criss-cross pattern before being detecting and forced to land.[10] Over the next days and weeks three million people die.

The Aum Shinrikyo attack served as a wake-up call, alerting officials that the once-unthinkable was not only possible, it might even be probable. This was no longer science fiction.

President Clinton promised the gathering that he would seek ways to strengthen the anaemic 1972 Biological Toxins and Weapons Convention, but there was little immediate satisfaction on that score—no one knew how to make violations of the treaty verifiable.[11]

The first genuinely tough attempt to enforce the treaty targeted Saddam Hussein's regime in Iraq. It demonstrated that controlling a government's use, or threatened use, of biological weapons was difficult if not impossible with available technical and diplomatic tools.

On August 2, 1990, an estimated force of 545 000 Iraq troops and tanks marched on neighbouring Kuwait, seizing Kuwaiti oil reserves and instituting martial law. Seven months later an allied force of some 690 000 combatants, led by the US administration of President George Bush, carried out an air and land war against Iraq's then million-man army, taking 175 000 Iraqi soldiers prisoner and inflicting some 85 000 casualties. The vanquished Iraqi leadership was compelled to sign a treaty guaranteeing that, among other things, all of Iraq's chemical and biological weapons and stockpiles would be destroyed immediately. This allowed United Nations inspectors, at least technically, the greatest investigational access to Iraq's war machine ever afforded under the Biological Toxins and Weapons Convention.

But the following year, on July 5, 1992, Iraq denied UN inspectors entry to a suspected bioweapons storage site. International tension rose, US sanctions of Iraqi trade were put in place, and three weeks later Baghdad yielded, allowing UN inspection of the contested site. No suspected materials were found; some inspectors claimed Iraq was playing a shell game, moving the weapons from one place to another, hiding the incriminating evidence.

The rationale for UN suspicion appeared strong. In 1989 the Iraqi Air Force had successfully launched its first orbital three-stage rocket, and appeared to have ballistic missile capability. With its $5 billion annual military budget Iraq spent heavily on acquisition of high-technology equipment. And in April 1990 Saddam Hussein had grandiosely announced that his forces had developed missile-loaded binary chemical weapons, mounted on modified long-range SCUD missiles. 'I swear to God that we will let our fire eat half of Israel if it tries to wage anything against Iraq,' Hussein declared in 1990.

Saddam Hussein had rarely levelled a political or military threat without following it through: in the 1980s Hussein obliterated every Iranian town and village he threatened.[12] The ensuing Iran/Iraq war lasted eight bloody years and claimed an estimated 240 000 Iranian civilian and military lives.[13]

Some of those casualties had been victims of Iraqi chemical weapons, inflicted from the first days of the war. Iran claimed, and UN inspectors had at least partially verified on site in 1984, 1986, and 1987, that mustard gas and a nerve gas called tabun were dispersed by aeroplanes and rockets. A UN team determined that Iraq was in violation of the Geneva Protocol.[14] It is estimated that 5 per cent of all Iranians who were exposed to these chemicals during the war died, but exact numbers of dead are not known.

Shortly after Iraq signed a cease-fire in 1988 Saddam Hussein refocused his attention on his country's Kurdish minority. On March 19, 1988, the Iraqi Air Force attacked the Kurdish village of Hallabja, killing nearly all its inhabitants. Though international observers didn't learn of the attack or reach the site for several days, Western intelligence experts concluded that the Kurds were victims of cyanide and mustard gas.[15]

Thereafter, Iraq began, by its own admission, an unprecedented chemical weapons build-up. And in 1996 Saddam Hussein's government conceded that biological weapons production had also commenced at that time.[16]

In the late 1980s Hussein acquired and developed chemical and biological weapons (CBW), with the complicity of US, Japanese, Austrian, British, Swiss, Dutch, and German commercial suppliers and technicians. Enormous chemical plants were built in Samarra, Falliyah, Al Muthanna, and just outside Baghdad. And, in collaboration with Argentina and Egypt, Iraq developed Condor missiles capable of delivering CBW to distant targets. Further, Iraq modified several SCUD missiles to give them very long-range capacity—capable of reaching targets in Israel.

For several years after the end of the Operation Desert Storm war, Iraq played a cat-and-mouse game with UN inspectors, hiding as much chemical and biological evidence as possible.

In 1994 Germany's BND intelligence unit (Bundenachrichtendienst, or Federal Intelligence Service) discovered a complex trail of acquisitions used by Iraq to obtain weapons and biowar materials, largely from Western European sources. Among the mountains of supplies obtained illegally by Iraq, despite international sanctions, were thirty-nine *tons* of bacterial growth medium, purchased mostly from Oxoid, a British subsidiary of Unilever.[17]

'It is absolutely inconceivable that Iraq could have had legitimate medical uses for that much growth medium,' Henderson insisted. 'Claiming legitimate use defies all boundaries of credibility.'

All of Iraq's medical and scientific laboratories had previously consumed less than 441 pounds of medium annually, or 0.5 per cent of the tons that were imported. Iraq was never able to account for the use or whereabouts of the seventeen tons of imported medium.[18]

Iraq's original seed sample of anthrax had been purchased above-board from American Type Culture Collection, then based in Rockville, Maryland, during the mid-1980s. The purchase was cleared by the US Department of Commerce during the Reagan Administration.

United Nations inspectors eventually concluded that Iraq had built an impressive biological weapons armamentarium before the Desert Storm war,[19] including about eight thousand pounds of anthrax, eight kilograms of concentrated botulinum toxin, and at least four other types of bacteria, five of viruses, and three other biotoxins. Just before the war broke out, the UN team concluded, Iraq had grown 340 litres of *Clostridium* for botulism toxin production. At numerous sites—particularly the Al Hakam Single-Cell Protein Plant, located a few miles south of Baghdad—stainless steel fermenters capable of holding 1450 litres of toxins or micro-organisms were found.

Though the Iraqi government eventually admitted to some of those findings, no one outside the Iraqi military leadership knew how much of the material had actually been turned into weapons. Growing bacteria or viruses was one thing; working out how to keep it alive aboard a flaming missile or bomb was quite another.

The Americans knew a fair amount about that problem.[20] During World War I US secret agents discovered that German laboratories were developing weaponized ricin toxin designed to be inflicted as a one-to-one weapon. (The protein ricin, found in castor beans, was a highly toxic neurological poison that would kill a human being who ingested as little as 180 micrograms of the compound. Though it was three hundred times less potent than botulism toxin, ricin was thirty times more potent than Aum Shinrikyo's sarin gas.) As far as is known these early weapons were never used. And at the war's end the League of Nations concluded that biological weapons were impractical and therefore did not pose a serious threat.

Twenty-seven years later in World War II, the US Army maintained that organisms and toxins remained impractical because they could never be used as weapons. But France, the United Kingdom, and Japan didn't agree: all three had substantial bioweapons programmes during World War II. And Japan had developed and used its bioweapons in Manchuria from 1933 to 1940. Using biobombs, it successfully caused outbreaks of typhus, cholera, and plague in China.[21] In addition, Allied investigations after the war revealed that Japan had used bioweapons for dysentery and paratyphoid.

A US biological weapons programme commenced in 1943 but was unable to convert any agents into weapons before the war's end.

With the Cold War came an escalation in American efforts to weaponize biology. In the 1950s special yellow fever-carrying mosquitoes were developed and tested. Unique bombs for release of pathogens were invented, as well as large-scale aerosols and submarine mines. Experiments were conducted, releasing microbes in New York, San Francisco, South Dakota, Minnesota, and, unintentionally, Canada.[22] A 1950 army experiment spraying bacteria from a boat sickened several San Franciscans, allegedly killing one.[23]

The most aggressive American biowarfare effort was conducted during the Korean War (1951–1953), and involved development and use of a variety of bacteria and disease-carrying mosquitoes. Though the US Joint Chiefs of Staff gave the military's scientists a green light to develop and use whatever bioweapons they could, the entire effort was hidden from the American people, even Congress. The military leaders were well aware that their deliberate creation of epidemics in Korea would be viewed as morally repugnant by US citizens.[24]

The offensive biological warfare programme continued, still shrouded in secrecy, for fifteen more years in the United States.

By 1966 the United States was spending $38 million a year on development of biological weapons, creating weapons from anthrax, *Pasteurella tularensis, Bacillus globigii,* and agricultural microbes such as stem rust, a fungus deadly to wheat. The weapons were stockpiled on a fifteen-thousand-acre site outside Pine Bluff, Arkansas—thousands of gallons of death, nestled inside rusting metal canisters. Like their nuclear counterparts that were mounted on missiles inside silos all over America the biobombs were Cold War weapons that few scientists or military leaders hoped to ever actually use. But the mentality of the capitalist-versus-communist era dictated a sort of historic suspension of rationality in favour of paranoia-driven technological development. If there were rumours of bioweapons developments in communist Korea, according to the mentality of the day, then surely capitalist America had better race toward technical superiority—even if the weapons of choice conjured up nightmares of mass civilian death, perhaps genocide.

But the 1960s were a bad time for the United States to be in the bioweapons game (if there ever was a 'good' time for such efforts): widespread antiwar demonstrations and public uncertainty about the veracity of American military statements put activities at Fort Detrick, Fort McClellan, and the Edgewood Arsenal under harsh political scrutiny.[25]

So in November 1969, President Richard M. Nixon announced that 'the United States of America will renounce the use of any form of deadly biological weapons that either kill or incapacitate. Our bacteriological programmes in the future will be confined to research in biological defence . . . and on measures of controlling and preventing the spread of disease.'

US stockpiles were destroyed over the following five years, and US offensive bioweapons programmes stopped abruptly. The experience, however, taught the Americans that it was one thing to grow trillions of deadly bacteria or viruses; it was quite another to create a means of delivering those pathogens, alive and lethal, effectively sickening enemy soldiers.[26]

Similarly, British and French military researchers abandoned bioweapons research not simply for moral reasons, but also because it proved so difficult to truly convert living microorganisms into weapons.

So as United Nations inspectors struggled in the 1990s to discern exactly what Iraq had developed, they paid closest attention to sorting out what might have been transformed into weapons. By 1994 the inspectors concluded that Iraq had, indeed, used botulinum toxins, but, as Dr Raymond A. Zilinskas put it: 'Though in possession of several hundred biological weapons, Iraq's tactical biological warfare capability during the Persian Gulf War actually was quite limited . . . [and] had Iraq's biological warfare munitions actually been used, their effect would have been limited to contaminating a relatively small area of ground surrounding the point of impact and exposing nearby individuals to pathogens or toxins in the form of aerosols.'[19]

The Iraqis, it seemed, were technological klutzes. They had loads of nasty germs, but little capability of delivering biobombs to designated targets. Further, Iraq's SCUD attacks in Israel were wildly off target due, the inspectors later determined, to an almost complete lack of inertial guidance systems. In 1992 Iraq could no more have tactically biobombed Tel Aviv than it could drop an A-bomb on Paris.

But subsequent years of investigation convinced UNSCOM—the United Nations special commission responsible for CBW inspections—that the Iraqi government was clandestinely continuing to develop biological agents as weapons throughout the 1990s. And Iraq had research and development collaborators, particularly in Libya. Zilinskas felt certain that Iraq could, within a matter of months, be capable of having 'remotely piloted vehicles, long-range fighter-bombers or cruise missiles equipped with tanks and sprayers and programmed to avoid detection by flying low and, following ground contours, could reach populations located within one thousand kilometres of Iraq's borders and disperse agents under conditions favourable for carrying out a successful biological attack.'

In the summer of 1995, Saddam's son-in-law who was in charge of Iraq's CBW effort, Lieutenant General Hussein Kamal al-Majid, defected to Jordan and was closely grilled by the CIA, UNSCOM, and European intelligence experts. Kamal told his interrogators that Iraq possessed vast stores of biological agents. Confronted by the truth, Iraq was compelled to destroy much of its postwar reserves, and Saddam admitted to having produced, among other things, a half a million litres of anthrax and botulinum toxin. Further, boxes of damning documents were turned over to UNSCOM. Based on these papers, UNSCOM concluded that Iraq had imported *more* than the thirty-nine tons of bacterial growth media originally estimated and experts were left to ponder the countless possibilities of its use.

Kamal, meanwhile, was lured back to Baghdad, along with another of Saddam's sons-in-law—both were soon assassinated.

UNSCOM director Richard Butler said Iraq had admitted that in 1992 it had seventy-five SCUD missiles loaded with either biological or chemical weapons. UNSCOM managed to destroy thirty of them but did not believe that Iraq had, as claimed, eliminated the other forty-five, Butler said. Increasingly in 1997 Iraq blocked UNSCOM activities. By November of that year President Bill Clinton was once again publicly prepared to wage a US/Iraq war over the matter—which would have constituted the first war in world history fought over the lack of transparency[27] in bio-weapons matters.

The US House of Representatives released a Task Force on Terrorism and Unconventional Warfare report on February 10, 1998. The report claimed that Iraq still then possessed forty-eight SCUD missile launchers and forty-five missiles, 'the majority' of which were loaded with bioweapons. Further, there were at least 8400 litres of anthrax and tons of chemical weapons in Iraq. The congressional report further charged that Iraq possessed ship-mounted drones capable of dropping biobombs on Europe and select spots in the Middle East. Biobombs and missiles were hidden from UNSCOM in Sudan and Libya. In Wau, Sudan, Iraqi scientists were once again manufacturing chemical weapons in the German-made Yarmook facility. And, the report also claimed, in Libya, Iraqi-made biological and chemical weapons were mounted on medium-range ballistic missiles capable of hitting targets up to 3000 kilometres from Tripoli. About a dozen Iraqi scientists were making anthrax and botulinum in the General Health Laboratories, located in Tripoli.[28]

Though many experts felt that much of the report could not be substantiated, it set a mood in Washington, and among US allies.[29]

Frustrated by an endless cat-and-mouse game between UN inspectors and Iraqi authorities the United States waged two crucial attacks in 1998. The first targeted Khartoum, Sudan, hitting a site the United States claimed was used by Iraqi-trained Sudanese to manufacture biological weapons. This alleged weapons factory was, according to the United States, used by the same terrorists who weeks earlier bombed US embassies in Nairobi, Kenya, and Dar es Salaam, Tanzania. The Sudanese government insisted that the targeted factory was a legitimate pharmaceutical plant.

As the House of Representatives debated impeachment of President Bill Clinton the US Air Force, on December 16, 1998, launched the second military assault: a series of bombing sorties aimed at alleged CBW manufacturing and storage sites in Iraq.

'Saddam Hussein must not be allowed to threaten his neighbours or the world with nuclear weapons, poison gas, or biological weapons,' Clinton said in a televised speech that day. 'I have no doubt today that, left unchecked, Saddam Hussein will use these terrible weapons again.'

What did Iraq, Libya, and Sudan actually have? No one outside those countries really knew; Iraq denied everything, and nobody in Khartoum or Tripoli was saying anything about the matter.[30] By mid-2000 renewed allegations surfaced, claiming Iraq was developing a new viral weapon, and doing so right under the noses of UN inspectors.[31]

The Iraqi situation made all too apparent the absurd weaknesses of the Biological Toxins and Weapons Convention of 1972. It was a toothless wonder, full of good intentions but utterly lacking in the key components of effective arms treaties: transparency, power of inspection, verification, and enforcement. For several years biologists from all over the world had been gathering in Geneva for meetings aimed at finding ways to strengthen the Convention. But none could deny that bioweapons treaty enforcement was, as Joshua Lederberg had told the White House, infinitely more complicated and difficult than nuclear arms control. It was too easy to make biobombs, and too hard to find them.

Opposition to inspection was by no means restricted to so-called rogue nations, such as Iraq. Worldwide the pharmaceutical industry protested provisions that would allow outsiders unannounced entry into drug manufacturing plants for purposes of inspection. Yet without such investigative power no one could ever enforce the Convention, as bioweapons production sites and pharmaceutical plants use the same sorts of equipment and personnel.[32] Gillian Woollett, spokesperson for the Pharmaceutical Research and Manufacturers of America, said such provisions would discriminate against legitimate businesses, yet fail to find anything because, 'a treaty is only for those who play cricket.'

Matters were only worsened by evidence that bioweapons production was, indeed, proliferating.

'Biological weapons may emerge as the principal proliferation concern of the next decade,' wrote analyst Brad Roberts.[33] 'Reports indicate that eleven countries are pursuing offensive-oriented biological warfare programmes, up from just four in the 1960s.'

Henderson only touched on such diplomatic issues when he addressed his colleagues in Atlanta. Nor did he say publicly what he had secretly told government officials: someone will inevitably cause a deliberate epidemic within a decade's time. His primary mission, at Osterholm's insistence, was to reveal details of possible bioterrorism, in hopes that he would inspire the public health community, spurring them to action. So Henderson turned to Iraq's admitted anthrax programme—one that made more than enough of the bacteria to kill every man, woman, and child living in the Middle East.

'Iraq acknowledges making 8000 litres [of anthrax],' Henderson said in his speech. 'The ramifications of even a modest release in a city are profound.'

He spun a tale of public health horror, by once again turning his Atlanta audience's attention to history: a Soviet Ministry of Defence anthrax experiment that went tragically awry on April 2, 1979, in a facility outside the city of Yekaterinburg.[15] An accident occurred in the weapons production facility, causing the release of an unknown quantity of dry anthrax spores. Some seventy-seven residents of the zone immediately south of the plant came down with the classic symptoms of inhaled anthrax: illness within one to six days of exposure, marked by muscle pains, fatigue, malaise, fever, and a non-productive cough. Sixty-six of those individuals, or 83 per cent of them, because much, much worse, developing infections in their brains or nervous systems, leading to meningitis and seizures; or had huge colonies of bacteria in their lungs that produced local haemorrhages and slowly caused them to suffocate; they usually died in shock. The Ministry of Defence realized the organisms had escaped their containment and distributed prophylactic antibiotics and vaccines. The local fire department was ordered to wash down the entire city. Hospitals, schools, and restaurants were scrubbed clean with disinfectants.[5] As days wore on, more succumbed, leaving a trail of death along the path of prevailing winds. Livestock found as much as fifty kilometres south-east of the military plant also perished. In some human cases symptoms didn't strike until six weeks after exposure.

The town nearest the bioweapons laboratory, Chkalovsky, was particularly hard hit, with perhaps one thousand deaths—all covered up by the Soviet government, only coming to international attention at the behest of environmental officer Sergei Volkov nineteen years later.[34] The US Los Alamos National Laboratory analysed lung biopsy material from several of those victims in 1997, concluding that at least four different strains were in the lethal mist that spewed out of the laboratory, and the concoction was resistant both to available vaccines and antibiotics. Thus, the Ministry of Defence's actions following the accident were useless, and it is possible that nearly every person who was exposed to the anthrax mixture succumbed.[35]

After the incident—which Soviet authorities originally denied was related to man-made anthrax—local medical experts tried to publish autopsy reports on forty-two victims, demonstrating that the massive internal haemorrhaging and lymphatic activity in the lungs was due to *inhaled* anthrax, not bacteria accidentally eaten from ailing sheep (as was claimed by the Soviet authorities). The report was suppressed until 1993.[36]

Finally, in 1992, the new Russian President Boris Yeltsin acknowledged that the accident had been part of a vast Soviet biological weapons programme. 'There will be no more lies—ever,' Yeltsin declared in a 1992 speech to the US Congress. Denouncing Soviet deceptions and the Communist beliefs behind them, Yeltsin swore 'that we will not let it rise again in our land.'

Harvard's Matthew Meselson calculated that Russia's lethal accident involved less than one gram of anthrax spores, an amount that could easily be hidden from inspectors, airport security guards, or police.

'So along comes [Yekaterinburg] and there you are with cases coming down what—forty-two days,' Henderson recalled. 'So I talked to [anthrax] experts and said, "What's the probability this is resuspended particles in the air?" And they were adamant that couldn't happen. Since that time Friedlander at USAMRIID[37] has exposed monkeys to low-dose anthrax. One monkey came down at fifty-nine days postexposure. And the more awesome thing: is it possible we don't have an endpoint for exposure?'[38]

So, Henderson reasoned, 'Suppose that somebody throws a little bit of anthrax into the subway. When do we decide that it's safe to go back into the subway?' How long might lethal spores drift about in the air, or nestle into nooks and crannies from where, under proper conditions, they might emerge years later, be resuspended in the air, and kill unsuspecting victims?

Henderson was convinced that even a minuscule, barely detectable quantity of anthrax spores would have a profound public health impact on a North American, Japanese, or European city. Though the spores could not be spread from person to person, those microbes could circulate in the air for days, perhaps months.

'Emergency rooms would begin seeing a few patients with high fever and some difficulty breathing perhaps three to four days following exposure,' Henderson told his public health colleagues. 'By the time they were seen, it is almost certain that it would be too late for antibiotic therapy. Essentially all would be dead within twenty-four to forty-eight hours. No emergency room physicians or infectious disease specialists have ever seen a case of inhalation anthrax; medical laboratories have virtually no experience in diagnosis. Thus, it is probable that a delay of at least three to five days would elapse before a definitive diagnosis.

'Once the diagnosis was made, one would be faced with the prospect of what to do over the succeeding six weeks. Should vaccine be administered to those who might have been exposed? Unfortunately, there is at present little [anthrax] vaccine available. ... Should antibiotics be administered prophylactically? If so, which antibiotics and what should be the criteria for exposure? What quantity would be required to treat an exposed population of perhaps 500 000 persons over a six-week period? Should one be concerned about additional infections occurring as a result of anthrax spores being subsequently resuspended and inhaled by others? Does one request everyone who has been anywhere near the city to report to his or her local physician for treatment at the first occurrence of fever or cough, however mild? Undoubtedly, there would be many persons with such symptoms, especially in winter. How does one distinguish these from the premonitory symptoms of anthrax, which may precede death within twenty-four to forty-eight hours? Can one imagine the reaction of a large population confronted with this array of problems?'

A year later officials from the Pentagon, several other federal agencies, and the New York City government were involved in an anthrax terrorism role-play event. Somebody placed aerosols inside Grand Central Station at rush hour, releasing anthrax spores. Two weeks later Gotham was a ghost town because millions had fled in panic, antibiotic supplies were long since depleted, more than a million people were dead or ailing, the New York Stock Exchange had collapsed, and law and order had broken down. It was, as one participant put it, 'a highly improbable event, but one with such horrible, catastrophic probable outcome that it simply had to be taken seriously.'

Botulinum toxin posed fewer uncertainties; its lethal power in minuscule doses was well understood. As was its ease of manufacture. The toxin was derived from a common bacteria, *Clostridium botulinum*, which is an anaerobic microbe that grows readily on fruits and vegetables stored at room temperature in airtight containers. The precise pathogenicity of the toxin could vary from one *Clostridium* strain to another, but botulinum toxin generally killed any untreated individual who ingested 10 ng of the substance: an invisible microfraction of a minuscule droplet. The same dose, multiplied by the number of kilograms an individual weighed, was guaranteed lethal when inhaled.

Antibiotics were useless if an individual was exposed to pure toxin. All medicines were worthless. Only the rarely available sera of botulinum toxin could prevent death due to botulism.

The toxin, a protein, directly attached itself to receptors on the surface of nerve cells, gaining entry to the neurons. Once inside, the toxin interfered in the biochemical processes essential to production of chemicals that transmitted signals among nerve cells. Unable to communicate, the neuronal system would break down. The medical result was an illness that initially looked a bit like the flu but increased in severity within twenty-four to forty-eight hours to include dizziness, slurred speech, difficulty walking, dulled and incoherent thinking, severe muscle weakness, uncontrollable drooling and nasal drips, difficulty breathing, inability to swallow, and loss of appetite. Eventually—in two to four days—the lack of signals in the brain and nervous system shut down one or more key body functions and the individual died.

Because the toxin was not a living organism, but a protein, it was easy to store and convert to an aerosol. A very small amount went a long way. About seventeen pounds of a concentrated liquid suspension of the toxin would be enough to kill about half the people living in a 27 710-acre area, assuming they were exposed. That wouldn't be many people if the target was the desert region of the Persion Gulf. But if it were Hong Kong, Tokyo, Los Angeles, New York City, or London, millions of lives could be lost.

Horrible as the impacts of anthrax or botulinum might be, D. A. Henderson's chief concern, he told the visibly agitated Atlanta audience, was the microbe he had defeated two decades earlier: smallpox. Smallpox, Henderson thought, was the ultimate weapon of mass destruction or, WMD. The possibility that samples of smallpox might fall into nefarious hands—indeed, might already have found their way onto the international arms market—was Henderson's obsession.

'You cannot really be sure,' Henderson said, that all the former Soviet samples of smallpox were accounted for and safely stashed inside Siberian freezers. Even assuming goodwill all-around, 'Virologists are such squirrels. A lot of this stuff goes in deep freezes...at no time could you ever say, no matter what you did, that there was no [smallpox] virus anywhere.'

Henderson asserted that he considered evil use of the virus a grave potential as long as any sample of smallpox remained in a freezer anywhere in the world. Yet elimination of all remnants of a biological species—even a lethal pathogen—was repugnant to many scientists, so by WHO agreement the American and Russian samples remained alive, in frozen limbo.

'I have no question I'd like to see it destroyed tomorrow,' Henderson insisted.[39]

Despite such fears, in April 1999 President Clinton revoked US support for destruction of the smallpox stocks.

The smallpox virus was highly contagious, both by contact and, under close conditions, through the air. Unvaccinated people were thought to have one-in-three odds of dying of the disease, and most survivors of the dreaded virus were physically scarred for life.

Few people in 1999 were particularly knowledgeable about humanity's former nemesis. Even Henderson conceded that such death toll estimates were matters of conjecture on his part. When he wanted hard facts Henderson called Australia and spoke to an eighty-six-year-old university professor named Frank Fenner.

Despite his age Fenner was a remarkably prolific author and advisor to numerous government committees, both in Australia and all over the world. His modest office in the University of Canberra was covered with stacks of unfinished manuscripts, photo-copied research papers, laboratory data, and the texts of speeches he'd recently de-livered. The walls were lined with arguably the best smallpox library in the world. And as he spoke with a visitor the spry Fenner often leapt to his feet, sprinting across the room to grab the perfect reference book or article to bolster a given statement. Ignor-ing shocks of white hair that fell across his face as he peered through manuscripts Fen-ner would periodically shout, 'Ah! There it is. Come look! Here are the bloody facts.'

He nonchalantly guided his visitor through the facts of the fearful virus—offering some of the same details he had given President Clinton and Australia's Prime Minis-ter John Howard when in 1998 he argued in favour of destroying the smallpox viruses. Though Fenner was one of the world's top virologists in his youth, and had devoted decades to the study of smallpox, he had no delusions about the danger that his pet research subject's continued existence posed.

'In the absence of the vaccine in London about 10 per cent of all deaths in any given year were due to smallpox,' Fenner began, referring to eighteenth-century documents. 'The death rate among those who got infected was 25 per cent for adults and 40 to 50 per cent in children. There was a time when they wouldn't give names to children unless they had survived smallpox.'

After vaccination became commonplace in Europe the 1870 Franco-Prussian War answered the question of how long immunity might last, because the Prussian Army revaccinated all its troops, but the French did not. The French suffered 125 000 small-pox casualties, 18.7 per cent of which were fatal. The Germans, in contrast, had only 8463 cases with a mere 5.4 per cent fatality rate.

Fenner stared from behind clear blue eyes, shrugged, and said, 'That tells you that immunity cannot be expected to last very long. You cannot expect that many people in the world today are still immune, given all vaccination ceased in 1980.'

When he had spoken to President Clinton in early 1998 Fenner told the American leader that he ought to support destruction of all smallpox viruses: 'Why don't you come out in the open and say you're scared of bioterrorism,' Fenner asked, arguing that would be the most honest rationale for destruction of the microbes.

The president said, 'But you can never be sure it's eradicated,' Fenner recalled. And unless every single virus were truly destroyed some stocks ought to be saved as research tools, Clinton had continued, in the event of a catastrophe—of a deliberate release.

Fenner lost the argument.

And in the summer of 1999 the US Congress released a report claiming that both Iraq and North Korea were in possesson of secret smallpox stockpiles.[40] The congressional public pronouncement drew from intelligence documents submitted a year previously to President Clinton.[41]

Fenner had not known of the report when he spoke with President Clinton. But it would not have swayed him: the Australian remained convinced that every single smallpox virus on earth had to be destroyed. Having seen firsthand what the virus could do to the human body, and knowing how rapidly it could spread, Fenner was adamant.

The disease process itself was the stuff of which nightmares were made. When enemies in old England cursed, 'A pox on you!' they knew whereof they spoke. So great were the early-twentieth-century death tolls that in 1995 it was estimated that vaccination programmes administered a generation previously were in the 1990s saving *$1 million a day* in the United States due to elimination of smallpox illnesses and deaths.[42]

The virus entered the cells lining human lungs and made its way from there to the lymph nodes all over the body. This usually took one to three weeks, during which the infected human felt fine, had no limits on his or her physical activity, and may have come in contact with dozens—even hundreds—of other people, possibly passing on the lethal virus.

Once billions of viruses were made and dispersed all over the infected body through the bloodstream, then fever, muscle pains, vomiting, headaches, and back pain set in. Two days later a rash appeared, spreading from the face and forearms down the trunk to the genitals and legs. After forty-two to seventy-two hours the rash would erupt into large, obvious poxes, some of which could have been haemorrhagic, bleeding out viruses. Two weeks into the illness scabs appeared over the poxes, which shed at week three, leaving acnelike scars all over the body and often grossly disfiguring the victim's face.[43]

No one in the world had been vaccinated since 1980, Fenner again reminded his visitor; some countries ceased smallpox immunization in the early 1970s. In the United States vaccinations stopped in 1972, rendering two generations of children and young adults at the turn of the century vulnerable to the virus. 'It is doubtful,' Henderson concluded, 'that more than 10 to 15 per cent of the population today have significant residual smallpox immunity.'

Until September 1997 Henderson had limited his discussions of biological weapons to unclassified arenas, fearing that such information was likely to provoke panic in some, and evil ideas in others.

'I was concerned, worried about copycats,' Henderson explained. But then Osterholm had persuaded him to rethink his position. 'What I think persuaded me was I found people in the defence community who could not get their superiors to look on this with more seriousness.'

A newfound sobriety on the issue first hit Western intelligence communities—especially in London and Washington—in the early 1990s, as news of the true scale and scope of the Soviet Biopreparat programme became known. Nobody in the West had previously realized the gargantuan scale of the Soviet biodeath programme.

Americans had their first chilling glimpses of Biopreparat in 1996, and this reporter was the first US journalist to gain entry to their facilities.

A gray pallor hangs over Siberia's largest city, Novosibirsk. In winter's twilighted sun a stern city yields on its outskirts to vistas of belching smokestacks and decaying concrete apartment complexes. Farther on the visitor encounters forests of white birch and pine trees. Stark and largely leafless in the winter chill, the trees beckoned viewers into a natural environment that was at once awesome and threatening. Even a late-winter chill was enough to remind visitors that wandering about in Siberia's version of nature was dangerous business, indeed.

About an hour outside the city, near a top secret town called Koltsovo, the forest yielded to an enormous complex of a hundred large concrete-and-steel buildings, surrounded by an eight-foot-tall concrete wall. Three rows of electric wires topped the wall. A bird landed on one and remained perched, harmlessly, on wires that once electrocuted unwanted guests.

A Russian Army guard, shivering inside a glass booth, acknowledged visitors, welcomed to VECTOR if they possessed proper credentials.[44]

Six years after the fall of the Soviet Union VECTOR, the USSR's premier virus weapons facility, had a seedy, has-been look to it. Weeds sprouted from long-neglected cracks in the pavements and streets. The roads had potholes big enough to challenge even 4×4 sports utility vehicles. Most exposed steel was covered in rust, and large cracks in the concrete facades of several buildings appeared to be more than mere eyesores. Some of the laboratories and offices seemed in danger of collapsing.

Broken windows went unrepaired, the bitter Siberian wind left to sweep into the now ghostly halls of research. Once a bustling minimetropolis dedicated to the scientific pursuit of perfect vectors of man-made disease, by the end of the 1990s VECTOR lay nearly silent; only the sound of the cold wind's relentless pummelling of the deteriorating buildings resonated in the otherwise empty air.

Scattered about, dressed in tattered uniforms, Russian soldiers idled away the long, cold, boring hours, guarding microscopic charges. In Building Number 1, for example, row upon row of industrial freezers housed Ebola, Lassa, smallpox, monkeypox, tick-borne encephalitis, killer influenza strains, Marburg, HIV, hepatitis A,B,C, and E, Japanese encephalitis, and dozens of other human killer viruses. And there were dozens of different strains of smallpox viruses—140 of them were natural, wild strains. Some were handcrafted by the bioengineers of VECTOR, giving them greater powers of infectivity, virulence, transmissibility.

The Russian Army guards didn't fully understand what was in Building Number 1. They called them 'superbugs.' But they did know that the bugs were terribly valuable—worth their weights exponentially in incalculable amounts of gold. These young men, and tens of thousands of their counterparts, were guarding more than three hundred once-secret cities, factories, and laboratory complexes in Russia—former places of plutonium production, nerve gas manufacture, uranium mining, and biological weapons development.

By 1996 the two million Russian soldiers, most of them conscripts, represented a disorganized, underpaid (or unpaid), demoralized horde, armed with military skills and weapons in a country rife with economic hardship. While its colonels and generals loudly lamented the grand days of Soviet global military power, Russia's young soldiers were simply killing time, staying off the country's swelling unemployment lists, and waiting for opportunities—other than combat—to present themselves. Meanwhile, corruption was rampant in all tiers of the military. The enlisted men smuggled drugs and guns, while high-level officers ordered their troops to build dachas for their mistresses, sold Soviet arms on the world armaments market, and siphoned off millions of roubles for personal use. Yeltsin's government made arrests—even jailed a deputy minister of defence and the leader of Russian ground troops. But the pillage continued.

Russian policy experts Daniel Yergin and Thane Gustafson noted that Yeltsin's attempts to reduce the size of the country's army resulted in an incredibly top-heavy military force: of 1.5 million personnel 690 000 were officers, 2200 of them generals.

'In many respects the Russian military and the security police remain states within a state,' Yergin and Gustafson wrote in 1995.[45] 'The military and the security forces still command large blocks of property in the form of parks, sanatoria, dachas, housing, clubs, bases, schools, and institutes. There have been many charges recently that senior officers have been selling these properties back into private hands—or their own. But Yeltsin has so far refused to open an investigation that would embarrass his senior officers. Both the military and the security forces have resisted internal reform, as time goes on this resistance is likely to grow.'

Russia's most popular military leader, General Lev Rokhlin, was murdered mysteriously in his holiday dacha in early July 1998, prompting rising discontent in army ranks. A host of other former generals, including General Alexander Lebed, quit the military for the world of politics.[46] In the summer of 1998 the Russian stock market collapsed, and for the sixth time since he came to power, Yeltsin watched his economy spiral into a tailspin, and his approval rating drop to just 2 per cent. By the summer of 1998 Russian soldiers were literally eating dog food: one thousand tons of processed animal parts originally manufactured for canine consumption. All heat and electricity was shut off at most barracks, and the streets of Moscow were lined with uniformed soldiers begging for money. One mentally ill sailor, driven over the edge by the Russian Navy's poverty, hijacked a nuclear submarine in September 1998.

In such an atmosphere of humiliation, economic chaos, and political instability, it would be no surprise if a handful of soldiers decided to smuggle one or two test tubes of hellish power—undetectable, as they would be—to whatever group offered an appropriate political agenda or large amounts of cash. With each passing day of chaotic activity in Russia, American and European analysts grew more anxious, openly worrying that the former USSR stockpiles might become sources of leverage— or worse—fall into the hands of political renegades or dissident soldiers.

However, the job of transferring bioweapons technology from a Siberian laboratory to freezers in some other belligerent nation—or to the control of a rebel faction within Russia—could best be handled not by a soldier but by a scientist. Indeed, biological weapons were almost unique in the 1990s in that the substance was perhaps of less value than the intellect behind it. A scientist who genuinely knew how to genetically enhance and turn a lethal virus into a weapon need not risk his life smuggling frozen test tubes, however minuscule they might be: all his buyers needed was the knowledge of molecular biology stored in his brain. At the onset of the Cold War nuclear physicists were in that position. But by the early 1980s biology had replaced physics as the intellectual property of greatest global value. And though Russia's civilian scientific enterprise was in shambles, no nation had more men and women with the intellectual knowledge of how to turn microbes into weapons.

In a 1992 meeting US President George Bush told Russia's Boris Yeltsin that the American government had learned of Biopreparat and wanted the programme stopped, its stockpiles destroyed. Yeltsin professed ignorance of all but the bare bones of the programme. He asked retired General Anatoly Kuntsevich to prepare a report on the Soviet Union's bioweapons programme. Kuntsevich reported later that year that the USSR's efforts were breathtaking in scope. Dozens of killers had been turned into weapons for missile, rocket, and aerial bomb delivery, including anthrax, Q fever, tularaemia, and a host of viruses. And over the years these weapons had been tested on Vozrozhdeniya Island, located in the middle of the rapidly receding Aral Sea.[47]

The Kuntsevich report described a complex web of bioweapons programmes, including Biopreparat and separate laboratories and test sites run by the Ministry of Defence. In addition to forty-seven Biopreparat sites, the Ministry of Defence had several bioweapons factories, laboratories—even in heavily populated Moscow—and missile test locations. Biopreparat, the Soviet government claimed, was merely a civilian pharmaceutical programme. And the Ministry of Defence's bioweapons programme did not, officially, even exist. Estimates are, however, that some seventy thousand scientists and technicians were employed in these efforts before 1992. But by 1997 most were no longer to be found working in the laboratories, bioweapons factories, or test sites. Where did they go?

'Nobody knows,' Dr Kanatjan Alibekov said. In 1992 Alibekov defected to the West, moved to Virginia, and Americanized his name, becoming Ken Alibek. The Kazakhstani biologist started doing bioweapons research in 1975, rising through the ranks of Biopreparat to become deputy chief of the Soviet programme in 1987 when he was just thirty-six years old.[48]

'Nobody can answer' the question of where all those workers went, Alibek continued. 'Some, like me, are in the United States. Some are in Europe. But, you know, there is a very high probability that some are in the Middle East. When you are suggested to make one thousand dollars a month—for them this is a huge amount of money.'

Alibek said that Biopreparat employed thirty-two thousand civilians/scientists in his day, and the bioweapons programme of the Ministry of Defence involved another ten thousand military scientists. In addition, thousands of test site personnel released sample biobombs at Yekaterinburg (where the 1979 anthrax accident occurred), Kirov, Sergiyev Posad, and Strizhi. Among the achievements that Alibek claimed this programme made were the weapons described above, and: antibiotic-resistant (incurable) plague, missile-mounted smallpox, mass scale production of the haemorrhagic fever viruses Ebola, Marburg, and Machupo, and antibiotic-resistant anthrax.

In their top secret Sergiyev Posad laboratory the Biopreparat scientists worked out how to mass-produce smallpox viruses, cultivating tons every year. At VECTOR in 1990—just one year before the collapse of the Soviet Union—Alibek led a team that worked out how to turn smallpox into a weapon, dispersing the deadly microbes in aerosols. And under orders from President Mikhail Gorbachev, Alibek insists, they manufactured eighty to a hundred tons of the horrible stuff yearly.

Ghastly as their work was, the Biopreparat scientists—including Alibek—were convinced that the United States had a comparable biological arsenal, and that a serious Cold War confrontation was inevitable. Fed paranoid and often false 'intelligence' by the KGB, the Soviet scientists felt certain that Americans would soon unleash equally abominable epidemic weapons, slaying innocent civilians from Vladivostok to Leningrad.

Alibek was one of the last Biopreparat defectors to reach the West—but the first to publicly reveal the programme's secrets. Alibek's claims received a lot of attention in Washington and came under attack in some circles for being exaggerations. But Henderson found Alibek 'quite impressive', and Osterholm said the Kazakhstani's information gave him nightmares.

In London's intelligence circles Alibek's assertions didn't appear too far off the mark. British intelligence debriefed Alibek's boss, Vladimir Pasechnik, in 1989 when he defected to the United Kingdom. From Pasechnik they learned that many apparently legitimate enterprises, such as plasma clinics and vaccine plants, were actually parts of the Biopreparat nightmare. And the Russian revealed that he had personally supervised modification of cruise missiles, making them bioweapons delivery systems.[49]

Alibek's defection a decade later and the information he provided disabused Western authorities of any hope that the Soviets had abandoned bioweapons development. President George Bush, in a report to Congress in 1993, decried Biopreparat, saying: 'The Russian offensive biological warfare programme, inherited from the Soviet Union, violated the Biological Weapons Convention through at least March 1992. The Soviet offensive bioweapons programme was massive, and included production, weaponization, and stockpiling.'

Why did tens of thousands of biologists eagerly participate in creating weapons of mass destruction out of life, itself? There was the paranoia—including KGB misinformation, of course. But there also were the perks, both personal and scientific. Biopreparat scientists ate tomatoes in January in Siberia, travelled widely, had decent apartments where such things were reserved for Communist Party bosses, got their children into the best colleges, and—perhaps most significantly for the biologists— had open, remarkably free access to Western scientific literature, even conferences. At a time when it was forbidden for physicians to read American, Western European, or Japanese medical journals and texts, Biopreparat researchers could study whatever they liked. While Soviet geneticists, molecular biologists, and agronomists struggled to recuperate from the tremendous damage wrought by Lysenkoism, the bioweapons scientists blithely rejected all of Lysenko's idiocy, devoured the writings of Watson, Crick, Monod, Berg, Bishop, Baltimore, and Varmus, and eagerly learned to manipulate DNA.

'There were two different worlds of science,' Alibek later explained. 'In 1973 the Soviet Union signed a decree to increase work in genetic engineering. A lot of money was put into development of this programme. A lot of work was secret. The final objective was to develop these weapons. And there was *no* contact between civilian and military scientists. We started from scratch, but we used all knowledge obtained by the West. A huge analytical system existed just to analyse the work of the West.'

When the Ebola epidemic broke out in Kikwit, Zaire, in 1995 a group of VECTOR scientists sent word that they had long-since developed a vaccine, and tested its use on human volunteers during the heyday of Biopreparat. VECTOR's deputy director Sergei Netesov didn't know, or wouldn't say, where the Russians originally obtained their Ebola samples, nor how they had been aware of unpublished findings in Western laboratories, but clearly he and his VECTOR colleagues were up to speed on Ebola when they attended the 1996 Antwerp meeting on the virus.[50] Stored in Russia, Netesov said, were supplies of Ebola antisera made by infecting sheep and goats in the BL-4 laboratory at VECTOR. Ten volunteers had received the antisera, with no ill effects, Netesov claimed. And when one of his colleagues was bitten by an Ebola-infected monkey at VECTOR repeated injections with the antisera saved the scientist's life.

Even more ambitious than Biopreparat's efforts were those of the Soviet military's Ebola programme, which also mysteriously obtained samples of the virus and of unpublished American laboratory findings. In military facilities Ebola antiserum was made in horses and tested repeatedly on human beings.[51]

As top physicians in the Soviet Union scrubbed their operating theatre walls, ignorant of all modern infection control practices, the scientists in Biopreparat approached molecular biology as if it were another Cold War race to the moon. For a bright young biologist in the 1970s, Biopreparat offered enormous intellectual advantages over just about any other Soviet options. As further enticement the USSR threw in chauffeured cars, priority A access to food supplies, state-of-the-art laboratories, almost unlimited supplies of experimental animals, and marvellous intellectual puzzles to solve. It was, by Soviet standards, an almost irresistible offer.

And it was all blown away in 1992. Poof! No more privileged status. No more research money. No more large Soviet salaries. With the stroke of a pen in late 1992, Yeltsin eliminated nearly all funding for bioweapons research. Or tried to.[52]

Suddenly there were in the world thousands of unemployed, humiliated bioweapons scientists. That worried Chris Howson, Colonel Dennis Duplantier, Alexis Shelokov, and their British counterparts enough that they hatched an unprecedented trilateral scheme to put some of the Biopreparat personnel on the US payroll. Beginning in 1997 the US Department of Defence and National Academy of Sciences, working in a trilateral arrangement with their counterparts in Russia and the United Kingdom, began, as Shelokov put it, 'trying to get [the Russian bioweapons laboratories] converted to peacetime work.'

Shelokov and Howson sat on a National Academy of Sciences committee that hatched the plan and helped run it. Howson explained that his interest in the effort was 'to get my hands on that wonderful expertise and put it to work on improving global health, not harming it.'

Handfuls of Russian scientists at VECTOR and other Biopreparat facilities were funded by the Pentagon to work on developing vaccines against the terrible microbes they had created. They collaborated directly with USAMRIID and the CDC. Under the scheme, some of the Russian scientists would have a chance to work in public health laboratories in the United States, and Americans would get inside Biopreparat.

American scientists who visited the Biopreparat facilities during the late 1990s had quite a shock. The crude quality of the laboratories—even, in some cases, primitive nature—demonstrated that very, very dangerous work and sophisticated molecular biology could be carried out in just about any facility, provided adequate intelligence was at the helm.

For example, in its heyday, VECTOR boasted more than four thousand scientists and thousands more support personnel, all working in relatively new facilities (built in 1974). It was a showcase for Russian talent during the 1970s. But by 1997 more than half the VECTOR scientists and workers were gone. And those that remained were a dispirited bunch working for little or no money inside a rapidly decaying infrastructure.

Deputy Director Sergey Netesov got a peptic ulcer trying to run the virtually unfunded VECTOR complex in 1997. It was hard to raise interest in VECTOR and its scientists. No one had heard of the facility, of Netesov, or of their work until 1992 when its existence was declassified. While recovering from surgery Netesov continued efforts to find funds for the faltering facility.

'We are trying to use any opportunity to make money for our institution,' Netesov said, his face drawn and pale. 'We tried to make vodka but we couldn't make money because the taxes were too high.'

To put Netesov's position in perspective, having VECTOR forced to consider vodka production as a last-resort means of financing was roughly equivalent to saying the Los Alamos National Laboratory in New Mexico should cease receiving funds from Congress and go into the manufacturing of robot toys to subsidize its scientific research programme.

Netesov, who was VECTOR's expert on the Ebola and smallpox viruses, was nearly brought down by simple garden-variety bacteria following his ulcer surgery. The widespread antibiotic resistance in Novasiask forced his doctors to prescribe expensive drugs, which Netesov had to purchase on his own.

Some distance away from Netesov's office, past several weed-choked lawns and fissured pavements, loomed Building Number 5: Molecular Biology. No guards blocked its entry. Yet on the eleventh floor Sergei Shchelkunov continued, to search for the gene responsible for virulence—in monkeypox. Shchelkunov, a recipient of the US Department of Defence funding, was sequencing smallpox, cowpox, and monkeypox viruses, he said, 'to get a picture of evolutionary interrelatedness of these viruses.'

At the request of the CDC and World Health Organization, Shchelkunov was working out the genetics of the strain of monkeypox that broke out in Congo in 1997.

The entry to nearby Buildings Number 6 bore a forbidding sign in Cyrillic: ATTENTION. THIS BUILDING OPERATES UNDER RESTRICTED CONDITIONS. ONLY THOSE IMMUNIZED FOR SMALLPOX MAY ENTER. But no security guards were present in 1997 to enforce the stricture. Down long, dark hallways, unlit with expensive electricity, were unoccupied laboratories, seemingly caught in time somewhere around 1975. Like a scene out of the *Twilight Zone* it appeared that work in most laboratories simply stopped one day, midway in experiments. Dusty laboratory benches were loaded with out-of-date equipment.

Upstairs Alexander Guskov worked by muted winter sunlight. His task, also funded by the CDC, was to preserve VECTOR's hundreds of smallpox samples, periodically venturing into the maximum containment facility to verify the vitality of the twenty- to fifty-year-old frozen viruses.

Biologist Valery Loktov was also a participant in the collaborative programme put together by the US National Academy of Science. He was heading studies of a river fluke that had contaminated all the fish in local Siberian rivers and was increasingly being found in Japanese and North American fish.

'Eighteen to nineteen per cent of the local [human] population is infected,' as a result of eating those contaminated fish caught in Novosibirsk's rivers, Loktov said. And in hamster studies the fluke caused liver cancer 100 per cent of the time.

While Loktov's work could be done in minimal security facilities, VECTOR was designed for study of Biohazard Level-4 microbes—those that could kill humans more than 50 per cent of the time and are both incurable and, so far, not affected by any known vaccine. Until 1996 VECTOR's BL-4 laboratories were filled with activity, including research on Ebola and several other haemorrhagic fever viruses, encephalitis viruses, and some unusual forms of hepatitis.

A year later, however, the BL-4 laboratories were silent, and the cages of the maximum containment animal colony were empty. Though it brought financial hardship into the lives of VECTOR scientists, the disuse of their BL-4 facilities was probably a good thing.

'We need to modernize the facility if we want to attain US BL-4 standards,' Loktov admitted, pointing out the ominous lack of proper exhaust air treatment filters to prevent escape of dangerous microbes. US scientists said that even more troubling was the fundamental design of the place—a sort of huge, hulking industrial mass that bore many of the same flaws seen in Soviet designs of factories and nuclear power plants. For example, enormous ducts criss-crossed the ceilings, and exposed heating and ventilation pipes wound around them. The net effect was a ceiling spaghetti of exposed iron and steel that would be impossible to decontaminate in the event of a microbial leak.

Close inspection revealed that most of the antimicrobial filters in the laboratory were installed in 1981 and were originally designed not for biological control but as nuclear radiation barriers. Washed latex gloves, ready for reuse, hung on a pipe in one laboratory. Most of the airlock and pressure doors were heavy iron portals first made for Soviet nuclear submarines.

The space suits Russian scientists used while working with lethal microbes were uncomfortable and heavy, grumbled one of Loktov's colleagues as he reluctantly climbed into one, demonstrating safety procedures. It was difficult to move around in the heavy rubber and steel suit, much less manipulate tiny syringes and test tubes full of deadly viruses.

'We've had no incidents of infection of our personnel who worked with such equipment,' Loktov insisted. 'But it is old equipment. Very old equipment. And now we have no funds for new equipment. It's very dangerous work.'

In Building Number 1 of the enormous VECTOR facility were row upon row of freezers, all on triply redundant electrical systems that supposedly ensured that even if the primary electricity grid for Novosibirsk Oblast went down, the freezers would remain colder than ice. Which was a good thing because inside of them were trillions of living viruses and bacteria, the mere names of which conjured fear in medical circles. Were they to escape their iced test tube surroundings, sneaking past old leaky seals and poorly maintained freezer insulations, many of the microbes could flood into the air, possibly infecting VECTOR personnel and starting an epidemic.

This extraordinary reservoir of human predators was comparable to the CDC's deadly warehouse in Atlanta. But the multilayered, intense security that protected the CDC cache was not mirrored in Novosibirsk.

'You can't preclude the fact that anyone can walk out with biological samples,' bioweapons expert Anthony Cordesman, of the Centre for Strategic and International Studies in Washington, said. Had someone already done so, taking microbes away from VECTOR to another, undisclosed location? 'If people in government were free to confirm or deny [the rumours] they probably would not confirm. But that does not imply that there is no evidence for concern.'

In a statement released by the US secretary of defence on November 25, 1997, William S. Cohen underlined this fear: 'The United States remains concerned at the threat of proliferation, both of biological warfare expertise and related hardware, from Russia. Russian scientists, many of whom are unemployed or have not been paid for an extended period, may be vulnerable to recruitment by states trying to establish biological warfare programmes. The availability of worldwide information exchange via the Internet or electronic post facilitates this process.'

Even beyond such sinister causes, microbial leaks could have occurred if the facilities and staff morale were not improved. The viruses and bacteria could not simply sit forever in Building Number 1 freezers. To remain viable they must occasionally be removed, thawed, and injected into animals or cells. Such passaging, as the process was called, had not been done for most of the samples for years—eventually Netesov and his staff would have to choose between allowing the samples to deteriorate beyond use, or risking their health and the safety of others by climbing into those old rubber space suits and going back inside the antiquated BL-4 laboratories.

Should something go wrong the scientists could have turned to their thirty-year-old rotary telephones, dialed through an old-fashioned manually manipulated Siberian switchboard, and called Novosibirsk for help. It would probably have been faster, however, to turn to their computers and send an E-mail to Washington.

In 1996 when Colonel Duplantier and the National Academy of Sciences (NAS) group planned their cooperation he thought that funding for about twenty researchers would be enough. But, Duplantier said later, 'When we went to visit, the magnitude overwhelmed us.'

At a workshop in Kirov in July 1997, Duplantier was stunned by the numbers for Biopreparat alone: 'Forty-seven institutes, forty thousand employees,[53] nine thousand scientists, eleven full-scale research institutes with two thousand people with special expertise in pathogens. That's how big it was!'

Clearly, then, the US/UK effort to make work for Biopreparat scientists was inadequate. Funding twenty could hardly halt the activities of forty thousand.

However there weren't forty thousand people working inside Biopreparat by 1997. Where did they all go?

'It's very difficult to discuss this topic. It's a very sensitive discussion,' Alibek said nervously. 'I know what kind of weapon could be developed just using regular rooms. For me, I need to have just a very simple laboratory, equipment. Even without any agent developed by any cell culture house. I can go outside, take just soil samples. I can manufacture weapons.'

Back in the summer of 1995 Western intelligence sources had accused the Russian military of continuing its bioweapons effort, and of assisting Iran in mounting a similar programme.[54] Amid allegations of misconduct—including continued bioweapons production and sale of expertise to other governments—among Russians funded by the US programme the congressional General Accounting Office attacked the effort in early 1999, and its future appeared precarious.[55] The White House, however, seemed committed to the programme, as signalled in President Clinton's 1999 State of the Union address, which pointedly referred to the importance of US/Russian cooperation to prevent spread of biological weapons.

Though Biopreparat opened its laboratories to the United Kingdom and United States, the Ministry of Defence did not. Henderson, for one, was thoroughly convinced that tremendous danger lurked in those MOD laboratories. So was Alibek.

In the spring of 1997, *Jane's Weekly*, a prominent British military publication, published a claim—based on information from sources in Britain's spy centre, MI6—that Russian scientists had developed a genetically modified strain of anthrax that was resistant to all vaccines and antibiotics. On the face of it the claim appeared preposterous to biologists acquainted with the bacteria.

But weeks later Chris Howson made one of several site visits to Biopreparat facilities and asked about the alleged anthrax superbug. He was told, 'Well, we do have strains here that are resistant to vaccines and antibiotics.' As rumours of that encounter spread around Washington, Henderson and Osterholm, as well as the army scientists working at the Fort Detrick biodefence laboratory, grew increasingly anxious. They all hoped that Howson had heard bravado, not truth.

However, at the beginning of 1998, came British publication of work by A. P. Pomerantsev and his colleagues at the State Research Centre for Applied Microbiology, a Biopreparat facility in Obolensk. Using advanced genetic engineering techniques the Obolensk team inserted virulence genes from a humanly harmless species, *Bacillus cereus*, into *Bacillus anthracis*, the organism that causes anthrax. In addition, the *anthracis* strain upon which this work was performed was bred for complete antibiotic resistance. The result was an entirely new form of anthrax resistant to penicillin and vaccines, and capable of residing dangerously inside human cells in ways never previously seen with anthrax.[56]

Lederberg was stunned.

'This, as far as I know, is the first example of an artificially contrived new pathogen,' the elder statesman of biology told his colleagues. 'The kind of obvious cat is out of the bag.... It's the thought of this kind of work going on sub rosa that is really the black cloud hanging over us.'

USAMRIID's Colonel Arthur Friedlander issued a statement saying that the American military felt that the Russians had developed 'a new potential biological warfare agent'. 'This new organism is based on anthrax and is reported to be resistant to the Russian vaccine,' Friedlander continued. 'It likely causes disease by a different mechanism than that used by naturally occurring anthrax strains. The development of genetically engineered new organisms using anthrax and other biological warfare agents is a potential threat which must be carefully evaluated.'[57]

Pomerantsev's group had obtained all that they needed from Western sources simply by exploiting the candid atmosphere of basic biology and public health research. The technique they had used to modify B. *anthracis* was borrowed from work published by cell biologist Daniel Portnoy from the University of California, Berkeley. Portnoy worked with a different organism—*Bacillus subtilis*. In 1990 he succeeded in forcing B. *subtilis* to express genes from another bacterial species—*Listeria monocytogenes*—resulting in new capacities for the organism. In particular, Portnoy crafted *Listeria* genes for destruction of red blood cells into B. *subtilis*, making a new bacteria that could punch holes in red blood cells and survive outside of the sort of soil milieu in which such organisms were usually confined. It was an innocent sort of study, of the type academic researchers in the West were most inclined to perform. Call it a 'proof of principle', the Portnoy effort simply showed that the more primitive bacterial organism possessed the necessary machinery for sophisticated activity, provided it got the right genetic blueprints.[58]

Pomerantsev's group paid homage to the Portnoy work: 'The cloning of the structural gene for the L. *monocytogenes* haemolysin into an asperogenic mutant of *Bacillus subtilus* resulted in conversion of a common soil bacterium into a parasite that can grow in the cytoplasm of a mammalian cell. According to this model an acquisition of haemolytic properties by B. *anthracis* strains can allow them to escape host immunity by means of penetrating host cells. The data presented in this study confirm the statement that "the evolutionary leap from an extracellular existence to an intracellular lifestyle may only require the acquisition of a limited number of genes."'

In other words, a literal garden-variety bug could be transformed into one that could thrive inside the human bloodstream.

Portnoy was aghast. It had never occurred to him that his work converting the B. *subtilis* soil bacteria into one that could live inside mouse cells could also apply to other soil organisms—including anthrax. When he first learned of the Russian experiment Portnoy tried to throw sceptical water on it, casting doubt on the veracity of Pomerantsev's publication. But as he pored over the paper Portnoy realized with horror what had been done: his work had been perverted: 'Now I'm getting scared,' he said.

Portnoy wasn't the only scientist whose work was used by the Obolensk group. In order to accomplish their anthrax conversion the Russians needed special *Bacillus cereus* genes—for insertion into the anthracis genome. Once again, they exploited the uniquely open atmosphere of basic biology research. In the days of active Biopreparat effort they turned to Dr Werner Goebel, a prominent biologist in Biozenthrun, located in Wurzburg, Germany. When Goebel was told of the use his genes were put to he was flabbergasted.

'I don't have any direct contacts to the Pomerantsev group,' Goebel E-mailed. 'I don't even know him personally. It is of course possible that I sent him (or more probably) a related person the genes which we cloned many years ago from *Bacillus cereus* as I did to many other people after its publication. He (or the other person) certainly did not mention that he wanted to put it into *B. anthracis.*

Former Biopreparat leader Alibek chuckled at Western science's naïveté.

'We started from scratch, but we used all knowledge obtained by the West,' Alibek explained. 'And Western scientists are very, very open people—it's not a problem to write a letter and get all you need.'

Decades earlier the need to share biological samples had led to the creation of special repositories of organisms, cells, and other biological material. As it was expensive to store such things in individual laboratories, these repositories maintained massive biological inventories and shipped requested samples to researchers all over the world.

Members of the US Congress expressed outrage in the late 1990s when it was learned that one such repository, American Type Culture Collection (ATCC) of Virginia, in 1995 had shipped anthrax samples to a laboratory in Iraq and plague to right-wing Ohio zealot Larry Wayne Harris—who was arrested outside Las Vegas in early 1998 with a supply of anthrax.

But in his defence to enquiring journalists ATCC Director Dr Raymond Cypress insisted that there was 'a tradition of exchange of materials in science, and we have no documentation of almost any of it.'

For example, twenty-seven research laboratories in America in 1997 published work on *Yersinia pestis*, which caused plague, 'but only four received cultures from us. So where did the rest come from?'

Well, there were 453 such repositories worldwide, according to the *World Directory of Collections of Cultures and Microorganisms*, 54 of which sold or shipped anthrax, 64 sold the organism that caused typhoid fever, and 34 offered the bacteria that produced botulism toxin. And 18 repositories, located in fifteen countries, traded in plague bacteria. These repositories were located not only in the United States and Europe, but also in China, Bulgaria, Iran, Turkey, Argentina, and sixty other nations. Some such repositories did business over the Internet, offering overnight shipment of microbes for nothing more than a credit card number—no proof of scientific credentials was required.[59] Like the open atmosphere of scientific exchange that allowed Pomerantsev access to Portnoy's and Goebel's work, the exchange of microorganisms had traditionally been fettered by little more than the prices dealers charged for their bugs. And such openness was thought to help public health, giving scientists speedy access to strains of bacteria and viruses for research use.

By Cypress's estimations 99.9 per cent of all research uses of such organisms were, indeed, in the interests of public health, basic science, or pharmaceutical development. And that emphasized the main problem with biological weapons verification and enforcement: dual use. Although there could be no legitimate civilian use for discovered VX gas supplies or pellets of weapons-grade enriched plutonium, both the equipment needed to produce bioweapons and, by and large, the biological agents themselves could be put to honest medical and research aims.

Unlike nuclear, conventional, or chemical weapons production, bioweapons required no dedicated facilities. Any pharmaceutical or medical laboratory and production site could be the source of manufacture. And bioweapons could be dispersed using standard agricultural equipment: pesticide sprayers or crop dusters.

Every step, then, in production of bioweapons involved materials and equipment that could be put to legitimate exploits: thus it was all, in national security parlance, 'dual use'. And the dual use dilemma lay at the heart of weapons inspection obstacles.

Some members of the intelligence community believed that the Biopreparat anthrax had made its way to Iraq—an allegation that could never be proven, even if samples of a vaccine and antibiotic-resistant strain of *B. anthracis* were found. The Iraqis could always assert that the bacterial strain arose naturally—on Iraqi, not Russian, soil. And whatever criminal proof the intelligence operatives claimed to possess implicating a Russian scientist or two was never made public—indeed, it probably never could be without compromising sources. These uncertainties made it possible to use the act of accusation as a diplomatic weapon, tarnishing the reputation of a nation without offering a shred of proof. It seemed almost as bad as the state of diplomatic affairs during the Cold War.

Allegations concerning an illness dubbed Gulf War Syndrome further underscored the tremendous difficulties in diagnosing an ailment and determining its cause in the context of war. Did thousands of Allied soldiers suffer a unique ailment caused by exposure to a chemical or biological substance during the Persian Gulf War? Several veterans groups and their physicians said yes, pointing to a long list of symptoms shared by many returning soldiers. A host of causes were suggested: pesticides, US Army vaccines, fumes from burning military vehicles, smoke from a bombed Iraqi chemical weapons depot, chronic fatigue syndrome, mass hysteria. Years after the war's end debate still raged in the United States, Canada, and the United Kingdom over every conceivable aspect of Gulf War Syndrome. The inability to resolve the public quarrel—even to reach consensus on whether Gulf War Syndrome existed— illustrated how difficult it would be to sort fact from fiction in any conflict if an unusual or subtle organism were inflicted on combat troops.

The Gulf War, coupled with news of Pomerantsev's superbug anthrax invention, prompted US Defence Secretary William Cohen in May 1998 to allocate $130 million for anthrax vaccination of 2.4 million active duty military personnel. Almost immediately resistance surfaced as recipients of the vaccine claimed the immunization had caused severe health problems, and more than a hundred servicemen and women faced summary courts-martial rather than be vaccinated. As protest spread among US soldiers, sailors, and airmen it became disturbingly obvious that Americans could no longer be counted upon to undergo mass immunizations willingly—even in the face of possible bioterror threats.

The anthrax vaccine was only one of many immunizations US military personnel were required to receive. The lengthy list included vaccines against cholera, Japanese encephalitis, plague, typhoid, and yellow fever. No soldiers risked courts-martial over those vaccines, even though some of them posed significantly greater health hazards or were of a far lower efficacy. For example, the cholera vaccine was no longer recommended by WHO or the CDC because it could actually cause cholera in some people and offered only marginal immunological protection. The CDC had abandoned the plague vaccine, finding that cheap, low-risk prophylactic doses of tetracycline offered good protection for individuals in Yersinia-infested areas. And the Japanese encephalitis vaccine produced severe allergic reactions in a several recipients. Yet no protests were raised against those vaccines.

Between May 1998 and March 1999 more than 630 000 US military personnel received the anthrax vaccine: forty-two of them, or 0.007 per cent, suffered adverse reactions, seven of which were severe enough to require hospitalization. All recovered fully.

Yet the antimilitarist peace organization Citizen Soldier waged a strong protest against the anthrax vaccination campaign. The group's attorney Todd Ensign said that there was 'good faith concern' about anthrax vaccination, boiling down to, 'what is the hurry here? Is there some other agenda? I think it's, Number One, this has connotations of warfare, so that concentrates the mind. Cholera, diphtheria—they're just not dramatic in the same way. It raises the question, ' "Wait, does this mean I'll be exposed to anthrax?" '

Via the Internet, Citizen Soldier spread the gospel of anthrax vaccine protest. The group's perspective was decidedly from the left. But there were plenty of other groups on the political right who used the Internet to raise concern about the vaccine. Human Life International, an anti-abortion group, alleged that the vaccine was laced with human chorionic gonadotrophin—a female pregnancy hormone—as part of a massive, top secret campaign to sterilize US soldiers. Behind the effort, the group claimed, were WHO, the World Bank, and the Rockefeller and Ford Foundations. At a Gulf War veterans Web site soldiers were advised that human fetuses were destroyed, and their body fluids used in the anthrax vaccines. In darker conspiratorial tones various fundamentalist Christian and far-right groups warned of a NATO plan to take over America by weakening US troops, giving them an anthrax vaccine that was filled with chemicals that would spark an autoimmune response, thereby turning the vaccinee's immune system against his own body. Similarly fantastic theories were espoused by Canadian opponents of that country's military anthrax vaccine programme.

Some members of the US Congress and its General Accounting Office were inclined to accept the notion that autoimmunity-inducing compounds were in the anthrax vaccine. And though there was absolutely no evidence to support the claims, GAO insisted that a chemical called squalene had been incorporated into the vaccine as an adjuvant. Further, GAO insisted that squalene sparked autoimmune responses.[60]

Social historian David Rothman of Columbia University saw a larger lesson in the suspicions and protests among active duty soldiers and veterans—one that he suspected would cloud all civilian and military vaccine campaigns aimed at offsetting bioterrorism. During World War II, he said, Americans had been very enthusiastic about the marriage of military and medicine, a union that produced mass penicillin use for bacterial diseases, refined blood transfusion procedures, and chloroquine prophylaxis for malaria.

With the advent of the Cold War after 1945, however, Americans began to feel uneasy about Pentagon medical efforts, particularly with rumours of cover-ups regarding radiation dangers.

'Fear of the mad, dangerous scientist is something ancient in American culture. We also have long had anxieties about our government, about the idea of government. And the military has evoked its share of anxieties,' Rothman explained. 'Until recently, however, all of these were separate suspicions. What you have now is something new.'

To accept that the anthrax vaccine was inherently more dangerous than, for example, the almost universally condemned cholera immunization, Americans had to reject the repeated, contrary assertions of the White House, an assortment of federal agencies, the Department of Defence, and the nation's medical science establishment.[61] It constituted seeds of doubt never previously expressed by Americans, Rothman insisted.

At Johns Hopkins University D. A. Henderson's Working Group on Civilian Biodefence carefully analysed all available information on anthrax, concluding that any plan to protect American citizens against terrorist use of the bacteria had to include vaccination.[62] Without either immunization or immediate prophylactic antibiotic use, inhalation of anthrax spores, the Group concluded, would be fatal to 80 per cent of those who were exposed. The Group strongly recommended vaccination of emergency response personnel.

But the anti-vaccination movement inside the military revealed how hard it might be to gain compliance with immunization from average Americans. This, despite mounting evidence that anthrax and other bioweapons were finding their ways into the hands of more rogue nations.

As the twenty-first century approached, the following nations possessed biological weapons, developed for missile or large-scale aerosol delivery to enemy targets: Iraq, Iran, Syria, Libya, China, North Korea, Russia, Israel, Taiwan, and possibly Sudan, India, Pakistan, and Kazakhstan.[63]

The list cut across power groups, ideology, political organization, and geography.[64]

In addition to these countries many non-governmental international political organizations were thought to be developing or seeking to purchase bioterrorist weapons. Intelligence sources in Europe and the United States, including retired Central Intelligence Agency Director John Deutch, insisted this was the case, though for security reasons details were not provided.[65]

Beyond advances in delivery capacities, the bioweaponry itself was expected to improve by leaps and bounds. Until 1985, all of the world's bioweapons manufacturers had the same limited list of agents that could be assured of killing thousands of

..nies and were deliverable with missiles or other systems. Each nation knew the list and stockpiled antidotes and vaccines. It was a standoff.

But as the Pomerantsev case illustrated, biology was intellectually to the 1990s what physics was in the 1940s and 1950s: a field of exponential discovery. What seemed impossible in 1980 was manageable by 1990 and easy fodder for high school biology classes in 1995. In 1993, the US congressional Office of Technology Assessment (OTA) predicted that:

> Genetic engineering is unlikely to result in 'supergerms' significantly more lethal than the wide variety of potentially effective biological agents that already exist, nor is it likely to eliminate the fundamental uncertainties associated with the use of microbial pathogens in warfare. However, gene-splicing techniques might facilitate weaponization by rendering microorganisms more stable during dissemination (e.g. resistant to high temperatures and ultraviolet radiation). Biological agents might also be genetically modified to make them more difficult to detect by immunological means and insusceptible to standard vaccines or antibiotics.

Biology moved along far more rapidly than even the OTA anticipated. A multinational effort in the 1990s to determine the sequence and identify all of the genes of the human genome charged ahead at a pace far exceeding expectations. And it inspired efforts to sequence the DNA or RNA of microbes. With that came unwitting identification of unique targets in humans, and weapons in microbes.

In a 1996 editorial the British medical weekly *Lancet* noted that 'a concern has slowly surfaced about biological weapons with selective ethnic targets. Anyone voicing such concerns at a meeting of molecular biologists or infectious disease specialists risks scorn. "That's the stuff of science fiction." But is it?'

Determining the genetic sequence of a virus, such as Ebola, was no longer much of a feat. John Mekalanos at Harvard Medical School worked out how to find genes in bacteria quickly that were responsible for virulence.[66] At Stanford University Stanley Falkow developed a way to see which genes in the organism that caused typhoid fever were switched on first, after the pathogen infected human cells.[67] This quick and dirty technique singled out virulence genes. Influenza researchers, in hopes of spotting a naturally emerging superflu before it caused a 1918-type pandemic, sequenced that virus and identified some of its key pathogenesis genes.[68] In 1998 scientists at the Frederick Cancer Research Centre in Bethesda determined, genetically, exactly how anthrax kills human cells.[69]

By the late 1990s the tools were in hand. There was a massive pool of bioengineers.[70] They had genetic blueprints to guide their efforts.[71] There were precedents. And there were stockpiles. Western militaries hardened their biodefences, vaccinating troops, stockpiling antitoxins, storing appropriate antibiotics, purchasing bioprotection suits

and masks, carrying out war games drills involving biological weapons, and supporting research on potential biodetection devices.

But protection of innocent men, women, and children was another matter.

'There's just been *no* looking at this on the civilian side,' Henderson lamented.

In his speech that spring morning in Atlanta, Henderson warned that no one had
a master plan for dealing with the collateral impact of bioweapons on civilians located
around a combat zone—or the deliberate impact of bioterrorist damage inflicted on
an unsuspecting community.

'To date, the focus of concern with respect to countering civilian terrorism has been
almost wholly on chemical and explosive weapons and a response which is, at most,
a modest extension of existing protocols to deal with a hazardous materials incident,'
Henderson intoned. 'A chemical release or a major explosion is far more manageable
than the biological challenges posed by smallpox or anthrax.'[72] Following an explosion
or a chemical attack, the worst effects are quickly over; the dimensions of a catastrophe
can be defined; the tolls of injuries and deaths can be ascertained; and efforts can be
directed to stabilization and recovery. Not so following the use of smallpox or anthrax.
Day after relentless day, additional cases could be expected—and in new areas.

Comparisons to the impact of nuclear weapons, once considered ridiculous, arose
in every 1990s policy discussion of biological warfare. The key similarities were their
lasting effects long after an initial explosion or release and the likelihood that nearly all
of the dead would be civilians. For example, national security analyst Brad Roberts felt
that biological weapons constituted the 'poor man's answer to the nuclear bomb,'
creating the possibility of asymmetrical strategies of conflict.

'In such strategies,' Roberts wrote, 'weaker states seek to pit their strengths against
the weaknesses of stronger ones in order to deter intervention or prevent the stronger
state from bringing to bear its full military potential.'[73]

The strategic superiority of biobombs over nuclear weapons, under such circumstances, would be greatly enhanced, Roberts argued, by the creation of what might be
termed 'designer bugs', genetically engineered for such strategic advantages as racial
targeting. With nuclear weapons there was always the risk that winds would carry
radioactive fallout toward the bomber's own troops, and no living creature was immune
to the mutational impact of ionizing radiation. But bioweapons designed to exploit
a specific genetic vulnerability might be harmless to the inflictor's troops while devastating not only opposing armies, but also entire civilian populations.

As writer Robert Wright put it, 'If someone asks you to guess which technology
will be the first to kill 100 000 Americans in a terrorist incident, you shouldn't hesitate;
bet on biotechnology.'[74]

When US Navy Commander James K. Campbell contemplated preparedness for
biological weapons attacks he spoke of 'the postmodern terrorist', who did not hesitate
to target civilians. Campbell said that 'of increasing occurrence is the ultraviolent
terrorist act followed by silence', such as the bombing at the 1996 Olympics in Atlanta.

Or the 1998 bombing of the US embassies in Dar es Salaam and Nairobi. Such events, he argued, 'suggest a shift in terms of the message the terrorist was supposedly sending. Where traditional terrorists used the event to gain access to a bully-pulpit to air their grievances, these silent terrorists send a silent message creating a superordering sense of overwhelming fear and vulnerability.'

An action that seemed unimaginably ghastly to most people, Campbell said, was precisely the kind of step the new 'postmodern terrorist' was likely to take. Unfettered by governmental restraints—indeed, unconnected to any government—this novel terrorist, Campbell argued, was likely to be so strongly motivated by religion or political issues that the damage inflicted by his or her actions could far exceed that caused in more traditional conflicts. The reason: the postmodern terrorist was often willing to take measures that were so dangerous as to be suicidal, as well as killing others.

In the 1990s in the United States, Senator Sam Nunn was the politician who appeared most knowledgeable about defence and national security issues. Following the Aum Shinrikyo attack in Tokyo, Nunn, echoing concern about postmodern terrorism, said: 'The number one security challenge in the United States now and probably for years ahead is to prevent these weapons of mass destruction, whether chemical, biological or nuclear, and the scientific knowledge of how to make them, from going all over the world to rogue groups, to terrorist groups, to rogue nations.'[75]

'As we enter the twenty-first century, we may well be facing weapons of mass destruction used not on the battlefield by warriors,' wrote US Air Force Lieutenant Colonel Terry Mayer, 'but among dense population centres by deranged nonnation states—a sobering perspective.'[76]

In May 1993, President Clinton echoed those sentiments in a key speech to the Annapolis Naval Academy, saying: 'Rather than invading our beaches or launching bombers, these adversaries may attempt cyber-attacks against our critical military systems and our economic base ... or they may deploy compact and relatively cheap weapons of mass destruction.'

Preparing to meet the challenges posed by the use of biological weapons at the hands of such groups or individuals was an enormous task that was only beginning to be tackled in Europe and the United States at the turn of the century.

Just ask retired Atlanta fire chief Don Hiett. In 1996 he was in charge of all emergency responses for the Olympics, and in preparation he saw FBI files on attempted and successful terrorist events never made public. When it came to bioweapons, Hiett said, 'We are far, far short of where we need to be. We're far, far short in detection. And as first responders we don't think in the big picture.'

For example, when a bomb exploded during an Olympic rock festival Hiett was one of the first responders on the scene.

'Honey, let me tell you,' Hiett said in a Georgia drawl, 'nobody had the mind-set to think of biological or chemical. And nobody will think of it until we start seeing the canaries dropping in the coal mine. ... There was some forethought, and it was mainly a chemical thing. Biologicals—first off, most people don't even think bombings happen in America. Well, let me tell you, there's twenty a day!' And increasingly, Hiett continued, terrorist threats and actions involve biological weapons. 'The potential is here, there's no doubt about it.'

Though twenty-seven American cities participated during the late 1990s Department of Defence-run training exercises, all of the nation's municipalities remained ill-prepared for such an eventuality. Henderson insisted that the focus of training was wrong: there needed to be a sustained, long-term effort to prepare emergency room and public health personnel, firefighters, or police.[77]

Were a terrorist to release what Henderson considered the ultimate weapon—smallpox—the once universally vaccinated population would be highly vulnerable. The US government had, two decades earlier, stockpiled enough vaccine for about 15.4 million people,[78] and the World Health Organization had 500 000 doses stored in the Netherlands. Various additional national stockpiles totalled about sixty million more doses, of varying quality and potency. Clearly, were smallpox released most of the world's population would be vulnerable and, given smallpox's 30 per cent kill rate, nearly two billion people could die.

Two *billion* human beings.

In 1999 the picture actually worsened, amid discovery that the US smallpox vaccines had severely deteriorated. Originally made in the 1970s by the Wyeth pharmaceutical company, the vaccines were stored at the CDC facilities in Atlanta, in the form of freeze-dried crystals, packaged in 100-dose quantities inside vacuum-sealed glass tubes. The tubes were further sealed with rubber stoppers held tight by metal clamps. To their dismay CDC investigators discovered that condensation had built up inside many of the glass tubes, indicating that the rubber stoppers had decayed and vacuum pressure had been lost.

The Food and Drug Administration said that the nation's smallpox vaccine supply 'failed quality assurance'. And that was only the first of several problems shocked government and private scientists discovered as they scrutinized America's smallpox vaccine stockpile. The checks only occurred because the White House, anxious about evidence that samples of the deadly virus might have been distributed beyond the two WHO-designated repositories, called for production of additional vaccine supplies for the US armed forces. Investigators thought it wise to first check the status of the original stockpile—one that six presidents had, apparently mistakenly, assumed would protect the population if ever needed. It was a good thing such eventuality hadn't arisen.

The condensation, it turned out, was simply problem number one. The second concerned a fluid, or diluent, that was supposed to be mixed with the freeze-dried crystals just before vaccination. The diluent had what was called a 'brilliant green' indicator in it that was supposed to help the vaccinators see the droplets passing out of the needle onto the recipient's arm.

But the 'brilliant green' had changed colour, and appeared to be deteriorating rapidly. And there was another problem: the needles. Smallpox vaccination is unlike other immunizations in that it cannot be administered as a simple shot. Rather, the droplets of vaccine must be scratched into the skin using a special instrument called a bifurcated needle. It turned out that the US stockpile contained fewer than one million such needles, and nobody in the world still manufactured them.

But the largest problem was what scientists called VIG, or variola immunoglobulin. Whenever a large number of people were, back in the 1960s, vaccinated against smallpox a handful of them—less than 1 per cent of all vaccinees—suffered severe adverse reactions. For them a quick shot of VIG was a lifesaver. In 1999 however, CDC investigators realized that there were only enough stockpiled VIG doses to handle 675 adverse reactions, or the number of such events that would typically occur if three million people were immunized. And even those few doses of VIG seemed compromised as they had taken on a pink hue, rather than the acceptable colourless status of freshly made supplies.

Were an emergency to occur, the US population would be completely vulnerable to smallpox. And though the other European and South African vaccine stockpiles hadn't undergone similar scrutiny there was little confidence in those, either. The last time a mass emergency vaccination had taken place in the United States was 1947, when a traveller from Mexico spread smallpox in New York City. Vaccines were then readily available, and 6.35 million New Yorkers were immunized in less than four weeks—a feat that a half century later US authorities would not be able to repeat should it become necessary. In 1961 a similar mass vaccination campaign was executed following appearance of smallpox cases in England: 5.5 million people were immunized in one month. A decade later the recognition of cases in Yugoslavia prompted rapid vaccination of 20 million people in that country. Were a smallpox crisis to emerge, in 2000, neither of these efforts could be repeated.

At the urging of the White House the Department of Defence had in 1997 awarded the small biotechnology company Dynport a $30 million contract to make 300 000 doses of smallpox vaccine for military personnel. It was as a result of queries from Dynport that the CDC and FDA had investigated the status of the old vaccine stockpiles. And upon learning of the sorry state of that supply the White House asked Dynport to look into the feasibility of making another forty million doses for civilian use.

Dynport looked into the question and came back with an offer—forty million doses for $1 billion.

'Outrageous,' hollered Henderson. 'I looked at what we paid at WHO in 1974 for vaccines we got from Switzerland, the US, the UK and Canada. It was between a half cent and 1.7 cents per dose. Now, allowing for inflation to, say, 10 cents, or heck, let's even say to $1 a dose, okay? You should only be talking about $300 000 to meet the DOD contract and, at most, $40 million for the civilian side.'

While the haggling continued between Dynport and federal officials the Wyeth company quietly set to work making fresh vaccine diluent. But no company stepped forward to manufacture the needed forty to fifty million bifurcated needles. And the Baxter pharmaceutical company was having a tough time working out what had happened to the VIG supplies it had made twenty years earlier.[79]

Large-scale stockpiling of smallpox vaccines in key civilian zones of the United States and Western Europe might, after all, be of limited value for two reasons: individuals would develop symptoms diagnosable as smallpox only several days after exposure, by which time thousands—even millions—would have been exposed; and only several days or weeks after vaccination would individuals have developed sufficient antibodies to stave off infection.[80]

For other vaccine-preventable microbes, such as anthrax, the lag time between inoculation and development of powerful antibodies could be far longer—up to a year, even with boosters. And of course vaccines would be of no value whatsoever if the culprits created vaccine-resistant killer germs. Further, a determined enemy could simply try a succession of microbial weapons—or use a cocktail at the outset—defying even the best organized population vaccine defences.

In the United States the federal model for civilian protection was essentially patterned after that of the military. Based on recommendations made in the spring of 1998 by a White House panel of scientific experts, President Clinton ordered hundreds of millions of dollars' worth of vaccine stockpiles, advanced biodefence training for National Guard troops, and accelerated urban preparedness based on a military response model.[81]

The strategy almost immediately came under fire from public health advocates.

'I look at it this way,' Henderson said following a 1998 US Senate hearing on bioterrorism. 'This is our main defence: state and local public health, local doctors. Here we are investing $300 million for fifty-plus twenty-two-man National Guard units, and what possible relevance are they to the problem? Why aren't we putting a billion dollars into strengthening what is actually our frontline response. Hell, we haven't even got a strategy!'

At the same Senate hearing,[82] Minnesota's Osterholm grew indignant when asked what it would take to get America's cities prepared to respond to bioterrorism: 'There is simply nothing that scares me like this issue. . . . Today you hit a major building in this country with an aerosolizing device with smallpox, it could quickly be all over the country. The orientation here in Washington, DC, is on chemical terror. But giving the National Guard $300 million does nothing for bioterrorism. The key is local public health.'

'What I'm trying to determine is how much money you need to spend on the three Ps: planning, preparedness, and prophylaxis,' CDC economist Martin Meltzer explained.

To work it out, Zimbabwe-born Meltzer imagined a small city of 100 000 people, a calm warm evening, and a crop duster. That plane was loaded with one of three deadly bacteria: anthrax, brucella, or tularaemia. A cloud of microbes enveloped the city, exposing everyone to its deadly contents. What would happen?

Meltzer discovered that in the case of such treatable bacterial diseases the severity of the attack, both in terms of lives lost and cost to the community, would depend on how quickly authorities recognized what had occurred and how rapidly they distributed prophylactic antibiotics to the population to prevent individual illnesses.

'The cost of delay—the cost of not being prepared, in the case of anthrax,' Meltzer explained, 'if you wait to day six [after the attack] before starting your prophylaxis programme the difference in deaths is five thousand if you start on day one versus thirty-five thousand on day six.'

The assumptions built into Meltzer's model were, if anything, overly optimistic. Doctors correctly diagnosed the exotic diseases, ideal treatments were administered, hospital costs were low, and if local authorities decided to administer prophylactic antibiotics to the population they, in their wisdom, selected the perfect drugs and had ready supplies on hand. Such assumptions were, Meltzer admitted, 'a bit on the rosy side'. Nevertheless, they revealed clearly that the costs of delay, and the numbers of lives saved with rapid response, were profound.

For example, if local officials in Meltzer's mythological city of 100 000 picked the correct antibiotic and administered it in the proper dose within twenty-four hours of an attack, about 5000 people would die and the total cost of medical care for the community would be $128 million. If, in contrast, it took six days for authorities to realize what had happened, correctly diagnose the microbial culprit as anthrax, and commence mass antibiotic prophylaxis with the appropriate drug, nearly 35 000 people would perish and treatment costs for the dead and ailing would total $26.2 billion.

In terms of fiscal costs the difference was exponential. If an anthrax attack was recognized within twenty-four hours and widespread doxycycline prophylaxis was administered to the entire exposed population the costs for treatment, hospitalization, and lost productivity due to illness or death would be $3.7 billion. If the prophylaxis didn't commence until day six, the attack would cost the community nearly $25 billion—a billion less than the cost of no response at all.

When asked what such an attack might cost a large metropolitan area such as New York and its neighbouring suburbs, Meltzer thought out loud: 'How much more difficult is it to aerosolize an agent to infect a population of fourteen million? Is it impossible? No. But there is some difficulty. If time isn't a factor, no problem.... Let's see, if 100 000 people were exposed would you have to prophylaxe fourteen million?'

Meltzer stopped his mental computation, concluding that a clever terrorist wouldn't even try to infect everyone. In a large, dense city, 'How much do they actually have to disperse in order to create an all-out panic?'

In a larger city centre, then, the true costs of a bioterrorist event might be secondary factors associated with panic, such as the collapse of the stock market in New York or commodities market in Chicago.

So, from Meltzer's point of view, cities large and small would be well advised to get ready, stockpiling supplies of relevant antibiotics, vaccines, and general medical supplies. Of these three, Meltzer concluded antibiotics were the most crucial. Of slightly less importance was preparing local police and military responders to contain order and forestall mass hysteria.

'Do you want to be so scared that you paralyse yourself,' asked Meltzer rhetorically. 'Or do you want to become alerted, informed, and prepared?... You have to be prepared to deliver postexposure prophylaxis to a large number of people. That is the challenge that bioterrorism represents.'

Meltzer was, of course, the first to admit that his scenario didn't address the potentials of either drug-resistant bacteria or viruses. Such agents, Meltzer asserted, were too frightening for even him to contemplate, as few potentially lethal viral illnesses were treatable or preventable with available vaccines.

The Meltzer study was one of the key influences on the Clinton administration's decision to develop antibiotic stockpiles for use in the defence of civilians. Former New York City Commissioner of Health Dr Margaret Hamburg was placed in charge, working inside the US Department of Health and Human Services. Her tasks were to determine which antibiotics could actually save lives should various bacterial agents be released in a US city, what the shelf lives of those drugs were, how they ought to be stored, and how in a crisis they could be equitably and rapidly distributed. It was, Hamburg said, 'an almost overwhelming challenge.'

Henderson asserted that, were a highly infectious virus released, the primary protection would be air-filtered quarantine units. But few hospitals had such facilities, as New York City discovered earlier in the decade when the super-drug-resistant group W strain of tuberculosis appeared on AIDS wards in several facilities.

Recognition that a bioterrorist event has occurred was the key, regardless of whether the agent was bacterial or viral. And if Navy Commander Campbell was correct, the modern bioterrorist wasn't likely to issue warnings, claim credit, or in any way acknowledge the event.

It would be a surprise.

Local authorities 'probably aren't going to be able to recognize it has happened... until the incubation period is over,' Clark Staten, executive director of the Emergency Response and Research Institute in Chicago, insisted.[83] 'And by then you've got it spread over a wide area. And it may take longer to recognize there's a pattern going on.'

It will begin, the experts say, with a couple of cases of 'flu' in one hospital, three in another, and so on. Hours or days may pass before health-care workers start wondering why there is so much 'flu'—and most of these diseases do begin with flulike symptoms—flooding into the hospitals. Eventually someone would call the local public health department, alerting officials that some sort of epidemic is occurring, or so authorities hope. Of course when an unusual encephalitis outbreak struck New York City during the summer of 1999 only one physician took note and made such a call to

Department of Health authorities. Retrospective investigation revealed that New Yorkers had been becoming ill and dying of encephalitis for weeks before the city realized what was going on. And once the existence of such an outbreak was known federal CDC scientists incorrectly diagnosed the cause as St Louis encephalitis. Weeks passed before academic researcher Dr Ian Lipkin of the University of California in Irvine correctly determined that the deceased patients were victims of, instead, West Nile virus, a North African microbe never previously seen in the Americas.

As the clock ticks away in an outbreak an epidemiologist would be dispatched to determine the cause of the cases. If the bioagent were a fairly common bacterium, such as *Clostridium botulinum*, local hospital laboratories should be able to identify the culprit.

But if a microbe not usually seen by local physicians, such as anthrax, Q fever, Ebola, smallpox, or plague appeared, local facilities probably would not be able to diagnose the problem. With precious time passing, people dying, and disease possibly spreading, local officials would then await word from the diagnostic laboratories at the CDC in Atlanta. And if any truly dangerous organism were the suspected culprit—such as smallpox—all CDC analysis would be handled in the Special Pathogens BL-4 laboratory.

During the summer of 1994 Dr Marcelle Layton started her job as New York City's chief of infectious disease control, learning that 'by the way, part of your job description is planning for biological warfare,' Layton said in a 1998 speech to her colleagues.

'It is easy to be overwhelmed by the more than sixty agents that the Department of Defense says have the capacity to be weaponized,' Layton continued, noting that 'for many of these agents there are very limited supplies of treatments . . . and capacity to do specimen analysis and autopsies. Panic and terror could be expected, even among the health-care providers, themselves.'

By order of New York City Mayor Rudolph Giuliani municipal employees like Layton were generally forbidden to discuss any details of the city's response plan publicly. When Office of Emergency Management Director Jerry Hauer did address the topic he deliberately spoke in dry, even boring, tones. The concern was that individuals with evil intent would spot fears and weaknesses, which they would exploit in a terrorist attack.

But Layton summarized the city's situation by saying, 'Most of us . . . have grave concerns about whether or not our current public health system has the capacity to respond. Are we prepared? No.'

In 1997 and 2000 New York City had actually undergone Department of Defense citywide bioterrorism drills. In 1996 Mayor Rudolph Giuliani created the Office of Emergency Management run by Jerome Hauer, a professional emergency manager and firefighter with ten years' experience in corporate and government preparation. Hauer travelled to Israel to learn how that country planned to respond should microbes be released by terrorists in Tel Aviv. He studied Pentagon plans. He conducted drills involving forty-one New York City hospitals, and declined to comment on most public queries or told the public that the city was ready for the worst. But in public meetings Hauer acknowledged that a bioattack involving a human-to-human transmissible agent would quickly overwhelm the city's hospital emergency rooms, require hasty construction of alternative care facilities, and if not handled extremely carefully, would provoke widespread panic that could not be controlled by the New York Police Department. In a 1999 role-playing anthrax drill, Hauer's staff and the New York City Police Department quickly lost control of the populace and Gotham descended swiftly into a hysterical, nightmarish scene unlike any seen in North America since the 1918 flu pandemic.

Osterholm scoffed at Hauer's confidence, and there was no love lost between the two government officials. Osterholm insisted that New York, or any other city, couldn't consider itself 'prepared' for a bioattack unless it had stockpiled of millions of doses of vaccines and antibiotics—which no city had. And he wasn't sure that Hamburg's anti-biotic stockpiles could ever reach New York or any other city and be distributed rapidly enough to stave off disaster.

'Look, suppose the president is coming to New York to speak at the UN,' Osterholm suggested. 'He gets out of the car. A plane flies down the East River. You know, the president and the bum on the street are breathing the same air. So that plane spews out anthrax. Are you going to tell me New York is ready for that?'

Could any city be ready for such an evil act? Perhaps not, Osterholm conceded. But the degree to which any municipality was prepared for such an abomination would depend not on emergency personnel such as police, but on the strength of the city's basic public health infrastructure.

Osterholm insisted that Hauer, and all other city emergency planners, were grossly underestimating the amount of panic such an event would provoke: 'I can tell you, a single case of meningitis in a local high school causes enough fear and panic to bring down a whole community.... Now imagine you're telling people, "This is going to unfold for eight weeks, and I can't tell you if you're going to die." And with every symptom people in the public feel, real or imagined, they're going to think, "I've got it! I'm gonna die!"'

'You don't think that's panic? Think again,' Osterholm continued. 'Part of my message has been sharpened because of a lack of response by these people who want to say, "We're prepared." Heck, it's like stealing sweets from a baby. Just ask, "So where are your vaccines?"'

If New York City wasn't prepared, how could its neighbouring towns and villages, from Newark to East Hampton, possibly be expected to know how to respond to such an attack?

Colonel David Franz, deputy commander of the US Army Medical Materiel Command, devoted years of his life to readying the military for bioweapons. He insisted that this tremendous American vulnerability 'underscores the need for a strong technical base that we cannot get away from in this nation. We need far forward capabilities.... The timelines are critical, even for a hoax. We've got to know what we're dealing with to treat people properly and to prevent panic.'

Though Congress directed the military to develop that technical base, the Department of Defence was understaffed. Until 1997, for example, Franz ran USAMRIID, located inside Fort Detrick. USAMRIID was the military's only BL-4 top security facility in which such superlethal microbes as Ebola and smallpox could be studied safely, and had responsibility for developing and testing treatments and vaccines for potential biological weapons.

Between 1991 and 1998, due to budget cuts, USAMRIID lost 30 per cent of its scientists and technicians, and they could no longer promote junior scientists.

'We're eating our seed stock,' said USAMRIID scientist Peter Jahrling. The budget situation froze all of the agency's scientists and physicians in tiers they had occupied for years. No one advanced, and no young, fresh scientists entered at the bottom level, training to take over the nation's vital laboratory in due course. USAMRIID became a laboratory full of ageing, demoralized men and women who collectively possessed most of the West's knowledge of biodefence.

If an emergency developed due to biological weapons use, Franz said, 'We would have ... to pull people in from all other divisions.'

So many federal, state, and local agencies were supposed to respond if a bioweapons event occurred in the United States that it was doubtful anyone would know precisely who was supposed to be notified first and which group would be in charge.

'We need a "wiring diagram" of how federal assets are requested,' Charlotte, North Carolina, Fire Chief Luther Fincher Jr declared. 'What is the federal emergency number? How is it activated? Who determines what assets will be spent? What are the defined roles for each federal agency dispatched? Do they understand that they will report to the local incident commander for assignment? ... There can be no hesitation or confusion about any of this after an incident occurs.'

Interestingly, the one federal agency that was *not* supposed to be in charge was the Department of Health and Human Services—public health. In most cases it was law enforcement that called the shots, despite the near certainty that federal and local police forces would know next to nothing about viruses, biotoxins, or bacteria. Law enforcement tended to be slow to recognize such threats, and then responded in classic police fashion, throwing every available weapon or tactic at the situation regardless of the scientific wisdom of its use.

On April 24, 1997, for example, events in Washington, DC, proceeded precisely by the book according to the FBI. But public health terrorism experts say what happened at the B'nai B'rith national headquarters that Passover day offered terrible evidence of the flaws and vulnerabilities in America's preparedness—or lack thereof—for a biological attack.

It was the third day of Passover and the Jewish human rights organization was closed, except for its security guards. Amongst the April 23 post was an eight-by-ten-inch padded envelope that sat for twenty-four hours in the B'nai B'rith post room.

On Friday morning one of the post room employees noticed that the package was leaking a red sticky substance—blood, perhaps. And written on the package—which had passed through the US postal system—were the words *Yersinia* and *anthrachs*. The first referred to *Yersinia pestis*, the bacterium that cause plague. The second was a misspelling of *anthrax*.

For the following nine hours the B'nai B'rith building was surrounded by the Washington, DC, fire department, police, FBI, and District of Columbia emergency management personnel. The air-conditioning system was shut down, and the post room was designated a 'hot zone', DC Fire Department Battalion Chief Alvin Carter recalled.

'The area was cordoned off. There's a hot zone, a warm zone, and a cold zone. Each zone required different protective equipment,' Carter explained. 'All civilians are in the cold zone.'

All of the people who were in the 'hot zone' post room were required to remain there until, Carter said, 'the area was decontaminated.' The suspect bioterrorist package was placed in an airtight HAZMAT, or Hazardous Materials Team, container and transported by car to the Naval Medical Research Institute in Bethesda, Maryland.

The sample was taken to G. W. Long's laboratory where, Long said, 'within minutes we were able to say it was negative for plague and anthrax,' the two agents the envelope claimed were enclosed.

As navy scientists worked to determine the actual contents of the package, DC authorities and the FBI took the following measures: the entire B'nai B'rith building and neighbouring structures were quarantined; fire department personnel dressed in Level A, fully encapsulated suits hosed down the 'hot zone' with chlorine; and a set of sheets were strung out in the Washington, DC, street and potentially exposed individuals were ordered to strip and submit to a spraying with a chlorinated water pounded at them by high-powered fire hoses.

'That's how you decontaminate,' Carter explained.

An FBI supervising Special Agent who asked not to be identified said that the emergency response 'went slowly, but everybody wanted to be careful. . . . There's a federal disaster response plan that kicks in and you follow certain protocols.' And key to the federal protocols were local HAZMAT teams: such fire department HAZMATs would, he said, play the leading role in any bioterrorist event.

'Pretty much any good metro fire department has materials for chemical hazards—same thing.'

Thankfully, the package contained a broken petri dish full of nothing but strawberry Jell-O, along with a note from the would-be assailant, Counter Holocaust Lobbyists of Hillel, an Orthodox Jewish group that stridently opposes liberal Judaism.[84]

Contrary to the FBI's view, public health experts say responses to chemical versus biological hazards should *not* be the same. They argue that several mistakes were made at B'nai B'rith that could have spread disease had the package contained anthrax or plague.

First, by orders of the local HAZMAT, which was trained to handle chemicals or explosives, the air-conditioning system at B'nai B'rith was shut down. But this didn't occur until emergency services were notified of the suspicious package—twenty-four hours after it had arrived in the building. Thus potential microbes could have circulated throughout the building, making the entire complex a 'hot zone', not just the post room.

The second concern was for the decontamination procedure used on one post room employee, a B'nai B'rith security guard, and two emergency personnel—the sprayed fire hoses. The FBI insisted that chlorine in the water 'kills everything. If it's biological, it will kill it. That's all you have to do.'

But biologists said that some organisms—such as anthrax spores—might well resist droplets of chlorine. And high-powered hoses could actually disperse the organisms into an aerosol mist that could rain down over the area.

Further, DC HAZMAT and the FBI benefited from their proximity to the navy's top—indeed, *only* —bioterrorism laboratory—Bethesda. When asked what would happen elsewhere were such an incident to occur, the navy's Long shrugged and said, 'I'm not aware of anything for the rest of the country. If somebody put up the money some of this could be used elsewhere. But I'm not willing to go testing all over the country.'

In other words, the rest of America would be on its own, unable to determine the contents of suspicious packages rapidly.

In 1997 to 1999 the FBI had the leading role in training local firefighters—HAZMATs—in the first response to biological weapons attacks. Nearly seventy thousand firefighters were trained in WMD (Weapons of Mass Destruction), operating in manners that equated chemical and biological attack responses. It was, Osterholm insisted, *the* fundamental flaw in all American plans for defending the nation's citizens against bioweapons attacks. Osterholm said that 'biological weapons cause diseases that exist in nature and may occur spontaneously in human populations. . . . The investigative steps for detection and identification of the agent would be the same as that for a naturally occurring agent. Therefore, the first and most fundamental strategy for dealing with bioterrorism was to develop effective means for combating all infectious diseases. . . . improving the public health infrastructure and biomedical research capacity.'

Long before it became chic in America to point out the possibility of a bioattack on US citizens, a religious cult did, indeed, use bioterrorism. And, underlining Osterholm's point, it was local public health that recognized what had happened and responded. It took place on September 17, 1984, in a remote corner of northern Oregon. Four days later patients contracted acute stomach pains, fever, chills, headaches, bloody stools, and vomiting; by September 24 more than 150 people in rural

Wasco County, Oregon, were violently ill. In the sparsely populated county of 21 000 people such a sharp increase in gastrointestinal cases drew attention from Oregon state authorities.

By the end of September, 751 cases of acute gastroenteritis had occurred in the county, representing 9 per cent of the total population. Laboratory tests showed that all the victims were infected with *Salmonella typhirium*.

'Usually the county sees less than five cases of salmonellosis a year,' Dr Michael Skeels, chief epidemiologist for Oregon's state health department, said. The incident sparked a large public health investigation because, 'it was the largest food-related outbreak in the US in 1984,' he added.

It took a year of intense study for Skeels's team, working with CDC and FBI experts, to work out what happened, and another twelve years to gain permission from state and federal investigators to publish the details in the *Journal of the American Medical Association*. Federal authorities feared that merely describing the incident would spark copycat crimes across the nation.

It all traced back to the Big Muddy Ranch, near the town of Antelope in Wasco county. A religious cult there planned to take over the county's political apparatus.

In the early 1980s Bagwan Shree Rajneesh was an Indian guru who claimed enormous numbers of followers in the United States, most of whom wore red, orange, or fuchsia clothing because the Bagwan said he loved the colours of sunrise. The cult bought Big Muddy Ranch and quickly outnumbered the local residents. In 1984 the Rajneesh group, having many grievances with county officials, pushed for a special election, which might have given them control of the county's affairs.

As the election approached, the Rajneesh group, led in these efforts by an American nurse who had taken the Indian name Puja, built a biology laboratory at Big Muddy and ordered samples of several microbes, including *Salmonella typhirium*, from American Tissue Type Culture, then located in Maryland. The laboratory, called Pythagoras Clinic, had actually been licensed by the Oregon State Health Department.

'I licensed it,' Skeels said with a shrug. 'The irony of that did not escape me.'

Following various books and medical articles readily available in libraries and bookshops, Puja's laboratory grew large supplies of *Salmonella*.

And on the eve of the county election, hoping to make hostile voters too ill to go to their polling booths, the Rajneesh followers put the bacteria in dressings at salad bars in the county's ten most popular restaurants.

Fortunately the religious cult lacked sufficient biological knowledge to breed drug-resistant strains of the bacteria, and all the illnesses responded swiftly to antibiotic treatment.

When Skeels and the FBI raided Big Muddy Ranch a year later, however, they discovered 'a bacteriological freezer-dryer for large-scale production' of microbes, Skeels said. They also found a library of such things as *The Anarchists Cookbook*, literature on manufacture and use of explosives, and military biowarfare articles.

'We lost our innocence over this,' Skeels said. 'We really learned to be more suspicious. . . . Obviously these pathogens are too easy to purchase.'

'These cases were first picked up by the Wasco County health department,' Skeels concluded, adding that 'the first significant biological attack on a US community was not carried out by foreign terrorists smuggled into New York, but by legal residents of a US community. The next time it happens it could be with more lethal agents. . . . We in public health are really not ready to deal with that.'

If Wasco County hadn't had an alert disease surveillance system, the sudden increase in salmonellosis would have gone unnoticed. The Rajneesh cult would have got away with it. And perhaps, emboldened by its success, the religious cult might—as Aum Shinrikyo did years later—have escalated their efforts. If the agent they used the next time were more toxic even Skeels's alert group would be at a loss to prevent mass murder.

'I'm concerned with, how are we going to make the diagnosis? Fire departments aren't going to play a role in this thing unless it's a hoax,' Osterholm insisted. 'For most of these illnesses what's going to get picked up is an undiagnosed illness that suddenly overwhelms doctors' offices, emergency rooms, and ambulances.'

In two chilling role-plays, public health and law enforcement officials staged responses to bioterrorism events, revealing critical flaws in the nation's safety net. At a December 1998 Biological and Chemical Weapons Conference at Stanford University public health officials failed to mount an effective response to the deliberate release of a superflu virus: in a few months one million Americans would have been dead, had it been real.

A more elaborate event was enacted in February 1999 in Crystal City, Virginia, by the Johns Hopkins Centre for Civilian Biodefence Studies. The details unfolded over an eight-hour period in a packed, tense room full of public health, military, and law enforcement personnel. In this instance the vice president of the United States visited a prestigious university located in a mythical town dubbed North-east. It's 1 April. Eleven days later a twenty-year-old student who had heard the vice president reports to the university hospital's emergency room with flu-like symptoms: high fever, muscle aches, fatigue, headache. She is sent home with aspirin and the old maxim: get plenty of rest and drink lots of fluids.

Two days later the young woman returned to the hospital, fighting for her life. A university janitor who had cleaned up after the vice president's speech also arrived with the same symptoms. By six o'clock that night, April 13, the hospital infectious diseases expert is gingerly ready to voice an outrageous conclusion: both patients have smallpox.

Since smallpox was officially eradicated from the face of the earth in 1977 and samples of remaining viruses are supposed to be under lock and key only in Atlanta and Siberia there can be but one conclusion: someone has stolen laboratory samples of the virus, and deliberately released them in a bioterrorist attack aimed at the United States vice president.

In this situation, within two months more than fifteen thousand people would have died of smallpox worldwide and epidemics would have been out of control in fourteen nations. All global supplies of vaccine would be depleted and it would take years to manufacture enough to save humanity. The global economy would be teetering on the brink of collapse as nations closed their borders and sank into nationalistic isolation, barring all Americans from entering their countries. In the city of North-east utter chaos would reign, and the National Guard would have imposed martial law over the two million residents.

Similarly, government authority would have either broken down or reverted to military-style control in cities all over the world as smallpox claimed lives and pitted terrified citizens against one another.

A top smallpox expert scribbled projections on the back of an envelope and gently slid it in front of the governor of his state: within twelve months eighty million people worldwide would be dead.

'We blew it,' declared California's top state public health laboratory expert Dr Michael Ascher. 'It clearly got out of control. Whatever planning we had . . . it didn't work. I think this is the harsh reality, what would happen.'

Although most of the public in North America and Europe remained ignorant of the sorts of issues raised in such situations, handfuls of Internet-hooked extremists, right-wing militiamen, psychiatrically imbalanced men of anger, and postmodern fascists were aware of the finer points of bioterrorism. Recipes for botulinum and anthrax production were on the Internet. Books describing biotoxin assassination techniques were readily available. Some private militia groups trained in the use of bioweapons.

For example, Uncle Fester, as he called himself, was a Green Bay, Wisconsin, devoted father of two. He was also the author of Silent Death, a book adorned with a skull and crossbones that purported to teach readers hundreds of ways to kill using chemical and biological poisons. While his youngest cried for attention, forty-year-old 'Fester', who declined to reveal his real name, bragged on the phone to a reporter that the book 'sells a couple thousand copies per year,' to people he imagined were 'holed up in their bunkers waiting for Armageddon to come. And then they will come out of their bunkers and use these skills.'

Fester's book told readers how to be a 'crafty executioner' by poisoning individuals with botulinum toxin, noting that 'once these symptoms of botulism appear, the anti-toxins that medical science has developed are completely useless.'

Fester, who said he had degrees in both biology and chemistry, told his readers how to manufacture and use several of the world's deadliest microbes, suggesting that they use the US postal service. One should 'have no contact with any delivery service,' Fester said, pointing out dozens of ways to ensure that no evidence turned up in victims' autopsies.

'Look around the world,' Uncle Fester challenged. 'There are multiple places in the world where the skills in this book could be used to good purpose. In the United States? Not as long as we have free speech. But there are rat holes all over the world.'

Asked if he had ever tested his 'recipes', the Wisconsin assassination guide was cagey. After all, under recent congressional law such activity would be illegal.

'Let's just say I know they work,' Uncle Fester said with a chuckle. And then he recommended his Web site on the Internet, where further 'cooking' details were available.

Ex-biker and former Klan member Kurt Saxon, aged sixty-six, also had a Web site that was full of the same sorts of things one could read in his books, *The Poor Man's James Bond*, Volumes 1–4. The books were full of ways to maim, kill, and torture victims, including with biological weapons. In the introduction of the first volume, Saxon told his readers that 'this book is power' and praised right-wing 'militants' who, he wrote, would be transformed by his book. Yet, he insisted, most would-be American terrorists were 'a bunch of hate-filled losers'.

When asked about Larry Wayne Harris, who had twice been arrested with plague and anthrax, Saxon chortled, 'The guy who was caught with anthrax in Vegas? Well, he was a member of Identity. And that means he's clinically insane.' But Harris had his mind straight enough in 1997 to be able to write a book: *Bacteriological Warfare: A Major Threat to North America*. In it, Harris cleverly avoids violating federal laws, telling readers how to make biobombs by describing actions he claims outsiders plan to use against the US.

Thus, the information was readily available to those who wanted it, and apparently many Americans did. In its 1998 annual report, the Southern Poverty Law Centre identified 474 so-called hate groups in America, representing a 20 per cent increase over the previous year. The largest, Identity, had fifty thousand members in 1998. It is estimated by some observers that there were eight hundred right-wing militia groups in the United States in 1999, some of which advocated the overthrow of the US government and conducted tight Green Beret-style training of their members, who carried sophisticated weaponry.

A Washington DC, FBI Special Agent, who would not be named, said the numbers of terrorist threats called into the nation's capital every year had increased steadily, exceeding five per day by 1998.

An unreleased White House 1995 report on terrorism had predicted that a terrorist could kill millions of residents of the nation's capital by dropping a hundred kilograms of a biological agent out of the back of a crop duster flown on a windless day over Washington, DC. They had also predicted that a virtual amateur could develop bioweapons which, if dispersed in the New York subway system, would claim tens of thousands of lives.

But were America's militants and fanatics ready to try biological terrorism? Law enforcement leaders claimed that religious cults and militant political groups were the *most* likely to try bioweapons. After all, they argued, the first domestic mass biological poisoning was carried out in 1984 by members of the Rajneesh religious cult. And the first bombing of a fully occupied government office building was in 1995 in Oklahoma City—executed by American political extremists.

It was, perhaps, the tone of their rhetoric that sparked the most concern. In *The Poisoner's Handbook*, for example, author Maxwell Hutchkinson told readers that they could poison or kill Internal Revenue Service workers by filling out fake tax return forms, lacing them with a mixture of ricin toxin and DMSO—a concoction that the author claimed was 100 per cent lethal.

'The purpose of all this is to disrupt the operations of the Internal Revenue Service,' Hutchkinson wrote. 'If done on a large enough scale, it would serve two purposes—it would make it more difficult for the IRS to operate efficiently, thus helping tax cheats and tax protestors. It might also awaken the politicians to the depth of resentment felt by the taxpaying public.'

Fortunately, Hutchkinson was a lousy chemist: DMSO only serves as a solvent, passing substances through the skin into the bloodstream, if a simple chemical is involved. Proteins, such as ricin, couldn't dissolve in DMSO.

But the depth of Hutchkinson's antagonism was unmistakable. He suggested that his readers kill Catholics by soaking their rosary beads in *Phytotoxin abrin*, a toxin derived from precatorious beans; he wrote that 'botulism is fun and easy to make'; and he urged survivalists worldwide to hone their skills, readying themselves for biological defences in the Armageddon.

In light of all this, the US Congress passed a number of laws aimed at making it harder for anyone—citizen or overseas agent—to attack America with bioweapons. In 1989 it passed the Biological Weapons Act, which made it illegal for any American to possess, trade, sell, or manufacture a biological substance 'for use as a weapon'. In 1991 it passed an export controls law, soon put in force against Iraq, that barred US companies from trading with countries believed to be developing bioweapons.

After the Oklahoma City bombing, Congress passed the Anti-Terrorism Act of 1996, which allowed federal authorities to arrest anyone who even 'threatens' to develop or use biological weapons. And the following year, by order of Congress, the CDC named twenty-four infectious organisms and twelve toxins as 'restricted agents' use or possession of which required a federal permit.

Congress sought technological solutions as well, allocating money for Department of Defence research on devices that might identify bugs and sanitize contaminated areas. The first in use was the navy's TagMan, a large gene scanner that could identify whether a liquid sample contained any of several known agents in less than half an hour. But the system had limitations: it was not portable, and could not be used for serious Biohazard Level-3 or BL-4 agents—precisely the most worrying microbes. Most significantly, it couldn't analyse air samples.

The DODs Defence Advanced Research Projects Agency, or DARPA, had $2 billion to fund wild and crazy science ideas—notions so far-out that standard civilian funding sources would not consider them. Among DARPA's many projects were $61.6 million of bioweapons defence efforts. The primary DARPA hope was that someone would develop a fast, cheap, safe, and portable way to sample air for the presence of nasty organisms. Most of the research focused on unique genetic attributes of bacteria and viruses.

One project involved trying to grow human nerve cells on microscopic chips that would change colour or light up if the nerves detected some sort of neurotoxic agent. Such a device—if ever practicably developed—could be a sort of early warning system that would sense the presence of nerve-damaging agents such as botulinum.

Several laboratories—notably Argonne National Laboratory in Chicago—were trying to develop chips that were lined with thousands of pieces of DNA from bacteria, to serve as probes. Argonne's goal was to have an air detection device that was small enough that it could be handheld, akin to a police radar gun. But research director Eli Huberman said such a thing 'is years away from mass production or for widespread use.'

Furthermore, neither the Argonne device nor any others in development considered sampling the air for viruses. Even the DARPA wild thinkers hadn't imagined how that could be done.

Even the simplest technological approach to bioweapons proved to be too much for DOD contractors. In the spring of 2000, Defense Department officials revealed that protective space suits US troops had relied upon in the Persian Gulf, and that still formed the basis of soldiers' defence against deadly microbes, were defective. At least 5 per cent of the 900 000 suits Department of Defense had purchased during the 1990s were useless, and the reliability of the entire inventory was suspect.

It seemed unlikely, then, that a quick technological answer would soon be found. Thus, the three immediate Western responses to bioterrorism appeared to be seriously flawed: military defence, HAZMAT reactions, and high-technology sensors.

For instance if the Red Army had succeeded in releasing drug-resistant anthrax spores in the Bourse Station of the Paris metro at 8:00 a.m. on a warm Wednesday in June, what would be the role of the French army, Sûreté, Paris police, or any number of high-tech sensor devices? None. The most important responders would be the doctors, epidemiologists, ambulance drivers, nurses, and bureaucrats of the Paris public health system. It is they who would note—days after the event—that large numbers of Parisians appeared to be ill, suffering similar symptoms. And with questioning they might realize that all the ailing individuals routinely took the same metro train, or stopped at the same station.

And regardless of whether or not anyone ever realized that the lethal biological mist was dispersed in the Bourse metro station—or caught the terrorists responsible—it is the public health system that would track down and treat the patients, determine who should receive prophylactic antibiotics and dispense the drug, conduct epidemiology that could determine whether the new anthrax outbreak was spreading from person to person, and analyse the organism to see what special attributes it might have.

Yet it was a military-style response that dominated government thinking. Legally the Department of Defence was on shaky constitutional ground in asserting its right to seize command in the event of a domestic bioterrorist event. Defence Secretary William S. Cohen announced on February 1, 1999, creation of a special command within DOD, designed to coordinate responses to domestic biological attacks. A popular 1995 film, *Outbreak*, had depicted such an event, in which the US Army declared martial law and took full control of an American city in order to limit spread of an airborne transmissible form of the Ebola virus. Such a clear violation of the United States Constitution might be alright for Hollywood, civil libertarians cried, but not for the real world.

In his January 22, 1998, speech to the National Academy of Sciences President Clinton said 'we will be aggressive. At the same time I want you to know that we will remain committed to uphold privacy rights and other constitutional protections, as well as the proprietary rights of American businesses. It is essential that we do not undermine liberty in the name of liberty.'

That day Clinton requested congressional approval for a $10 billion antiterrorism programme, including $86 million for improving public health surveillance, $43 million for research on vaccines for anthrax, smallpox, and other potential biological warfare agents, and $300 million for stockpiles of essential drugs and vaccines. The proposed expenditure marked a doubling in the previous year's bioterrorism budget.

In an interview the previous day with the *New York Times* President Clinton acknowledged that he had 'spent some late nights thinking a lot about this and reading a lot about it ... For example, we know that if all of us went to a rally on the Mall tomorrow with ten thousand people, and somebody flew a low-flying crop duster and sprayed us all with biological agents from, let's say, two hundred feet, that, no matter how toxic it were, half of us would walk away for reasons no one quite understands. You know, either we wouldn't breathe it, or we'd have some miraculous resistance to it. And the other half of us, somebody would have to diagnose in a hurry and then contain and treat.'

The job of building the nation's drug and vaccine stockpile fell to Hamburg. In her new capacity as assistant secretary of health for the US Department of Health and Human Services, she was racing to catch up with the Department of Defence and the FBI. Public health was a late entrant into the bioterrorism field, she said, and significant dangers lurked in the developing antiterrorist infrastructure. Beyond the already voiced civil liberties issues Hamburg worried that 'the danger is we don't want public health identified with the CIA and FBI activities. Particularly in terms of global infectious disease surveillance. We in public health need to have public trust and confidence.'

Already local public health departments were having a hard time striking that balance in responding to fake bioterrorism events. It seemed that claiming to have placed or shipped an anthrax-containing device had suddenly become chic. Jessica Stern of the Council on Foreign Relations had counted forty-seven such hoaxes in the United States since 1992. In all forty-seven cases local fire and police authorities had reacted seriously, decontaminating two thousand people in these incidents and appearing on the scenes dressed in full body protection suits. And Stern's list was by no means comprehensive.

Secretary of the Navy Richard Danzig warned that panic, in and of itself, was becoming the new terrorist tool, adding that 'only through a new union of our public health, police, and military resources can we hope to deal with this dangerous threat.'

But Hamburg was worried that the hoaxes were occurring precisely *because* the police and FBI were responding. It seemed bioterror hoaxes attracted some of the same sick individuals as enjoyed watching fire departments douse buildings that they had set afire.

'When an envelope comes in saying "This is anthrax," we don't need the fire department in full protective gear on site,' Hamburg insisted. 'What we need is to discreetly move the envelope to a public health laboratory for proper analysis. Mass decontamination and quarantine only added fuel to the fire of the hoax perpetrators and it's totally unnecessary in terms of public health.'

It was obvious that public health, law enforcement, and defence had very different priorities. For public health the paramount concerns were limiting spread of disease, identifying the causative agent, and, if possible, treating and vaccinating the populace. Law enforcement, however, was in the business of stopping and solving crimes, and the scene of any bioterrorist incident was primarily, a source of evidence. Managing an outbreak response would, for the FBI and police, constitute a conflict of interest, as they would be focused on detaining witnesses and obtaining evidence even if their efforts ran counter to public health.

The primary mission of the Department of Defence is to protect the United States against military foes. Secondary to that is defending the health of its troops. How that squared with intervening—indeed, *commanding*—responses to domestic bioterror incidents wasn't clear.

When public health needed to intrude upon individuals' lives in order to protect the larger community it did so in limited ways and usually under the promise of confidentiality. For example, during an epidemic individuals might be asked to submit to blood tests and medical examinations, and their medical charts might be scrutinized.

On a more long-term basis public health protects the community by monitoring disease trends, logging who is suffering or dying from what diseases. Again, the information is generally stored in confidential or anonymous form.

Globally the World Health Organization and a variety of other groups kept similar count of nations' diseases, monitoring for emergence of new epidemics. After the 1995 Kikwit Ebola epidemic WHO sought to create a more rigorous surveillance system and encouraged countries to be more open about epidemics in their populations.

All these functions, in all tiers of public health from villages to global levels, required maintenance of a crucial social contract: the individual or country agrees to disclose information for the sake of the health of the larger community. And in return public health authorities promise never to abuse their trust, maintaining discretion and protecting patient privacy.

But the fear of bioterrorism threatened to destroy that vital social contract, as it was not one shared by law enforcement or defence. The closer public health drew to the other two, the greater the danger that it would lose all trust and credibility in the eyes of the public it served.

Some public health advocates were convinced that no marriage between their profession and law enforcement could ever work, and denounced all efforts to increase bioterrorism concerns. One prestigious group argued that 'bioterrorist initiative programmes are strongly reminiscent of the civil defence programmes promoted by the US government during the Cold War... fostering the delusion that nuclear war was survivable.'

For many older public health leaders the bioterrorism issue at the turn of the century brought up nasty memories of Cold War cover-ups and suppression of science. By adopting the issue, they warned, public health was buying into a framework of paranoid thinking. And, indeed, in 1999 biologists for the first time found their work facing censorship in federal laboratories in the wake of allegations of Chinese espionage at the Los Alamos National Laboratory. The Department of Energy, which ran the national laboratories, clamped down so hard in 1999 that the National Academy of Sciences warned that the future of the US scientific enterprise could be imperiled. Though the DOE's primary concern was computer and nuclear secrecy, the threat of bioterrorism prompted the agency to broaden its new security restrictions to embrace basic biology research as well.

'This is a truly pernicious list' declared Nobel laureate Burton Richter, director of the Stanford Linear Accelerator centre in Palo Alto, addressing the National Academy of Sciences.

Overall, many advocates argued, public health's role in the bioterrorism issue could only be a comfortable one if it were an equal partner with the military and law enforcement. Or, perhaps, better than equal.

In his historic speech in Atlanta during the winter of 1998 D. A. Henderson had beckoned public health to jump on board a train already in motion, conducted by the defence, intelligence, and law enforcement communities. Less than a year later public health was on board the train, but clearly not in the conductor's seat. Some public health advocates gleefully confided that concern about bioterrorism might be the political trigger that restored funding for their collapsing infrastructures. But the wiser among them recognized that dollars earmarked for bioterrorism issues would never be applicable to such essential programmes as syphilis monitoring, well-baby programmes, HIV counselling, immigrant TB screening, or cardiovascular disease surveillance.

Osterholm knew that he had instigated the public airing of previously secret biological weapons fears. And he took no satisfaction in that—not so long as the essential role of public health remained unresolved.

'I use this analogy,' Osterholm explained. 'It's like riding giant waves in Maui. You can't be an inch farther out than the data. But you can't wait to act, either. For three years I was almost the lone voice on biological terrorism.'

He rode his Maui big wave, Osterholm said, dreaming of surfing while Arctic winds blasted the walls of his office. Now the trick would be to keep public health from being wiped out. Hunched over his phone the Minnesota State epidemiologist was watched over by a sign on the wall behind him.

It read THE BUG STOPS HERE.

CHAPTER 6

Epilogue

The changing face of public health and future global prophylaxis.

Responsibility requires freedom.
—Amartya Sen, 1999[1]

The poor, we're told, will always be with us. If this is so, then infectious diseases will be, too—the plagues that the rich, in vain, attempt to keep at bay.
—Dr Paul Farmer, 1999[2]

There is a chain that runs from the behaviour of cells and molecules to the health of populations, and back again, a chain in which the past and the present social environments of individuals, and their perceptions of those environments, constitute a key set of links. No one would pretend that the chain is fully understood, or is likely to be for a considerable time to come. But the research evidence currently available no longer permits anyone to deny its existence.
—*Why Are Some People Healthy and Others Not?* Robert Evans, Morris Barrer, and Theodore Marmor 1994[3]

In 1346 a particular set of circumstances occurred, in a peculiar sequence, resulting in what may have been the first true global epidemic. Perhaps only the Americas and Antarctica were spared humanity's globalized Black Death.

The event involved no dark, conspiratorial forces concocting evil means of deliberate spread. It simply entailed the right mix of human social evolution, weather, and ecology occurring simultaneously with a force that was devastating to *Homo sapiens* of Europe, Central Asia, the Indian subcontinent, Indochina, the South Seas, the Middle East, northern Africa, and the Arctic.

With epidemics, timing is everything.

Yersinia pestis had undoubtedly been infecting fleas and rodents for centuries, occasionally affecting a human who mysteriously fell victim to the bacterium's lethal force. But by the 1300s the human race had scattered across the globe, many of them—perhaps a fifth of the population—living in cities and trading posts. Caravans loaded with goods were making their way across the most forbidding terrains, from the Gobi Desert to the Sahara. Sailing ships carried goods from port to port, continent to continent. It was an era of profound globalization in which cooks in Venice were discovering the wonders of pepper and cinnamon, London's tailors were sewing wondrous silk garments, and the emperors of China witnessed the chemicals they used for fireworks exploited effectively in the West as gunpowder.

In that earlier age globalization brought riches and wonders to some, sparked an intermingling of cultures and languages with sprinklings of ideas from faraway places, and forever changed the nature of economics, politics, and warfare.

It also created new opportunities for *Yersinia pestis*. At some point in 1345 to 1346, weather conditions favoured large flea and rat populations in Mongolia, giving *Yersinia* ample opportunities to reproduce and spread between the insects and rodents. The weather must also have been favourable for the horses and camelback caravans that wended their ways from Mongolia, through China, and along the Silk Route of Asia.

Stowaways also made the journey: fleas, rats, and *Yersinia*. And within eighteen months the Black Death was claiming millions of lives across the Old World.

In the fourteenth century, as a response to the Black Death, some of the basic tools and laws of public health were created: quarantine, ship inspections, leprosariums, mass burials during epidemics. These were applied crudely, without any understanding of the causes of the scourges sweeping through the fourteenth and fifteenth centuries. All too often such methods of epidemic control were accompanied by ruthless, brutal repressions of the populations thought to be responsible for given diseases, such as the Jews of Europe and Infidels of the Ottoman Empire.

Wherever globalized trade went, disease hitchhikers went too, taking their tolls on Incas, Aztecs, Maoris, Polynesians, Russians, Laotians, French, and Moroccans. A price, it seemed, had to be paid for the first internetting of human beings, connecting Iroquois via English ships indirectly to Hawaiians, and Irish via the Dutch armada to Papua New Guineans. Even such slow-motion fourteenth-century globalization came at a cost.

In the twentieth century global economics and power were the causes of three world wars, two fought on battlefields, and one 'cold' one, involving the constant threat of thermonuclear weapons. (Only a handful of people realized that the world also lived under the peril of biowarfare catastrophe at the time.)

With the 1989 fall of the Berlin Wall and 1991 collapse of the Soviet Union the nations of the world suddenly faced three unshakable new facts. First, the capitalist market system was the basis for all trade and economics, and Marxist approaches to economic equity or distribution were dead. Second, the old alliances were no longer meaningful, and superpower protection of corrupt, dictatorial proxy state leaders was over. And third, the price hundreds of millions of people had paid for the Cold War and its subsequent global structural readjustments was their health and well-being.

It may seem paradoxical that there are voices of discontent—including my own—decrying the global state of public health, claiming that the triumphs of our time are transient, under siege, even doomed. At the close of the twentieth century, life expectancies are soaring, not just in wealthy industrialized nations, but in many of the world's poor countries, as well. The World Health Organization forecast in 1999 that average life expectancy globally in 2025 will be seventy-three years—up from just forty-eight in 1955. In 1955, some twenty-one million children died before their fifth birthdays; in 1995, only eleven million did.

Yet these promising overall trends disguised local and regional reversals that were profoundly disturbing to health experts. The double epidemics of TB and AIDS set sub-Saharan Africa's hard-fought health advances spiralling backwards towards the nineteenth century: life expectancies shot downward regionally in the 1990s, and infant mortality rates jumped upward. By 1998, for example, Malawi's average life expectancy rate had fallen below its pre–World War II levels, thanks almost entirely to the human immunodeficiency virus. So dire was the situation by 2000 that the World Bank declared the AIDS pandemic its 'number one priority' and Bank president James Wolfensohn vowed that 'no sensible AIDS programme would be stopped for lack of money.' Never before had a public health issue been given such prominence in the Bank's portfolio.

Advances made in poor countries proved frighteningly fragile. They were easily reversed by wars, corruption, global economic shifts, new epidemics, or refugee movements.

In the former Communist world—particularly in the nations that once made up the Soviet Union—life expectancies had reversed course with such rapidity and drama as to exceed anything seen in the absence of war over five previous centuries. Indeed, some regional downturns were proportionally greater than anything witnessed during peacetime since the pneumonic plague reached Moscow in the fourteenth century.

In 1955 the world was deeply divided: Communist bloc versus capitalist West. The roughly 2.5 billion people living on earth in 1955 grew up in an explosively prosperous economy. In 1973, however, the world's economy fell into a twenty-year-long sluggish recession that was most strongly felt in developing countries. By 1994, when global economic recovery began, there were 5.8 billion mouths to feed, most of them left malnourished.

In the wealthy world the artificial trade and currency alliances in the capitalist market economies—united by their opposition to communism during most of the twentieth century—turned competitive with a vengeance after the fall of the Berlin Wall. There was no longer any need for concern that European workforces would embrace socialism or communism, so government handouts didn't have to be used as lures to an obedient proletariat. Western European economies, long taxed by national and cultural commitments to social welfare, found their national health systems were baggage too weighty to carry during the competitive sprint for global economic power. As health-care costs inflated, physicians throughout Europe reduced the numbers of procedures, medications, and treatments they administered to their patients.

Nevertheless, national health systems sank into debt, physicians failed to receive full reimbursement for their services, and government calls for managed care resonated from Lisbon to Oslo. With the twenty-first century approaching, Europe prepared to merge into a single economy, lean and strong, ready for fiscal showdowns with American, Japan, China, even the new Russia.

Russia staggered, however, seemingly unable to transform itself into a viable, first world market economy without succumbing to the tragedies of the developing world: corruption, political instability, capital centralization, and the complete collapse of social service infrastructures.

Some of the same frailties, long masked by stupendous capital growth and productivity, brought the economic powerhouses of Asia to their knees just two years before the millennium. In rural Japan and South Korea the crash of 1998 signalled the greatest public revenue health hardships since World War II.

And in the poorest countries of the world the already difficult became impossible. As former Tanzanian President Julius Nyerere put it: 'When the world sneezes we catch pneumonia.' The economic gap between the world's richest and poorest nations widened from 1961 to 1997 from about a twelvefold difference to a thirtyfold one. The sharpest widening took place between 1994 and 2000—at the same time as the inequalities in life expectancies and infant mortality rates grew most disparate. By then Nobel laureate Amartya Sen was no longer a lonely voice: his was echoed by a chorus of economists and public health experts who showed that the wealth of nations, and the degree of fairness with which that wealth was distributed within nations, determined countries' infant mortality rates. Poverty, they declared, killed babies.

In contrast, at the eve of the twenty-first century Americans enjoyed a phenomenal boom; their economy was the strongest on the planet. Though artificialities also plagued the US economy—notably the investment character of its stock exchanges—Americans had so much cheap food that more than half of the population was medically obese.

But beneath the veneer of America's political and economic world domination problems lurked. By 1997 some 43.4 million Americans—more than 15 per cent of the population—had no health insurance. In 1998 that figure jumped to 44.3 million, or 16.3 per cent of the population. Since 1993, when the Clinton administration first initiated the US health care reform debate, the uninsured population had grown by 4.5 million, among them one out of every four children in the country. An additional 71.5 million Americans lacked health care insurance for at least part of 1997, with a disproportionate percentage of the uncovered drawn from Hispanic, African-American, and poor white populations. The government's safety net—Medicaid and Medicare—didn't reach to protect a third of all Americans living below the poverty line. And many who were insured had coverage under plans that put a straitjacket on their care, limiting patients to the medical practices deemed cost-effective within a profit-making paradigm.

'Two-thirds of all deaths under the age of sixty-five are now postponable, if not preventable,' American Public Health Association President Dr Joyce Lashoff declared in 1991. Yet, with each passing day more and more Americans put off vital health care needs, clogged public hospital emergency rooms, or went bankrupt trying to pay their medical bills.

America had reached a critical health juncture, the seriousness of which was written in the numbers. Studies in 1997 showed that 56 per cent of the uninsured put off treatments due to lack of funds, and 47 per cent found it difficult or impossible to obtain medical care when needed.

Most insured Americans were covered through their employers, a victory that had been won decades earlier through labour union collective bargaining. But the end of the twentieth century had brought significant changes in the American workplace resulting in millions of fully employed Americans having no health insurance. And millions more were covered, the costs having been docked from their pay: in other words, they were paying some or all of their medical cover themselves.

By the end of 1998 a third of all Americans favoured some form of radical reconstruction of their health-care system, registering the highest level of dissatisfaction seen in any major industrialized society. They were spending twice as much annually on their out-of-pocket health needs as Canadians, and more than triple the $1347 annual per person payments made by citizens of the United Kingdom. The average American in 1997 spent $4090 on personal health care, compared to $2339 for a typical German.

Americans were, by the late 1990s, nearly matching out-of-pocket every uninsured dollar spent on medical care with another dollar for treatments delivered outside the system. From use of acupuncture to herbal remedies, quartz bedtime crystals to magnet therapy, Americans lacked faith that mainstream medicine could adequately meet their needs, and spent billions of dollars on alternative health remedies, to the tune of more than $2000 per capita annually.

Despite spending more on their health than any other peoples, citizens of the United States had the slowest rate of improvement in life expectancy of any industrialized nation. Americans born in 1960 had a life expectancy of 69.7 years, and in 1996 of 76.1 years, a gain of 6.4 years. In contrast, Japanese born in 1996 could expect to live 80.3 years, a gain of 12.6 years since 1960. The Japanese paradox directly challenged US health assumptions, as that country's populace had experienced the most rapid increase in life expectancy seen anywhere in the world during the second half of the twentieth century. Yet Japanese per capita spending on health ranked the lowest of any industrialized nation. The biggest health spender—the United States—ranked far behind Japan on every significant health index.

Another crucial public health indicator—maternal deaths—was on the rise in America, after a fifty-year decline. In 1987 the rate of maternal deaths associated with pregnancy was 7.2 per 100 000 women in the United States. Three years later it was 10 per 100 000, according to the Centers for Disease Control and Prevention. On a global scale, young children in the United States were certainly better off than their counterparts in Central Africa, India, or the former Soviet nations, but they fell well behind twenty-nine other nations when ranked by UNICEF for under-five mortality. Among the countries whose children had better 1996 survival rates were Slovenia (just four years after its war of secession from Yugoslavia), the Czech Republic, South Korea, and all of Western Europe. The Children's Defense Fund argued that most of the comparatively poor health of America's youngsters was a function of poverty and lack of health insurance, noting that half of the country's children lived in single-parent homes, a quarter were poor, and one out of twenty-four was born to a mother who lacked any prenatal care.

The twenty-first century opened on a new age of market globalization, joyfully embraced by some, dreaded by others. Massive, rapid change could irrefutably be forecast.

It posed interesting and troubling questions for public health.

At a time when the former Soviet public health infrastructure was moribund, when HIV was devastating sub-Saharan Africa, when impoverished India was spending a fortune on nuclear weapons development at the expense of its populations health, and when long-antagonistic groups were taking advantage of the end of Cold War policing to slaughter ethnic enemies, public health was in a shambles. It could not meet its basic twentieth-century core duties, that is, to ensure the public's safety at the community level, much less handle the new challenges posed by twenty-first century globalization. The safety of individual communities was eroding amid dwindling commitments to protection of the air, water, food supply, and hygiene systems. The drugs and pesticides that had insured miraculous improvements for the Northern Hemisphere during the sixth and seventh decades of the twentieth century were losing effectiveness by the final decade.

Risk increased. Though HIV surfaced in 1981 it might better be considered the first great pandemic of the twenty-first century. It spread swiftly from country to country, continent to continent in a retrovirus form that used human DNA as its vehicle and hideaway. Globalized sex and drug trades ensured HIVs ubiquity. And HIV, in turn, facilitated the circumnavigation of new, mutant forms of tuberculosis, the one taking advantage of the weakened human state caused by the other.

In the fourteenth century global travellers were few and slow. By the seventeenth century European nations were amassing wealth through global conquest and trade, conducted at the behest of kings, queens, and royally sanctioned companies. No European nation could hope to have power without spreading its tentacles to the south, east, and Americas.

The nineteenth and early twentieth century saw shifts in power and the end of colonialism, but trade remained encumbered by Cold War restrictions and the great costs of maintaining those far-flung corporate tentacles. Telecomputerization and the fall of communism erased such barriers, for the first time making the world a potential oyster for hundreds of millions of holiday makers, immigrants, entrepreneurs, speculators, and home television viewers. Cars were assembled from parts made in a dozen different countries; Indians made software that was programmed into computers made in South Korea, Sri Lanka, California, and Mexico; air travel became so popular that few of the world's major airports in 2000 could handle the traffic.

Once the world was globalized for kings and queens, then for wealthy industrialists. In the twenty-first century globalization would be ordinary, accessible not just to the patricians but also to plebeians.

Millions on the move.

Billions of humans on earth.

Shipping trillions of tons of cargo, crops, and animals.

And, by doing so, increasing everybody's risks, from Guadalajara to Guangzhou.

And ahead lurked new global risks that could exact painful prices from the public's health.

The world's population was ageing, most significantly in North America, Western Europe, Japan, Korea, and China. This would have two important effects on public health: first, on economics, and then on infectious diseases. In financial terms the wealthy West and Asia were approaching crisis points as their national tax and productivity bases were soon to shrink considerably, placing enormous burdens on their smaller, young adult populations. For the West this would be the result of the retirement of its Baby Boom generation, leaving behind two much smaller adult generations to carry the societies' fiscal burdens. In Japan, Korea, and China a combination of shrinking birth rates and phenomenal longevity meant that many Asians would live well into their nineties but be financial burdens to their families or states.

Part of the 'problem' was that these people had embraced concerns about a population explosion and come to understand that smaller families were healthier and financially more stable households. Instead of having six children and hoping two would be males who survived into their thirties, taking care of their ageing parents, the late twentieth century saw these societies recognize a new concept: have two children, both of whom survive, and the parents try to make enough money so that they can care for themselves in retirement.

By 1999 the United Nations Population Fund proudly announced that, yes, the global population had grown from one to six billion during the twentieth century. But its swelling was slowing, and it would only hit 7.5 billion by 2040, then actually begin to decline. If true, that would mean that wise government and careful management of Planet Earth's resources could allow humanity and nature to coexist without horrendous damage to the globe's biodiversity and ecological integrity. It just *might* be possible.

But the generation born between World War II and 1970 would pay a price in their old age for not leaving a large tax base in their wake. In the United States, for example, the over-sixty-five-year-old population grew from 26 million elderly people to 38.6

million between 1977 and 1997, and their health costs to the federal government climbed from $21.5 billion to $214.6 billion. By 2020 the individual medical costs per pensioner were expected to have risen from $9200 on average in 1995, to more than $25 000. And there would be 69.3 million elderly people in the United States requiring Medicare coverage possibly requiring $1.7 trillion for care.

Globally in 1998 there were 580 million over-sixty-year-olds, 355 million of whom lived in the world's poorest countries. By 2020, predicted the World Health Organization, there would be a billion elderly people on earth with 700 million of them residing in developing countries.

And the World Bank forecast that the number of elderly people living in developing countries by the mid-twenty-first century could, for the first time in human history, exceed the numbers of children under fifteen years of age.

Beyond economics, this radical restructuring of the global population, from an overwhelmingly youth-dominated demography in the mid-twentieth century to an ageing one less than eighty years later, posed an interesting and potentially dangerous herd immunity issue.

As people age their immune systems erode, replacing white blood cells and lymphatic tissue at a slower pace and in a less diverse repertoire over time. As a result, elderly bodies are more vulnerable to disease than young ones. Their immune systems are less able to scavenge for aberrant cells, thereby blocking tumour development. Regulatory mechanisms break down with age so that elders suffer more autoimmunity as their antibodies attack bone (arthritis), glands (Graves' disease), and vital organs. And the ageing defences fail more frequently when confronted with microbial diseases. That is why influenza and pneumonia, for example, are often lethal infections in old people, whereas the identical microbes may produce little more than a few days' discomfort in young adults.

Herd immunity was a well-known, but remarkably poorly understood, concept in the twentieth century. Vaccinologists had long realized that unless a crucial threshold of immunization was crossed—say, 90 per cent of a given community was vaccinated—the disease-causing microbes would continue to lurk and kill vulnerable individuals. Few scientists could predict what would occur when the percentage of societal pools with weakened immune systems increased and the efficacy of their childhood vaccinations waned. HIV offered some clues, albeit in the context of young adults and children. Wherever the percentage of HIV-positive adults exceeded 10 per cent of a given society waves of opportunistic secondary epidemics followed, notably of tuberculosis.

But HIV depletion of youthful immune systems wasn't a clear mirror of what transpired in the ageing process; like all body functions, the immune system decayed over time at different rates in every individual, usually unpredictably. What would happen with epidemic disease in the twenty-first century? Would moderately virulent influenza strains claim millions of lives, spreading among the elderly? Would drug-resistant bacteria emerge at an accelerated pace, transmitted readily with nursing homes and centres of older populations? Nobody could predict empirically what might occur when a given society's older population exceeded 30 per cent in wealthy countries or 10 per cent in poor ones. There simply weren't any precedents from which to derive estimates.

For twenty-first century public health leaders, the prospect of diminished herd immunity due to societal ageing posed significant challenges. To reduce the threat of contagion, microbe surveillance both locally and globally would need to be significantly better than it had been at the close of the twentieth century; it needed to be more widespread, based on far more sophisticated laboratory capabilities, and far more vigilant. Public health scientists would also need to learn more about how ageing bodies responded to vaccines, perhaps designing immunizations tailored to older people much as nearly all twentieth-century vaccines had been designed specifically for children under twelve years of age. Only in the 1990s were influenza vaccines created especially with the elderly in mind. Would it be necessary after 2010 to design special vaccines for measles, diphtheria, polio, pertussis, and the other ancient child killers in order to stave off waves of ancient microbial pandemics amongst the elderly?

Water supplies, too, would pose a particular public health challenge in the twenty-first century because such microbes as *Cryptosporidium* and *Legionella* were most dangerous to older people. As the sheer numbers of older people in global communities rose the need for ever purer water would also increase.

And the forecast called for more pain.

At the close of 1998 the US Health Care Financing Administration projected a doubling in health-care costs, jumping from $1 *trillion* in 1996—already a staggering figure—to $2.1 trillion in 2007. Per capita the world's highest spending on health—13.6 per cent of personal income—would soar to 16.6 per cent by 2007, and annually costs would rise by 6.5 per cent. According to government projections, the burden of those increased costs would fall directly on the shoulders of average Americans, as federal and state expenditure was expected to shrink.

How in the world could Americans pay for their personal and collective health? By 1990 one out of every six Americans, or 13 per cent, lived below the poverty line. In 1999 the US Census Bureau redefined poverty, pushing the line from the roughly $16 000 income annually for a family of four to $19 500. With that definition 17 per cent of the US population was impoverished.

And a worrying wealth gap was swelling in the United States. From 1989 to 1998 the poorest fifth of American society lost an average of $587 in real annual income whereas the richest 5 per cent of the country gained $29 533. During the 1990s median American family income increased by $600, and thanks to personal property and investment values net family worth jumped $11 900. But debt also rose during the decade, driving more families to the edge. The number of families classified as 'very poor'—those living on less than $8018 per year—increased, and as the Children's Defense Fund put it, 'We have five times more billionaires but four million more poor children.'

The net effect was increasing poverty, decreasing expenditure on social and health services, and rising housing costs. History clearly demonstrated the critical import- ance of a strong middle class to the maintenance of public health. Yet most of America was witnessing both a shrinkage of its middle class and greater financial pressure on the strata of society between the expanding ranks of the poor and the enlarging bank portfolios of the superrich.

If America was so rich in 2000 where was all the money going? The top 5 per cent of the society saw its wealth, compared to poorest Americans, expand from a ten-fold differential in 1970 to a twenty-fold one in 1996. In 1998 elite business executives earned 419 times more than their office and factory workers, compared to a forty- two-fold difference in 1980.

A key study carried out by Fordham University found that despite overall US economic growth the American social-health index had fallen steadily since its peak in 1973. The index annually evaluated sixteen social factors (such as numbers of impov- erished children, adults lacking health insurance, and average weekly earnings in real income terms), rating them on a scale of 0 to 100. In 1973 the US index topped at 77.5. By 1993 it was down to 40.6. And it kept falling thereafter.

In 1999 the World Bank concluded that there were more people living in dire poverty at the close of the twentieth century than at any time since World War II. Of course, overall there were more human beings; but a greater percentage of them in 1999 were surviving on less than one dollar a day than had since the 1950s: 1.5 billion in all. The surge in global poverty was largely credited to the collapse of the 'Asian Miracle' an economic calamity for much of South Asia and the western Pacific region. In some Asian countries the percentage of the population living on less than one dollar a day doubled in a single year (1997 to 1998). And within nations the wealth gap had caused the middle class to shrink or disappear.

With the very notable exceptions of Singapore and the United States, the wealthiest nations in the world, all of them democracies, had large middle classes, and their richest citizens controlled less than 30 per cent of the country's wealth. In most— notably the northern European countries—the wealthiest fifth of the societies con- trolled less than 23 per cent of the national wealth.

The reverse was the case in the poorer nations of the world, where more than a third of national wealth was concentrated in the hands of a small societal elite. In most cases these figures underestimated the true proportions of the developing and post- Communist nations' wealth gaps, as they reflected only disparities in the official eco- nomies. If corruption and black market economies were included in these estimates then the concentrations of wealth in such countries were even more severely skewed toward the elite, often just to a handful of families or clans.

In 1996 just 358 super-rich individuals controlled as much personal wealth as the combined income and assets of the 2.3 billion poorest people in the world. Three men—Bill Gates, Warren Buffett, and Paul Allen—had a combined 1999 wealth of

$156 billion, or $20 billion *more* than the combined GNPs of the forty-three poorest nations. Global critics charged that this signalled a sort of capital lawlessness; globalization, they said, was really about an effort to concentrate the planet's wealth in the hands of perhaps one-hundredth of a per cent of its population. Less radical critics pointed to the need for stronger national governments and rules of law to protect the integrity of the marketplace and ensure free access to trade for entrepreneurs and small businesses. Limiting lawlessness and monopolies, they argued, was the key to more equitable distribution of wealth in the twenty-first century globalized community. Regardless of the macroeconomic finger-pointing it was clear in 2000 that the gap between rich and poor nations was widening.

The United Nations Development Program decried what it called this 'dangerous polarization' insisting that it was being driven by the telecomputer age. And finance giant J. P. Morgan said that by the close of 1999 only $119 billion worth of capital would have flowed from the richer nations to the poorer ones—less than half the sum that moved from rich to poor in 1997.

A comparison of key nations worldwide at the close of the twentieth century demonstrated the factors most responsible for the health of citizens. If the observer began with the small Central American nation of Costa Rica it seemed that a relatively poor nation, with average per capita shares of GDP (gross domestic product) at just $2640 a year, could achieve remarkable health for its people, even though its climate was tropical and environment rife with parasitic and mosquito-born disease potential. On a scale of 1 to 188, with 188 being best, Costa Rica ranked an impressive 144 for child mortality rates, its infant mortality was low at 12 per 1000 live births, and average life expectancy was seventy-seven years.

In contrast, Russia, with almost equal per capita GDP earnings, ranked only 115 in child mortality, had an infant mortality rate of 20 per 1000 births, and life expectancy of just sixty-five years. And the United States, with an impressive per capita GDP of over $28 000 a year, ranked 159 in child mortality, had an infant mortality rate of 7 per 1000, and life expectancy of seventy-seven years—equal to Costa Rica.

What did that mean? Why would the wealthy United States and poor Costa Rica have roughly equal public health indicators, while nearly fiscally equal Costa Rica and Russia had markedly variant health statuses? The answers lay in other tell-tale figures, such as the percentage of GNP spent on health (8.5 per cent in Costa Rica versus 4.8 per cent in Russia), though after a point excessive spending (such as 14 per cent of US GNP) offered no added benefit. Classic public health mainstays were also crucial, such as access to safe drinking water—nearly every Costa Rican could trust the safety of water coming from his or her tap, but fewer than half of all Russians could be so confident.

A careful reading of the data also demonstrated that adult literacy rates correlated more closely with life expectancy and infant mortality than did GDP per capita.

Zambia and Zimbabwe offered striking evidence of the complexities of public health. Once called Northern and Southern Rhodesia, the nations shared much common culture, were divided by the Zambezi River along a lengthy common border, and both ranked as nations with greater than 20 per cent adult HIV rates. Yet Zambia, which provided safe water to only a third of its people and spent only 3.3 per cent of its GNP on health, had an infant mortality rate more than double Zimbabwe's, an average life expectancy of forty-three years, and ranked appallingly as 12 in the world for child mortality.

Next door, Zimbabwe was hardly a picture of perfect health, with life expectancy of a mere forty-nine years. But it offered safe drinking water to 79 per cent of its population, spent 6.2 per cent of GNP on health, and ranked 58 for child mortality. It was AIDS that brought Zimbabwe's life expectancy down to forty-nine—the nation's chief premature death toll was among its young adults, not, as was the case in neighbouring Zambia, its babies and infants.

In the 1950s famed public health advocate René Dubos admonished his colleagues to 'think globally, act locally'. Fifty years later the reverse was also wise: global efforts were needed to protect local public health. The 1977 eradication of smallpox signalled worldwide recognition that a grave global threat could *never* be eliminated locally unless it was knocked out of every nook and ecological cranny of the planet. The world rallied then but failed to follow through afterwards, by mixing global and local public health action across the board.

Global public health action on a continuing basis would, if it truly existed, constitute disease prophylaxis for every locality, from rich nation to poor. New York City need not worry about its inability to stop plague at JFK Airport if India's infrastructure could do the job in Surat, preventing spread beyond that Gujarati city. And Tokyo need not fear Ebola if Congo's hospitals were sterile environments in which the virus could not spread. Safety, then, is as much a local as international issue. In public health terms every city is a 'sister' with every other city on earth.

But for such an international system of health to exist every nation needs to demonstrate political and economic will. In 1999 the World Bank, under the leadership of James Wolfensohn, and World Health Organization under Dr Gro Harlem Brundtland scolded national leaders, telling them that the age of handouts from the rich was over. If a national government failed to make good faith efforts to improve the health of its people it could not expect assistance from the United Nations agencies or the wealthy West.

Public health infrastructures were remarkably delicate entities. The instant crash of public health in the former USSR nations offered striking proof of their fragility. And the hospital-acquired and hospital-spread epidemics of Ebola in Kikwit, MRSA in Manhattan, and multidrug-resistant tuberculosis in Russian institutions proved that a poorly maintained medical infrastructure could in some ways be worse than no system at all, undermining public health.

Public health is a bond—a trust—between a government and its people. The society at large entrusts its government to oversee and protect the collective good health. And in return individuals agree to cooperate by providing tax monies, accepting vaccines, and abiding by the rules and guidelines laid out by government public health leaders. If either side betrays that trust the system collapses like a house of cards.

Many factors contributed to the diminution of the public health trust worldwide at the close of the twentieth century: some were related to the erosion of old systems of protection; others reflected a failure to address the new attitudes towards health for the globalized twenty-first century.

In terms of the classic, older systems in 1990, the US Department of Health and Human Services released its 675-page *Healthy People 2000*, a manifesto of public health goals for the millennium. At the time, the report stated, Americans were spending annually $65 billion on smoking-related illnesses, $4.3 billion on AIDS treatment, and $16 billion on drug- and alcohol-associated ailments. The 1990 report was an update of the original one, released in 1979, and reflected failure to meet most of the timetable of health improvement then laid out, during the Carter administration. Noting that health-care spending had risen from 5 per cent of GNP in 1960 to 12 per cent in 1990, and lost productivity due to death and illness had risen, the official report estimated that 'injury alone now costs the nation well over $100 billion annually, cancer over $70 billion, and cardiovascular disease $135 billion.'

The report detailed an extremely long list of health goals for America, most of which were to be achieved not through expenditure on government regulation and services, but on 'health promotion' a catchall phrase for public education efforts aimed at convincing the nation that it should eat less and more healthfully, exercise more, stop smoking, have fewer (but healthier) children, avoid violent behaviour, and cease abusing alcohol and recreational drugs.

The report recognized that none of its goals could be reached unless the then thirty-one million uninsured Americans had access to primary care, and it stipulated that *Healthy People 2000* goals wouldn't be attainable until all Americans could afford to see doctors regularly.

Sadly, the draft *Healthy People 2010 Objectives* noted little improvement in basic health indicators, such as life expectancy. It reflected utter defeat in improving access to health care for Americans. The disparity between white and non-white American health widened during the 1990s. And the numbers of Americans who were losing work and leisure time due to illness rose, from 18.9 per cent in 1988 to 21.4 per cent in 1995. The report noted a startling series of deficiencies in basic public health information, and chart after chart was filled with 'not available' in place of numbers for such things as percentages of diabetics receiving primary care, oral cancer death rates by race, and blood cholesterol levels in poor Americans. This dearth of data reflected what the report identified as America's primary problem: its declining public health infrastructure:

This report made clear that the infrastructure upon which the national public health system functions requires definition, coordination, and strength to realize the universal public health mission. The documents continued deterioration of the national public health system: health departments are closing; technology and information systems are outmoded; emerging and drug-resistant diseases threaten to overwhelm resources; and serious training inadequacies threaten the capacity of the public health workforce to address new threats and adapt to changes in the health care market.

While the federal government worried about the nation's weakening public health infrastructure academic public health veered into new territory, far removed from its traditional role: based on large epidemiological surveys—some of which were of shoddy design—academics issued strong recommendations regarding personal behaviour and health.

If health could not be purchased by individuals, some argued, society as a whole could improve its status through non-medical interventions. And certainly there were American public health victories during the last quarter of the twentieth century which contributed to the country's rising life expectancy. Anti-smoking campaigns and litigation could be credited with a tremendous decline in tobacco use, which, in turn, prompted annual 1 per cent decreases in cancer deaths from 1970 to 1995 and was the key factor in reducing heart disease. Another contributor to America's healthier hearts was the nation's changing diet, away from saturated fats. Seat belts and drink-driving campaigns lowered the car accident death rates. And an enormous national campaign during the 1990s brought teenage pregnancy rates down from the highest in the industrialized world in the mid-1980s to about the OECD median by 1998.

As academic researchers sought to refine their recommendations, particularly regarding diet and lifestyle, contradictions surfaced. Confused Americans worried, for example, about heart disease lowered their consumption of fatty foods but increased their overall caloric intake, increasing the national rate of obesity—also a contributor to heart disease.

The credibility of the public health message was further undermined by racial stigma, as those diseases most prevalent in minority communities were commonly linked to African-American, Native American, or Hispanic diets and behaviours. When the messenger was perceived as the 'white government' the message was viewed with suspicion, even hostility. The Tuskegee legacy haunted absolutely every public health effort aimed at black Americans during the 1990s.

During the 1980s and 1990s public health seemed to be in a 'blame the victim' mode: if diseases were personally preventable through proper diet, exercise, and lifestyle, it was axiomatic that the presence of cancer, atherosclerosis, and other potential killers was indicative of poor personal behaviours. Some insurance companies took the logical step of financially penalizing individuals who defied such public health messages as 'stop smoking' and 'lower your cholesterol level'.

This did not endear public health to its public.

In March 1999 the Centers for Disease Control and Prevention conducted an opinion poll, finding that 57 per cent of questioned Americans could not define public health properly, even when given clear descriptions from which to select. Most said that they had 'negative evaluations' of the public health system. And, in order of their ranking, the survey group said contaminated drinking water, toxic waste, air pollution, bacterially contaminated food, and pesticides represented their greatest health fears.

For many Americans the 'blame the victim' perspective of the last decade of the twentieth century flowed from the same science that throughout the 1970s had issued nearly daily warnings about cancer-causing substances in the nation's food, water, environment, and workplaces. Many of the chemicals viewed with panic and trepidation in the 1970s proved to be only marginally hazardous in environmental doses a decade later. Nevertheless, fear of environmental carcinogens had created a tough and expanded federal regulatory apparatus involving the Environmental Protection Agency, Food and Drug Administration, Occupational Safety and Health Administration, and continued to dominate public concern three decades later.

In this environment of restrictions, amidst strong business antipathy to public health regulatory programmes, Ronald Reagan swept into the presidency in 1980. His two terms in that office were marked by the dismantling of public health's regulatory powers. Within eight years the Reagan administration had so thoroughly defeated its regulatory adversaries that public health was forced into defeat, even on issues of bona fide community health threats, its most outspoken voices of environmental concern sidelined along the margins of academia and political activism.

As the twenty-first century approached, the combined impact of mounting numbers of uninsured Americans, slashed public health budgets, and widespread antigovernment sentiment could be felt in the rundown county health offices, clogged public hospital emergency rooms, and mounting squabbles over which diseases were most deserving of federal research dollars.

Public health became increasingly political, forcing its advocates to defend not only their policies but also the role of government itself. To be fair, public health had always been a very political pursuit: its budgets were politically controlled, and implementation of public health principles invariably came up against one interest or another. But now public health in much of the richest country in the world was fighting for its life.

Medicine, too, was struggling. In 1999 the always conservative American Medical Association voted to support unionization of doctors—a move so radically different from the organization's historic stances as to prompt jaw-dropping gasps from the health industry. The AMA's vote reflected rising anxiety among doctors in the United States, who feared their profession was losing not only income but also dignity, power, and respect. American physicians were not, at the close of the twentieth century, a happy lot. Physician dissatisfaction was topped only by the angst among American nurses, and by health consumers.

In response to this collective anxiety, optimists within the health-care industry referred to the turn of the century as a transition period that, like so many times of change, might be a bit rocky before the envisioned Nirvana was reached. But the future, they insisted, would usher in a glorious age of New Medicine, drawing from the tools of New Biology. Just as antibiotics had vanquished the bacterial scourges that had plagued humanity for centuries, so New Biology would conquer the chronic killers—cancer and heart disease—as well as mental disorders and addictions.

Would cancer still be a major killer of Americans in the twenty-first century? Probably not, forecast the director of the National Cancer Institute, Dr Richard Klausner, because Science was entering an era of 'dramatic, unimaginable change' in which cancerous cells, and even cancerous genes, would be spotted and controlled or eliminated long before tumours even developed.

'I think that's the scenario,' a clearly excited Klausner exclaimed. Revolutionary breakthroughs made in biology over the previous twenty years opened up the possibility of developing an actual strategic plan for elimination of cancer in the United States, Klausner said, and 'we've decided on a path and we're already heading down it.'

For heart disease, too, a light shone brightly at the end of a new treatment tunnel, predicted pharmaceutical industry insider Randall Tobias, and the millennium offered 'truly miraculous possibilities' that would, he insisted, include 'an end to surgery.'

An end to open-heart surgery and invasive oncology? Had the former CEO of Eli Lilly pharmaceutical company turned into a hopeless optimist? No, insisted Tobias, because 'in the not-so-distant future ... the life sciences will have accomplished the biological equivalent of putting a man on the moon.'

At the root of Klausner's and Tobias's grand optimism were three key areas of basic science innovation: human genetics, protein chemistry, and nanotechnology. The Human Genome Project was racing to the finish line, having nearly completed the delineation of the entire code contained within the DNA of all twenty-three human chromosomes. Hundreds of private and public laboratories were hard at work deciphering the newly discovered code sequences, working out what genes actually coded for, how to turn them on and off, and what sorts of mutations led to particular diseases.

The Holy Grail of medicine (and, by inference, public health) in the next millennium was prevention of chronic diseases—cancer, strokes, Alzheimer's, schizophrenia, diabetes, and hundreds of others—through intervention either at the genetic or protein levels. Since all life functions and malfunctions usually boiled down to protein interactions, 'nothing is too *Star Trek*kie' Klausner insisted.

For example, cancer cells usually bore proteins on their surfaces that were different from those found on normal cells, and resulted from expression of certain genes. In the future, scientists planned to inject microscopic detectors into outwardly healthy people, and these nanoprobes would 'seek out cancers. It's absolutely possible.' Klausner continued, 'We're working on it with NASA. It's really exciting. If we can think of stellar probes where the signal-to-noise ratio is much, much greater, we're going to be able to find a cancer cell in the human body.'

And the next step, Klausner predicted, was 'why not arm those little molecular machines? Send them into the body to seek and destroy cancer cells. So I can actually envision treating cancer before it happens,' long before anybody has tumours, when cellular change is still in the 'precancerous pseudodiseases' phase, as Klausner put it. And that, in Klausner's vision, constituted high-tech public health, focusing prevention not on the carcinogenic environment and diets of the community, but on the appearance of aberrant cells in individuals. It moved the very concept of public health from outside of the human body deeply inward.

Similarly, a number of genetic factors appeared to play roles in the build-up of cholesterol and other physical sources of vulnerability to heart disease and stroke. By 1998 researchers had already manipulated the cells and DNA of mice to make them skinnier versus fat, smart versus Alzheimer's-like, and cancer-free for a variety of malignancies. There were genetically manipulated mice that had human immune systems, were drug addicts (or not), and suffered a range of human diseases. Cloned cells could grow into tissues, perhaps in the future into whole replacement parts. Need a new heart? Clone it. Or better yet, inject seed cells into the damaged heart to grow replacement tissue and strengthen the organ.

As the secret code of human DNA was deciphered the next step was translation. Having the alphabet soup was one thing: knowing what signals and proteins it encoded was quite another. There were two basic ways to get at that mystery: through the front door or the back. Using massive high-speed computers 'front door' analysts took random sequences of DNA and scanned all available protein databases in search of matches. Once a match was found, the position of that particular protein's DNA code within human chromosomes might reveal something about how production of that compound was regulated—switched on or off. And neighbouring DNA sequences might contain other vital proteins that carried out related functions in the human body.

The back door approach started with cells and vital hormones, receptors or activators (such as chemokines or neurotransmitters). Scientists used superpowerful magnets or X-rays to tease out the three-dimensional structures of these vital proteins and manipulated those shapes to guess the nature of a compound that normally fitted into the bends, folds, and pockets of the targeted protein. Those clues would lead to construction of chemicals designed to block or stimulate crucial proteins in the body. In such a way, it might be possible to switch on or off hormones, enhance vitamin effectiveness, block addiction-triggering nerve cell receptors in the brain, or turn off cancer-promoting chemicals.

'In thirty to fifty years we'll have it *all* done,' predicted Nobel laureate Dr David Baltimore, president of Caltech. 'And we will have the value of that research in terms of drugs in a continual pipeline of discovery. Chemistry is the key to all of this—computorial and structural chemistry is just so powerful. . . . The number of protein structures we'll get a year will be measured in the thousands.'

The twentieth century began with a revolution sparked by the microscope, which opened humanity's eyes upon the world of gyrating, fiercely active germs. The Germ Theory was the engine that drove biology for half a century of published health discovery and triumph. With the 1953 discovery of DNA and, perhaps more critically, the early 1970s inventions of genetic engineering techniques, biology entered the Genome Era.

As the new century dawned, the Genome Era was passing its baton to the Age of Proteomics, promising an upheaval in pharmacology and medicine that proponents argued would be every bit as dramatic as had been Pasteur's and Koch's discovery of microbes, Fleming's finding penicillin, and Salk's and Sabin's polio vaccines. Surgeons would be on the unemployment lines, along with psychologists and drug rehabilitation workers. Doctors of the twenty-first century would practice an elegant new protein-based preventative medicine.

A sort of 'public health, if you will'. That's what industry leader Tobias called it: public health. And Glaxo Wellcome's Vice President Dr Allen Roses agreed.

'People are going to come in to their doctors with computerized medical records, genetic blueprints, embedded on small plastic strips, like credit cards,' Roses predicted. Those cards would represent a new marriage of sorts, between public health and medicine. Each card would carry the individual's entire genetic blueprint, and 'medicine will shift to true family medicine, based on a family's genes'.

In the twenty-first century, predicted the National Institutes of Health's Mark Boguski, physicians' textbooks 'will be our genes'.

But long before such fantasies could be fulfilled a few serious, sobering public health realities needed to be faced. The paramount one for the United States was a question of race and, perhaps, class. African-Americans consistently since the Civil War had lagged at least a decade behind whites of all economic brackets in achievement of such public health milestones as life expectancy, infant and maternal mortalities, and adult premature deaths. It was not that they had been more likely to become ill—although in some cases that was the case. Rather, they were more apt to die of their illnesses. And there was little evidence, US Surgeon General David Satcher argued, that African-Americans' DNA was to blame. Rather, a complex set of social and behavioural factors, combined with a lack of access to care on a par with that provided for whites, were the roots of the chasm that separated black and white health.

Similar disparities in health existed between whites and Asian-Americans on the one side, versus African-Americans, Native Americans, and Hispanics on the other, insisted Dr Phil Lee, former undersecretary of the US Department of Health and Human Services.

'For example, American Indians who come into contact with a different culture—what's the impact? Diabetes,' Lee said. 'That's not because their genes changed. Their diet changed. And the answer isn't to change their genes—it's change the lifestyle.'

Nobody could argue with the desirability of discovering means—genomic or otherwise—of intervening to prevent dreadful disabilities and chronic disease, even death. But would such high-technology approaches as genomic and proteomic drugs get at the core of global public health? If Russia's drinking water was still heavily contaminated in 2020 would proteomic nanoprobes constitute wise public health interventions? At the core of the biotechnology industry's use of the term 'public health' in reference to their genomic innovations was the word *prevention*. Public health leaders, unable to reach a consensus on the definition of their field during the 1990s, were ill-prepared at the millennium to debate New Biology's usurpation of their nomenclature. Was prevention, on an *individual* basis, equivalent to public health?

There was certainly plenty of money invested in genomic medicine, both by wealthy nations' governments and by the pharmaceutical industry. Even 'small' biotechnology companies were spending more than $1 billion in research and development of genomic and proteomic products by 2000. For the larger pharmaceutical giants billions of dollars spent on research and development in the genomic arena was a routine annual expenditure.

The excitement was at fever pitch in the industry. Investors commonly claimed that biotechnology would be in 2010 what cyberspace, the Internet, and computers were for the 1990s. The global economy, they argued, would go from the silicon age to the DNA era. Former Eli Lilly Chief Executive Tobias grinned as he pronounced, 'Something truly amazing is happening in medicine.'

In anticipation of these radical changes mammoth chemical, drug, and foods companies merged or formed partnerships during the 1990s, creating behemoth companies that controlled chemical, drug, and food manufacture on scales exceeding $100 billion. For example, two New Jersey corporations—Warner-Lambert and American Home Products—prepared to merge in late 1999. In the previous year each had revenues exceeding $10 billion and combined market capital of $150 billion. United, the companies were huge pharmaceutical and veterinary product manufacturers, controlled numerous vaccine and biotechnology spin-off companies, and manufactured some of the biggest-selling over-the-counter drug and hygiene products in the United States.

In the mid-1990s, the US Congress changed laws that previously regulated the boundaries among medicine, food, and dietary supplements. The lines were so blurred by the close of the decade that more Americans were already taking 'preventive medicine' in the forms of vitamin pills and modified foods than were taking prescribed prophylactic drugs. Between 1990 and 2000 the dietary supplement market for everything from orange juice enhanced with echinacea, vitamin C, and zinc to vitamin D plus calcium-enriched milks soared from $3.3 billion in the United States to more than $14 billion. In an odd state of affairs, companies could almost without regulation add a long list of physiologically active chemicals to foods but would be required to undergo extensive FDA approval tests in order to be permitted to sell the same blend of chemicals in pill form.

'For the first time in the 1990s you got a food product where you say, "If you eat this you live longer," and that's fibre for your heart,' Harvard University's Juan Enriquez explained. 'We're beginning to understand the biochemistry of foods. It's not that you're going to pay $20 000 for surgery at the end of your life. In the future you'll pay $20 000 for nutraceuticals over twenty years.'

Long life wasn't, of itself, the goal of residents of the wealthy world: they wanted those many decades to find them sexually adept, slim, in possession of a full head of hair, and, overall, youthful. In the early sixteenth century Juan Ponce de Léon risked a fortune and the lives of himself and a crew of men to sail from Spain to Florida in search of an elixir of youth. Youth-seekers of the twenty-first century will travel inwards, to their genes, in pursuit of elusive immortality. As the global population aged, so did collective vanity. No price—or profit margin—seemed too high to preserve the vanities of youth. Thus by the late 1990s the biggest-selling drugs were those that promised the individual a cheery personality (e.g. Prozac), plenty of hair on their head (e.g. Propecia), and staying power during sexual intercourse (Viagra). Each of these drugs when released proved wildly popular, were sold at enormous profit margins (Viagra at a 98 per cent annual profit), and pushed up stock market values for the relevant manufacturers. Indeed, the same Baby Boomers of the West who were the targets of these so-called lifestyle drugs were also betting their pensions and retirement years on stocks and mutual funds, with pharmaceutical companies ranking among the most popular in which to bank their futures.

In 1998 the pharmaceutical industry earned $99.5 billion in profits in the United States, alone: an 11 per cent increase over 1997. In 1999 drug sales profits rose another 16.6 per cent. Spending on pharmaceutical drugs nearly doubled in the United States between 1993 and 1998, rising from $50.6 billion in 1993 to $93.4 billion in 1998.

Global sales were also up, rising 7 per cent in just a single year (1997 to 1998) and making pharmaceuticals the fastest-growing and highest-profit legitimate industry in the world.

Soaring gross sales mirrored astounding net profit growths industrywide as well. During a time in 1997 to 2000 when typical successful corporations had annual profit growths of 4 to 7 per cent the average pharmaceutical company's profits grew by 14 to 18 per cent annually, and such expansion was expected to continue, if not quicken in pace, after 2000.

The result was fantastic price increases for medicines, making pharmaceuticals the new engine of health-care inflation at the dawn of the twenty-first century. Just a decade earlier it had been hospitals that drove inflation: by 1999 the real question facing policy makers was no longer whether insurance companies, governments, and individuals could afford the costs of hospital stays, but whether they would be able to afford to buy the drugs intended to prevent these hospitalizations. Drug companies not only increased the average price tags of newly released drugs, claiming such high costs were necessary to reimburse their research and development investments, but also boosted prices on older and generic drugs. And they were getting away with it, charging as much as $15 *per pill* for some medications.

Consumers searched frantically for sources of cheaper drugs, often bypassing doctors and pharmacies in favour of purchasing off the Internet or their local black market. The result was a deterioration of physician control, a rise in side-effects and drug-associated deaths, and a potential public health calamity due to antimicrobial self-medication and consequent promotion of drug resistance.

The drug industry responded to rising criticism of its high profits and prices by say-ing, as Enriquez had put it, that the future would witness *not* a net increase in health costs, but a shifting of those costs from hospital stays and treatments to preventive medications. And this would shift expenditures from the late-twentieth-century norm of predominantly the last decade of an individual's life to a trend more evenly distributed throughout life.

At Boston University attorney and ethicist George Annas found any notion of such cost shifting 'hilarious' noting that 'the major ethical pitfall is going to be how are we going to pay for this? What's the point? They say all expense will be at the front end— that's ridiculous! There's no way to get rid of the back end,' Annas insisted. 'Short of suicide or euthanasia there's no way to get rid of those last years of really compromised life.'

Everybody will die someday, of something. And few, Annas argued, were fortunate enough to feel terrific for decades and then one day simply fall down dead. Most people—even in the brave new world of genomic medicine—would slowly deteriorate and suffer an eventual degeneration and costly time in hospital.

Boguski of the National Institutes of Health said that in the future every single far-out idea was possible, and the only limits 'were social and economic'.

Most difficult was the world outside the United States. Assuming, for example, that the great breakthroughs forecast for mental illness were realized for the 400 to 500 million residents of North America and Western Europe, what would be available to the six to seven billion other human beings on planet Earth? Christopher Murray, from the World Health Organization, calculated that by 2020 depression would jump ten notches to rank as the second-most common debilitating illness in the world, driven by an ageing and increasingly frustrated human population.

While Americans in the 1990s obsessed over their neuroses and flights of blues the United States ranked comparatively low on the depression scale, with just 5 per cent of the population at some time in their lives being so diagnosed. And there were already medicines available that dramatically improved the lives of depressed Americans. The annual bill for treatment of depression and lost national productivity due to time away from work or suicide exceeded $44 billion.

But in France a staggering 16.4 per cent of the population was clinically depressed at some point in their lives, 19 per cent in Lebanon. And in many countries, notably China and India, millions suffered undiagnosed depressions that WHO's Murray predicted would draw both attention and demand for treatment by 2020. But how could countries such as Lebanon, China, and India afford to spend their equivalents of $44 billion a year on the disease? And assuming the predicted fruits of New Biology appeared in the coming decades, would they be affordable for mental patients in Brazil, Egypt, South Africa, and Thailand?

Even in the wealthy world the burden of depression hit hardest among the poor—precisely those least likely to be able to afford mood elevators and antidepressants. For the most part, it wasn't rich depressed or psychotic Americans who wandered the streets of New York City, homeless and babbling to unseen voices. If the poor of America couldn't afford access to the innovations of psychiatric medicine, certainly the even poorer populaces of the rest of the world could not.

Drug research and development was moving at a feverish pace at the close of the twentieth century. In the United States alone, the drug industry spent $17 billion on research and development in 1998, and some of the National Institutes of Health's $13.6 billion budget went toward pursuit of new medicines. Between 1975 and 1996 nearly 1240 new drugs were licensed—a very promising figure.

Except that of those 1240 drugs only 379 were for therapeutic interventions—for treatment of disease states. And just thirteen were for diseases that were the world's leading killers, primarily afflicting residents of tropical and poor countries. Dr Patrice Trouiller of the Centre Hospitalier Universitaire de Grenoble, argued that 'pharmaceutical firms operate like any private industry, they have no specific social welfare mission and respond to economic rather than social or human imperatives. All things considered, drug development for tropical diseases may not have a promising future in the current context. The profit-driven system is not responding to tropical medicine needs.'

It was a position with which Dr Harvey Bale Jr, head of the International Federation of Pharmaceutical Manufacturers, had little disagreement. He asserted that there was no marketplace to speak of in the poor world. And where any glimmerings of a market—purchasing power—existed, the World Trade Organization's Trade-Related Aspects of Intellectual Property Rights, or TRIPS, was routinely violated by local patent-busting drug companies. Only strong patent protections, coupled with improved local purchasing powers, could serve as true incentives for research, development, and distribution of drugs aimed at the health needs of the developing world, he argued.

Trevor Jones, director of the Association of the British Pharmaceutical Industry, insisted that it cost, on average, $500 million to research and develop a new drug, and a drug company expected to earn back that investment within the first three to five years of sales, thereafter making a profit. Estimates of drug research and development costs per licensed product varied wildly, from that $500 million figure to an incredibly low figure of $16 million. Regardless of how much a company invested in research and development of a new drug, Jones insisted, the manufacturer and its stockholders had a right to expect a full return on that investment within three to five years. Bale and Jones neatly sidestepped the question of how much pharmaceutical research was actually funded by American and European taxpayers, both through government support of basic science and tax exemptions granted to the drug industry. When such subsidies were incorporated into the R&D equation industry claims of justifiable profit margins withered. Even more challenging to the industry's economic calculus was mounting evidence that drugs were deliberately marketed in the US at prices significantly higher than those demanded of medical consumers in Europe and Canada. By 2000 American taxpayers and politicians were questioning why, if the US paid the lion's share of tax-supported global medical research, should its consumers also be paying the most exorbitant prices for the fruits of that scientific mission.

But the drug access problem extended well beyond new products just emerging out of the R and D pipeline. Some 150 nations had drawn up essential drugs lists, naming products considered to constitute their minimum pharmacological needs. About 90 per cent of the drugs on such lists were no longer covered by TRIPS or any form of patent protection—and the original manufacturers had long since earned back their R and D investments. Nevertheless, these drugs remained unobtainable in much of the world because of global distribution problems, local corruption that funnelled such purchases directly to black markets, and still-high costs. The lowest-priced drugs were often unavailable, as no manufacturer found reason to continue producing such things as the valuable antibiotic streptomycin to combat tuberculosis; five drugs used against African sleeping sickness; aminosidine for the parasitic disease leishmaniasis; uninterrupted supplies of cheap insulin for diabetes treatment; even the great post–World War II public health innovation, the polio vaccine.

The push for record-breaking profits 'leaves you focused on 300 to 400 million people in rich countries. But on a human rights level, of course, this is unacceptable,' Dr Bernard Pécoul of the Nobel Prize-winning Médecins Sans Frontières insisted.

'Our role is to organize a fight against this effort to reduce the pharmaceutical market to a very small population. We cannot accept . . . that for most of the world the essential drugs list is things from the 1950s and 1960s, many of which cause drug resistance.'

Among the many examples cited by Pécoul and his Médecins Sans Frontières colleagues was the deadly diarrhoeal disease shigellosis, which claimed hundreds of lives in Rwanda following that country's 1994 civil war. The *Shigella* bacteria developed resistance to all but one drug, ciprofloxacin, which cost more than Médecins Sans Frontières or other humanitarian organizations could afford. Médecins Sans Frontières negotiated a price break with the manufacturer, Bayer, ultimately saving thousands of lives. But Bayer's willingness to cut costs in order to stop an African epidemic was not, Pécoul insisted, typical. More commonly people simply died for lack of affordable medicine.

Further exacerbating the problem was poor, even fraudulent local production of drugs, usually in violation of TRIPS international patent laws. In some cases locally produced products were as good as the patented American-made ones, and simply cost local consumers 50 to 90 per cent less. But in all too many cases, Pécoul said, the results were substandard, even dangerous. The most egregious example cited in their study occurred in Nigeria during a massive West African meningitis epidemic in 1996 to 1998. A Nigerian company counterfeited vaccine labels for Pasteur Merieux and SmithKline Beecham products and sold sixty thousand doses of nothing but contaminated water. Injected into sixty thousand Nigerians, the dummy vaccines constituted a public health catastrophe that perpetuated the country's epidemic and cost thousands of lives, Pécoul charged.

What was to be done? The Médecins Sans Frontières group offered a list of recommendations, beginning with changes in global treaties that protected patents and pharmaceutical trade and allowing 'realistic pricing of potential drugs' sold in developing countries in exchange for local patent enforcement.

The group also called for a far more activist role in these issues on the part of the World Health Organization. And insisted that strong financial incentives would be needed to propel the otherwise dismal state of research and development on tropical diseases. The Médecins Sans Frontières group concluded that access to life-saving medicine was a human right.

When the World Trade Organization met in Seattle in November 1999 riots broke out, pitting an array of protestors from around the world against the gathering political and corporate leaders. Among the dissidents were public health advocates enraged over pharmaceutical pricing and health-care access inequities. Five weeks later President Bill Clinton addressed the elite Trade Forum in Davos, Switzerland, promising tax benefits to pharmaceutical companies that manufactured drugs for poor countries, and calling for reduced pricing on essential drugs. And when the World Bank convened its annual meeting in Washington, DC, in April 2000, protestors again rioted, many of them denouncing pharmaceutical pricing and inequity. Inside the Bank meeting, as well, the gross disparities between life-and-death drug needs versus availability for most of the world's population were the subjects of lengthy, often heated, discussion.

Although the drug companies applauded Clinton's promised tax breaks, they were loath to accept any responsibility for lack of equitable medication access worldwide.

Glaxo's Roses said that 'it's not the drug companies that are inhibiting getting the right drugs to the right patients. For a fraction of the cost of peacekeeping in those countries we could get people all the drugs they need.'

Consider, Tobias and Roses said, the example of antibiotics. These drugs were widely available and sold in every country in the world, yet the infectious diseases they targeted remained rampant. That was not because of the costs of drugs, they argued, but due to lack of proper health delivery infrastructures: doctors, nurses, hospitals, and clinics.

Not so, countered Pécoul. He argued that drug-resistant microbes were appearing in the wealthy world, where the problem was usually handled by simply switching to secondary or tertiary newer drugs—all of which were more expensive, in some cases more than ten times costlier. And at the bottom end of the market drug companies had stopped making such stalwarts of infectious diseases control as penicillin, streptomycin, and chloroquine. Thus, the world's poor faced a squeeze play in which their old drugs were no longer available, the midpriced 1960s and 1970s drugs were losing effectiveness due to drug resistance, and the super new drugs were completely unaffordable.

At stake, Pécoul insisted, was 'a time bomb' that would explode not just in the world's poorest countries, but in Europe and America as well. A time bomb of resurging infectious diseases, most of which would acquire phenomenal drug resistance capacities due to improper use and insufficient availability of antimicrobial agents.

A University of California, San Francisco, forecast predicted that by 2070 the world would have exhausted all antimicrobial drug options, as the viruses, bacteria, parasites, and fungi would have evolved complete resistance to the human pharmaceutical arsenal. That apocalyptic nightmare was, remarkably, shared by many of the world's top microbiologists and infectious diseases experts.

Although several laboratories are working on new ways to kill bacteria and viruses, most do not anticipate that fundamentally new approaches will emerge within the next ten years. Even if such drugs did eventually reach the marketplace, they would undoubtedly follow the financial pattern set with antibiotics: each newer drug costing far more than its predecessor. And the newer agents are usually more toxic, fraught with fiercer side-effects.

'The biggest concern is staphylococcus, where only one drug is left,' Stanford's Stanley Falknow said, referring to vancomycin. 'If that were incurable it would be devastating.'

Dr Anthony Fauci, director of the US National Institute of Allergy and Infectious Diseases, warned that mutated microbes, resistant to hosts of drugs, were the real crisis looming for the twenty-first century. 'There is more of a chance of a virulent influenza A wiping out whole populations than you and I getting a gene card,' he declared, dismissing the genomic future vision.

Examples of such lurking microbial threats, and humanity's apparent impotence to deal with them, abounded at the millennium, the three most potentially catastrophic being HIV, malaria, and tuberculosis. Combined in 1998 the three microbes claimed five million lives, according to the World Health Organization.

By the close of 1999 HIV was a lightning rod for protest against pharmaceutical companies, TRIPS, and global inequities in public health. The forecast for the future of the global pandemic was very grim. Already, according to the UNAIDS Programme, the virus's impact on Africa was 'catastrophic, and the scenario will only worsen unless global leaders work together to invest more—much more—in prevention efforts and programmes to address the multitude of social and economic problems that AIDS has wrought.'

Experts pictured nations obliterated by the world's newest plague, held out little (if any) hope of a cure for the viral disease, and differed significantly at the end of the century only on one point: how many more decades would pass before an effective, affordable HIV vaccine could be used worldwide.

The National Institutes of Health reached the conclusion that an HIV vaccine was the only thing that could slow the virus's seemingly relentless expansion around the world. By 1999 half of the agency's $1.5 billion HIV budget was aimed directly, or indirectly, at the search for a vaccine, offered Office of AIDS Research director Neal Nathanson. 'We're in it for the long haul,' he said with a sigh. But he argued that the private sector lacked similar long-term commitment to the vaccine problem, and 'none of the big players are seriously involved in developing a vaccine because they don't see the profit in it.'

When AIDS first surfaced in 1981 the global response was a medical, not public health, one: resources were skewed to the search for a cure. Fifteen years later Science offered up HAART, or highly active antiretroviral therapy. But in the long run HAART clearly was not the answer. Its price tag—$10 000 to $60 000 a year for the drugs alone—rendered HAART unusable for more than 90 per cent of the world's HIV population, estimated in 1999 by the United Nations AIDS Programme to number forty million people.

And in North America and Western Europe, where hundreds of thousands of people were on HAART in 1999, trouble was brewing. Many patients—about 50 per cent, depending on which studies were cited—had failed their initial rounds of HAART either because they could not tolerate the drugs' toxic side-effects or they had difficulty adhering to the rigorous daily schedules of medicine ingestion that HAART necessitated.

With the bloom clearly off the HAART rose AIDS advocates were calling for rapid development of drugs that hit new targets on HIV, possibly outwitting the virus's frightening mutation capacities. But Merck's vice president, Emilio Emini, said that there wasn't much in the drug development pipeline and it was 'impossible to answer' when such new agents might be ready: 'It's the temporal zone of chaos.'

'Where will we be in ten, twenty years?' Dr Peter Piot, Director of UNAIDS, asked. 'It's really, really hard to say. We haven't done [forecasts] going out more than to 2005. We've learned that projections turn out to be awfully wrong.'

Wrong, in that the epidemic had consistently outpaced worst case scenarios, particularly in Africa and Asia.

The key question for forecasters was the proverbial bell-shaped curve. Most, if not all, epidemics started at a low level, rose rapidly claiming large numbers of human victims, and then naturally slid back down the bell-shaped curve, ending up permanently at a modest, endemic level in the population. The reasons for that downward curve were multitudinous, and they varied from epidemic to epidemic. But the curve was always there.

Was there evidence of a bell-shaped curve for HIV, or would the epidemic continue to claim even more lives, ascending its death toll year after year well into the twenty-first century?

Piot believed that by 2005 HIV might hit the top of its bell in some hard-hit African countries, such as Uganda, Tanzania, Zambia, and Zimbabwe. But what a bell it was! The peak was only reached when upwards of a third of all adults under fifty years of age were infected in most parts of those societies, meaning a third of each generation would perish.

'What you have is a kind of modern conflagration. It's the modern equivalent of the great Plague,' said Larry Gostin, professor of law at Georgetown and expert on AIDS human rights. 'And that's what you're going to get in all of the developing world. It's going to be losses of whole generations. We're on the verge of the twenty-first century with all this modern technology and yet we're as vulnerable to pathogens as we were decades ago.'

'The critical difference,' Gostin continued, 'is that at those times we as a world community sat by and cried because we couldn't do anything. And now we stand by and watch, expressionless, because we choose not to do anything. And that's a clear measure of how far we as a species have moved, from compassion to disinterest, or self-interest.'

Piot said that reaching what appeared to be the top of the bell in some African societies had meant national bankruptcy, 'pushing households into poverty and starvation, people ending up on the streets. And then we'll be giving food aid, instead of investing in [HIV] prevention.'

The first community to reach an HIV bell curve was San Francisco's gay population, where the bell peaked in the mid-1980s when the infection rate exceeded 50 per cent. Since that time, due largely to the gay community's own education campaigns, the HIV rate has declined steadily, yet it still claimed a terrible 20 per cent of the remaining San Francisco gay population in 1998.

For more than a decade retired epidemiologist Jim Chin executed HIV forecasts for the World Health Organization and UNAIDS. He believed that 'there will continue to be from twenty-five to thirty million persons with HIV alive each year for the next twenty-five years, and hopefully by then (or before) the African countries can get their act together and begin to significantly reduce their annual incidence of new infections so that from twenty-five to fifty years from now, when my grandchildren become parents and then grandparents, the global prevalence of HIV infections will begin to drop to about ten to twenty million.'

Grim as that situation was, Chin conceded that India, with a population of one billion people, was the 'wild card' that could throw off all his forecasts. It was one thing for Botswana, for example, with a population of 1.4 million people, to have a 32 per cent infection rate among its young adults, or about 200 000 HIV cases. It was quite another for 32 per cent of all young adult Indians, or about 200 *million* people, to be infected. Piot said that Asia, particularly China and India, where two out of every five human beings lived, was the key to the future of the planet's HIV bell curve.

A 1998 joint publication of the World Health Organization, Harvard School of Public Health, and the World Bank entitled, 'Health Dimensions of Sex and Repro-duction,' sought to forecast HIV bell curves region by region for the world. The team predicted that much of Africa wouldn't see its HIV epidemic peak until 2005 to 2010. Asia's epidemics, they said, wouldn't peak until a decade later.

If true—and if an adult infection rate of more than 30 per cent was fated to con-stitute societies' HIV bell peak, by 2020 the world could have nearly half a billion people living with HIV and AIDS.

Some studies suggested the elusive bell curve might be unimaginably high. A US national security analysis of African armed forces found 1999 prevalence rates among soldiers ran as high as 60 per cent—a staggering figure unmatched by any other infec-tious disease of the twentieth century except, perhaps, the 1918 swine influenza. Well surpassing any flu toll were HIV levels seen in the South African armed forces— infection rates as high as 90 per cent, according to a March 2000 United Nations survey.

Given such a dire backdrop it came as no surprise that the arrival of HAART for wealthy countries sparked rage in poor, HIV-plagued nations. They could not afford the drugs, even when pharmaceutical companies reduced the prices. And various donor schemes for providing HIV drugs to poor nations, particularly in Africa, floun-dered on the rocky shores of long-neglected public health. If, after all, doctors in the United States were finding it extremely difficult to administer HAART to patients without prompting hard-to-treat side-effects and drug resistance, how could impov-erished clinics such as Kikwit's General Hospital do the job? The HAART dilemma proved the cases of both Pécoul and Roses: for poor countries the wrong sorts of drugs had been developed; and even free drugs could not be used properly in countries lack-ing viable public health infrastructures.

In most of the world the only viable solutions to HIV in the long run were a safe, 100 per cent effective vaccine; a cheap pill that in one or a very few doses completely elim-inated infection; or a vaginal and rectal microbicide that was very cheap (less than 10 cents per use), non-toxic, and highly effective in blocking HIV sexual transmission. In 2000 none of these solutions were at hand. And, more importantly, none were in the research and development pipelines of large pharmaceutical companies, mainly because of a lack of perceived future profitability.

The HAART model opened a set of profitable doors for the pharmaceutical indus-try. First, it allowed an acute infection to be treated as a chronic disease, dragging out treatment (and drug sales) for decades. Second, it escalated the level of socially accept-able public health disparity in the world, finding the companies and wealthy world governments facing remarkably little criticism for sparing the lives of European and North American citizens while witnessing obliteration of populations elsewhere.

Third, the treatment was based on a class of drugs, called protease inhibitors, that were very costly and difficult to produce; patent violation was minimized by the sheer scale of production obstacles. And fourth, even an extraordinarily expensive set of drugs could prove profitable within targeted wealthy nations if the sense of urgency was high enough to commit governments to their subsidized purchase. That Brazil, a developing country, committed to purchasing HAART drugs and dispensing them for free to its entire HIV population testified to the scale of acceptable pricing in a perceived national crisis.

Finally—most importantly—the HIV/HAART model showed that a public health problem could be 'acceptably' brought under medical control: even public health authorities bowed before the HAART model though, in truth, it offered more obstacles than solutions for HIV prevention and control.

Malaria had been controllable since chloroquine had been invented. As the parasites acquired drug resistance new drugs were used. But resistance to those emerged, too. By the late 1990s some three thousand children were dying daily of malaria, 90 per cent of them in the same African countries that were struggling against HIV. The parasites had acquired tremendous powers of drug resistance, rendering prophylactic therapy useless in much of the tropical world and treatment perilous. And global climate change brought warming trends that made higher elevation regions of Africa, Asia, and Latin America newly hospitable to malaria-carrying mosquitoes.

In 1998 the World Health Organization launched the Roll Back Malaria campaign, working with UNICEF and the World Bank to find incentives for development of new anti-malarial drugs. Though there were promising potential drugs in the research pipeline, no pharmaceutical company in 1999 had an internal malaria research programme.

Tuberculosis offered the most startling case of the failure of the medical model of public health. The catastrophic TB epidemic of Russia and neighbouring formerly Soviet nations was out of control by 2000, despite considerable efforts to rein it in through the use of antibiotics. In 1997 and 1998 the World Health Organization stuck to its DOTS mantra, repeating over and over again that the region's governments should adopt the directly observed short course therapy approach to TB control.

But it didn't work.

Drug-resistant TB swept over the Russian region, even in areas where authorities obediently followed WHO's protocols.

Far away in the Andes Mountains of Peru Dr Paul Farmer and his colleagues were working with residents of Carabayallo, the poorest neighbourhood of Lima. They discovered in 1997 that many of these Peruvians were suffering from tuberculosis, despite having received DOTS at local clinics. The Harvard group collected sputum samples from the TB patients and submitted them for analysis at a Massachusetts laboratory. In an urgent 1997 letter to colleagues and financial backers, Farmer and his partners described the situation:

A number of these patients we have identified have been found to have strains with resistance patterns more alarming than those documented in any other setting. None of these patients has been receiving appropriate treatment, since the medications necessary to cure their resistant disease are not available through the public health programme. This restrictive policy is in sharp contrast to the provision of free 'first-line' medicines for patients with the more usual, drug-susceptible strain of TB.

It became evident to us that these impoverished patients were neglected and at about the same time infecting a large number of individuals, including family members, co-workers, neighbours, and even casual contacts. Through in-depth interviews with these patients, we have been able to identify the processes by which poor Peruvians become sick with drug-resistant TB: inequalities in access to effective treatment are producing a vicious cycle which permits the emergence and transmission of this deadly disease.[4]

Farmer and other DOTS critics were increasingly uneasy. They argued that by 1999 multidrug-resistant strains of TB had emerged in more than one hundred countries, as the microbes stubbornly defied WHO's prescribed treatment. Further, most developing countries lacked a public health infrastructure that could effectively distribute the WHO-recommended drugs, especially to their poorest citizens.

In 1998 the World Health Organization brought together top pharmaceutical leaders, hoping to gain their support for the development of some form of pill that, taken alone, would have the impact of the complicated schedule of multiple drugs that formed the basis of DOTS. If a sufficiently inexpensive formulation could be found, combining several drugs that were then made by competing companies, TB control would be far easier. But the meeting was a disappointment. The companies told WHO that their targets were $1 billion 'big hitters' in the United States, not drugs that might sell for pennies in poor countries. There was no TB drug in the research pipelines of any large pharmaceutical or biotechnology company, anywhere in the world. The reason: no drug company was interested in pursuing *any* project that could realistically yield profits of less than $350 million a year, for five or more years. Even if all of the roughly estimated eight million TB sufferers worldwide went on the new superpill, each taking the medication for six months at an average total cost of eleven dollars per patient, the profit numbers simply wouldn't add up, the companies said.

Though WHO continued its optimistic DOTS chanting, its own dire reports forecast that 200 million people alive in 1998 would eventually develop tuberculosis, which far exceeded the total estimated number of worldwide tuberculosis cases that occurred over the course of the entire nineteenth century.

It was time to take stock: what was an appropriate strategy for TB control? Could catastrophe—globalization of completely drug-resistant, incurable tuberculosis—be averted without new drugs? Or an effective vaccine? In late 1999 the Centers for Disease Control and Prevention issued its recommendations, which boiled down to elimination of the one-size-fits-all WHO/DOTS approach, in favour of tailor-made strategies on a country-by-country basis. No strategy would work, the CDC warned, in the absence of a strong public health infrastructure. Thus, the US federal agency concluded, the only way residents of Los Angeles, Minneapolis, Paris, Tokyo, and London could truly be sure that their children wouldn't grow up in a world of threatening, incurable tuberculosis was by joining in a global commitment to basic public health.

The most condemning, most sobering report of all came from the auspices of billionaire George Soros in October 1999. Harvard's Farmer, the scientists in New York City's Public Health Research Institute, Soros's Open Society Institute, and researchers from all over the world collaborated on the massive report. They concluded that multidrug-resistant TB *already had spread around the world*, with strains having surfaced in at least one hundred nations. In horrifying detail the 258-page report documented failure after failure to control TB, and the enhancement of resistance as a result of inappropriate use of antibiotics. The worst examples were in Russia and the former Soviet Union nations, but the scientists documented terrifying death tolls due to antibiotic-resistant microbes all over the world.

'The best way to work toward elimination of TB is to provide effective treatment to all patients with active disease,' the report argued. 'Had DOTS been established before the emergence of resistance to antituberculosis drugs, DOTS alone might have been sufficient for TB control. But MDR-TB "hot-spots" have been identified on four continents, and the transmission of *M. tuberculosis* continues apace, as yet unchallenged by any coherent strategy.'

The report called for 'DOTS-Plus,' a strategic approach that involved use of still more drugs for longer periods of time, coupled with laboratory monitoring for resistance and strict supervision of patients to ensure compliance. It estimated a price tag of $1 billion a year to bring the global cataclysm under control. Soros had personally committed millions of dollars for such efforts in Russia, but far more was needed.

'If new money isn't made available immediately the epidemic may become virtually impossible to contain,' Farmer warned.

Malaria, tuberculosis, and the new scourges of hospitals (MRSA, VRE, VISA, and the like[5]) shared one critical feature: all had at some point been treatable or preventable with medicines that now were failing due to microbial evolution and inadequate public health. Would the list lengthen in coming years? Definitely, biologists warned. Would industry supply alternative drugs? Probably not—certainly not within an urgent time frame.

The drug companies were banking on vaccines. They said innovative products, such as vaccines made from the DNA of viruses or bacteria, would be available for tuberculosis, malaria, schistosomiasis, and other killers within twenty years. And, they promised, these vaccines would be affordable.

Affordable to societies such as those in sub-Saharan Africa, that spent less than ten dollars per citizen per year on all health-care needs?

'Here we are, one hundred years after Pasteur identified the cause of rabies and Koch the cause of tuberculosis,' former Health and Human Services Assistant Secretary Lee said. 'Yet we did more to control TB by social factors,' in Koch's day than through antibiotics a century later.

'Here we are,' Lee continued, 'one hundred years out and we still don't have a vaccine for tuberculosis or malaria.'

Meanwhile the opportunities for emergence and spread of such microbes will increase in coming years as the density, mobility, and relative poverty of the human population grows.

In the end, he argued, humanity was left with a disturbing, contradictory picture of the New Medicine. On the one hand, true miracles were ahead. On the other, a grim global social context challenged all optimism.

In Gostin's nightmarish vision of 2040, 'you'll have a population with virtual absence of disease and disability. And another overwhelmed by disease and disability.'

At the dawn of the twentieth century the Western world fused the ideas of civic duty and public health. Conquering disease was viewed as a collective enterprise for the common good.

'And now we end the century really rejecting the right of the health of societies in favour of the individual,' Gostin said sighing.

Where did we go wrong? Why had the sense of collective good disappeared? On a microscale, it seemed neighbours were less willing at the dawn of the twenty-first century to take minute risks or pay taxes on behalf of the health of the overall community. And on a macroscale, the wealthy world in 2000 seemed to be less willing than they had been during the days of colonialism a century earlier to come to the aid of African, South Asian, Eastern European, and Latin American populations. Why?

One obvious answer—perhaps *the* answer—was the very success of the medical approach to public health. Antibiotics, vaccines, antivirals, pesticides, antiparasitic drugs—these had been triumphs when first introduced. And they had worked, pushing the microbes into retreat and allowing whole societies to relieve themselves of the collective burden of plagues and childhood deaths. For societies that had full access to these boons—these genuine scientific miracles—it was possible for individuals to shift their thoughts from concern for the collective well-being to personal concerns about cancer, heart disease, diabetes, and countless other noncommunicable chronic ailments and killers.

It would be unfair to characterize such thinking as selfish. True, microbial death and disabilities continued to stalk the poor throughout the twentieth century, despite these great advances. But for those fortunate enough to grow up without such threats in their surroundings, pure practicality dictated a shift in focus. It is hard to fear that which doesn't visibly threaten when other worries and killers are lurking.

But the individual and medical approaches no longer made sense by the close of the twentieth century, amid global travel, international economic trade, rising drug resistance, and a widening wealth gap.

What did? In the late 1990s the World Health Organization was accused of having no strategy or sense of mission for global public health. It had for decades focused on provision of medicines—on the medical model of public health—leaving such basics as clean drinking water, decent primary health care, and safe, abundant foods up to local governments. And governments displayed a remarkable range in senses of responsibility for their populaces, from the Scandinavian cradle-to-grave all-inclusive health model down to the level of gross negligence, such as existed in Mobutu's Zaire.

In 1999 WHO Director-General Brundtland set out a new strategy for the global health organization, focused on those governments that seemed to shirk responsibility for their people. Under the scheme government and business leaders were presented evidence of the deleterious economic consequences of having a population that was in poor health. It was, in short, an appeal to the corrupt nature of such leaders, arguing that ignoring their people's public health needs would eventually hurt their financial balance sheets.

But as Lenin would no doubt have noted, this was not a strategy, but a tactic. And though it might constitute a clever approach toward raising concerns and dollars from the world's powerful, it did not supply a strategic plan for the expenditure of those resources.

More challenging was the task of forecasting, providing policy makers with a glimpse of humanity's medical future that might help make tough decisions about whether, for example, to build two new neonatal intensive care units, a few dozen rural clinics, or one large geriatrics centre with scarce government funds.

The amazing thing, Harvard public health expert Christopher Murray argued, was that no one really knew how many people in the world died or suffered from *any* disease or injury.

'If you go to WHO offices and ask, "How many young adults die of your respective diseases?" TB, or HIV, or cancer, whatever, the total when you add them all up exceeds the number of human beings who die annually by two- to three-fold,' Murray said.

About fifty million people died on earth every year in the late 1990s: only fourteen million deaths were ascribed to any cause in formal death certificates. An additional unknown number of people—probably a quarter of the world's six billion living human beings—suffered some form of illness, injury, or disability every year that was serious enough to warrant a day or more off from work or school. If the cause of humanity's deaths remained obscure, Murray said, its non-lethal illness burden was an utter black hole, largely because 'problems are brought to the attention of the world through the lenses of advocates. And despite everyone's best intentions you get distortion as a result. As much as possible we have to separate epidemiology assessment from advocacy.'

Diseases common to well-educated, well-heeled Westerners had their constituency groups that lobbied hard for medical research and treatment dollars. Key to that political effort was demonstration of need—and need equalled a death toll. So cancer advocacy groups, for example, rounded their numbers upwards to claim the maximum percentage of the world's annual death toll as theirs.

Lost in the numbers game was the most obvious fact: most deaths and illnesses in the world occurred among the poorest citizens of the planet, and their biggest killers simply didn't have powerful advocacy groups in Geneva, Washington, London, or Moscow. Malaria, tuberculosis, malnutrition—these were not ailments with formidable lobbies.

Murray headed a team of 150 scientists and physicians from throughout the world aimed at filling in the vast data gap and, as he put it, separate advocacy from epidemiology. The effort began under the direction of the World Bank in 1992 and had expanded to include the involvement of World Health Organization and the Harvard School of Public Health. By the time it was completed early in the twenty-first century ten volumes of information on the burden of human disease and several policy implication documents had been published.

And they were quite controversial. The World Health Organization's reports painted grim pictures of humanity's efforts to stave off infectious diseases such as HIV, tuberculosis, and malaria. They forecast a resurgence of old scourges, including those that were then vaccine-preventable.

The Harvard group's *Investing in Health*, in contrast, viewed the future as one rife with chronic disease, mental illness, cancer, and heart disease. By 2020, the report argued, microbes would be responsible for only 40 per cent of the burden of disease. Most illness and death would be due to cancer, heart disease, stroke, clinical depression, and car accidents.

As a result, the report stated, research and development spending should move towards the search for cheap ways to treat then-costly ailments such as myocardial infarction, breast cancer, acute depression, trauma, and stroke.

Murray's group concluded that the single biggest force pushing health priorities of the future was the ageing of the world's population. In Japan, Europe, and North America most of the population would by 2020 be over sixty-five years old.

Forecasting was a dangerous business, of course. Health planners in the United States had been absolutely certain in the late 1960s that more than 85 per cent of all deaths in America by the close of the century would be due to such chronic diseases as cancer and heart disease. In 1900 nearly 800 Americans out of every 100 000 died annually of infectious diseases. By 1980 that number was down to 36 per 100 000. That certainly seemed to bear out the forecasts. But then infectious diseases deaths started rising again in the United States, hitting 63 per 100 000 in 1995.

In an extensive, largely classified study the US Central Intelligence Agency scrutinized the Harvard and WHO forecasts, deciding that both captured 'some real trends' but 'overstate the progress achievable, while underestimating the risks.' The intelligence group concluded that the most likely situation was one of future deterioration in global health, followed in the mid-twenty-first century by limited improvement. Key to the CIA's pessimism were 'persistent poverty in much of the developing world, growing microbial resistance and a dearth of new replacement drugs, inadequate disease surveillance and control capacity, and the high prevalence and continued spread of major killers such as HIV/AIDS, TB, and malaria.'

In 1999 the World Health Organization settled for the following breakdown of global deaths: 53.9 million people died in 1998; 31 per cent suffered cardiovascular diseases, 25 per cent infectious diseases, 13 per cent cancer, and the remainder was comprised of deaths due to accidents, respiratory and digestive diseases, maternal childbirth fatalities, and 6 per cent other.'

Better data for policy makers would result from vastly improved disease surveillance systems, vital statistics reporting, and primary health infrastructure.

It was hard to escape that word—*infrastructure*. Such a deceptively banal-sounding term utterly failed to convey the millions of lives that might be long and healthy, or short and tragic, based on whether or not infrastructure existed.

During the Great Depression Paul de Kruif, who had been a true believer in the medical strategy of public health, witnessed the dreadful death toll that preventable and treatable diseases were taking on America's poor children. Embittered, prone to sarcasm, he asked in 1936:

> When you think that this science is really the right of all humanity, should be owned by humanity, by the living, by all who, half-dead, have a chance for life—
> Then what, fundamentally, could be more hopeful?
> Because when they understand that all their own babies can be brought to this strong and beautiful life, the people of the world will at last rise up and ask: Are or are not all of our children really going to live?
> And if not, then in the name of misery, why keep them alive.

Nearly seventy years later the question remained relevant. Science had, indeed, offered humanity a treasure trove of discoveries of public health significance. But at the close of the century everything seemed up for patent grabs, even the genomes of killer microbes that, once deciphered, were placed under corporate locks and keys, away from the utility of public health advocates.

Yet de Kruif's question contained a glimmer of an idea: democracy.

It's impossible as an individual to believe in a future if you don't believe in your power to influence the present. Making choices and taking actions to prevent theoretical future catastrophes or better the lives of your children, or grandchildren, are formidable steps to take for those who feel impotent in their day-to-day lives.

Public health in the twenty-first century will rise or fall, then, with the ultimate course of globalization. If the passage of time finds ever-widening wealth gaps, disappearing middle classes, international financial lawlessness, and still-rising individualism, the essential elements of public health will be imperiled, perhaps non-existent, all over the world. Capital would be skewed away from social service infrastructures, particularly those that meet the needs of the poor. Few public health barriers would be in place to prevent global spread of disease, and ever more drugs would be rendered useless by microbial resistance. United Nations agencies, including the World Health Organization, would witness further deterioration in their funding and influence. And political instability would foster increasingly irrational nation-state and rogue activities including, perhaps, bioterrorism.

There was another potential for the future. It didn't cast the world in a bed of aromatic roses, but neither did it forecast hell on earth.

The people of the world were coming to know a great deal about one another at the millennium, thanks to worldwide distribution of films, the Internet, television, and twenty-four-hour-a-day broadcast news. In the short term the global population witnessed one another's miseries with powerful impact in the 1990s. Earthquakes, carnage, ethnic cleansing, hurricanes, famines—these once-remote events filled living room TV screens and blared headlines from Cape Town to Moscow.

In the longer run, perhaps on a more subtle level, humanity also began to see the scale of planetary inequities. The writer was reminded of an experience in Harare, Zimbabwe, watching the film *Ruthless People* in a neighbourhood cinema. Bette Midler and Danny DeVito's amusing performances, curiously, drew no laughter from the audience, though the Zimbabweans did enjoy the film immensely. Rather than guffaw at Midler's slapstick virtuosity the crowd loudly sighed, 'oohed' and 'ahed' over the cars, stereos, houses, clothing, jewelery, electronic devices, and lifestyles displayed on the silver screen. They revelled in a sort of jealous fantasy state, gasping at the amazing and wonderful lives that they imagined all Americans enjoyed.

In American films and internationally distributed television shows no modern characters ever fretted over their diphtheria-slain child or malarial toddler. Life was free of such care, filled instead with gun-toting Clint Eastwood cops, glamorous Julia Roberts love affairs, and madcap Robin Williams adventures.

In the future was it not possible that, faced with such glaring evidence of the shortcomings in their own existences, more and more of the world's poor would demand accountability from their governments? Was it optimistic to imagine that in coming years politicians and government leaders who denied clean drinking water, safe foods, ample medicines, and basic public health to their constituencies would pay a price for such negligence and arrogance?

And one could hope that in the future violations of that trust would be punished.

That was the essence of US foreign policy in the post-Cold War period. The Agency for International Development, for example, devoted most of its resources to what it called 'democracy building'.

Perhaps, such proponents argued, the day would come when Indians would demand that their government spend 5 per cent of its GDP on non-corrupt public health activities. Perhaps the Zairois would one day cease their civil war and ethnic battles, face their national leaders, and cry out for health for their children. Perhaps African leaders who failed to place HIV prevention at the top of their priority lists would be drummed out of office by millions of grown-up AIDS orphans. Perhaps Russian voters would one twenty-first-century day come to believe in the power of the ballot and opt for candidates that espoused not tired ideological and nationalistic rhetoric but concrete programmmes for provision of social services.

And perhaps—indeed, probably—Americans would become fed up with their irrational public health and medical systems, demanding the long overdue, bold reappraisal of the nation's priorities for the health of its people. By 2000 there were already organizations forming all over the United States, as well as internationally, demanding that the pharmaceutical and health insurance industries shift their priorities away, at least incrementally, from profits toward Humanity's most urgent public health needs.

Health, broadly defined, may not qualify as a right for every human being. But the essentials of public health most assuredly were human rights. Every government in the world knew by 2000—irrefutably—that an unfiltered, unclean drinking water system could kill children. Every government knew that black market sales of antibiotics fuelled emergence of deadly drug-resistant microbes. No political leader could deny knowledge that allowing unfettered tobacco advertising and sales in his or her country would destroy the lungs, hearts, and other vital organs of the smoking citizens. Leaders could no longer deny that an HIV-loaded syringe, passed from one person to another, was every bit as dangerous as a loaded gun. Ignorance might have protected world leaders in the mid-twentieth century, but after the millennium it would be difficult to dodge a charge of negligent murder against a national leader who deliberately shunned provision of safe drinking water in favour of military or grandiose development expenditures. Trust and accountability: above all else, these were the pillars of public health.

After the Persian Gulf War the US government demanded global accountability regarding biological weapons. Together with its European allies the United States called for complete transparency in the manufacture and distribution of agricultural chemicals, pharmaceuticals, and petrochemicals. Only in an atmosphere of openness and accountability, the Clinton administration argued, could there be truth.

But *no* drug or chemical company, whether located in Baghdad or Baltimore, wanted outsiders inspecting its plants and operations. Trade secrecy, alone, necessitated barriers and blocked transparency. Resorting to typical law enforcement solutions in confronting such obstinacy, the United States funded research on high-tech solutions, such as devices that could 'sniff out' nasty microbes in the air or detect them in the water supply.

It was just another example of a public health threat confronted with technological solutions. There was not demonstrable justification for placing public trust in such options.

Were a biological attack to occur, or a naturally arising epidemic, the public would only have one viable direction in which to place its trust: with its local, national, and global public health infrastructure. If such an interlaced system did not exist at a time of grave need it would constitute an egregious betrayal of trust.

To build trust there must be a sense of community. And the community must collectively believe in its own future. At the millennium much of humanity hungered for connectedness and community but lived isolated, even hostile, existences. Trust evaporated when Tutsis met Hutus, Serbs confronted Kosovars, African-Americans worked with white Americans, or Estonians argued with Russians.

The new globalization pushed communities against one another, opening old wounds and historic hatreds, often with genocidal results. It would be up to public health to find ways of bridging the hatreds, bringing the world towards a sense of singular community in which the health of each member rises or falls with the health of all others.

Notes

Introduction

1 'Risky economies.' *The Economist* (November 13, 1999): 114.
2 Committee for the Study of the Future of Public Health. 'The future of public health.' Washington, DC: National Academy Press, 1988.
3 Callahan, D. *False Hopes: Why America's Quest for Perfect Health Is a Recipe for Failure.* New York: Simon & Schuster, 1998.
4 'Support for some public health programs increased in appropriations for FY 1997.' *The Nation's Health* (November 1996): 5–6; and 'Appropriations process tough on public health.' *The Nation's Health* (August 1995): 1.
5 Editorial. 'WHO: Where there is no vision, the people perish.' *The Lancet* **1350** (1997): 749.
6 Al-Mazrou, Y., Berkley, S., Bloom, B., *et al.* 'A vital opportunity for global health.' *The Lancet* **350** (1997): 750–1.
7 McKeown, T. *The Origins of Human Disease.* Oxford, UK: Basil Blackwell, 1988.
8 McKinley, J. B. and McKinley, S. M. 'The questionable contribution of medical measures to the decline of mortality in the United States in the twentieth century.' In *Health and Society. The Milbank Memorial Fund Quarterly* **55** (1977): 405–28.

Chapter 1

1 I was in Surat, as well as much of the rest of India, during the plague outbreak of 1994.
2 Sardesai, R. 'Black death.' *The Telegraph* (September 25, 1994).
3 Chakravartty, N. 'The rats will play...' *Economic Times* (Bombay) (October 4, 1994).
4 Dixit, J. N. 'Controlling crisis.' *Indian Express* (Bombay) (October 4, 1994): 8.
5 'Reaping a grim harvest.' *India Today* (October 15, 1994): 4.
6 For earthquake details and photos, see Nayar, R. 'Latur revisited: One year later.' *Sunday* (September 25, 1994): 23–38; and Unhale, S. 'Unending tragedy: A year after the Marathwada quake.' *Frontline* (October 21, 1994): 28–30.
7 Hinnebusch, B. J., Perry, R. D., and Schwan, T. G. 'Role of the *Yersinia pestis* hemin storage (hms) locus in the transmission of plague by fleas.' *Science* **273** (1996): 367–70.
8 Brown, R. 'Is behavioural thermoregulation a factor in flea-to-human transmission of *Yersinia pestis?*' *Lancet* **345** (1995): 931.
9 An excellent summary of the type III secretion can be found in Baringa, M. 'A shared strategy for virulence.' *Science* **272** (1996): 1261–3.
10 From 1995 to 1997 India's growth increased to 6 per cent a year, but the Asian crash of '98 put brakes on Indian growth. See: 'Time to let go: A survey of India.' *The Economist* (February 22, 1997), Special Supplement; and 'When China and India go down together.' *The Economist* (November 22, 1997): 41–4.

11 Modi, K. 'Surat textile and diamond industries grind to a halt.' *Business Standard* (New Delhi) (September 26, 1994): 1.

12 'The plague within.' *Business Standard* (Bombay) (September 27, 1994): 11.

13 Robboy, R. 'IDA extends record health sector credit to India.' *World Bank News* (March 28, 1996): 1–2.

14 Kumar, S. 'Non-governmental report spells out failings in India's health care.' *Lancet* 352 (1998): 380.

15 'Surat "fever" claims 45.' *Mid-Day* (September 22, 1994): 1.

16 Express News Service. 'Plague rages on; a death every hour in Surat.' *Indian Express* (September 24, 1994): 1.

17 In 1995 a strain of multidrug-resistant *Yersinia pestis* did surface in a fifteen-year-old boy in Madagascar. The strain was resistant not only to tetracycline, but also to all anti-*Yersinia* antibiotics, save, fortunately, trimethoprim. The case may have been related to a small Mozambican bubonic plague outbreak that occurred in September 1994—at the same time as India's outbreak. Or it could be part of Madagascar's July–October 1995 bubonic plague outbreak, which involved 348 cases, five deaths. Because there are many Indians living in both Madagascar and Mozambique and trade and travel between the countries is frequent, there is no way of knowing where this boy's ominous drug-resistant *Yersinia* originated. See: Rasolomaharo, M., Rasoamanana, B., Andrianirina, Z., *et al.* 'Plague in Majunga, Madagascar.' *Lancet* 345 (1995): 983–4; and Bonn, D. 'Multidrug-resistant plague case causes concern.' *Lancet* 350 (1997): 788.

18 For a flavour of this, see the front page of Calcutta's *The Telegraph* for September 27, 1994, and Pfizer ads such as 'Don't Get Plagued with Fear,' on page 19 of the *Sunday Times of India*, October 2, 1994.

19 All travellers bound for the United Kingdom from India were given a leaflet offering 'advice to passengers arriving in the UK by air from India.' It detailed information for physicians, calling for immediate tetracycline therapy, laboratory work, and notification of the UK's Communicable Disease Control Office.

20 Press Trust of India. 'Indian harassed at Heathrow.' *Times of India* (October 3, 1994): 1; and Agencies. 'U.K.-bound passengers found plague-free.' *Times of India* (October 4, 1994): 13.

21 A CDC assessment two years after the plague outbreak in India would find that 'it is unrealistic to expect any system effectively to screen all travellers returning from areas of recognized disease outbreaks. It is impossible to assess the sensitivity of the described surveillance system since no cases of pneumonic plague were identified either within or outside the system. In retrospect, the risk for an imported plague case was quite small, since the epidemic in India was limited in time and space and had far fewer cases than originally suspected. The WHO investigative team found no evidence of transmission in metropolitan areas other than Surat. Most of the patients with suspected plague in Surat came from poor neighbourhoods, residents of which would be unlikely to travel internationally. In addition, the short incubation period and severe symptoms of pneumonic plague and the rapid deterioration of the patient's condition substantially limited the contagious period and the opportunity for secondary transmission.' Fritz, C. L., Dennis, D. T., Tipple, M., *et al. Emerging Infectious Diseases* 2 (October 2, 1997): 1–9.

22 For details related to laboratory efforts and controversies see: Assorted letters and authors. 'Plague in India.' *Lancet* 345 (1995): 258–9.

23 Dr Jacob John, president of the Indian Association of Medical Microbiology, favoured the notion that another bacterial disease, tularaemia, was the culprit. 'I am not declaring that the epidemic was tularaemia without laboratory evidence,' John said. 'But I am stating that the epidemic has not yet been aetiologically diagnosed. It is by no means confirmed to be plague. In all probability it is not plague. Alternate diagnosis must be considered, for example tularaemia.' John went on to attack the lack of epidemiological detective work executed by authorities in

Surat, Maharashtra's Beed District, or anywhere else in the country, concluding: 'Has anyone heard about the case definition, we cannot accept that there was an epidemic.'

24 Kimball, A. M. Speech to the Centre for International Studies, University of Toronto, October 30, 1998.

25 'Was it the plague?' *The Economist* (November 19, 1994): 38–40.

26 On October 10 the Indian Ministry of Health issued this breakdown of cases:

Suspected cases		Confirmed cases	
By Oct. 9		*By Oct. 8*	*New on*
Cases	*Deaths*		*Oct. 9*
6344	55	272	16

27 'Were Ultras responsible for Surat plague?' *Hindustan Times* (July 9, 1995): A1.

28 It first assumed that any unusual features in Surat's *Yersinia* could not possibly have arisen naturally. The last Indian *Yersinia* strain available for comparison was from Karnataka in 1963, and it did not possess this genetic sequence. Several scientists—notably a biotechnologist from AIIMS and a virologist from Pune—claimed that it was 'categorically impossible' for such change to occur as a result of natural evolution. One went so far as to assert that there were no known examples of evolution adding, versus deleting, genes.

29 UNICEF, Information Statistics/India. UNICEF Web site: www.unicef.org/statis/country_1page81.htmlŕil, 1998.

30 Kumar, S. 'India has the largest number of people infected with HIV.' *Lancet* 353 (1999): 48.

31 Krishnan, E. Letter to *Lancet* 344 (1994): 1298.

Chapter 2

1 Translated from Kibari, N. and Lungazi, M. 'Le virus ebola à Kikwit: mythe, mystère ou réalité.' Editions Baobob, Kinshasa, Democratic Republic of Congo, 1998.

2 For descriptions of the Kikwit people's perception of the events during the 1995 Ebola epidemic I have relied on a combination of my own observations on site at the time, numerous local interviews conducted in May 1995 and March 1998, and on the seminal work of University of Bandundu professors Kibari N'sanga and Lungazi Mulala, 1998.

3 Garrett, L. 'Yambuku.' In *The Coming Plague. Newly Emerging Diseases in a World Out of Balance.* New York: Farrar, Straus & Giroux, 1994.

4 UNICEF. *The State of the World's Children 1998.* New York: Oxford Press, 1998. The eleven worse-ranked nations were, in order of greatest child mortality rates, Niger, Angola, Sierra Leone, Afghanistan, Liberia, Guinea-Bissau, Mali, Malawi, Mozambique, Somalia, and Guinea. All but three of the thirty-two highest child mortality nations were in 1995 in Africa. Those three exceptions were Afghanistan, Pakistan, and Cambodia.

5 Estimates of maternal death rates are hard to come by, as coroner records typically list other causes of mothers' demises in Africa. A survey of autopsies in Brazzaville, Congo, found rates so high as to mean that one out of every twenty-five women in that city died prematurely due to complications in pregnancy. Given that Brazzaville is the capital, where medical services are concentrated, this certainly indicates rural mortality rates are far higher. See LeCoeur, S., Pictet, G.,

M'Pelé, P., and Lallemont, M. 'Direct estimation of maternal mortality in Africa.' *Lancet* 352 (1998): 1525–6.

UNICEF estimates that across the Congo river in Zaire maternal mortality was higher, still, in the late 1990s. They say 870 mothers annually of every 100 000 pregnant women died, which is 14 per cent higher than the LeCoeur estimate for the Congo.

6 Muyembe, T. Speech to the International Colloquium on Ebola Virus Research, Antwerp, September 4–7, 1996.

7 The sorry history of Lumumba's assassination and Mobutu's rise to power is well documented. I refer readers to several sources, including: Kalb, M. G. *The Congo Cables: The Cold War in Africa— From Eisenhower to Kennedy*. New York: Macmillan, 1982; Fanon, F. *Toward the African Revolution*. New York: Grove Press, 1967; Nkrumah, K. *Africa Must Unite*. New York: International Publishers, 1963; Western Massachusetts Association of Concerned African Scholars. *U.S. Military Involvement in Southern Africa*. Boston: South End Press, 1978; and Winternitz, H. *East Along the Equator*. New York: Atlantic Monthly Press, 1987.

8 American, French, Belgian, and South African troops, as well as mercenaries, fought on behalf of the Mobutu regime, quashing rebellions against the dictator's brutal government. Occasionally these interventions were financed by Saudi and Israeli sub-rosa government funds. From his first days in office, Mobutu was unable to fully control Shaba and Katanga provinces, even his eastern flank bordering Rwanda, Burundi, and Zambia, which were always hospitable to rebel troops. When Cuba sent soldiers in support of the MPLA in Angola and the government of Ethiopia the Carter administration widened its backing for Mobutu. The French government's position, particularly during the François Mitterand years, was even more adamantly in support of Mobutu. In 1978 alone, fifteen thousand French troops fought in Zaire, defending the Mobutu regime in a *corps d'intervention*.

9 To get an idea of the scale of wealth lying beneath Zaire's soil consider these points, gleaned from the 1997 annual stockholders report for the Canadian mining company Melkior Resources, Inc.: '2800 square kilometres of the World's richest known copper-cobalt deposits, in an area that has already produced over 14 million tonnes of copper and 560 000 tonnes of cobalt since the beginning of the century and is poised to be the world's biggest supplier of these minerals. The region has also yielded uranium and gold.'

This statement refers to a single mining site in Zaire, and even with its obvious bravado cannot come close to expressing the scale of gem, mineral, and petroleum reserves nationwide.

10 Garrett, L. 'Plague Warriors.' *Vanity Fair* (August 1995): 85–161.

11 For details in this and the following section of this chapter I refer the reader to my many reports at the time, appearing in *Newsday* between March–September 1995.

12 'Quatre-vingt' is *Eurapatorium odoratum*, or *Hepathorium odorantrum*, a weed found in the tropics of Africa, Asia, and even Latin America. Where it originated is unclear. It was noted well to the north of Congo, in Nigeria, in 1963. (See Adams, C. D. *Flora of West Tropical Africa*. 2nd Edition, 1963.) It is, as local Kikwitians noted, a very aggressive weed, and a member of the daisy family. I thank Roy E. Gereau of the Missouri Botanical Garden and Clifford W. Smith of the University of Hawaii for assistance in determining the identity of 'quatre-vingt.'

13 Charlotte Kilesa and Augustin Bisambu were Gaspard Menga's grandparents, or the parents of his father, Innocent Menga. When Gaspard elected to be a Jehovah's Witness his older brother, Philémon, changed his own surname to Nseke as a sign that he remained a Catholic. As had his wife, Marie-José, Philémon died of Ebola.

14 At the time there was concern that Ebola, Marburg, or other deadly haemorrhagic fever viruses might break out in Goma. See: Garrett, L. 'Few drills—or skills—to foil a super plague.'

Newsday (July 31, 1994): A7; and Garrett, L. 'Refugee crisis worsens as aid is sent to Goma.' *Newsday* (July 24, 1994): A14.

15 Pécoul, B., Chirac, P., Trouiller, P., *et al.* 'Access to essential drugs in poor countries: A lost battle?' *Journal of the American Medical Association* 281 (1999): 361–7; and Paquet, C. and Van Soest, M. 'Mortality and malnutrition among Rwandan refugees in Zaire.' *Lancet* 344 (1994): 823–4.

16 The use of patient names is a very serious matter. Obviously, all patients, regardless of their nationality, have a right to full confidentiality. I have chosen, however, to use Kimfumu's name, as well as those of other Ebola patients, for two reasons. First, most of these names were widely published all over the world during the epidemic, and appear fully listed in Zairois publications. And secondly it seems important to humanize the epidemic and conditions in the African country. I hope that by personalizing such things residents of wealthy countries can identify more closely with the conditions under which their African counterparts live—and die.

17 His leader, Pastor Eloi Mulengamungu, would later declare Kikwit to be a Sodom upon which God was levying revenge in the form of Ebola.

18 Muyembe was one of the first scientists in Yambuku in 1976, arriving when that Ebola epidemic was peaking and out of control. Since that time Ebola had been one of the primary foci of his professional life.

19 It's worth asking what would have happened in Brazzaville if one of these reporters had been carrying Ebola. In the context of the 1995 epidemic, given the very brief amount of time the journalists were in Kikwit and the rather superficial nature of their interaction with the epidemic it would seem a near impossibility. But at a time when the movements of Zairois people were so terribly restricted and when Zaire nationals were being detained at international airports out of fear of spreading the frightening virus, the apparent free mobility of the media seems inconsistent. Detaining reporters would make no sense either. What would be appropriate policy in future epidemics? Clearly it would depend on the organism, its mode of transmission, the nature of journalists' contact with the situation, and WHO policies.

    All of this would be far easier to sort out, and policies of containment would make more scientific sense, if trained media liaisons were on the ground from day one of epidemics, carefully balancing reporters' needs for access against the greater exigencies for epidemic control. Some journalists, convinced that they would ultimately be placed under quarantine, booked passage on local boats, crossed the wide, muddy Congo River, and made their ways to Brazzaville, capital of the Congo. Lacking appropriate visas they were stuck in Brazzaville for considerable amounts of time.

20 While I was in Kikwit I followed, for the most part, the same hygienic precautions I observe throughout the poor, tropical world. I washed in liquid recyclable soap and drank two to three litres daily of bottled water or water that I filtered myself. I followed the old maxim of tropical medicine: don't eat it unless you can boil it, peel it, shell it, uncan it, or burn it. I was careful not to shake hands with anyone. And when eating in villages, where food is drawn with bare hands from a collectively used bowl or pot, I distributed disposable latex gloves, instructing my hosts and fellow diners that during an epidemic this was a wise precaution for all of us. To my distress, however, after sharing meals with a man known to have been exposed to Ebola I realized that latex was not protective against the oils used locally in food preparation, and the gloves leaked.

21 Kelly, M. J. 'Research on Ebola virus.' *Lancet* 347 (1996): 691; Jaax, N. K. 'Author's reply.' *Lancet* 347 (1996): 691; Jaax, N., Jahrling, P., Geisbert, T., *et al.* 'Transmission of Ebola virus (Zaire strain) to uninfected control monkeys in a biocontainment laboratory.' *Lancet* 346 (1995):1669–71; and Johnson, E., Jaax, N., White, J., *et al.* 'Lethal experimental infections of rhesus monkeys by aerosolized Ebola virus.' *International Journal of Experimental Pathology* 76 (1995): 277–86.

The design of Jaax's experiment is important. Six rhesus monkeys were placed in separate cages about three metres apart. Two received sprayed doses of interferon, which here was a placebo. These were the controls. Four others received a moderate aerosolized dose of Ebola (2.6 $log_{10}0PFUs$). The animals were exposed while they were fully anesthetized and laid inside airtight boxes. The solutions were pumped into these boxes, and the monkeys breathed that contaminated air for ten minutes. All four Ebola-exposed animals became infected and died of the disease within twenty-two days. Critics challenged the experiment's applicability to human exposure, as few people might be expected to remain in an airtight room for ten minutes with a patient. And, more difficult, they charged, was the assumption that ailing patients exhale or cough up such high doses of viruses.

22 Zaki, S. R., Greer, P. W., Goldsmith, C. S., *et al.* 'Ebola virus haemorrhagic fever: Immunopathological and ultrastructural study.' International Colloquium on Ebola Virus Research, September 4–7, 1996, Antwerp.

23 '2nd Ebola fever case suspected in Liberia.' Reuters (December 11, 1995).

24 Amblard, J., Obiang, P., Edzang, S., *et al.* 'Identification of the Ebola virus in Gabon in 1994.' *Science* 349 (1997).

25 'Neuf personnes décédés après avoir consommmé de la viande de chimpanzé.' *Agence France Press* (February 10, 1996); 'South African Ebola scare eases; case tied to Gabon.' *New York Times* (November 19, 1996): A15.

26 In South Africa concern about Ebola and other rare but deadly viruses is far from abstract. South Africa has faced its own frightening outbreaks—including one of Ebola—and the new openness with her African neighbours means the continent's most prosperous and internationally connected nation could well face further microbial dangers.

  Prior to 1994 South Africa was cut off from its African neighbours, who opposed the nation's apartheid policies, which separated the races and gave the white minority population virtually absolute control over every facet of the society. But with the election of Nelson Mandela to the presidency and elimination of all apartheid policies South Africa has become the darling of the continent, and the number one destination for young fortune seekers from every corner of Africa.

  The position of the new government is that South Africa has plenty of its own diseases that might also travel northwards. For example, some 160 000 people suffer from active tuberculosis, which kills 10 000 South Africans yearly. And the HIV/AIDS crisis has reached nightmarish proportions in the country, with some areas showing HIV-positive rates as high as 30 per cent among young adults. A report from the National Assembly says 1500 South Africans are newly infected with HIV every day.

27 See note 22.

28 Heymann presented these data on the Ebola outbreaks:

Site	Date	Cause of Viral Amplification? Or Control?	Deaths
Yambuku	1976	Poor infection control measures; reused nonsterile syringes	280
Tandala	1977	Good infection control measures in hospital	1
Kikwit	1995	Poor infection control nursing	245
Mayibout	1996	Good infection control measures in hospital	21*

*None were hospital-acquired cases.

29 United Nations Childrens Fund. *The State of the World's Children*. New York: UNICEF, 1998.

30 The infectable bats were the insect-eating little free-tailed bat and Angola free-tailed bat. And the Wahlberg's epauletted fruit bat was readily infected. These animals made billions of Ebola viruses in their bodies.

31 Phillips-Conroy, J. E., Jolly, C. J., Petros, B., *et al.* 'Sexual transmission of SIV agm in wild grivet monkeys.' *Journal of Medical Primatology* 23 (1994): 1–7; and Chen, Z., Telfer, P., Reed, P., *et al.* 'First simian immunodeficiency virus from a free-ranging sooty mangabey is equidistant from SIV and HIV-2 suggesting a new subtype.' *Annual Symposium on Nonhuman Primate Models for AIDS* 10 (1994).

32 Gao, F., Bailes, E., Robertson, D. L., *et al.* 'Origin of HIV-1 in the chimpanzee Pan troglodytes troglodytes.' *Nature* 397 (1998): 436–41; Garrett, L., 'Save the Chimps.' *Newsday* (February 1, 1999).

33 Environmental groups estimate the Congo Basin/Tai Forest logging rate is eleven million cubic metres of wood per year. The equivalent for all of Asia is ninety-two million; for all of Latin America it's twenty-eight million. See: World Society for Protection of Animals. 'Slaughter of the Apes.' London: WSPA, 1995; and McRae, M. 'Road kill in Cameroon.' *Natural History* 2/ 1997: 36–75.

34 Studies of bushmeat consumption throughout the region show that ungulates, such as dykers, are the main targets for hunters and account for between 58 to 95 per cent of all bushmeat consumed by people. Further, bushmeat accounts for upward of 75 per cent of all protein consumed by people living in and around Africa's equatorial rain forests. See: Wilkie, D. S. and Carpenter, J. F. 'Bushmeat hunting in the Congo Basin: An assessment of impacts and options for mitigation.' *Biodiversity and Conservation* (1999), in press. This is a comprehensive review of the literature.

35 Sources on the overthrow of Mobutu and subsequent Kabila regime include: 'A continent goes to war.' *The Economist* (October 3, 1998): 47–9; 'New Congo, same old ways.' *The Economist* (May 2, 1998): 41–2; 'War in the heart of Africa.' *The Economist* (August 22, 1998): 35; Chiahemen, J. 'Congo's Kabila sacks outspoken minister.' Reuters (November 11, 1998); Duke, L. 'Congolese seethe over Tutsi presence among Kabila forces.' *Washington Post* (November 11, 1998): A1; Edwards, M. 'Central Africa's cycle of violence.' *National Geographic* (June 1997): 124–33; Fisher, I. and Onishi, N. 'Congo's struggle may unleash broad strife to redraw Africa.' *New York Times* (January 12, 1999): A1; French, H. W. 'Congo leader losing luster.' *New York Times* (May 21, 1998): A1; and McNeil, D. G. 'A war turned free-for-all tears at Africa's center.' *New York Times* (December 6, 1998): WK5.

36 'Africa's economies.' *The Economist* (September 19, 1998): 126.

37 Breman, J. G. and Henderson, D. A. 'The authors' reply.' *Lancet* 339 (1998): 2027; Centres for Disease Control and Prevention. 'Human monkeypox—Kasai oriental, Zaire, 1996–97.' *Morbidity and Mortality Weekly Report* 46 (1997): 304–7.

38 The World Health Organization was deprived of its logical Nobel Prize for elimination of smallpox because of these protests. For more than a decade teams of scientists combed Central Africa in search of monkeypox epidemics. No evidence was found at that time of significant human-to-human transmission of the virus.

39 The allegation is not entirely fair. WHO did set up a surveillance communications network that would allow physicians in Kikwit to notify authorities swiftly, were Ebola or other microbes to resurface. It is, however, interrupted by local warfare.

   As for the health infrastructure, itself, WHO does not, under its United Nations mandate, get involved. The construction of hospitals and provision of supplies is somebody else's problem— a bilateral donor, a humanitarian organization, the World Bank. Unfortunately, at the time of writing no moneyed group anywhere in the world was, as a matter of priority, dedicated to health infrastructure development.

40 'The cost of Kabila.' *The Economist* (October 2, 1998): 48–9.

Chapter 3

1 Sinyavsky, A. *The Russian Intelligentsia*. New York: Columbia University Press, 1997.

2 Shkolnikov, V. and Meslé, F. 'Health crisis in Russia, Parts I and II.' *Population and Society* 8 (1996): 123–90.

3 Primary Russian demography sources include: 'Russian mortality double that in West.' *Russia Today Online*, November 13, 1998; Belaeyev, E. *Role of Sanitation and Epidemiology Service in Maintaining the Sanitation, Epidemiology and Well-being of the Russian Federal Population*. Perm: Tyniga Publishing House, 1996; Centres for Disease Control and Prevention. 'Vital and health statistics: Russian Federation and United States, selected years 1980–93.' US Department of Health and Human Services, Washington, DC, June 1995.

4 Chernobyl authorities claim that the nuclear material inside that sarcophagus is no longer in danger of escape or explosion. They even dispute the need to fortify the hastily constructed concrete shroud.

But Ukraine's substantial, independent physics community, as well as foreign experts, disagree. They say that the material inside the shroud is still in danger of undergoing an uncontrollable chain reaction, setting off a catastrophic nuclear explosion that could rain radioactive fallout over an area larger than that originally affected in April 1986. There are 200 tons of radioactive fuel inside the sarcophagus, 135 tons of which have the consistency of molten lava. That's enough to create an explosion greater than the Hiroshima bomb blast.

The sarcophagus was showing signs of weakening under the growing fuel pressure inside. And in the other reactors inexplicable auto-shutdowns and electronic problems were common. On the tenth anniversary of the disaster *Science* published several unsettling findings in its April 19, 1996, issue.

5 Sources on the environmental impact of the Chernobyl disaster include: numerous interviewees, and: Zakharov, Y. M. and Krysanov, E. Y. (eds.) *Consequences of the Chernobyl Catastrophe: Environmental Health*. Moscow: Centre for Russian Environmental Policy, 1996; and Feshbach, M. *Russia in Transition: Ecological Disaster*, A Twentieth Century Fund Report, New York, 1995.

6 Feshbach, M. *Environmental and Health Atlas of Russia*. Moscow: PAIMAS Publishing House, 1995.

7 Adult 1998 cancer incidence in Irkutsk was 14.5 times more than in the United States.

8 World Health Organization. 'Dramatic increase in thyroid cancer among children in Belarus and Ukraine after Chernobyl accident.' Press Release WHO/84, October 19, 1993.

9 Mitchell, P. 'Ukrainian thyroid-cancer rates greatly increased since Chernobyl.' *Lancet* 354 (1999): 51.

10 Bard, D., Verger, P., and Hubert, P. 'Chernobyl, 10 years after: Health consequences.' *Epidemiology Reviews* 19 (1997): 187–204.

11 United Nations Children's Fund. *Children at Risk in Central and Eastern Europe: Perils and Promises*. New York: UNICEF, 1997, 16.

12 'Russia's fear-worse factor.' *The Economist* (June 1, 1996): 45–6.

13 'Competitiveness.' *The Economist* (April 22, 2000): 98; and Soros, G. 'Who Lost Russia?' *The New York Review of Books* (April 13, 2000): 10–16.

14 Kohlmeir, L., Mendez, M., Shalnova, S., et al. 'Deficient dietary iron intake among women and children in Russia: Evidence from the Russian Longitudinal Monitoring Survey.' American Journal of Public Health 88 (1998): 576–80.

15 Drakulić, S. Café Europa: Life After Communism. New York: W. W. Norton, 1997.

16 Romania's AIDS epidemic was sparked by a very similar incident, eventually involving more than 2000 babies who were injected with HIV-contaminated, bloody needles. See Garrett, L. The Coming Plague, 1994, pages 505, 612, 701, footnotes 105–7; Dressler, S. 'Let the children die: AIDS in Romania.' AIDS Newsletter (London) 11 (10) (1996): 1; and Apetrei, C., Buzdugan, I., Mitroi, I., et al., 'Nosocomial HIV-transmission and primary prevention in Romania.' Lancet 344 (1994): 1028–9.

17 Russia AIDS Centre. 'HIV-infection surveillance in Russia in 1987–1996 (statistics).' Moscow: Russia AIDS Centre, 1997.

18 After 1991 most of the former Soviet states enacted tough AIDS laws that were sharply denounced by the international AIDS community. For a sense of what, in Western terms, is considered appropriate HIV-related legislation see: Gostin, L. O. and Lazzarini, Z. Human Rights and Public Health in the AIDS Pandemic. New York: Oxford University Press, 1997; and Mann, J. and Tarantola, D. AIDS in the World II. New York: Oxford University Press, 1996.

19 Ernberg, G. 'HIV outbreak among injecting drug users in Sveltogorsk.' UNAIDS letter to Pavel Kral, July 25, 1996; van der Laan, N. 'HIV crisis in Belarus "worse than Chernboyl."' Electronic telegraph (www.telegraph.co.uk), December 2, 1996.

20 Lilitsola, K., Tashkinova, I., Korovina, G., et al. 'HIV-1 genetic subtype A/B recombinant strain causing an explosive IDU epidemic in Kaliningrad.' Twelfth International Conference on AIDS, Geneva, June 28–July 3, 1998.

21 For more on the genetic diversity of HIV-1 strains in the ex-USSR see: Kozlov, A. P., Emeljanov, A. V., Verevochkin, S. V., et al. 'Characteristics of early phase of HIV/AIDS epidemic.' Russian Journal of HIV/AIDS and Related Problems 1 (1997): 225.

22 Zmushko, E. and Bolekhan, V. N. 'HIV-infection in the Russian Federation military forces.' Twelfth International Conference on AIDS, Geneva, June 28–July 3, 1998.

23 Daigle, K. 'Exposing the face of sex in Moscow.' The Moscow Times (April 4, 1997): 20; and multiple street interviews with prostitutes.

24 The line between organized crime and prostitution in the area profoundly limited public health access to these women. See, for example: Pyroyshkina, E. Presentation to the Twelfth International Conference on AIDS, Geneva, June 28–July 3, 1998; Stanley, A. 'A tale of murder and sex slaves to stun Dostoyevsky.' New York Times (August 28, 1997): A3; and Stanley, A. 'With prostitution booming legalization tempts Russians.' New York Times (March 3, 1998): A1.

25 See World Health Organization. 'Task force to curb sexually transmitted disease epidemic in Europe.' Press Release EURO/03/98, Copenhagen, April 1998.

26 Whitehead, C. 'The remaking of Czechoslovakian science.' New Scientist (March 3, 1990): 26–9; and Stone, R. 'Civil war leaves once-proud Georgian science in tatters.' Science 272 (1996): 1581–2.

27 Holden, C. 'Russia's science spending diving toward new low.' Science 283 (1999): 31.

28 Chuprikov, A. P., Linyov, A. N., and Martsenkovsky, I. A. Lateral Therapy. Kyiev: Zdorovie Publishers, 1994; and Merskey, H. 'The Chuprikov file: Documents evaluating the scientific work of Professor A. P. Chuprikov.' Geneva Initiative on Psychiatry, Amsterdam, 1994.

29 The reader is referred for details to the Geneva Initiative's journal, Mental Health Reforms, published quarterly out of Amsterdam since 1996. Available from gip@euronet.nl.

30 'Psychology has practically disappeared in Russia since [World War II], and in the fall of 1948 physics was under fire. Statisticians dare not publish conclusions unpalatable to the Central Committee. It is possible that authoritarianism simply cannot allow the existence of the intellectual

standards of free scientific inquiry.' Zirkle, C., ed. *Death of Science in Russia*. Philadelphia: University of Pennsylvania Press, 1949.

31 Ostrander, S. and Schroeder, L. *Psychic Discoveries Behind the Iron Curtain*. New York: Bantam Books, 1970.

32 Polavets, V. and Bilynska, M. 'Psychiatry problems related to religious boom in Ukraine in late '80s–early '90s.' In documents on the Abolition and Prevention of Political Abuse of Psychiatry, Geneva Initiative, August–September 1995, Amsterdam.

33 Soyfer, V. N. 'New light on the Lysenko era.' *Nature* 339 (1989): 415–20; Medvedev, Z. A. *The Rise and Fall of T. D. Lysenko*. New York: Columbia University Press, 1969.

34 Malia, M. *The Soviet Tragedy: A History of Socialism in Russia, 1917–1991*. New York: The Free Press, 1994.

35 'Another refuge from Lysenko?' *Nature* 329 (1987): 797.

36 The point was stated succinctly by Zirkle in 1949: 'When intellectual freedom does not exist, intellectual honesty becomes a liability, and the consequences for science are disastrous' (Zirkle, C., 1949).

And C. D. Darlington, two years earlier, summarized Lysenko's impact in stark terms: 'after thirteen years of persecution, the great fellowship of Russian biological research, formed in the revolution, had been crushed and broken. . . . Never before has science been offered so many martyrs to its cause, men, too, honoured and beloved throughout the world' (Darlington, C. D. 'Genetics in Russia after ten years of cold official warfare.' *Nineteenth Century* 142 (1947): 157–68).

37 Stone, R. 'Estonian researchers lead the way in science reform.' *Science* 274 (1996): 29–30; and Martinson, H. *The Reform of R & D System in Estonia*. Tallinn: Estonian Science Foundation, 1995.

38 Holden, C. 'Eastern Europe's social science renaissance.' *Science* 283 (1999): 1620–2.

39 See, for example, Hammond, A. *Which World? Scenarios for the 21st Century*. Washington, DC: Island Press, 1998.

Chapter 4

1 Callahan, D. *False Hopes: Why America's Quest for Perfect Health Is a Recipe for Failure*. New York: Simon and Schuster, 1998.

2 Caldwell, M. *The Last Crusade: The War on Consumption 1862–1954*. New York: Atheneum, 1988.

3 The burden of viral nosocomial infection was difficult to calculate. The CDC felt confident that blood screening and basic hospital hygiene had eliminated nosocomial spread of the AIDS virus, HIV, by 1985. But other blood-borne viruses, particularly hepatitis types B, C, and D, and herpes viruses, continued to spread in medical settings well into the 1990s. Vogt, M., Lang, T., Frösner, G., *et al.* 'Prevalence and clinical outcome of hepatitis C infection in children who underwent cardiac surgery before the implementation of blood donor screening.' *New England Journal of Medicine* 341 (1999): 866–70.

4 Blau, S. P. and Shimberg, E. F. *How to Get Out of the Hospital Alive*. New York: Macmillan, 1997.

5 Tenover, F. C. and Hughes, J. M. 'The challenge of emerging infectious diseases.' *Journal of the American Medical Association* 175 (1996): 300–4.

6 Jones, R. N. and Verhoef, J. Presentation to the 37th Interscience Conference on Antimicrobial Agents and Chemotherapy, Toronto, September 29, 1997.

7 Raad, I. and Darouiche, R. O. 'Catheter-related septicemia: risk reduction.' *Infection and Medicine* 13 (1996): 807–12; 815–16; 823. And Raad, I. 'Intravascular-catheter-realted infections.' *Lancet* 351 (1998): 893–8.

8 Patterson, J. E. 'Making real sense of MRSA.' *Lancet* 348 (1996): 836–7.

9 Boyce, J. M., Opal, S. M., Chow, J. W., *et al.* 'Outbreak of multidrug-resistant *Enterococcus faecium* with transferable *vanB* class vancomycin resistance.' *Journal of Clinical Microbiology* 32 (1994): 1148–53.

10 Blau, S. P. and Shimberg, E. F. 1997, op. cit.; Bolognia, J. L. and Edelson, R. L. 'Spread of antibiotic-resistant bacteria from acne patients to personal contacts—a problem beyond the skin?' *Lancet* 350 (1997): 972–3.

11 Senate Committee on Investigations. *The Growing Menace of Bacterial Infections*. Albany: New York State Senate, 1999.

12 In addition to the Senate report, see Roberts, R., Tomasz, A., and Kreiswirth, B. *Antibiotic Resistance in New York City: A Growing Public Health Threat and a Proposal for Action*. New York: Bacterial Antibiotic Resistance Group, 1995.

13 Notably, 'Account of the climate and diseases of New York.' See Duffy, J. *The Sanitarians: A History of American Public Health*. Illini Books Edition. Chicago: University of Illinois Press, 1992; and Duffy, J. *A History of Public Health in New York City*. New York: Russell Sage Foundation, 1968.

14 During the same period, New York City passed its own tough quarantine laws, opened New York Hospital, built a dispensary (located on the corner of Beekman and Nassau streets in Manhattan) for delivery of health care to the poor, and witnessed the opening of Bellevue Hospital, which came under city control in 1805.

15 Between 1840 and 1860, 4.5 million of Europe's poor landed in the US's eastern ports, swelling the already densely populated tenements and slums. More than 3.5 million of them never left New York.

16 In New York City, for example, typhoid fever claimed 1396 lives in 1847; cholera killed another 5071 (possibly 8000) in the summer of '49; smallpox and typhoid fever both hit in 1851, killing 1600 people; and cholera struck again the summer of '54, killing 2501. These epidemics, coupled with alarmingly increasing maternal and child death rates, by 1855 drove the New York City mortality rate upwards to forty-eight deaths per year per one thousand people.

17 An excellent rendition of Chadwick's contributions can be found in the chapter entitled 'Public Medicine' in Porter, R. *The Greatest Benefit to Mankind: A Medical History of Humanity*. New York: Norton, 1998.

18 Details can be found in Duffy, J. *The Sanitarians: A History of American Public Health*. Illini Books Edition. Chicago: University of Illinois Press, 1992.

19 This was not so clearly the case in Europe at the time. In the mid-nineteenth century, Americans were far more moralistic and uncaring in their approaches to public health than were their European counterparts. For example, Porter tells us that Rudolf Virchow called upon German physicians to become 'attorneys for the poor', and France's Jules Guérin announced the need for what he labelled 'social medicine'. In general, European public health leaders were far less judgemental of the sick and more politically engaged than were their American colleagues.

20 Ludmerer, K. M. *Learning to Heal*. Baltimore: Johns Hopkins University Press, 1985.

21 Jordan, P. D. *The People's Health: A History of Public Health in Minnesota to 1948*. St Paul: Minnesota Historical Society, 1953.

22 In his landmark paper, 'Aetiology of Tuberculosis,' Koch not only offered evidence that *Mycobacterium tuberculosis* was the cause of TB but also laid out the modes of transmission of the germ (which he mistakenly called a virus) and strategies for control of its spread.

23 Evans, R. J. *Death in Hamburg: Society and Politics in the Cholera Years 1830–1910*. Oxford: Clarendon Press, 1987.

24 'Lung Block' was bordered by Catherine, Cherry, Hamilton, and Market Streets.

25 See Sanger, M. and Russell, W. *Debate on Birth Control.* Girard, Kans.: Haldeman-Julius Company, 1921.

26 This period marked the beginning of toilet seat phobias, which, in the twentieth century, extended to include polio and all sexually transmitted diseases, allowing syphilitics to tell their spouses they 'got it from a public toilet.' With the appearance of AIDS in the 1980s, toilet seat phobia also embraced HIV.

   This is hardly a solely American phenomenon. In the 1990s—one hundred years after the introduction of indoor plumbing—most families living in formerly Soviet countries deliberately disconnected toilet seats, preferring to squat to avoid alleged contagion.

27 The massive water and sewer projects undertaken in Chicago, for example, are described in Cain, L. P. 'Raising and watering a city: Ellis Sylvester Chesbrough and Chicago's first sanitation system.'

28 New York City Department of Health. *Annual Report of the Department of Health of the City of New York*, 1905 (for 1870–1895), 1915 (for 1900–1915). Note that there is debate on these figures. See Free, E. and Hammonds, E. M. 'Science, politics and the art of persuasion.' In Rosner, D. (ed.), *Hives of Sickness*, Rutgers University Press 1995. By measurements focused on Manhattan's tenement areas, the change in diphtheria death rates was from an 1894 high of 785 deaths per 100 000 to just 300 deaths per 100 000 in 1900.

29 Hiscock, I. V. 'A survey of public health activities in Los Angeles County, California.' *American Public Health Association*, 1928.

30 A Board of Health that would execute the duties of public health for the entire region was created for Los Angeles County in 1915, when the population was approaching 700 000 people. Though nowhere in the United States had a county-level health department until 1911, few had as crying a need for one as did Los Angeles.

31 In 1900 some 40 per cent of all deaths annually in New York City involved children under five years of age. A 1918 survey by Josephine Baker also found that 21 per cent of all New York City schoolchildren were malnourished.

32 See Soper, G. 'Curious career of Typhoid Mary.' *Bulletin of the New York Academy of Medicine* 15 (1939).

33 Mallon, indeed, turned out to be a lifelong typhoid carrier as later studies revealed.

34 Baker, J. 1939; Fee, E. and Hammonds, E. M. 'Science, politics, and the art of persuasion.' In Rosner, D. (ed.), 1995, op. cit.; Leavitt, J. W. *Typhoid Mary* Boston, Beacon Press 1996; Soper, G., 1939, op. cit.; and Sufrin, M. 'The case of the disappearing cook.' *American Heritage* (August 1970): 37–43.

35 Hookworm disease is caused by any of three parasites indigenous to North America, particularly in subtropic ecologies. Hookworm larvae can infect people by entering cuts on bare feet. Once inside the body, hookworms can cause anaemia, weakness, and mental retardation.

   In 1906, when the Rockefeller campaign began, experts already recognized that though treatment options were poor, prevention was fairly simple. Shoes, socks, and long trousers were sufficient barriers, in most cases. Hookworm was a disease of extreme poverty.

36 By 1916 there were fewer than five schools of public health in the United States, but there were more than 160 medical schools—demonstrating that curative medicine was already a more attractive pursuit than populationwide disease prevention.

37 Stevens, R. *In Sickness and in Wealth: American Hospitals in the Twentieth Century.* Baltimore: Johns Hopkins University Press, 1989.

38 Ben-David, J. 'Scientific productivity and academic organization in nineteenth century medicine.' *American Sociological Review* 25 (1960): 830.

39 Golub, E. S. 1994. Adult cases of polio were rare, presumably because over decades of life, older individuals were naturally immunized by sequential exposures. In 1916 all but the wealthiest of

adults would have been exposed during childhood, having consumed less than ideally filtered water.

For this section on polio, see New York City Department of Health, *Annual Report of the Department of Health of the City of New York for the Calendar Year 1917*. New York, 1918.

40 Polio probably waned in 1917 because it had saturated the nonimmune population, causing disease in the most vulnerable and naturally vaccinating the rest. Over subsequent decades, scientists offered many explanations for the cyclic nature of polio, generally failing to recognize the salient feature.

41 As quoted in Kyvig, D. E. *Repealing National Prohibition*. Chicago: Chicago University Press, 1979.

42 Gray, M. *Drug Crazy: How We Got into This Mess and How We Can Get Out*. New York: Random House, 1998; and Ramirez, J. S. 'The tourist trade takes hold.' In Beard, R. and Berkowitz, L. C., 1993.

43 In New York City, for example, the going bribery rate was $400 a week to be divided among a list of officials for protection of a speakeasy and $40 a week to the local beat policeman.

44 Duffy, J. 1974, op. cit.; and New York City Department of Health, *Annual Report of the Department of Health of the City of New York for the Calendar Year 1920*. New York, 1921.

45 In its 1920 annual report the department also noted that, 'With the advent of Prohibition, a number of cases of wood alcohol poisoning were discovered,' offering a clear rationale for the involvement of medical, versus criminal, authority.

46 Because one of the larger early outbreaks surfaced in Spain, the 1918 epidemic was labelled 'Spanish Influenza' by all but the Spanish. If a geographic moniker was necessary, 'Kansas Flu' might have been more appropriate.

47 For this section, see Beveridge, W. I. B. 'The chronicle of influenza epidemics.' *History and Philosophy of Life Sciences* 13 (1991): 223–35.

48 Eyler, J. M. 'The sick poor and the state.' In Rosenberg, C. E. and Golden, J. (ed.), *Framing Disease: Studies in Cultural History*. New Brunswick, NJ: Rutgers University Press, 1992.

49 The nation's gross national product was soaring, from $16 billion dollars in 1860 to $65 billion in 1890. And by 1921 it topped $300 billion. During that period—a time of 19-fold growth in national wealth—average per-capita income rose only 5.8-fold. Why? Because it wasn't really America that got richer but an elite stratum at the top that amassed astonishing wealth.

50 Smith, D. B. *Health Care Divided: Race and Healing a Nation*. Ann Arbor: University of Michigan Press, 1999.

51 Dublin, L. I. 'The health of the Negro.' *Annals of the American Academy of Politics and Social Science* 140 (1928): 77–85.

52 White, R. *It's Your Misfortune and None of My Own: A New History of the American West*. Norman: University of Oklahoma Press, 1991.

53 Average life expectancy for a white boy born in the United States in 1925 was 57.6 years; for a white girl, 60.6 years. For 'Negroes and others' as they were then classified by the US Census Bureau, life expectancies that year were far lower: 44.9 years for boys and 46.7 years for girls. That figure was, of course, affected by their far greater infant mortality rates: 110.8 per 1000 for 'Negroes and others' versus 68.3 per 1000 for white babies. See US Bureau of the Census, 1976.

54 By 1920 public hospitals were the population's main medical providers nationwide, with charitable private hospitals playing a secondary role. In theory, all of these facilities were available equally to everyone. But that was not the case.

55 Starr, P. *The Social Transformation of American Medicine*. New York: Basic Books, 1982.

56 Paul De Kruif's 1920s books extolling the praises of science and public health were *Microbe Hunters, Hunger Fighters, Men Against Death, The Fight for Life, Why Keep Them Alive?* Hopkins, H. L. 'Hunger is not debatable.' *New York World Telegram* (July 30, 1935).

57 For these and other Depression-era basic facts, see Badger, A. J. *The New Deal: The Depression Years, 1933–1940.* New York: Macmillan, 1989; Heckscher, A. *When La Guardia Was Mayor: New York's Legendary Years.* New York: W. W. Norton and Company, 1978; and McElvaine, R. S. *The Great Depression.* New York: Random House, 1984.

58 The Hoover administration supported the deportations and sent federal officials to the West to deport an additional 82 000 men of Mexican heritage between 1929 and 1933. The effort failed, of course, as would all such deportation campaigns: bad as the economy of the West was in the 1930s, Mexico's was worse. And during those years an estimated 500 000 Mexicans crossed the border to El Norte, settling in California, Arizona, New Mexico, Texas, and Colorado. In California, these immigrants crowded in among the estimated 300 000 dust bowl refugees who also became targets of discrimination and political strife. Kleppner, P. 'Politics without parties: The western states, 1900–1984.' In Nash, G. D. and Etuliaian, R. (ed.), *The Twentieth Century West.* Albuquerque: University of New Mexico Press, 1987.

59 The 'iron lung' had been invented in 1928 by Philip Drinker of Harvard University.

60 San Francisco had a very sorry track record vis-à-vis the health of its Chinese population. During the 1870s to 1890s, when nearly every other locality in the country saw its death and disease rates go down, San Francisco's rose, primarily due to a sequence of epidemics of smallpox and diphtheria. Part of the problem—perhaps the paramount mistake—was the policy of the city's department of health of blaming Chinese immigrants for every single epidemic.

Chinatown was like a walled-off city within a city, ignored by the department except as a target for vilification. The Chinese, understandably, resented the finger-pointing and grew increasingly hostile toward the department. By 1900, department officials were complaining about hostile Chinese, while Chinatown's elders were instructing their community not to trust the government representatives. This, against the background of often brutal anti-Chinese sentiments that sparked lynchings and other violence against the Asian immigrants. It was a classic paradigm of social bigotry and mistrust serving to promote the spread of disease.

61 The epidemic ultimately ended not through the intervention of Science, but of Nature. The great San Francisco earthquake and fire of 1906 levelled the rodents' hiding places and drove the surviving rats to starvation. But feral rodents continued to harbour plague-infested fleas. Periodically throughout the twentieth century squirrels, in particular, became sources of isolated bubonic plague human illnesses and deaths. Thus, it could be argued that Gage's determined opposition to antiplague action allowed *Yersinia pestis* to become newly endemic in California rodent populations.

62 Two agencies were created within USPHS: in future years they transformed into the National Institutes of Health and the Centres for Disease Control.

63 Dubos, R. *Mirage of Health.* Garden City, New York: Doubleday Anchor, 1961.

64 The term *venereal* disappeared from public health terminology in the 1970s and was replaced by the phrase *sexually transmitted disease,* or STD. The word *venereal* was derived from the Latin word *venereus,* or 'of Venus', and referred specifically to heterosexual intercourse. By the 1970s the highest incidence rates of nearly every sexually transmitted infection in the United States were seen not among heterosexuals, however, but among gay men. Thus, public health leaders stopped using the limiting expressions VD and venereal, replacing them with the broader term.

65 Sexual diseases were, according to Harvard medical historian Allan Brandt, defined as 'a uniquely sinful disease . . . of moral decay. Behaviour—bad behaviour at that—is seen as the cause of venereal disease. These assumptions may be powerful psychologically, and in some cases they may influence behaviour, but so long as they are dominant—so long as disease is equated with sin—there can be no magic bullet.' Brandt, A. M. *No Magic Bullet: A Social History of Venereal Disease in the United States Since 1890.* New York: Oxford University Press, 1985.

66 This sorry state of affairs persisted throughout the twentieth century, and limited STD control programmes for decades. By the 1990s the moralistic American society for example, had a gonorrhoea rate of 150 cases per 100 000. In contrast, the sexually far freer and less moralistic Swedish society at the same time had a rate of only 3 per 100 000—fifty times lower. See Institutes of Medicine, *The Hidden Epidemic: Confronting Sexually Transmitted Diseases*. Washington, DC: National Academy Press, 1996.

67 For further information on the Tuskegee syphilis experiment and its ramifications, see Annas, G. J. and Grodin, M. A. 'Apology is not enough.' *Boston Globe* (May 18, 1997): Focus C-1; Bowman, J. E., Corbie-Smith, G., Lurie, P., Wolfe, S. M., Caplan, A. L., Annas G. J., Fairchild, A. L., and Bayer, R., Letters in response to 'Tuskegee as metaphor.' *Science* 285 (1999): 47–50.

On May 16, 1997, President William Jefferson Clinton apologized to the nation for the USPHS syphilis experiment. In his apology, presented at Tuskegee University, President Clinton said: 'The eight men who are survivors of the study are a living link to a time not so very long ago that many Americans would prefer not to remember but we dare not forget. It was a time when our nation failed to live up to its ideals, when our nation broke the trust with our people that is the very foundation of our democracy.... An apology is the first step.... We need to do more to ensure that medical research practices are sound and ethical, and that researchers work more closely with communities.'

68 Another World War II US military innovation was the use of chloroquine for treatment of malaria, coupled with DDT and 2,4-D pesticides for eradication of disease-carrying mosquitoes and lice. Both technologies initially proved as miraculously successful as had penicillin and were immediately put to vigorous civilian use. In the malarial southern states the double dose of pesticides and chloroquine was phenomenally successful. By 1952 the USPHS declared the disease eradicated from North America. For a detailed history of US malaria control efforts, see Garrett, L. 1994, op. cit.; Institute of Medicine. *Malaria: Obstacles and Opportunities*. Washington, DC: National Academy Press, 1991; and Wernsdorfer, W. H. and McGregor, I. *Malaria: Principles and Practice of Malariology*. Edinburgh: Churchill Livingstone, 1988.

69 Goodwin, D. K. *Lyndon Johnson and the American Dream*. New York: Harper and Row, 1976.

70 By 1970 average life expectancies at birth were 59.9 years for men and 63.9 for women. Remaining years for sixty-year-old Americans averaged 31.9 for men and 38.3 for women. In 1995 average life expectancies at birth were 72.5 years for men and 78.9 years for women. Men had gained 11.7 years since 1970; women, 13.7 years.

71 Hilts, P. *Smokescreen: The Truth Behind the Tobacco Industry Cover-Up*. Reading, Mass: Addison-Wesley, 1996; Kluger, R. *Ashes to Ashes: America's Hundred-Year Cigarette War, the Public Health and the Unabashed Triumph of Philip Morris*. New York: Alfred A. Knopf, 1996; and Orey, M. *Assuming the Risk: The Mavericks, the Lawyers and the Whistle-Blowers Who Beat Big Tobacco*. Boston: Little, Brown, 1999.

By the mid-sixties more than half of all men and a third of all women in the United States were cigarette smokers.

72 For example, Larry Agran's 1977 bestseller *The Cancer Connection* (New York: Houghton Mifflin) makes *no* references to tobacco or smoking, attributing 90 per cent of all US cancer incidence to environmental and occupational pollutants.

The cigarette versus pollution dilemma was better stated in 1973 by chemist Jeanne Stellman and physician Susan Daum. See Stellman, J. M. and Daum, S. M. *Work Is Dangerous to Your Health*. New York: Vintage, 1973.

73 Koop, C. E. *Koop: The Memoirs of America's Family Doctor*. New York: Random House, 1991.

74 In the 1980s California and Massachusetts pioneered the most successful anti-smoking campaigns, deploying Madison Avenue techniques. Both states levied heavy taxes on tobacco sales

and used the revenue to purchase prime television time and billboard space for highly sophisticated, often ironic, ads. The ad campaigns proved effective in reducing smoking levels in the two states below those in the rest of the United States, and in reducing the numbers of new smokers emerging annually among teenagers. See Centres for Disease Control and Prevention, 'Cigarette smoking before and after an excise tax increase and antismoking campaign.' *Morbidity and Mortality Weekly Report* **45** (1996): 966–70.

75 For a very accessible delineation of the biology of tobacco addiction, see Goldstein, A. *Addiction: From Biology to Drug Policy*. New York: W. H. Freeman, 1994.

76 Centers for Disease Control and Prevention, 'Cigarette smoking—attributable mortality and years of potential life lost—United States, 1990.' *Morbidity and Mortality Weekly Report* **42** (1993): 645–9. The CDC also estimated that if 1990 smoking levels continued, the generation born between 1978 and 1995 would eventually suffer 5 million deaths due to smoking, costing $50 billion a year in medical treatment and $1.4 billion annually in lost productivity and other indirect costs.

77 It is beyond the scope of this book to detail the long list of frustrations, monetary problems, political intrigues, and intellectual obstacles responsible for the utter failure in the pursuit of an HIV vaccine. Despite many highly optimistic statements over the years, made by authorities to the general public and to Wall Street, by the end of the century nobody had a product in hand that held the promise of doing for HIV what Salk's vaccine had done for polio. To understand some of the reasons why, see Cohen, J. 'Glimmers of hope from the bottom of the well.' *Science* **285** (1999): 656–657; Cohen, J. *Shots in the Dark: The Wayward Search for an AIDS Vaccine*, to be published in 2000, manuscript shared by author; Institute of Medicine, *The Potential Value of Research Consortia in the Development of Drugs and Vaccines Against HIV Infection and AIDS*. Washington, D.C.: National Academy Press, 1988; and various authors, 'AIDS: The Unanswered Questions.' *Science* **260** (1993): 1219–93.

78 On January 6, 1988, Governor Cuomo ordered all prenatal treatment sites across the state to encourage pregnant women to have HIV tests. This followed recognition that mandated anonymous screening of newborns statewide showed that in 1987 1 per cent were born HIV positive.

79 Carroll, M. 'To combat AIDS, New York may order bathhouses shut.' *New York Times* (October 25, 1985): B1.

80 Between 1983 and 1988, New York City's excess mortality rate increased by 5 per cent due to AIDS. In 1988 in the city 3739 people died of the disease. It was just the beginning. As of November 1989, some 22 200 AIDS cases had been reported in New York City since the epidemic's beginning, and AIDS was the leading cause of death for men aged thirty to forty-nine years and women aged twenty to thirty-nine years.

See Smith, P. F., Mikl, J., Hyde, S. *et al.* 'The AIDS epidemic in New York State.' *American Journal of Public Health* **815** (1991): 54–60.

81 These figures come from the 1998 and 1999 annual reports of the United Nations AIDS Programme, based in Geneva, Switzerland.

By the close of 1998, according to UNAIDS, the pandemic broke down as follows:

People living with HIV/AIDS	33.4 million
Newly HIV-infected in 1998	5.8 million
Deaths due to HIV/AIDS in 1998	2.5 million
Cumulative HIV/AIDS death toll since 1979	13.9 million

82 Gao, F., Bailes, E., Robertson, D. L., *et al.* 'Origin of HIV-1 in the chimpanzee *Pan troglodytes troglodytes*.' *Nature* **397** (1999): 436–41; and Weiss, R. A. and Wrangham, R. W. 'From *Pan* to pandemic.' *Nature* **397** (1999): 385–6.

83 Baltimore, Miami, New Orleans, Houston, Denver, and Los Angeles.

84 Brown, D. 'Triple-drug therapies are changing patterns, costs of AIDS treatment.' *Washington Post* (January 27, 1997): A4; Dunlap, D. W. 'Hype, hope and hurt on the AIDS front lines.' *New York Times* (February 2, 1997): E3; Garrett, L. 'A home run: Detectable traces of HIV gone from patients' bodies in short-term clinical trials.' *Newsday* (January 30, 1996): A5; and Martone, W. J. and Phair, J. P. 'HIV protease inhibitors: When and how they should be used.' *Infections in Medicine* Supplement, 1996.

85 Garrett, L. 'Miracle Backlash.' *Newsday* (December 17, 1996): B19; and Garrett, L. 'New AIDS cocktails: What we fear—experts say resistance could develop.' *Newsday* (July 2, 1996): B19.

86 Garrett, L. 'AIDS drugs fading: New prevention approach sought.' *Newsday* (August 31, 1999): A4; and Wainberg, M. A. and Friedland, G. 'Public health implications of antiretroviral therapy and HIV drug resistance.' *Journal of the American Medical Association* 279 (1998): 1977–83.

87 For example, in New York City in 1994 nearly seven thousand people died of AIDS. By the end of 1996 that number had fallen to five thousand. Europeans had seen an even more dramatic trend: between 1994 and 1998 death rates for HIV patients fell an astonishing 80 per cent. The greater successes in Europe may be functions of both wider access to health care (there were more than forty-three million uninsured Americans, Western Europe had near-universal health care), and greater initial conservatism there in use of experimental anti-HIV drugs during the period 1980–1995. (The latter could explain the relatively lower rates of multidrug-resistance seen in European, versus American, HIV patients.)

88 One explanation for the seemingly mysterious tendency of HAART drugs to lose their effectiveness over time was simple human physiology. Anybody who took five to ten even mildly toxic drugs a day was giving his liver, kidneys, intestinal tract, and bowel a real beating. Over time, these vital organs became less able to absorb and process the medicines, so the antiviral agents never reached their targets. The patients might be compliant with doctors' orders, but the liver or duodenum was not.

89 Standard HIV ELISA tests measured the presence in the blood of antibodies against the virus. Refined, highly tuned ELISAs could pick up even minute numbers of antibodies present in the first days of infection, before the immune system mounted a full response to the virus. Detuned ELISAs did the reverse, picking up only the large antibody presences that typically appeared three to five months after infection. By administering both the standard and detuned ELISAs, laboratory technicians could tell in which stage of infection an individual might be.

Chapter 5

1 Fenn, E. A. 'Biological warfare, circa 1750.' *New York Times* (April 11, 1998): A11.

2 Part of the problem Osterholm and others faced was a lack of scientific expertise inside the agencies. For example, the Department of State had virtually no one on staff with genuine expertise in science and technology. See: Solomon, A. K. 'The science and technology-bereft Department of State.' *Science* 282 (1998): 1649–50.

In 1998 President Clinton appointed Dr Kenneth Bernard to the National Security Council, marking the first time that an individual with science and medical expertise sat on that crucial advisory group. John Gannon, chair of the National Intelligence Council, openly sought such expertise from university scientists. In a 1998 speech at Stanford University, for example, he said, 'When I look at this distinguished audience, I can spot just the kind of talent we need to attract . . . to contribute to the defence of our country against the mounting biowarfare threat.' See: Gannon, J. Speech, Stanford University, November 16, 1998.

3 A brilliant account of these events can be found in Remnick, D. *Resurrection: The Struggle for a New Russia*. New York: Random House, 1997.

4 Lederberg, J. Speech to the International Conference on Emerging and Infectious Diseases, Atlanta, Georgia, March 8, 1998.

Lillibridge, S. 'Public health preparedness and response roles for CDC related to bioterrorism.' International Conference on Emerging and Infectious Diseases, Atlanta, Georgia, March 10, 1998.

5 This account was drawn from many interviews and printed sources. For further details the reader is referred to: Falkenrath, R. A., Newmann, R. D., and Thayer, B. A. *America's Achilles' Heel: Nuclear, Biological and Chemical Terrorism and Covert Attack*. Boston: Massachusetts Institute of Technology Press, 1998; Hoffman, B. *Inside Terrorism*. New York: Columbia University Press, 1998; Schweitzer, G. E. and Dorsch, C. C. *Superterrorism: Assassins, Mobsters, and Weapons of Mass Destruction*. New York: Kluwer Academic, 1998.

6 There are many sources for the details presented on the Aum Shinrikyo cult and its activities. In addition to interviews, the following sources were used: 'Congress probes Japanese cult.' Military Newswire, 1996; NSTC Committee on International Science and (CISET) Working Group on Emerging and Re-Emerging Infectious Diseases. 'Global microbial threats in the 1990s.' The White House, 1996; 'Japanese cult member gets life.' Associated Press (May 26, 1998); 'Japanese guru will hear litany of nerve-gas victims.' Associated Press (April 20, 1996); Lewthwaite, G. A. 'Terrorist attacks in US expected.' *Baltimore Sun* (November 1, 1995): A1; Morita, H., Yanagisawa, N., Nakajima, T., *et al.* 'Sarin poisoning in Matsumoto, Japan.' *The Lancet* **346** (1995): 290–3.

7 Some authorities in 1998 were convinced that Aum Shinrikyo not only continued to exist, but was at that time also actively recruiting new members. See Miller, J. 'Some in Japan fear authors of subway attack are regaining ground.' *New York Times* (October 11, 1998): A12.

8 A year previously, on June 27, 1994, Aum Shinrikyo had conducted their first successful attack, releasing sarin gas in the central Japan city of Matsumoto.

9 John Sopko, an advisor to the US Senate, told *New Scientist*'s Robert Taylor that 'the actions of the Aum . . . create a terrifying picture of a deadly mix of the religious zealotry of groups such as the Branch Davidians, the antigovernment agenda of the US militia movements, and the technical know-how of a Doctor Strangelove.'

10 Office of Technology Assessment. *Technology Against Terrorism: The Federal Effort*. Washington, DC, 1993.

11 Excellent review of the limitations inherent in the Biological Toxins and Weapons Convention can be found in: Johnson, S. E. (ed.). *The Niche Threat: Deterring the Use of Chemical and Biological Weapons*. Washington, DC: National Defense University Press, 1997. Roberts, B. (ed.). *Biological Weapons: Weapons of the Future?* The Centre for Strategic and International Studies, Washington, DC, 1993.

I covered the Persian Gulf war for *Newsday*, along with *Newsday* reporters Tim Phelps, Susan Sachs, David Firestone, Ron Howell, Josh Friedman, and Pat Sloyan.

12 The Iran/Iraq war began with diplomatic tensions between the two countries in 1980.

13 No one really knows how many people were wounded or died in the Iran/Iraq war. Neither government felt it in their interests to release real numbers. The figures cited in the text come from US intelligence estimates. But these are surely conservative. One estimate puts Irani deaths, alone, as high as one million, including elimination of 20 per cent of all eighteen to thirty-year-old men. Another estimates 250 000 Irani dead and 100 000 Iraqi. The Iraqi Ministry of Defence claimed one million Iranians were killed; three million injured and maimed. Whatever the case, the carnage was horrendous. And it was reified in Teheran with the famous fountain of martyrs, flowing with human blood.

14 United Nations. 'Report of the mission dispatched by the Secretary-General to investigate alle-
    gations of the use of chemical weapons in the conflict between the Islamic republics of Iran and
    Iraq.' New York: UN Security Council, March 12, 1986; and Dingeman, J. and Jupa, R. 'Chemical
    warfare in the Iran–Iraq conflict.' *Strategy and Tactics* 113 (1987): 51–2.
        Sidell, F. R. and Franz, D. R. 'Overview: Defense against the effects of chemical and biological
    warfare agents.' In Zajtchuk, R. *Textbook of Military Medicine*. Bethesda, MD: Office of the
    Surgeon General, United States, 1997.

15 Manngold, T. and Goldberg, J. *Plague Wars: The Terrifying Reality of Biological Warfare*. New
    York: St Martin's Press, 1999.

16 Two events seem to have propelled Iraq in the CBW (chemical/biological warfare) direction. In
    1981 the Israeli Air Force had bombed and destroyed Iraq's Osirak nuclear reactor—a gift from
    the French government. Israel claimed Hussein's government was obtaining weapons-grade
    nuclear material and making atomic bombs at the site. Israel's credibility in such matters was
    tainted by its own 1990 admission that it had a chemical weapons programme—details of which
    were not forthcoming.
        Interestingly, there is no evidence in the public record that the United Nations demanded
    right of inspection of the acknowledged Israeli chemical weapons, despite the fact that their use
    would violate at least two international treaties to which Israel is party. Further, intelligence
    sources agree that Israel has bioweapons capabilities and may have stockpiled some offensive
    biological agents. But Israel has never been compelled by the UN or any Western government to
    provide an accounting of its CBW efforts or submit to a UNSCOM inspection.
        Though Western military experts were certain that Israel's claim was exaggerated, they had no
    doubt at the time that Hussein was, indeed, trying to make Iraq a nuclear nation.
        McKay, S. and Baker, J. 'Weapons proliferation after the storm: What implications should the
    United States draw from the Iraqi experience?' Conference on Arms Control and Verification,
    Williamsburg, Virginia, June 1–4, 1992.

17 George, A. 'Saddam bought germ warfare chemicals in UK.' *Evening Standard* (London) (July
    11, 1995): 23; Butcher, T. 'Iraq crisis: Germ warfare "jelly" sold to Iraq until 1996.' *The Daily Tele-
    graph* (London) (February 19, 1998): 19; Beal, C. 'How to spot a killer cloud.' *New Scientist*
    (April 8, 1995): 24; and Bone, J. 'Chemical agents.' *The Times* (London) (December 13, 1997),
    Features.

18 Tucker, J. B. 'Hide-and-seek, Iraqi style.' *New York Times*, (November 22, 1997) Op Ed page.

19 Zilinskas, R. A. 'Iraq's biological weapons: The past as future?' *Journal of the American Medical
    Association* 278 (1997): 418–24.

20 Regis, E. *The Biology of Doom: The History of America's Secret Germ Warfare Project*. New York:
    Henry Holt and Company, 1999.

21 Scientific and Technical Advisory Section, US Armed Forces, Pacific, 'Biological warfare.' Vol. 5
    (1945).

22 Smart, J. K. 'History of chemical and biological warfare: An American perspective.' In Zajtchuk,
    R., op. cit., 9–86.

23 Cole, L. A. 'The worry: Germ warfare. The target: Us.' *New York Times* (January 25, 1994): A19;
    and Hersh, S. M., *Chemical and Biological Warfare: America's Hidden Arsenal*. New York:
    Doubleday and Company, 1969. Regis, E., 1999, op. cit.

24 For an exhaustive, hair-raising account of US chemical–biological weapons use in Korea see:
    Endicott, S. and Hagerman, E. *The United States and Biological Warfare: Secrets from the Early
    Cold War and Korea*. Bloomington, Indiana: Indiana University Press, 1998.

25 For a litany see Broad, W. J. and Miller, J. 'Once he devised germ weapons; now he defends
    against them.' *New York Times* (November 3, 1998): F1.

26 Though there have been allegations to the contrary, I can find no evidence that the United States used biological weapons in Indochina during the US/Vietnam War. For details on yellow rain and Soviet use of mycotoxins in Laos and Afghanistan, see: Cole, L. A. *The Eleventh Plague: The Politics of Biological and Chemical Warfare*. New York: W. H. Freeman & Company, 1997, 179–81.

27 *Transparency* is a classic term used in national security circles. It refers to the willingness of a nation to leave its weapons programmes 'transparent' to outsiders concerned with treaty verification or international security issues. Any weapons treaty must allow outsiders to verify claims a participating nation makes—a process that can only be completed if the given country makes its programmes 'transparent'. For example, no nuclear arms treaty can possibly be enforced if one of the parties lies, hides its weapons, refuses inspection, or otherwise obfuscates. The lack of Iraqi transparency, alone, constituted a treaty violation even if the country wasn't hiding anything.

It should be noted, however, that neither Iraq nor Libya had signed the Biological Weapons Convention.

28 Bodansk, Y. 'The Iraqi WMD challenge—Myths and reality.' Task Force on Terrorism and Unconventional Warfare. US House of Representatives, February 10, 1998.

29 A month later British Prime Minister Tony Blair ordered all his nation's air and sea ports placed on full alert following word that Iraqi agents were smuggling various disguised products containing anthrax into the United Kingdom. No such contaminants were found, but, as in Washington, a new mood of bioweapons concern took hold in London. The British alert followed on the heels of Baghdad's arrest of microbiologist Nassir al-Hindawi, considered the mastermind of Iraq's biological weapons programme. UNSCOM inspectors speculated that Hindawi's arrest was intended to keep the scientist sequestered from inquiring investigators.

30 Crossette, B. 'Iraq still trying to conceal arms programs, report says.' *New York Times* (January 27, 1999): A8; and Broad, W. J. and Miller, J. 'The hunt for germs and poisons.' *New York Times* (December 20, 1998): Section 4, 1.

31 Crossette, B. 'Iraq suspected of secret germ war effort.' *New York Times* (February 8, 2000): A14.

32 Monath, T. P. and Gordon, L. K. 'Strengthening the Biological Weapons Convention.' *Science* 282 (1998): 1423–4; Roberts, B. 'New challenges and new policy priorities for the 1990s.' In Roberts, B. 1993, op. cit.; and 'Bioweapon threat seen rising but treaty talks far from results.' Daniel J. Denoon's Insider Newsfile, December 28, 1998.

33 Roberts, B. 'Between panic and complacency: Calibrating the chemical and biological warfare problem.' In Johnson, S. E. 1997, op. cit.

34 There are many press accounts of Volkov's statements and corroboration. The most to the point is Englund, W. 'New questions raised about '79 Russian anthrax outbreak.' *Baltimore Sun* (February 20, 1998): A8.

35 Untreated pneumonic anthrax normally has a 90 per cent kill rate. Even if diagnosis is swiftly made antibiotic treatment is tricky and death rates of 10 to 20 per cent can occur.

36 Abramova, F. A., Grinberg, L. V., Yampolskaya, O. V., *et al.* 'Pathology of inhalation anthrax in 42 cases from the Sverdlovsk outbreak of 1979.' *Proceedings of the National Academy of Sciences* 90 (1993): 2291–94. Please note that Yekaterinburg was in Soviet times called Sverdlovsk. References may be coded under that name. See also Guillemin, J. *Anthrax: The Investigation of a Deadly Outbreak*. Berkeley: University of California Press (1999).

37 Colonel Arthur Friedlander of the US Army Medical Research Institute on Infectious Diseases, located at Fort Detrick, Maryland.

38 During World War II the British military had performed anthrax experiments on Gruinard Island, Henderson noted. Fifty-five years later the soils of Gruinard were still toxic, loaded with potentially lethal anthrax spores.

39 But significant debate over destruction of the remaining smallpox stocks persisted. For key components of that debate see: National Academy of Sciences, *Assessment of Future Scientific Needs for Live Variola Virus*. Washington, DC: National Academy Press, March 15, 1999; and Garrett, L. 'Smallpox as tool adds to destruction debate,' *Newsday* (March 16, 1999): A18; Shalala, D. E. 'Smallpox: Setting the research agenda,' *Science* 285 (1999): 1011.

40 Commission to Assess the Organization of the Federal Government to Combat the Proliferation of Weapons of Mass Destruction, *Combating Proliferation of Weapons of Mass Destruction* (1999), 104th Congress, Washington, DC, Government Printing Office.

41 Broad, W. I. and Miller J. 'Government report says 3 nations hide stocks of smallpox,' *New York Times* (June 13, 1999): A1.

42 Wirth, T. Speech to the CISET Conference on Emerging Diseases, US State Department, Washington, DC, July 25, 1995.

43 Downie, A. W. 'Smallpox', in Mudd, S. (ed.) *Infectious Agents and Host Reactions*. New York, W. B. Saunders, 1970.

44 Information about VECTOR and Biopreparat was obtained during an on-site visit in March 1997. And see: Adams, J. 'Iran: Russia helps Iran's bio-warfare.' Reuters (August 27, 1995).

45 Yergin, D. and Gustafson, T. *Russia 2010 and What It Means for the World*. New York: Vintage Books, 1995.

46 In 1998 Alexander Lebed was elected governor of Russia's Krasnoyarsk State, which includes numerous former bioweapons facilities. Krasnoyarsk is potentially the richest of all Russian states, as within its borders are among the world's greatest reserves of gold, silver, high-grade coal, oil, diamonds, and precious minerals.

47 Soviet health expert Murray Feshbach, of Georgetown University, considers Vozrozhdeniya Island one of the most dangerous places on earth. Once controlled by the Soviet military, the island now straddles the Aral Sea territories of Kazakhstan and Uzbekistan, neither of which have armed forces capable of defending Vozrozhdeniya. Further, the Aral Sea, as a result of inane Soviet water policies and pollution, is rapidly shrinking. Twenty years ago, Vozrozhdeniya was easily defended, as it took several hours to reach the island by boat. Today it is possible to get within spitting distance of the 'island' by driving a high-chassis vehicle across the 'lake'. Feshbach says several mass die-offs of wild fish and animal populations near the island since 1976 were probably the result of exposure to bioweapons.

48 Alibek's chilling autobiography, rich in details of the Biopreparat and Soviet military bioweapons programmes, was published in 1999. See Alibek, K. and Handelman, S. *Biohazard*. New York, Random House, 1999.

49 And Pasechnik's information jibed nicely with evidence obtained ten years earlier by British intelligence following the assassination of Bulgarian defector Georgi Makrov. The Bulgarian stood at a London street corner awaiting a bus when an unseen man approached, carrying a most unusual umbrella. The man, a KGB operative, had a tiny canister filled with high-pressure gas, attached to a pellet of the deadly biotoxin ricin hidden inside the umbrella. That canister was connected at one end to a spring lock system triggered by tapping a button located near the umbrella's handle. At the opposite end of the umbrella the tip was bored, creating a barrel through which the lethal pellet was propelled. The KGB agent simply strolled up to Markov, tapped the naive Bulgarian with his umbrella, and disappeared in a British crowd. Markov died, but another Bulgarian defector, Vladimir Kostov, survived being assaulted by a similar device. Kostov came out of a Paris metro station on a cold winter day. He felt a sudden pain and saw a man, carrying an umbrella, run away. French physicians successfully removed the pellet from Kostov's back, and he survived, probably because his heavy winter clothing slowed the pellet's entry into his body, preventing ricin from getting into his bloodstream. US intelligence claims

there were at least six other ricin assassination incidents of this kind, including one in a shopping mall in Virgina. Eitzen, E. M. and Takafuji, E. T. 'Historical overview of biological warfare.' In Zajtchuk, R. 1997, op. cit.

50 Kudoyarova-Zubavichene, N. M., Chepurnov, A. A., Sergeyev, N. N., *et al.* 'Preparation and use of Hyperimmune serum for therapy of filoviruses'; and Ryabchikova, E., Kolesnikova, L., Netesov, S. Y., *et al.* 'An analysis of filovirus pathogenesis on animal models'; both were presentations at the International Colloquium on Ebola Virus Research, Antwerp, Belgium, September 4–7, 1996.

51 As described in Chapter 3, VECTOR's Elena Ryabchikova had also done studies comparing responses to Ebola infection in various animal species, including rhesus monkeys, baboons, African green monkeys, and guinea pigs. By passaging the virus through successive generations of guinea pigs she successfully increased the virus's virulence, eventually making a form of Ebola that was, after eight generations, 100 per cent lethal to guinea pigs. Besides being an interesting piece of virology this study could have indicated that Biopreparat was trying to determine how to make Ebola more deadly to human beings.

52 Alibek insists that some elements of the old Biopreparat and military bioweapons programmes continue today. And he claims that his former bosses continue to conduct genetic engineering of pathogens. He even claims that these Russian scientists have attempted his assassination on at least one occasion in Virginia. See Alibek, K. and Handlemas, S., op. cit., 1999.

53 The careful reader will note that the personnel estimates for Biopreparat and the Russian Ministry of Health's bioweapons programme are variously reported over a range of some 10 000. It appears that even those Russians who were in leadership positions in those programmes cannot recall precisely how many people were in the biowar machine.

54 According to a disputed *New York Times* account some top Biopreparat scientists have turned up in Iran. See: Miller, J. and Broad, W. J. 'Bio-weapons in mind, Iranians lure needy ex-Soviet scientists.' *New York Times* (December 8, 1998): A1; Broad, W. J. 'Iranian denies seeking biological arms in Russian.' *New York Times* (December 12, 1998): A3; and Miller, J. 'Russian biologist denies work in Iran on germ weapons.' *New York Times* (January 19, 1997): A7.

55 Miller, J. 'Bombs-to-plowshares program criticized.' *New York Times* (February 22, 1999): A8; Stout, D. 'US imposes sanctions on tech labs in Russia.' *New York Times* (January 13, 1999): A7; and Miller, J. and Broad, W. J. 'Germ weapons: In Soviet past or in the new Russia's future?' *New York Times* (December 28, 1998): A1.

56 As the paper's authors wrote: 'acquisition of haemolytic properties by *B. anthracis* strains can allow them to escape host immunity by means of penetrating [human] host cells.' This, the authors continued, constituted 'an evolutionary leap'.

57 An august team of anthrax experts wrote in 1999: 'Whether our medical system would be able to provide appropriate prophylaxis and therapy in the event of a large-scale exposure to pathogenic endospores remains uncertain, even doubtful.' See Dixon, T. C., Meselson, M., Guillemin, J., and Hanna, P. C. 'Anthrax'. *The New England Journal of Medicine* 341 (1999): 815–26.

58 Bielecki, J., Youngman, P., Conelly, P., and Portnoy, D. A. '*Bacillus subtilis* expressing a haemolysin gene from *Listeria monocytogenes* can grow in mammalian cells.' *Nature* 345 (1990): 175–6.

59 For a discussion of possible ways to limit such access versus its deleterious impact on science, see: Roberts, B. 'Export controls and biological weapons: New roles, new challenges.' *Critical Reviews in Microbiology* 24 (1998): 235–54.

60 Some Gulf War veterans insisted that squalene had been in the anthrax vaccines they were given during the Persian Gulf conflict and was the basis of Gulf War Syndrome.

61 The only precedent for such disbelief was the Vietnam War use of Agent Orange, a herbicide later implicated in a wide range of health defects in Vietnam veterans, Vietnamese civilians, and their

children. In the Agent Orange case, however, government and the medical community were divided in their interpretation of data, and those who doubted official DOD safety claims had widespread support in establishment circles. Such was not the case with protest over the anthrax vaccine.

62 Inglesby, T. V., Stephenson G., *et al.* 'Medical response to anthrax attack'. *Journal of the American Medical Association* **281** (1999): 1735–45.

63 This list has appeared in numerous places, cited from a variety of sources. See in particular, Office of Technology Assessment, August 1993.

64 Complex biological warfare alliances formed in the 1990s. North Korea's most lucrative export was the SCUD missile, in some cases adapted for delivery of chemical or biological weapons. Among North Korea's buyers were Egypt, Cuba, Iran, Syria, Iraq, and Libya. (See: Grubb, J. 'Nonproliferation "progress" in Korea: Next steps'. Conference on Arms Control and Verification Technology, Williamsburg, Virginia, June 1–4, 1992.)

65 Typically the evidence publicly offered for allegations that international terrorists were already in 1999 in the business of making biobombs is strategic, rather than concrete. The groups of concern have steadily escalated both their weaponry and kill rates. In the 1990s the World Trade Center in New York City and US Embassies in Nairobi and Dar es Salaam were bombed, signalling, intelligence sources say, just this sort of escalation.

They also point to a general proliferation in the number of international groups that are willing to resort to terrorist tactics. The Rand Corporation estimates, for example, that there were eleven such organizations in the world in 1968; fifty-five in 1978, and steady growth thereafter. (See Hoffman, B. 1998, op. cit.). An even more startling estimate for 1997 was offered by Glenn Schoen: one thousand terrorist organizations worldwide. (See Schoen, G. 'Understanding contemporary terrorism'. Georgetown University, 1997, and Schweitzer, G. E. and Dorsch, C. G. 1998, op. cit.) The spectre of organizations not under the control of any government gaining weaponized microbes was the driving force of concern in most policy circles, despite the lack of publicly available, concrete evidence that any such organization was, indeed, contemplating such a horrific tactic to meet its political ends. Given the sudden urgency bioterrorism attracted in the US White House, DOD, and counterparts in Europe in 1998 it must be assumed that secret information gathered by intelligence agencies did, indeed, then point to such activities and intentions in terrorist circles.

66 Landau, M. 'How the cholera bacterium got its virulence'. *Focus*, Harvard Medical School, July 19, 1996, 1.

67 Valdivia, R. H. and Falkow, S. 'Fluorescence-based isolation of bacterial genes expressed within host cells'. *Science* **277** (1997): 2007–11.

68 Some further examples of work in the genetics of virulence include: Cotter, P. A. and Miler, J. F. 'Triggering bacterial virulence'. *Science* **273** (1996): 1183–4.

69 Duesberg, N. S., Webb, C. P., Leppla, S. H., *et al.* 'Proteolytic inactivation of MAP-kinase-kinase by anthrax lethal factor'. *Science* **280** (1998): 734.

70 From 1975 to 1991 the numbers of people who obtained PhDs in the United States in biology increased by 30 per cent, reaching 5700 per year. Some 60 000 biologists were employed in the United States by the 1990s. And the number of biotechnology companies went from zero in 1975 to more than 1800 in the United States and Europe in 1992. See: Taylor, R. 'All fall down'. *New Scientist* (May 11, 1996).

71 By the late 1990s scientific tools were developed that might allow for genetic targeting of microbes against specific human races, and finding ways to turn a contact-transmissable agent (such as HIV) into an airborne one (e.g. influenza). See: Eickoff, T. 'Airborne disease: Including chemical and biological warfare'. *American Journal of Epidemiology* **144** (1996): S39–S46; and Reany, P. 'Ethnically targeted weapons may not be far off'. Reuters (January 21, 1999).

72 Note Nass, M. 'Biological warfare.' *Lancet* 352 (1998): 491.

73 Also 'Such strategies appear increasingly likely at a time when some states seek to enforce norms through collective security operations. For the former, biological weapons may be deemed useful in blunting the front edge of an invasion, when interventionary forces are at their most vulnerable, or in creating a political backlash against intervention within the major powers. In circumstances short of war, biological weapons may be deemed less useful; nuclear weapons continue to operate more fundamentally on perceptions than do biological weapons, especially given the outlaw status of the latter. But a state brandishing biological weapons as an instrument of last resort or threatening to unleash them in terrorist strikes would gain important leverage in times of crisis. The leaders of such states may also reckon that the threat or actual use of biological weapons would be less likely to incite a powerful counter response by the stronger adversary than would nuclear use.' See: Roberts, B. 'Controlling the proliferation of biological weapons.' *The Nonproliferation Review*, ISSN 1073–6700, Monetary Institute of International Studies, 1994, 55–60.

74 Wright, R. 'Be very afraid.' *The New Republic* (May 1, 1995): 19–27.

75 The targets of such rogue attacks, also in Nunn's parlance, were likely to be civilian: national landmark symbols, dense centres of economic activity, crossroads of vehicular or mass transport, commercial planes, national parades, sporting events that drew international audiences. In the 1990s the following examples of Nunn's thesis were targeted by domestic or foreign terrorists: the World Trade Center in New York City, the Tokyo subway system, Pan Am flight 103, the Oklahoma Federal Building, numerous sites in Israel, several civilian localities in England and Ireland hit by the IRA, the Olympics pavilion during the Atlanta competition, Buddhist sanctuaries attacked by Tamil nationalists in Sri Lanka, abortion clinics throughout the United States, a Jewish cultural centre in Argentina, the training headquarters of the Saudi National Guard in Riyadh, American consulate officials in Pakistan, and opponents of the Bhagwan Shree Rajineesh cult in Oregon. See also Hoffman, B. 'Terrorism today and tomorrow.' In *Inside Terrorism*, 1998, op. cit.

76 Mayer, T. N. 'The biological weapon: A poor nation's weapon of mass destruction.' At www.cdsar.af.mil/battle/chp8.html.

77 Henderson, D. A. 'The looming threat of bioterrorism.' *Science* 283 (1999): 1279–82.

78 Although twelve million doses are stored in CDC freezers—as of 1998—the quality of several lots is considered highly suspect. It is possible that less than five million doses remain of viable immunogenicity. See Breman, J. G. and Henderson, D. A. 'Poxvirus dilemmas—Monkeypox, smallpox, and biological terrorism.' *Lancet* (August 20, 1998): 556–9.

79 Garrett, L. 'Smallpox vaccine tainted.' *Newsday* (April 13, 1999): A6; Altman, L. K., Broad, W. J., and Miller J. 'Smallpox: the once and future scourge?' *New York Times* (June 15, 1999): F1.

80 Though Henderson thought it wise for the United States and other nations likely to be targeted by biobombers to rebuild vaccine stockpiles, his primary position was that 'all known stocks of variola [smallpox] virus should be destroyed as soon as possible,' including identified samples at VECTOR and the CDC. See Breman, J. G. and Henderson, D. A. 1998, ibid.

81 For an excellent description of the politics behind this American decision, see Broad, W. J. and Miller, J. 'Germ defense plan in peril as its flaws are revealed.' *New York Times* (August 7, 1998): A1.

82 Appropriations Hearing on Epidemics and Bioterrorism, US Senate Committee on Appropriations, Subcommittee on Labor, Health and Human Services, June 2, 1998.

83 Staten's organization and database may be accessed at www.emergency.com.

84 Thomas-Lester, A. and Wilgoren, D. 'In the B'nai B'rith building, some waited in fear, others prayed.' *Washington Post* (April 25, 1997): A20.

Chapter 6

1 Sen, A. *Development as Freedom*. New York: Knopf, 1999.

2 Farmer, P. *Infections and Inequalities: The Modern Plague*. Berkeley: University of California Press, 1999.

3 Evans, R. G., Hodge, M., and Pless, I. B. 'If not genetics, then what?' In Evans, R. G., Barrer, M. L., and Marmor, T. R. *Why Are Some People Healthy and Others Not?* New York: Aldine De Gruyter, 1994.

4 Kim, J. Y., Farmer, P., and Dahl, O. Letter to Partners in Health, September 18, 1997.

5 MRSA: methicillin-resistant *Staphylococcus aureus*; VRE: vancomycin-resistant *Enterococcus*; VISA: vancomycin-insensitive *Staphylococcus aureus*. See Chapter 4 for details on these organisms.

Index